Manual of I.V. Therapeutics

Manual of I.V. Therapeutics
2nd edition

Lynn Dianne Phillips, RN, MSN, CRNI
Instructor of Nursing
Butte Community College
Oroville, California

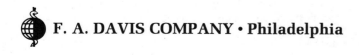

F. A. DAVIS COMPANY • Philadelphia

F. A. Davis Company
1915 Arch Street
Philadelphia, PA 19103

Printed in the United States of America

Last digit indicates print number: 10 9 8 7 6 5 4 3 2 1

Acquisitions Editor: Joanne Patzek DaCunha, RN, MSN
Cover Designer: Steven R. Morrone

As new scientific information becomes available through basic and clinical research, recommended treatments and drug therapies undergo changes. The author(s) and publisher have done everything possible to make this book accurate, up to date, and in accord with accepted standards at the time of publication. The authors, editors, and publisher are not responsible for errors or omissions or for consequences from application of the book, and make no warranty, expressed or implied, in regard to the contents of the book. Any practice described in this book should be applied by the reader in accordance with professional standards of care used in regard to the unique circumstances that may apply in each situation. The reader is advised always to check product information (package inserts) for changes and new information regarding dose and contraindications before administering any drug. Caution is especially urged when using new or infrequently ordered drugs.

Library of Congress Cataloging-in Publication Data

Phillips, Lynn Dianne, 1947–
    Manual of I.V. therapeutics / Lynn Dianne Phillips. — 2nd ed.
        p.   cm.
    Includes bibliographical references and index.
    ISBN 0-8036-0131-X
    1. Intravenous therapy—Handbooks, manuals, etc.   I. Title.
    [DNLM: 1. Infusions, Intravenous—methods—handbooks.   2. Infusions,
Intravenous—nursing—handbooks.   3. Infusions, Intravenous—examination
questions.   WB 39 P561m 1997]
    RM170.P48   1997
    615'.6—dc21
    DNLM/DLC
    for Library of Congress   96-40183
                                                                                    CIP

To the women who have enriched this passage of my life
My sister, Peggy
My daughter, Christa
My dear friends, Mary Van Mierlo, Leslie Baranowski, DiAne
Fischer, Darlynne Giorgi, Laurie Scheall, and Hillary Cook

To my husband
Don, for his support and love

To my parents
Larry and Margie Schuetz

To all my students
This is for you.

PREFACE

I.V. related skills, according to an *American Journal of Nursing* 1991 survey, are performed by 85 percent of the nurses in the acute setting. During many years of educating nurses about techniques in I.V. therapy, I have heard this question asked over and over again: "Why don't we have more of this information in nursing school?" Another common question is, "Why doesn't our staff development department have more classes so that we can keep up our competency skills in I.V. related therapies?" Lack of time is the response. Using time as a valued resource, this manual can be used by student and novice nurses in the hospital or alternate setting where I.V. therapy skills are necessary, or as a resource for the expert practitioner.

My unsuccessful search for a self-paced comprehensive text for students and educators, along with my quest for a research book for practitioners, has resulted in the modular-experiential approach to learning I.V. therapy skills presented in this text. *Manual of I.V. Therapeutics* provides a text from which instruction builds from simple to complex, incorporating theory into clinical application. The skills of recall, nursing process, patient education, along with detailed summaries, provide the foundation to produce a knowledgeable practitioner. The psychomotor skills associated with I.V. therapy are presented in step by step procedures based on standards of practice. Competency criteria is presented at the end of each chapter detailing cognitive and performance criteria, with suggestions for evaluation of competency.

This book uniquely combines a workbook, text, and pocket guide. Each chapter in Units Two and Three has accompanying objectives, defined glossary terms, a pre-test and a post-test, worksheets, competency criteria and a critical thinking activity. Nursing process, in a table format, is presented at the end of each chapter with a strong emphasis on assessment and interventions. Included in this new edition is focus spots on home care issued and patient education. Standards of practice are emphasized using Occupation Safety and Health Administration (OSHA) guidelines and Centers for Disease Control and Prevention (CDC) 1995 revised standards for Intravascular Device-Related Infections.

This manual is divided into three units: Unit One lays the foundation for practice, Unit Two covers basic I.V. therapy, and Unit Three covers advanced practice. Unit One provides two chapters designed to introduce the reader to the legal responsibilities, risks, and steps of continuous quality assessment and competency criteria. The history includes past, present, and future trends that contribute to the changing clinical practice of I.V. therapy.

Unit Two provides the essential eight chapters for a foundation in I.V. therapy practice. This edition, besides the original seven chapters, has a new chapter on infection control. Unit Two emphasizes a modular approach covering fluid and electrolytes, parenteral solutions, equipment, techniques for peripheral venipuncture; complications, special needs of pediatric and geriatric populations, and infection control concepts.

Unit Three includes five chapters covering content specific to central line management, administration of medications, transfusion therapy, nutritional support with an additional new chapter on antineoplastic therapy.

The appendixes include reference charts for physical and chemical compatibility, normal reference laboratory values, and the guidelines for controlling occupational exposure to hazardous drugs and dilution rates for I.V. drugs. Due to the changing role of the Licensed Practical/Licensed Vocational Nurse (LPN/LVN), a list of states that have expanded the role of I.V. therapy in the LPN/LVN practice is provided.

I hope this new edition provides you, whether a practicing health care provider or nursing student, with valuable insight into the safe practice of I.V. therapy and a reference for this rapidly advancing field.

Lynn D. Phillips

ACKNOWLEDGMENTS

The author would like to acknowledge the following:

Timothy David Mitas, my son, for his artistic talent and contribution to this project.

The nurses in the speciality practice of I.V. therapy.

The nursing department at Butte Community College for their support and encouragement during this revision.

Joanne P. DaCunha, Nursing Acquisitions Editor, who assisted in the final development of this manual.

Robert G. Martone, Publisher, Nursing, whose foresight brought the project to F.A. Davis.

Ruth De George, Executive Editorial Secretary, who always greeted me with a warm, friendly voice.

Herbert Powell, Director of Production, and Robert Butler, Assistant Director of Production, for guiding my manuscript through the production process.

CONTRIBUTING AUTHOR

Leslie Baranowski, BSN, CRNI
Infusion Therapy Services Program Manager
Sutter/CHS Central Area
Sacramento, California

CONSULTANTS

Leslie Baranowski, BSN, CRNI
Infusion Therapy Services Program Manager
Sutter/CHS Central Area
Sacramento, California

Beth Fabian, BA, RN, CRNI
Director of Clinical Services
Ivonyx
17197 Larrel Park Drive, Suite 540
Lavonia, Michigan

Pamela Hockett, RN, BSN, OCN, CRNI
Clinical Educator Medical Oncology
Enloe Hospital
Chico, California

Brenda Bradley Johansson, RN, C, BA, MSN, CNRN, CCRN
Acute Care Educator
Enloe Hospital
Chico, California

Anna Marinelli, RN, BSN, OCN
Hospice Case Manager
Enloe HomeCare and Hospice
Chico, California

Roxanne Perucca, RN, BSN, CRNI
I.V. Therapy Clinician
University of Kansas Medical Center
Kansas City, Kansas

Christine Pierce, RN, MSN, CS, CRNI
Manager, Home Infusion and Perinatal Services
Meridia Health Systems
Cleveland, Ohio

Alivia Strawn, ASN, RN, CIC
Infection Control Coordinator
Enloe Hospital
Chico, California

CONTENTS

Lists of Tables xvii

UNIT ONE
Introduction to the Practice of Intravenous Therapy

CHAPTER 1
Intravenous Therapy: Past, Present, and Future Trends........ 3
Renaissance Era (1438 to 1660), 4
The 19th Century, 4
The 20th Century, 7
Advances and Trends in the 90s, 11
Trends for the 21st Century, 11

CHAPTER 2
Risk Management and Quality Patient Management 17
Glossary, 17
Risk Management, 18
Quality Patient Management, 33

UNIT TWO
The Basics: Foundation for Practice

CHAPTER 3
Fundamentals of Fluid Balance 45
Glossary, 45
Body Fluid Composition, 48
Fluid Distribution, 48
Fluid Function, 50
Homeostatic Mechanisms, 53
Physical Assessment, 55
Fluid Volume Imbalances, 59
Patient Education, 63

xiii

Home Care Issues, 63
Patient Education, 64
Home Care Issues, 64

CHAPTER 4
Fundamentals of Electrolyte Balance 73
Glossary, 73
Basic Principles of Electrolyte Balance, 76
Electrolytes: Function, Deficit, Excess, and Treatment, 76
Patient Education, 95
Home Care Issues, 95
Acid-Base Balance, 99
Major Electrolyte Imbalances, 100

CHAPTER 5
Parenteral Solutions 115
Glossary, 115
Rationales and Objectives of Parenteral Therapy, 118
Key Elements in Parenteral Solutions, 123
Hypotonic, Isotonic, and Hypertonic Solutions, 124
Types of Parenteral Solutions, 125
Patient Education, 142
Home Care Issues, 142

CHAPTER 6
Infection Control 149
Glossary, 149
Immune System Function, 153
Basic Principles of Epidemiology, 156
Strategies for Prevention of Infection, 161
I.V.-Related Infections, 163
Patient Education, 172
Home Care Issues, 172
Technologic Advances, 172

CHAPTER 7
Equipment 183
Glossary, 183
Infusion Delivery Systems, 186
Administration Sets, 190
Peripheral Infusion Devices, 195
Inline I.V. Solution Filters, 204
Blood Filters, 206
Electronic Infusion Devices (EIDs), 207
Accessory Equipment, 215
Patient Education, 219
Home Care Issues, 219

CHAPTER 8
Techniques for Peripheral Intravenous Therapy 229
Glossary, 229
Anatomy and Physiology Related to I.V. Practice, 232

Approaches to Venipuncture, 239
Summary of Steps in Initiating I.V. Therapy, 249
Recommendations for Use of Peripheral Venous Catheters, 253
Discontinuation of I.V. Cannula, 253
Latex Resealable Lochs (PRN Devices), 254
Heparin Flush Versus Saline Flush, 254
Controversial Practices, 256
Patient Education, 259
Home Care Issues, 259

CHAPTER 9
Complications of Intravenous Therapy 269
Glossary, 269
Local Complications, 272
Systemic Complications, 291
Erratic Flow Rates, 300
Patient Education, 302
Home Care Issues, 302

CHAPTER 10
Intravenous Therapy: Special Problems...........................313
Glossary, 313
Pediatric I.V. Therapy, 316
Geriatric I.V. Therapy, 330
Special Problems, 334
Patient Education, 338
Home Care Issues, 338

UNIT THREE
Advanced Practice

CHAPTER 11
Administration of Intravenous Medications......................349
Glossary, 349
Advantages of Intravenous Medication, 353
Disadvantages of Intravenous Medication, 353
Drug Compatibility, 357
Methods of Intravenous Medication Administration, 358
Anti-Infective Administration Considerations, 372
Narcotic Infusion Considerations, 375
Investigational Drugs, 378
Patient Education, 380
Home Care Issues, 380

CHAPTER 12
Central Venous Access Devices 391
Glossary, 391
Anatomy of the Vascular System, 394
Central Venous Catheter Materials, 395
Short-Term and Long-Term Access Devices, 396
Occluded Central Venous Devices, 421
Patient Education, 427
Home Care Issues, 427

CHAPTER 13

Transfusion Therapy 439

Glossary, 439
Basic Immunohematology, 443
Blood Donor Collection Methods, 448
Blood Component Therapy, 451
Colloid Volume Expanders, 461
Alternative Pharmacologic Therapies, 462
Administration of Blood Components, 466
Complications Associated with Blood Component Therapy, 474
Patient Education, 480
Home Care Issues, 480

CHAPTER 14

Antineoplastic Therapy 491

Glossary, 491
Role of Clinician, 495
Cellular Kinetics, 496
Antineoplastic Agents, 499
Common Side Effects of Chemotherapy, 509
Routes of Administration, 521
Patient Education, 529
Home Care Issues, 530

CHAPTER 15

Nutritional Support 543

Glossary, 543
Concepts of Nutrition, 547
Nutritional Assessment, 548
Nutritional Requirements, 551
Modalities for Delivery of Nutritional Support, 559
Parenteral Nutrition in the Pediatric Patient, 567
Complications and Nursing Considerations, 568
Standards of Practice for Nutritional Support, 578
Patient Education, 581
Home Care Issues, 582

Appendices 593

Appendix A: Nomogram of Body Surface Areas, 594
Appendix B: Physical and Chemical Compatibility Chart, 597
Appendix C: Normal Laboratory Reference Values, 602
Appendix D: OSHA Guidelines 1995: Controlling Occupational
Exposure to Hazardous Drugs, 604
Appendix E: Dilution of Intravenous Drugs, 612
Appendix F: Resource List of National Organizations, 616
Appendix G: Survey of Scope of Intravenous Practice by State for
Licensed Practical and Vocational Nurses, 617

Index 619

TABLES

1–1. Summary of Key Advances in I.V. Therapy in the
Renaissance Era 5
1–2. Summary of Key Advances in I.V. Therapy in the 19th
Century 8
1–3. Summary of Key Advances in Transfusion Therapy 9
1–4. Summary of Key Advances in I.V. Therapy in the 20th
Century 11

2–1. Strategies for Risk Management 19
2–2. Agencies Influencing Standards of Practice 22
2–3. I.V. Therapy Risk Management Screens 24
2–4. Key Components of Informed Consent...................... 25
2–5. JCAHO Competency Requirements 28
2–6. Educational Three-Part Competency Program Model 30
2–7. JCAHO 10-Step Monitoring and Evaluation Process 35
2–8. Quality Management Model: Catheter-Related Sepsis....... 37

3–1. Percentages of Total Body Fluid in Relation to Age and
Sex 48
3–2. Water Balance: Intake and Output.......................... 50
3–3. Mechanisms of Transport 51
3–4. Quick Assessment Guide for Fluid Imbalance 59
3–5. Extracellular Fluid Disorders: Deficit and Excess 60

4–1. Positive and Negative Ions in Body Fluids.................. 76
4–2. Comparison of Electrolyte Composition in Fluid
Compartments 77
4–3. Critical Guidelines for Administration of Potassium 83
4–4. Critical Guidelines for Removal of Potassium 84
4–5. Critical Guidelines for Administration of Magnesium....... 90
4–6. Summary of Electrolyte Imbalance 96
4–7. Summary of Acute Acid-Base Imbalances................... 104

5–1. Sample Schedule for Restoration Therapy for Nasogastric
Suctioning 121
5–2. Contents of Available Intravenous Fluids 126
5–3. Quick-Glance Chart of Common I.V. Fluids 137

6–1. Organs of the Immune System 154
6–2. Strategies to Improve Antibiotic Use 159
6–3. Antimicrobial Agents Effective Against Certain
Nosocomial Pathogens 160
6–4. Risk Factors for Infusion Phlebitis in Peripheral I.V.
Therapy. 164
6–5. Microorganisms Most Frequently Found in I.V.-Related
Infections 165
6–6. Nursing Procedure: Steps in Catheter Culturing. 168
6–7. Three Cutaneous Antiseptics Used for Prevention of I.V.
Device-Related Septicemia 168

7–1. Advantages and Disadvantages of the Glass System 187
7–2. Advantages and Disadvantages of the Plastic System 189
7–3. Comparison of Peripheral Infusion Devices. 196
7–4. Guide for Over-The-Needle Catheter Use 198
7–5. Function of Filters 205

8–1. Comparison of Artery and Vein 233
8–2. Selecting an Insertion Site for the Superficial Veins of the
Dorsum of the Hand. 234
8–3. Selecting an Insertion Site for the Superficial Veins of
the Arm 235
8–4. Phillips 15-Step Venipuncture Method 238
8–5. Tips for Selecting Veins 240
8–6. Two Methods of Performing a Venipuncture 244
8–7. Troubleshooting Difficult Veins. 245
8–8. Stabilizing the Catheter. 245
8–9. Conversion Chart: Rate Calculation 249

9–1. Local Complications 272
9–2. Steps for Checking Slowed Infusion 275
9–3. Factors Affecting Phlebitis Formation 277
9–4. Infusion Phlebitis Scale 277
9–5. Frequently Administered I.V. Drugs: pH and
Recommended Dilution 279
9–6. Factors Affecting Risk for Extravasation Injury 284
9–7. Antidotes for Extravasated Drugs 287
9–8. Risk Factors Associated with Septicemia 291
9–9. Removal of Air from Primary Set. 295

10–1. Normal Laboratory Values for Children 317
10–2. Components of the Pediatric Physical Assessment 318

10–3. Nursing Interventions for the Child Requiring I.V. Therapy as Related to Physical and Psychological Development 325
10–4. Assessment Guidelines for Fluid Volume Disturbances in the Elderly 332
10–5. Special Problems 334

11–1. Advantages of Intravenous Medication Administration 353
11–2. Disadvantages of Intravenous Medication 354
11–3. Drugs that have Increased Absorption in PVC Containers .. 355
11–4. Medications Used for Intraspinal Narcotic Administration 371
11–5. Categories of Antibiotics 374
11–6. I.V. Antifungal Medication Guidelines 375
11–7. I.V. Antiviral Administration Guidelines 376
11–8. I.V. Narcotic Administration Guidelines 377

12–1. Comparing Central Venous Catheters 399
12–2. Care of Central Venous Catheters 407

13–1. ABO Blood Grouping Chart 443
13–2. ABO Compatibility Chart 444
13–3. Summary of Testing Donor Blood 446
13–4. Summary of Blood Components 463
13–5. Steps in Administration of a Blood Component 466
13–6. Risks of Transfusion Therapy 478

14–1. Oncology Patient Assessment 496
14–2. Timing of the Cell Cycle 498
14–3. Classes of Antineoplastic Drugs and Biologic Response Modifiers 501
14–4. Alkylating Agents 501
14–5. Antimetabolite Agents 502
14–6. Natural Products 503
14–7. Hormones and Hormone Antagonists 505
14–8. Common Adverse Effects of Chemotherapy 509
14–9. Pharmacologic Management of Diarrhea 511
14–10. General Procedure for Extravasation 514
14–11. Recommended Extravasation Kit Contents 514
14–12. Agents for Oral Care 515
14–13. Antiemetics Commonly Used for Prevention and Treatment of Chemotherapy-Induced Nausea and Vomiting 517
14–14. Methods of Delivering Antineoplastic Agents 522
14–15. Advantages and Disadvantages of IP Management Methods 525

15–1. Components of a Nutritional Assessment 549
15–2. Physical Findings Associated with Deficiency States 552

15–3. Dextrose Solutions for Total Parenteral Nutrition 554
15–4. Lipid Emulsions for Total Parenteral Nutrition.............. 555
15–5. Amino Acid Solutions for Total Parenteral Nutrition 557
15–6. Daily Vitamin Recommendations from the AMA 558
15–7. Daily Trace Elements Recommended by the AMA 558
15–8. Indications for Total Parenteral Nutrition.................... 561
15–9. Standard Peripheral Vein Nutrition Solutions/Liter......... 563
15–10. Standard Central Parenteral Nutrition Solution 564
15–11. Specialized Parenteral Formulas............................ 566
15–12. Complications of Parenteral Nutrition....................... 569
15–13. Summary of Monitoring of Parenteral Nutrition Therapy .. 580

UNIT ONE

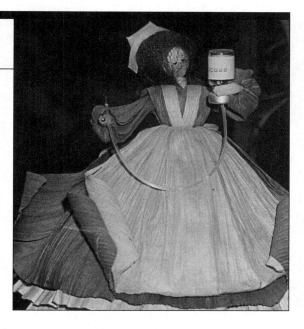

INTRODUCTION TO THE PRACTICE OF INTRAVENOUS THERAPY

CHAPTER 1
Intravenous Therapy: Past, Present, and Future Trends

CHAPTER 2
Risk Management and Quality Patient Management

Intravenous Therapy: Past, Present, and Future Trends

CHAPTER CONTENTS

LEARNING OBJECTIVES
RENAISSANCE ERA (1438 to 1660)
THE 19TH CENTURY
Transfusion Advances
Infusion Advances
Aseptic Technique Advances
Nutritional Support Advances
Medication Advances
THE 20TH CENTURY
Transfusion Advances
Infusion Advances
Nutritional Support Advances

Medication Administration Advances
Advances in Education
ADVANCES AND TRENDS IN THE 90S
TRENDS FOR THE 21ST CENTURY
Health Care Reform
Bloodborne Pathogens
Technology
Education
KEY POINTS
REFERENCES

LEARNING OBJECTIVES

Upon completion of this chapter, the reader will be able to:

- Identify strategic events in the evolution of intravenous therapy.
- Discuss the impact of these events on current intravenous therapy.
- Recognize the need for further investigation into more effective ways to deliver intravenous therapy.

*In the beginning, God created nursing. He (or She) said, I will take a solid, simple, significant system of **education** and an adequate, applicable base of **clinical research** and on these rocks, will I build My greatest gift to Mankind—nursing practice. On the seventh day, He threw up His hands. And has left it up to us.*

MARGRETTA M. STYLES

The foundation for intravenous (I.V.) therapy began slowly with contributions from chemists, physicians, and architects. The specialty practice of I.V. therapy as we know it today has many heroes and heroines who have made an imprint on this area of medicine. The history of I.V. therapy is woven with individuals aided by advances in technical development. Five hundred years have elapsed from the discovery of the circulation of blood to today's state-of-the-art tunneled catheters, implanted ports, and blood component therapy. A review of the roots of I.V. therapy precedes the study of the theoretic and practical applications of I.V. therapy.

RENAISSANCE ERA (1438 to 1660)

The history of I.V. therapy began with the discovery by Sir William Harvey of the circulation of blood. Until the late Renaissance period it was known that the arteries and veins both contained blood, but it was believed that the blood ebbed and flowed "like the human breath." The essential parts of the circulatory system and the capillary networks were unknown, and for centuries this fundamental error was accepted as truth. Harvey was the first to discover that the heart is both a muscle and a pump, and he lectured extensively in Europe to educate other physicians.

Sir Christopher Wren, the famous architect of St. Paul's Cathedral in London, worked with a chemist and produced the first hypodermic needle. Wren inserted a hollow pipe in the blood vessel of a dog and injected wine, ale, opium, scammony, liver of antimony, and other substances directly into the bloodstream and studied their effect. He was thus credited for using a quill and bladder to inject the first I.V. substance.

A German physician, Johann Majors, was the first to use Sir Christopher Wren's discovery of the hypodermic needle and injected unpurified compounds into humans. The disastrous consequences of this early experimental work were compounded by the fact that infections occurred at the site of injection, resulting in death.

In 1667, the first well-documented transfusion from an animal to a human was performed. The Parisian physician John Baptiste Denis infused lamb's blood directly into the circulation of a 15-year-old boy. The boy died quickly. This early experiment was not well received, and in 1687, by edict of the church and parliament, animal-to-human transfusions were prohibited in Europe (Schmidt, 1959, pp 59–62). Because of this edict, 150 years passed before injecting substances into the circulation again became of interest, in the 19th century. Table 1–1 summarizes the key advances in I.V. therapy during the Renaissance era.

THE 19TH CENTURY

Transfusion Advances

During the 19th century, there were many advances in medicine. One of the first was man-to-man transfusion first performed by Dr. James Blundell in London in 1834.

4

TABLE 1–1. SUMMARY OF KEY ADVANCES IN I.V. THERAPY IN THE RENAISSANCE ERA

Year	Key Advances
1543	Andreas Vesalius published written account of his work on anatomy and surgery based on dissections.
1616	Sir William Harvey discovered circulation of blood.
1628	Sir William Harvey published theories on circulation, considered to be the beginning of modern I.V. therapy.
1660	Sir Christopher Wren invented the first hypodermic needle.
1662	German physician Johann Majors injected compounds into human, using Wren's needle.
1667	First well-documented transfusion from animal to human performed in Paris by John Denis. This led to the edict from the church and parliament prohibiting all further work on transfusion therapy.

Dr. Blundell is credited with the correlation between blood loss and hyoxemia during hemorrhage (Rutman & Miller, 1985).

Infusion Advances

In 1831, the Anatomy Act was designed to regulate human dissection. Florence Nightingale was 8 years old and Joseph Lister was 4 years old. An outbreak of cholera, the second pandemic, was spreading across Asia and Europe from India. In that same year, Dr. Brooke O'Shaughnessy, a recent Edinburgh graduate, age 22, wrote his first paper on cholera. He became engrossed in the cause and cure of cholera. O'Shaughnessy described cholera and studied the blood drawn from patients with the disease. He wrote to *The Lancet* on February 4, 1832:

> The blood drawn in the worst cases . . . is unchanged in its anatomical or globular structure . . . It has lost a large proportion of its water . . . It has lost also a great proportion of its neutral saline ingredients . . . Of the free alkali contained in healthy serum, not a particle is present . . . Cited in Cosnett, 1989

The first practical application of O'Shaughnessy's observations was by Dr. Thomas Latta, who used infusions of saline to treat the intractable diarrhea of cholera. He published his results in *The Lancet* on June 2, 1832. However, there were no previous records of water and salts being given deliberately to restore constituents of the blood. Of the first 25 reported cases treated by saline, eight patients survived. There was severe criticism of this method of treatment, and when the pandemic spread to America in 1852–1863, the use of intravenous saline was not accepted (Cosnett, 1989).

Aseptic Technique Advances

During the latter part of the 19th century, advances were made in medicine. Accelerated knowledge regarding bacteriology, pathology, and pharmacology revealed new approaches to problems of medicine.

One new approach was the use of nitrous oxide and ether as a form of anesthesia by Horace Wells. A chemist, Charles Jackson, assisted W.T.G. Morton in his first surgical operations with ether at Massachusetts General Hospital in Boston on October 16, 1846. This method of anesthesia quickly spread throughout America and Europe, but chloroform soon came to be preferred to ether.

5

In 1847, a Viennese obstetrician, Ignaz Semmelweis, noted that physicians moving from autopsies to the obstetrical unit were communicating highly pathogenic substances between the two departments. He was the first to require physicians to wash their hands in a solution of chlorine before examining an obstetrical patient. Semmelweis reduced the death rate in the maternity wards by over 90% between 1846 and 1848 through this simple procedure of cleanliness.

Louis Pasteur, a chemist, later demonstrated the scientific basis for Semmelweis's theory, proving that bacteria were living microorganisms. However, Pasteur's ideas were challenged, and it was not until Lister's work in 1867 that the germ theory was accepted and the war won. Lister's work focused on sterility in the operating room and led to the practice of asepsis. His aseptic technique came to replace older antiseptic methods, and was universally accepted.

In 1889, the use of gloves for surgical procedures was introduced by William Halsted of Johns Hopkins Hospital in cooperation with the Goodyear Rubber Company. By 1899, the use of rubber gloves became popular, not only to protect the patient but to protect the practitioner from the corrosive hand rinse being used.

The primitive state of medical knowledge and practice in the 1880s had an influence on the morbidity or mortality of infants and young children of the time. Infant mortality rate during this time varied from 250 to 500 of 1000 live births. The high morbidity and mortality rates of the late 19th century accounted for the average life span staying at 35 to 38 years. Enteric disorder, malnutrition, and common respiratory and contagious diseases constituted the major causes of death during the 19th century.

Nutritional Support Advances

Claude Bernard, a French physiologist, experimented with injecting sugar solution into dogs in 1834. He continued his work for the next two decades, injecting egg whites and milk into animals, with some success. Bernard also discovered that cane sugar, injected intravenously, soon appeared in the urine, whereas ingested sugar did not because of breakdown by the digestion process (Rombeau & Caldwell, 1986).

Further advances in nutritional support came in 1869 when Menzel and Perco of Vienna wrote a paper on the use of fat, milk, and camphor injected subcutaneously (Grant, 1992). By 1878, the use of oil and protein extract to treat patients suffering from anorexia nervosa was reported, and cow's milk was being injected for nutritional support. In Canada, Hodder experimented with use of cow's milk to correct fluid and nutritional losses caused by cholera. The results were considered good; however, Hodder was barred from practice of medicine by his colleagues, and further work in nutritional support was abandoned (Grant, 1992).

Medication Advances

Medications during the turn of the century were limited primarily to coal tar products, which were used to treat febrile illnesses and influenza. The following is a list of the 10 most commonly administered compounds during the 19th century:

1. Ether
2. Morphine
3. Digitalis
4. Diphtheria antitoxin
5. Smallpox vaccine
6. Iron
7. Quinine
8. Iodine

9. Alcohol
10. Mercury (Kalisch & Kalisch, 1995)

Table 1–2 summarizes the key advances in I.V. therapy in the 19th century.

THE 20TH CENTURY

Transfusion Advances

In 1900, Karl Landsteiner proved that not all human blood was alike with the discovery of three of the four main blood groups. This led the way to compatible blood transfusions and the development of blood banks. In 1911, Dr. Ottenberg of New York demonstrated that it was safe to use a donor person whose serum agglutinated the recipient's red cells but unsafe to use a donor whose red cells were acted upon by the recipient's serum. This work originated the idea of the universal donor. Until 1914, there was no way to prevent the coagulation of blood, and every transfusion was performed via the direct method, recipient to donor. However, with the discovery of sodium citrate, blood could be stored and blood banking began.

Many advances in transfusion practices occurred during wartime. Between 1936 and 1939 during the Spanish Civil War, the practicality of supplying stored blood from the civilian population to wounded men on the front was proved. During World War I, criteria for transfusion were established. During World War II, the donor criteria were established and the closed collection system used.

Additional advances include use of packed red blood cells in the United States during the 1940s, discovery of the Rh factor on red blood cells in 1940, and the establishment of the American Association of Blood Banking (AABB) in 1947 to meet civilian needs (Rutman & Miller, 1985).

Component therapy began when Cohn designed the first cell separator in 1951. In 1970, blood components and the prescribing of selected components for individual situations, such as packed cells for the anemic patient, were instituted. Table 1–3 summarizes the key advances in transfusion therapy in the 20th century.

Infusion Advances

Until Dr. Florence Seibert discovered pyrogen substances in distilled water, there were many problems related to pyrogens (proteins foreign to the blood) within solutions. Researchers worked to eliminate those pyrogens, and the administration of parenteral solutions became safer. Until 1925, the most frequently used parenteral solution was 0.9% sodium chloride solution because of its isotonic relationship to blood. After 1925, dextrose was used extensively to provide a source of calories. I.V. solutions, however, were used only for the critically ill patient.

Great strides were made at Massachusetts General Hospital, where nurses were first assigned to be I.V. nurses. The services of the I.V. nurse consisted of administering I.V. solutions and transfusions, cleaning infusion sets, and cleaning and sharpening needles. The role of the nurse changed primarily because of the shortage of physicians during World War II. Nurses took over jobs that physicians had always done: injections, suturing wounds, taking blood pressure readings, and drawing blood, as well as administering infusion therapy. Nurses were trained in I.V. therapy by the anesthesiologist in the operating room.

In the mid-1950s, I.V. therapy was used for two main purposes: major surgery and dehydration. Solutions of 5% dextrose and water or 0.9% sodium chloride for surgical patients were infused over 3 to 4 hours and discontinued at night.

Less than 20% of hospital patients received I.V. therapy in the mid-1950s. The

7

TABLE 1–2. SUMMARY OF KEY ADVANCES IN I.V. THERAPY IN THE 19TH CENTURY

Year	Key Advances
1818	English obstetrician James Blundell revived the idea of transfusions for hemorrhage during childbirth. He proved that animal blood was unfit to inject into man, and that only human blood was safe.
1831	The Anatomy Act, designed to regulate human dissection, was debated. An outbreak of cholera, the second pandemic, spread across Asia and Europe from India.
Dec. 1831	Dr. William Brooke O'Shaughnessy wrote a paper on cholera and applied chemistry to its cure. He cited detailed descriptions of blood from cholera patients. He recommended restoring blood to its natural specific gravity, and restoring the saline matter of blood.
June 1832	Dr. Thomas Latta of Scotland used intravenous saline on cholera patients, successfully based on Dr. O'Shaughnessy's work on cholera.
1834	Dr. Blundell performed the first man-to-man transfusion. Claude Bernard experimented with injecting sugar solution into dogs.
1852–1863	Despite further pandemics, I.V. saline was not widely used.
1845	Horace Wells demonstrated the use of nitrous oxide and ether for anesthesia.
1846	W.T.G. Morton, with assistance from a chemist, used ether in the first surgical operation with this agent at Massachusetts General Hospital in Boston.
1847	Dr. Ignaz Semmelweis noted that infection was transferred from postmortem patients to obstetrical patients. He was the first to require physicians to wash hands in solution of chlorine before the examination of maternity patients.
1857	Dr. Louis Pasteur demonstrated the scientific basis for the Semmelweis theory.
1867	Lord Joseph Lister achieved success with meticulous attention to sterility during surgical procedures.
1878	Oil and protein extract were used to treat anorexia nervosa. Dr. Hodder experimented with the use of cow's milk to correct fluid and nutritional losses caused by cholera in Canada and was barred from the practice of medicine.
1889	Dr. William Halsted, in cooperation with the Goodyear Rubber Company, developed the first rubber gloves.
Late 1800s	Dr. Edward Robinson Squibb founded a pharmaceutical company and manufactured products, including talcum and ether anesthetic, in tins.

site most frequently used by nurses during this period was the antecubital vein. A 16- to 18-gauge steel reusable needle was used and stabilized with leather restraints. Disposable plastic sets became available and replaced reusable rubber tubing, and frequent infiltrations with metal needles led to the development of the flexible plastic catheter for insertion by the cutdown method (Crossley & Matsen, 1972).

In 1950, the Rochester needle was introduced. This device consisted of a resinous catheter on the outside of a steel needle; the catheter was slipped off the needle into the vein and the needle removed. In 1958, the Intracath (Deseret Pharmaceutical Co.), a plastic catheter lying within the lumen of the needle, was introduced in individual sterile packaging. This type of catheter reduced the need for surgical cutdown for placement of the 1940s catheter (Weinstein, 1993). The first change in the steel needle appeared in 1957, when McGaw Laboratories introduced small vein sets with foldable wings as grips.

The momentum for change in the I.V. therapy field occurred during the 1960s. A variety of solutions were marketed, expanding the choice to approximately 200.

TABLE 1–3. **SUMMARY OF KEY ADVANCES IN TRANSFUSION THERAPY**

Year	Key Advances
1876	Blood groups had not been discovered.
	Transfusion devices were crude.
	All transfusions were direct, blood could not be stored.
1900	Landsteiner described the ABO blood group system.
1911	Ottenberg of New York used donor selection and originated the idea of universal donor.
1918	ABO blood group system was first used.
(World War I)	Anticoagulant was first used.
	Pretransfusion testing was not routinely performed.
	Widespread use of plasma began.
1936–1939	Shock was treated with plasma.
	Hemorrhage was being treated with red blood cells.
1941–1945	Blood was drawn in closed system.
(World War II)	Blood airlifted overseas instead of being drawn locally.
	Shelf life is extended.
	Packed red blood cells are widely used.
	Filters are used for plasma infusion.
	Fresh frozen plasm (FFP) received some limited used.
	Relationship of transfusions to hepatitis was realized.
1947	American Association of Blood Banking (AABB) was established.
1950	Closed-system bottle with acid-citrate dextrose (ACD) was used.
	Methods sterilizing plasma was attempted.
	Storage and transportation studies were being conducted.
1965–1973	High risk of hepatitis was found in Vietnam.
(Vietnam War)	Blood was drawn in Japan and shipped to Vietnam.
	Blood could be stored 31 days.
	Work was conducted on preservative ACD-adenine.
1972	National Blood Policy was established.
1973	National Blood Policy was announced by Health, Education and Welfare (HEW).
1975	American Blood Commission was formed.
1989	FDA approved use of epoetin alfa (EPO) for treatment of anemia associated with chronic renal failure.

Piggyback medications were used, and filters and electronic infusion devices flooded the market.

Since the 1980s tunneled catheters, such as Hickman-Broviac and Groshong, have provided a means of central venous access for delivery of total parenteral nutrition (TPN) and cytoxic therapy. In the past 5 years, totally implanted access devices, consisting of a subcutaneous reservoir connected to a catheter positioned in the central circulation, provided alternatives for patients requiring long-term access. The changes in management of patients needing long-term I.V. therapy with permanent central venous lines have expanded the field of I.V. therapy.

Nutritional Support Advances

The first I.V. hydrolyzed protein and fat were administered to animals during the early 20th century, leading the way to today's nutritional support solutions. In 1937, Dr. W.C. Rose identified amino acids, which were essential for growth in rats and led to the development of protein hydrolysates for infusion into humans.

9

In 1963, at the Harrison Department of Surgical Research at the University of Pennsylvania, a young surgical resident, Stanley Dudrick, conducted the first experiment to determine definitely whether or not long-term total I.V. nutrition was feasible. Dudrick's experiments were quickly applied to starving adult patients, who would probably not have survived without total parenteral nutrition (Dudrick & Rhoads, 1972).

In 1967, the first TPN was given to patients at Children's Hospital in Philadelphia. In 1968, RhoGAM was manufactured and available to the physician for Rh-negative mothers to prevent hemolytic disease of the newborn.

During the 1970s, fat emulsion (Intralipid; Abbott Pharmaceuticals) was instituted as an adjunct to nutritional support. In 1977, the formation of nutritional support teams began. The American Society for Parenteral and Enteral Nutrition (ASPEN) was formed and held its first clinical congress in Chicago.

In the 1980s, TPN evolved into a science, providing nutrients by vein in sufficient amounts to achieve anabolism. Disease-specific formulas were developed to address particular needs of patients with renal, cardiac, or hepatic disease. In 1983, TPN moved to the home (HPN) (Weinstein, 1993).

Research continues in this sophisticated field, with further work on the role of amino acids; indications for medium-, short-, and long-chain triglycerides; and the use of antioxidants or "free radical scavengers" (Fischer, 1991).

Medication Administration Advances

Medications were not routinely administered by the I.V. route, but sometimes intramuscularly. For seriously ill patients with diseases like meningitis, penicillin or chloraphenicol was given by continuous I.V. drip. When patients required medication added to their infusions, an intern carried out this procedure, often using medication that had been unrefrigerated for long periods of time. When blood was needled, the patient received whole blood in a glass bottle, and the blood was administered by the intern with assistance from the nursing staff.

Cutdowns continued to be used until the mid-1970s for severely ill patients to prevent the complication of infiltration. Cathether sites were changed only when they were not functioning. It was not until the early 1970s that the Centers for Disease Control (CDC) developed recommendations for infection control related to I.V. therapy.

During the 1970s, the administration of pain medication was expanded by alternative routes. In 1976, successful administration of morphine directly into the subarachnoid space of animals was demonstrated by Yaks and Rudy. In 1977, Wang proved that an intrathecal injection of morphine provided profound relief of pain in humans (Zenz, 1984). Today the intrathecal and epidural routes have proved effective for administration of specific medication therapies.

Advances in Education

In the 1970s, there was a scarcity of I.V. information in nursing journals, and I.V. therapy journals were nonexistent until the late 1970s. Nursing schools presented I.V. therapy in a limited manner, with more theory than practical management.

The past 10 years have been the fastest in growth for the I.V. therapy field. The National Intravenous Therapy Association (NITA) published recommendations for practices in the early 1980s. On October 1, 1980, the US House of Representatives recognized and nationalized I.V. Nurse Day throughout the country. It was *resolved, that I.V. Nurse Day be nationally celebrated in honor of the National Intravenous Therapy Association Inc. on January 25 of each year . . .*

according to a portion of the proclamation as presented by the Honorable Edward J. Mackey from the Fifth Congressional District of Massachusetts (Gardner, 1985).

NITA's first national Certification Examination for Intravenous Nurses was offered in March 1985. In 1987, NITA changed its name to the Intravenous Nursing Society (INS). Table 1–4 summarizes the key advances in I.V. therapy in the 20th century.

ADVANCES AND TRENDS IN THE 90S

A 1990 *American Journal of Nursing* survey found that 81% of nurses performed I.V. skills over 75% of their time (Griffith, Thomas, & Griffith, 1991). The role of the nurse has also changed in home care settings, with patients requiring home care monitoring of I.V. therapy. Today 90% of hospitalized patients receive I.V. therapy. Hospitalized patients in the year 2000 will be those needing highly intensive and sophisticated treatment. Looking ahead to the 21st century, it is inconceivable that nurses will be limited to the responsibilities that they hold today. By the turn of the century, nurses will be assuming more and more health care responsibilities. Changes in expenditures for health care, hospital costs, and seriously ill patients all will make an impact on the nursing profession.

TRENDS FOR THE 21ST CENTURY

Health Care Reform

By the mid-1990s the US health care industry employed more than 10 million people, including 2,200,000 nurses. This industry, now the nation's largest, is the leading labor sector in the entire United States. In 1994, almost 100,000 registered nurses (RNs) were considered advanced-practice nurses with special clinical expertise (Kalisch & Kalisch, 1995).

TABLE 1–4. **SUMMARY OF KEY ADVANCES IN I.V. THERAPY IN THE 20TH CENTURY**

Year	Key Advances
1900	Karl Landsteiner discovered three of four main blood groups.
1914	Sodium citrate was used to preserve blood.
1914	Hydrolyzed protein and fats were first given intravenously to animals.
1923	Dr. Florence Seibert discovered pathogens in distilled water. Sterilization practices for infusion therapy changed.
1937	W.C. Rose identified amino acids essential for growth in rats leading to development of protein hydrolysate for infusion.
1940	Drs. Landsteiner and Weiner discovered the Rhesus factor (Rh).
1940	Work by Tocantins and O'Neil led to the use of intraosseous infusions.
1945	A flexible plastic intravenous catheter inserted by cutdown was developed.
1950	The Rochester needle was introduced.

Continued on following page

11

TABLE 1–4. SUMMARY OF KEY ADVANCES
IN I.V. THERAPY IN THE 20TH CENTURY (*Continued*)

Year	Key Advances
1958	Deseret Pharmaceuticals introduced the Intracath.
1960	First hyperalimentation experiment on animals began.
1960	Peripherally inserted central lines began to be used in critical care units.
1963	Researchers at University of Pennsylvania conducted the first experiment to determine long-term total I.V. nutritional support feasible by Stanley Dudrick.
1968	RhoGAM was used to treat Rh hemolytic disease.
1970	Blood components became available for use in specific situations.
	Centers for Disease Control (CDC) guidelines for I.V. therapy were published.
	Occupational Safety and Health (OSH) Act created three agencies:
	Occupational Safety and Health Administration (OSHA)
	National Institute of Safety and Health (NIOSH)
	Occupational Safety and Health Review Commission (OSHRC)
1972	Concept of accessing an implantable port was introduced.
1973	First central venous tunneled catheter was developed. Broviac right atrial catheter was designed and introduced.
1976	Fat emulsions were used for nutritional support
1977	National Cancer Institute (NCI) began testing intraperitoneal chemotherapy in selected patients.
	American Society for Parenteral and Enteral Nutrition (ASPEN) held its first clinical conference.
1980	NITA published recommended practices for I.V. therapy.
1980	US House of Representatives recognized I.V. Nurse Day.
1981	CDC revised guidelines for management of intravascular catheters
1982	Implantable ports were developed for long-term access.
1983	Resurgence of interest arose in intraosseous infusions in children.
1985	First credentialing examination was offered by NITA.
1986	Resurgent use of peripherally inserted central lines (PICC).
	Patient controlled analgesia was used.
	OSHA published guidelines for the management of cytotoxic durgsin in the workplace.
1987	NITA became the Intravenous Nurses Society (INS).
	OSHA enforces CDC guidelines on Universal Precautions.
1990	Safe Medical Device Act. Home infusion therapy was well established.
	INS revised standards of practice.
1992	Colony stimulating factors were introduced.
	OSHA Bloodborne Pathogens Standard (BBPS) was established.
	FDA issued safety alert warning of the risks of needlestick injuries associated with hypodermic needles and I.V. equipment.
	NIOSH set controversial recommendations for health care worker use of powered air-purifying respirators (PAPRs).
1995	OSHA revised guidelines for management of controlling occupational exposure to hazardous drugs in the workplace.
	CDC revised guidelines for intravascular catheters, administration sets, and parenteral fluids.
1996	INS offers first credentialing examination to LPN/LVN.
	INS published revised standards of practice.

The current health care reform package continues to be debated. The focus of the reform is the quality and accessibility to care for 37 million Americans who lack health insurance. Nurses will play a major role in the health care reform because 60% to 80% of primary health care traditionally provided by physicians can be provided by nurses.

A shift in focus from high-tech, hospital-based care to primary health care has already begun. This trend will only accelerate toward the 21st century. Nurses in the next decade will need to be cognizant of terms such as "global budgeting," "managed care," and "total quality management" (Larkin, 1993).

Bloodborne Pathogens

Occupational exposure to bloodborne pathogens is a risk to nurses, especially those working in I.V. therapy. Safety will continue to be an issue with focus on product features such as recessed or needleless systems. Legislation on product design for practitioner protection may also affect clinical standards of practice.

Technology

Technology will continue to evolve in health care. Patients will find treatment in noninstitutional settings such as outpatient centers, diagnostic centers, self-care centers, and health-related shopping centers. It is projected that the patient will be more capable of matching his or her disease or illness with the appropriate care setting and will have more autonomy in the prevention and treatment of the illness. Satellite telemedicine and video network hookups will be in common use. Nurses will routinely provide services outside hospitals, addressing patient's relatively minor problems in noninstitutional ways (Kalisch & Kalisch, 1995). Nurses will manage catastrophic cases and work through insurance agencies as independent practitioners.

Growth and expansion of the nurse's role are both necessary and desirable. The changing role of the nurse is leading to the development of many new programs designed to prepare the nurse to use new skills and assume new responsibilities. New roles are emerging, with nurses developing interdependent, collaborative, and peer relationships with physicians. I.V. therapy is just one of the interdependent roles needing a sound foundation in basic as well as advanced theory.

The role of the RN is well defined in the initiation, maintenance, and therapeutic modalities as identified in each state's nursing practice act. Standards of practice established by the INS and the CDC have set guidelines for the role of the RN in all aspects of I.V. therapy and nutritional support.

Education

Because of the shortage of licensed personnel in many settings, the role of the licensed practical/vocational nurse (LPN/LVN) as an integral part of the I.V. therapy team is in the process of evaluation.

The role of the LPN/LVN has been expanded in 26 states to encompass the initiation, maintenance, and delivery of solutions, antibiotics, blood components, and peripheral nutritional support. Each of the 26 states has established the expanded role of the LPN/LVN with clear guidelines for practice. Another 19 states delegate the role of I.V. therapy to the institution in which the LPN/LVN is practicing. Four states have elected to deny I.V. therapy in the scope of the LPN/LVN. Refer to Appendix F for the survey on the expanded role of the LPN/LVN.

The INS has recognized that the LPN/LVN has a place in the scope of I.V. nursing and is preparing a credentialing examination for the LPN/LVN to be initiated in September of 1996.

KEY POINTS

INTRAVENOUS THERAPY: PAST, PRESENT, AND FUTURE TRENDS

Renaissance era (1438–1660)
Major advances
Discovery of the circulatory system
First hypodermic needle invented
First documented transfusion from animal to human—led to the edict from the church and parliament prohibiting all further work on transfusion therapy
19th Century
Major advances
1818 transfusions revived to treat hemorrhage during childbirth—human to human only
Anatomy Act regulated human dissection
Paper written on cholera and recommendations for restoring blood with saline
Use of I.V. saline on cholera patients
Use of nitrous oxide and ether for anesthesia
Hand washing noted to reduce transmission of infection
Dr. Pasteur and Lord Lister work on cleanliness and sterility
Use of cow's milk to correct fluid and nutritional losses caused by cholera in Canada
First rubber gloves
First pharmaceutical company
20th Century
Major advances
1900–1920
Discovery of three of four blood groups
Sodium citrate used to preserve blood
1920–1945
Rh factor discovered
First work in 1940 on intraosseous infusions
First hyperalimentation
Flexible plastic I.V. catheter inserted by cutdown
1940–1960
First hyperalimentation experiments
PICC used in critical care units

1960–1970
>First work on long-term TPN
>RhoGam used to treat Rh hemolytic disease
>Blood components become available for use
>CDC publishes guidelines for I.V. therapy

1971–1980
>Concept of implantable port introduced
>First central venous tunneled catheter developed
>Fat emulsions used for nutritional support
>First standards of practice published by NITA

1981–present
>CDC revised guidelines for management of intravascular catheters
>Implantable ports developed for long-term access
>Resurgence of interest in intraosseous infusion in children
>PICC begin to be used
>Patient controlled analgesia used
>OSHA enforces CDC guidelines on Universal Precautions
>Safe Medical Device Act—Home infusion therapy well established

1991–1997
>Colony stimulating factors were introduced
>OSHA Bloodborne Pathogens Standards established
>FDA issued safety alert warning of risks of needle-stick injuries associated with needles and I.V. equipment

REFERENCES

American Journal of Nursing. (1990). LPN's widen their role, disagreement grows. Controversies in care. *American Journal of Nursing, 90*(2), 16–17.

Cosnett, J.E. (1989). Before our time: The origins of intravenous fluid therapy. *Lancet,* (4), 768–771.

Crossley K., & Matsen, M. (1972). The scalp-vein needle. *J.A.M.A., 220,* 985.

Crow, S. (1993). Sterilization processes. *Nursing Clinics of North America, 28*(3), 695.

Dudrick, S.J., & Rhoads, J.E. (1972). Total intravenous feeding. *Science American, 226,* 73–80.

Fischer, J.E. (1991). *Total parenteral nutrition.* Boston: Little, Brown.

Gardner, C. (1985). United States House of Representatives honors the National Intravenous Therapy Association, *National Intravenous Therapy Association, 14*(1), 5.

Grant, J.P. (1992). *Handbook of total parenteral nutrition* (3rd ed). Philadelphia: W.B. Saunders.

Griffith, H.M., Thomas, N., & Griffith, L. (1991). MDs bill for these routine nursing tasks. *American Journal of Nursing, 91*(1), 22–27.

Jackson, M.M., & Lynch, P. (1990). Infection control: In search of a rational approach. *American Journal of Nursing, 90*(10), 65–73.

Kalisch, P.A., & Kalisch, B.J. (1995). *The advance of american nursing* (3rd ed). Philadelphia: J.B. Lippincott.

Larkin, M. (1993). Chief executive officer's report. *Journal of Intravenous Nursing, 16,* 210.

Millam, D.A. (1987). I.V. therapy 30 years ago. *National Intravenous Therapy Association, 10,* 118–121.

Rombeau, J.L., & Caldwell, M.D. (1986). *Parenteral nutrition,* vol. 2. Philadelphia: W.B. Saunders.

Rutman, R.C., & Miller, W.V. (1985). *Transfusion therapy principles and policies* (2nd ed). Rockville, MD: Aspen.

Schmidt, J.E. (1959). *Medical discoveries who and when.* Springfield: Charles C. Thomas.

Thomas Spitzer, R. (1987). Catch the wave of nursing in the '90s. *Nursing 87,* 8–10.

Sutcliff, J. (1992). *A history of medicine.* New York: Barnes & Noble.

Viall, C.D. (1990). Your complete guide to central venous catheters. *Nursing 90,* (2), 34–41.

van Heyningen, W.E., & Seal, J.R. (1983). *Cholera: The American scientific experience 1947–1980.* Boulder, CO, Westview Press.

Weinstein, S. (1993). *Plummer's principles and practices of intravenous therapy* (5th ed). Philadelphia: J.B. Lippincott.

Zenz, M. (1984). Epidural opiates for the treatment of cancer pain. *Recent Results Cancer Res 89,* 107–114.

Risk Management and Quality Patient Management

CHAPTER CONTENTS

GLOSSARY
LEARNING OBJECTIVES
RISK MANAGEMENT
Sources of Law
Standards of Care
Product Problem Reporting System
Documentation
Competency Standards
Occupational Risks
QUALITY PATIENT MANAGEMENT
Approaches to Quality Management
Types of Standards
Intravenous Therapy Nursing Teams
KEY POINTS
REFERENCES

GLOSSARY

Audit   A review of care using defined criteria

Civil law   Laws that affect the legal rights of private person or corporation

Competent   Being capable or able; knowing how to function

Competency   Integrated behaviors, derived from explicit set of desired outcomes

Corrective action   A defined plan to eliminate deficiencies

Criminal law   Offense against the general public; effects on welfare of society as a whole

Criteria   Elements necessary to define and measure quality

Data collection   Gathering information through interviewing, observation, and inspection

Documentation   A recording, in written or printed form, containing original, official, or legal information

Evaluation   Inspection, examination, and quality judgment

Expert testimony   Witness from the same professional specialty explaining to the court what the standard of care should be in the situation at hand

Goal   Broad statement

Implementation   Carrying out a plan

Intervention   Interference that may affect outcome

Liable   Legally responsible for damages, answerable

Malpractice   Negligent conduct of a professional person

Negligence   Not acting in a reasonable or prudent manner

Nursing standard   Specific statement about the quality of some facet of nursing care

Outcome   The result of the performance (or nonperformance) of a function or process(es)

Performance improvement (PI)   Performance is what is done and how well it is done to provide health care

Process A goal-directed interrelated series of actions, events, mechanisms, or steps

Quality Comprehensive positive outcome to a product

Quality assurance (QA) The determination of the degree of excellence through monitoring and evaluation to detect and resolve problems

(QA) Quality assessment

(CQI) Continuous quality improvement

(TQM) Total quality management

Quality management An ongoing, systematic process for monitoring, evaluating, and problem solving

Risk management Process that centers on identification analysis, treatment, and evaluation of real and potential hazards

Statutes Written laws enacted by the legislature

Structure Standard that refers to conditions and mechanisms that provide support for the delivery of care (e.g., policy and resources)

Tort Private wrong, by act or omission, which can result in a civil action by the harmed person

LEARNING OBJECTIVES

Upon completion of this chapter, the reader will be able to:

- Define the terminology related to risk management and quality patient management.
- Identify the sources of laws.
- Summarize the evolution of standards of care.
- Identify the three types of standards in nursing.
- Identify the areas of breach of duty in I.V. nursing.
- State the key points in an incident report.
- State the definition of quality management.
- State the three parts to a competency based education program.
- Differentiate between continuous quality improvement and total quality management.
- Identify the nursing responsibilities of an I.V. therapy team.

The world, more especially the Hospital world, is in such a hurry, is moving so fast, that it is too easy to slide into bad habits before we are aware.

FLORENCE NIGHTINGALE 1873

RISK MANAGEMENT

In the 1930s, nurses were required to almost blindly follow every doctor's order. By the 1960s, the courts began to recognize that nurses were exercising more independent judgment in caring for patients and therefore should accept legal responsibility for their own actions. The 1980s launched the formation of new health care delivery options. These changes have led to increased specificity of clinical standards for all types of health care providers. The Intravenous Standards of Practice (1996) define risk management as "a process that centers on identification, analysis, treatment and evaluation of real and potential hazards."

Risk management concepts include the concerns organizations face with exposure to losses. The chances of loss or risks are treated in an organization by financing,

TABLE 2–1. **STRATEGIES
FOR RISK MANAGEMENT**

Understanding of laws that govern practice
Establishment of nursing standards of practice
Use of incident reports
Informed consents for patients
Developing and participating in product evaluation
Developing nursing competency standards
Documentation
Identification of occupational risk
Quality patient management

purchase of insurance, or practicing loss control. Loss control is preventive and protective activities that are performed before, during, and after losses are incurred. Prevention of patient injury and employee injury, reduction of losses, and survival of the organization are the key concepts supporting risk management (Goldman, 1991). Understanding risk management requires an understanding of the sources of laws and standards of care guiding practice.

Risk management can be divided into five categories:

1. Identifying patterns and trends of risk through internal audits and tracking of claim
2. Reporting individual risk-related incidents and attempting to reduce the liability related to them
3. Developing and participating in the product evaluation system with appropriate "safe-guards" (informed consent)
4. Monitoring patient care setting to identify risks
5. Preventing those events most likely to lead to liability (Wilkinson & Moore, 1990)

The Joint Commission on Accreditation of Healthcare Organizations (JCAHO) advocates the establishment of an integrated risk management and quality assurance program (Wilkinson & Moore, 1990). The strategies for risk management related to I.V. therapy are in Table 2–1.

Sources of Law

In the United States, there are four primary sources of law: (1) the Constitution, (2) statutes, (3) administrative law, and (4) common law. The Constitution is the basic framework upon which our government is built. The Constitution, however, has little direct involvement in the area of *malpractice.*

Statutes are laws enacted by the legislature and passed by the House of Representatives and the Senate as basic rules for society. There were a minimal number of statutes dealing with malpractice before the malpractice crisis of the mid-1970s. Today only a few federal statutes deal with malpractice; however, there are many such state statutes.

Administrative law is a form of law made by administrative agencies, such as the National Labor Relations Board and the Interstate Commerce Commission. These agencies have limited effect on malpractice.

The final source of the law is common law. This is court-made law. Most law in the area of malpractice is court-made law. The courts are responsible for interpreting the statutes. Most malpractice law is not addressed by statute, but is established by the courts (Fiesta, 1988).

Legal terms that nurses should become familiar with are (1) criminal law, (2) civil law, (3) tort, (4) malpractice, and (5) rule of personal liability. Criminal law relates to an offense against the general public because of its harmful effect on society as a whole. Criminal actions are prosecuted by a government authority, and punishment includes imprisonment, fine, or both. The administration of I.V. therapy, if performed in an unlawful manner, can involve the nurse in a criminal offense. Violation of the Nurse Practice Act or the Medical Practice Act by an unlicensed person is considered a criminal offense.

Civil law affects the legal right of the private person or corporation. When harm occurs, the guilty party may be required to pay damages to the injured person.

A private wrong, by act or omission, is referred to as a tort. This can result in civil action by a harmed person. Common torts related to the nursing practice include negligence, assault and battery, false imprisonment, slander, libel, and invasion of privacy. When dealing with a rational patient who refuses treatment, it is best to explain the treatment, verbally reassure the patient, and then notify the physician of refusal.

✎ **NOTE:** Coercion of a rational adult patient to place an I.V. cannula device constitutes assault and battery.

Negligence occurs when a nurse does not act in a reasonable and prudent manner, with resultant damage to a person or that person's property. Malpractice is the negligent conduct of a professional person. However, carelessness is not synonymous with negligence. Medical malpractice is generally defined as "a departure from the accepted standards of practice which the average qualified health care provider of the same or similar specialty as the defendant would deliver at the time and under the circumstances with consideration for the resources available and advances in medical science" (Lumsden, 1990).

✎ **NOTE:** If an act of malpractice does not create harm, legal action cannot be initiated.

The rule of personal liability is "every person is liable for his own tortuous conduct" (his own wrongdoing) (Bernzweig, 1981). A physician cannot protect the nurse from an act of negligence by bypassing this rule with verbal assurance. Nurses are liable for their own wrongdoings in carrying out physicians' orders. This rule is relevant to nurses in the areas of medication errors (the most common cause of malpractice claims) and administration of I.V. fluids. Nurses have a legal and professional responsibility to be knowledgeable regarding the I.V. fluids and medication that are administered (Weinstein, 1993).

Standards of Care

Evolution of Standards

In 1912, the Third Clinical Congress of Surgeons of North America resolved that "some system of standardization of hospital equipment and hospital work should be developed. Institutions having the highest ideals may have proper recognition before the profession, and those of inferior standards should be stimulated to raise the quality of their work. In this way patients will receive the best type of treatment, and the public will have some means of recognizing those institutions devoted to the highest ideals of medicine." From 1919 to 1970, the adopted standards referred to the minimum level "considered essential to proper care and treatment of patients in the hospital" (Roberts, Coale, & Redman, 1989).

At the national level, the standards of nursing practice are established by the American Nursing Association (ANA) and the JCAHO, along with various specialty organizations. At the state level, the various Nurse Practice Acts are the authority by which nurses can practice. At the local level, specific standards are set forth in the hospital/agency procedure manual (Creighton, 1987).

A nursing standard is a specific statement about the quality of some facet of nursing care. This statement contains the criteria by which the effectiveness of that facet can be evaluated. Standards are the criteria for measuring performance against the optimal achievable degree of clinical excellence. Standards are formulated to communicate expectations of nursing practice.

The Food and Drug Administration (FDA) regulates products in the United States, including over-the-counter and prescription drugs and pharmaceuticals, food, cosmetics, veterinary products, biologics, and medical devices. Nurses use many medical devices and usually are the primary reporters of device problems.

In 1990, the Medical Device Act was amended and clearly places responsibility for ensuring that medical devices in domestic commercial distribution are safe and effective for their intended purposes.

The nurse is the best judge of product integrity by inspection of equipment prior to use. Examples of medical device problems related to I.V. therapy practice are:

- Loose or leaking catheter hubs
- Occluded cannulas
- Defective infusion pump tubing
- Contaminated infusates
- Misleading labeling
- Inadequate packaging
- Cracked or leaking I.V. solution bag

Several agencies are influencial in developing standards of practice. Table 2–2 lists the most important standards.

Nursing Standards

Standards of nursing care reflect the mission, values, and philosophy of the agency. Nursing process, professional accountability, fiscal responsibility, and other areas of care are included within these standards. Standards should reflect the type of care that the patient will receive on a given unit or within a service. These are called performance standards and should (1) include the minimum acceptable behavior for the nurse congruent with department standards and standards of practice; (2) define performance in observable, measurable behaviors; (3) be specific to the staff nurse role and job description; (4) include all aspects of the nurse's role, including leadership and organizational expectations; and (5) serve as the basis for employee selection decisions and performance appraisal system (Porter, 1988). There are three types of standards in nursing:

1. Standards of structure, which consider organizational framework.
2. Standards of process, which encompass patient procedures in health care setting.
3. Standards of outcome, which consider the objectives or goals of patient care.

All must be given equal weight and scrutinized with the same degree of diligence to ensure quality of care (Meisenheimer, 1992).

Breach of Duty

After the standard of care has been established and legal duty shown in negligence cases, the injured party must prove that breach of duty has occurred. In negligence

21

TABLE 2–2. **AGENCIES INFLUENCING STANDARDS OF PRACTICE**

Year	Agency	Task
1970	Joint Commission on Accreditation of Hospitals (JCAH)	Revised its focus and published a manual for hospitals that defined optimum achievable standards.
1974	ANA	Published generic and specialty standards for nusing care.
1978	CDC	Set standards for infection control practice regarding infusion therapy.
1980	National Intravenous Therapy Association (NITA)	Set standards of practice for I.V. therapy.
1987	JCAHO (formerly JCAH)	Mailed "Agenda for Change," which changed the commission's focus from evaluating a health care of organization's capability of delivering quality care to helping institutions provide quality health care.
1987	Omnibus Budget Reconciliation Act (P.L. 100-203)	Set standards for accreditation of home care.
1989	JCAHO	Issued standards regarding what constitutes high-quality home care services.
1990	Food and Drug Administration (FDA)	Amended Medical Device Act.
1991	Occupational Health and Safety Administration (OSHA)	Passed final rule on bloodborne pathogens.
1992	OSHA (implementation of bloodborne pathogen standards)	Engineering and work practice controls must be in place. Personal protective equipment must be available. Free hepatitis B vaccination program must be in place. Hazardous material labeling must be in place.
1990	Intravenous Nursing Society (INS; formerly NITA)	Published revised Standards of Practice for I.V. therapy.

cases, breach of duty often involves the matter of foreseeability. Forseeability is the legal requirement that the case must be judged on the unique facts as they were at the time of the occurrence, since it is always easier to state what should have been done in retrospect. Certain events may foreseeably cause a specific result. The following is a list of breach of duties related to I.V. therapy nursing:

1. Delay in administration of medication
2. Unfamiliarity with drug
3. Route of administration not clarified
4. Failure to qualify orders
5. Negligence in patient teaching

Also, the nurse must be aware at all times that failure to observe, failure to intervene, and verbal rather than written orders are potential risks for all nursing areas. Nurses must assess the patient and formulate a nursing diagnosis to meet the patient's needs. Courts have not extended the concept of nursing diagnosis to the liability of the nurse's practice at this time.

Malpractice cases are most frequently based on negligence in physical care. There are many documented cases of malpractice related to all procedures performed on patients. Sometimes the breach of duty occurs because a nurse fails to perform a procedure according to proper standards of care.

✎ **NOTE:** Because of the risk of malpractice, policy and procedure manuals are vitally important in all aspects of physical nursing care. Practicing and performing specific physical care based on the policies and procedures ensure quality care.

The practice of verbal orders rather than written orders potentially places the nurse at higher liability risks. Most states require that verbal orders be countersigned by the physician within 24 hours (Fiesta, 1988).

Nurse's Role as Expert Witness

Studies indicate that 70% to 80% of all civil litigation involves medical and scientific evidence and the testimony of experts (Wecht, 1979). In the profession of nursing, especially the specialty of I.V. therapy, the likelihood of being involved in some legal matter, directly or indirectly, is great (Masoorli, 1995).

In every negligence or malpractice proceeding, the injured party or plaintiff must prove that the defendant did not act in the way that a reasonably prudent professional would have acted in the same or similar circumstance. An expert is required to explain the appropriate standard of care and to indicate the deviation from standard care.

The role of the expert is *not* to establish standards of care. Rather, the expert's role is to educate the judge and jury regarding the standards already established by the profession. Expert nursing testimony increases with the technical complexity of a case. An expert witness is usually selected from the same area of experience as the defendant nurse. Additional expertise, such as national I.V. certification or research experience is also important (Fiesta, 1991).

✎ **NOTE:** The specialty area of I.V. therapy is a high-risk technical area.

Unusual Occurrence Reports

Unusual occurrence reports should be filed every time there is a deviation from the standard. Unusual occurrence reports are simply records of an event and are considered an internal reporting mechanism for quality assurance. They should be reported to the superior and the episode must be objectively charted, but reference to the report should not appear in the legal patient record. The occurrence report should contain the following 10 key points:

1. Patient's admitting diagnosis
2. Date incident occurred
3. Patient's room number
4. Age of patient
5. Location of incident
6. Type of incident
7. Nature of incident (medication error, mislabeling, misreading, policy and procedure not followed, overlooked order on chart, patient identification not checked). It should be noted (on the unusual occurrence report) if a physician's order was needed after the occurrence
8. Factual description of incident

TABLE 2–3. I.V. THERAPY RISK MANAGEMENT SCREENS

1. Medication error
2. I.V. fluid error
3. Anaphylaxis or severe allergic reaction
4. Severe irritation or breakdown at site
5. Site infection
6. Phlebitis stage +2 or +3 (INS standards)
7. Needlestick to patient, family member, or health care personnel
8. Neurologic deficit, sign or symptom not present prior to I.V. therapy
9. Patient withdraws consent for treatment or refuses treatment
10. Equipment failure or malfunction with potential impact on patient care
11. Patient complaint related to I.V. therapy
12. Other adverse or unexpected event (specify)
13. Break in policy/procedure (specify)
14. Particulate or other observable contaminant of I.V. fluid or medication
15. Severe infiltration or extravasation of vesicant agent

For home infusion services add the following screening for risk management:

1. Diarrhea, fever, dysrhythmia, sudden weight loss or gain, and infections other than site infections.
2. Questioned safety of home environment for continued home I.V. therapy
3. Rehospitalization for I.V. therapy

Source: Adapted from Tan, M.W. (1990). Occurrence screens: A risk and quality control tool for intravenous nurses. *Journal of Intravenous Therapy, 13*(5) 308–311, with permission.

9. Patient's condition before incident
10. Results of the incident or injury

✎ **NOTE:** Unusual occurrence reports are meant to be nonjudgmental, factual reports of the problem and its consequences (Gardner, 1987).

Unusual occurrence reports are useful for identification of patterns of I.V. medication errors or potentially dangerous situations. Trend analysis monitors patterns of their occurrences. Nursing staff must feel free to file reports; a report is not an admission of negligence. These reports have the potential for saving lives by identifying unsafe practices. More than ever before, risk may be managed by prevention. The JCAHO in 1996 will implement five indicators on medication use for its Indicator Measurement System, a performance measurement system intended to help to evaluate the performance of health care organizations as part of its survey and accreditation process. Table 2–3 presents risk-management screens for I.V. therapy.

Informed Consent

One of the most effective proactive strategies taken in risk management is the informed consent. The purpose of informed consent is to provide patients with enough information to enable them to make a rational decision regarding whether to undergo treatment. The focus is on a patient's understanding of the procedure not just signing a consent to perform a procedure (Goldman, 1991).

For a consent to be valid according to Hogue (1986), three conditions must be met: (1) the patient must be capable of giving consent; (2) the patient must receive the necessary information to make an informed decision; and (3) the consent must not be coerced. Getting the consent form signed may be the nurse's responsibility

TABLE 2–4. **KEY COMPONENTS OF INFORMED CONSENT**

Process
1. Accurate and complete information
2. Including an understanding of:
Risks
Benefits
Alternatives
3. Understanding of:
Language idioms
Intelligence
Hearing loss
4. Opportunity for dialogue
Consent
1. After consideration of all options
2. Agreed in verbal and written word
3. Documentation of consent obtained

Source: Kathleen Sazama, MD, J.D. Associate Medical Director, Center for Blood Research, Sacramento, California, with permission.

and is defined by policy. If the patient does not give informed consent, there may be grounds for liability. The consent form is actually a *risk-management* tool designed to avoid charges of malpractice, along with protecting the consumer. Table 2–4 identifies the necessary component parts to informed consent.

Informed consents are used when inserting peripheral central lines and placing implanted ports or tunneled catheters.

✎ **NOTE:** The consent form helps to establish a good relationship with the patient and to protect everyone—the nurse, the doctor, the hospital and the patient.

Product Problem Reporting System

When to Report

Inappropriate use of medical devices also may contribute to pain and suffering. The FDA evaluates approximately 2000 medical devices a month. Devices are inspected on three levels:

1. Good manufacturing controls
2. Application for a device existing before 1976 and is in common use
3. Implantable or hazardous devices

The simple act of "gerryrigging" or otherwise manipulating a device to overcome a small problem results in the liability for that piece of equipment residing with the institution (Weinstein, 1996). The law states that the responsibility shifts to the institution when a practitioner interferes with the design of a piece of equipment (Abbey, 1993).

Report any problems with medical devices, if the event observed involves, or has the potential to cause, a death, serious injury, or life-threatening malfunction. In

25

1992, a congressional hearing focused on needle safety and needleless system and safe medical devices. Since this hearing, OSHA and the CDC along with the FDA have been collaboratively reviewing the issue of safe medical devices. OSHA expects hospitals to have an ongoing system in place to evaluate safer medical devices (Williams, 1995).

What to Report

A complete description of the problem and information regarding the device needs to be submitted, including:

- Product name
- Manufacturer's name and address
- Identification numbers of the device (lot number, model number, serial number, expiration date)
- Problem noted
- Name, title, and practice specialty of the user of the device

How to Report?

Problems are reported in writing to:

> Medical Device and Laboratory Product Problem Reporting Program (PRP)
> United States Pharmacopeia
> 12601 Twinbrook Parkway
> Rockville, MD 20853
> (800) 638-6725

✎ **NOTE:** It is the health care professional's responsibility to report medical device problems (Scott, 1990).

Documentation

Another strategy for risk management is documentation, which should be an accurate, timely, complete written account of the care rendered to the patient. The health care record charts the patient's history, health status, and goal achievement (Baker, 1990). It should be objective and completed promptly. Documentation should be legible and include only standard abbreviations. Nurses and other health care providers should keep charting free of criticism or complaints. There should be no vacant lines in charting, and every entry should be signed. In an office or home care environment, chart dates of return visit, canceled or failed appointments, all telephone conversations, and all follow-up instructions (Creighton, 1987).

In the 1990s, the emphasis is on quality improvement, with a focus on evaluating organizational and clinical performance outcomes. Documentation is one way of evaluating outcomes. The many formats for charting include problem-oriented medical record, pie charting, focus charting, narrative charting, and charting by exception. Regardless of the format developed for documenting I.V. therapy, basic requirements of the plane of care exist, including goals, actual and potential problems, and nursing interventions and outcomes.

✎ **NOTE:** Patient complaints of vascular access device discomfort should include date and time, name of vein-specific insertion location, gauge and length of the device, brand and style of the device, the I.V. solution or intermittent injection device infused by gravity or pump, rate of flow and patient comments (Masoorli, 1995).

Competency Standards

Competency has been defined as integrated behaviors, including possession of knowledge, skills, abilities, and basic professional requirements that nurses must meet. A competent nurse in I.V. therapy is well qualified by education and capable of performing I.V. therapy in an exact and effective manner using the appropriate knowledge of nursing, technical expertise, and specialized skills (Dugger, 1993). Within the educational context, competency may be defined as a simultaneous integration of the knowledge, skills, and attitudes that are required for performance in a designated role and setting (Alspach, 1992).

In developing standards, it is important to have a clear understanding of such terms as competent and competency. Competency is a level of care used to determine whether grounds exist for disciplinary action by a state licensing board. Competency is also used to assess civil liability against a nurse in a malpractice case.

The practice setting for I.V. therapy delivery is as varied as the patient populations served by this specialty practice. From the hospitalized neonate to the elderly in an extended care facility or the home, the competencies of the nurse—that combination of knowledge, skills, and abilities necessary to fulfill the role of a nurse administering I.V. therapy—spans all ages and disease processes. Basic competencies are intended to serve as guidelines for the practicing nurse and to assist in design of orientation and continuing education programs (Pierce, 1995).

I.V. nursing is defined as using the nursing process relating to fluids, electrolytes, infection control, oncology, pediatrics, pharmacology, quality assurance, technology and clinical applications, parenteral nutrition, and transfusion therapy. The practice of I.V. nursing encompasses the nursing management and coordination of care to the patient in accordance with:

1. State statues
2. INS standards of practice
3. Established institutional policy
4. JCAHO requirements (Table 2–5)

Competency-Based Educational Programs

Competency-based educational programs establish specific goals, accountability, individualization, and behaviors for practitioners by defining clear expectations for levels of performance (Bazinet, Erickson, & Thomas, 1989). According to Scrima (1987), the licensing examination required for all nurses cannot be expected to accurately reflect knowledge in a profession in which the knowledge base exhibits a half-life of 5 years. Therefore, the responsibility of ensuring a competent staff often falls to the institution in which the nurse is practicing. McGregor (1990) has developed a framework for developing staff competencies and ensuring that the institution is delivering safe care. This framework includes:

- Development of standards
- Development of skills test
- Assessment of learning needs
- Planning educational programs
- Presentation of educational programs
- Evaluation of learning outcomes

TABLE 2–5. JCAHO COMPETENCY REQUIREMENTS

A. HR. 1 The organization's leaders define for their respective areas the qualifications and job expectations of staff and a system to evaluate how well the expectations are met
    1. Job descriptions that include the required qualifications and competencies are developed and used in the competence-assessment process
        a. Performance evaluations
        b. Competency-assessment mechanisms
        c. Staff development plans
        d. In-service and continuing education records

B. HR. 2 The organization provides an adequate number of staff whose qualifications are commensurate with defined job responsibilities and applicable licensure, law and regulation and or certification
    1. Appropriate knowledge and experience for assigned responsibilities
        a. Job descriptions
        b. Orientation curriculum
        c. Staff development plans/in-service records

C. HR. 3 Processes are designed to ensure that the competence of all staff members is assessed, maintained, demonstrated, and improved on an ongoing basis
    1. HR 3.1 The organization has established methods and practices that encourage self-development and learning for all staff
    2. HR 3.2 A staff orientation process provides initial job training and information, including an assessment of an individual's capability to perform specified responsibilities
    3. HR 3.3 On-going in-service and or other education and training maintain and improve staff competence
    4. HR 3.4 The organization collects aggregate data on an ongoing basis regarding staff competence patterns and trends to identify and respond to staff learning needs

D. HR. 4 The organization assesses an individual's ability to achieve job expectations as stated in his or her job description
    1. Competence assessment activities exist and are documented for each staff member

Source: From the Joint Commission on Accreditation of Health Care Organizations (1996). *Accreditation manual for hospitals, 1996.* Section 2, Human Resources, pp 355–371.

The following statistics on health care providers supports the growing need for competency-based education.

CURRENT STATISTICS ON HEALTH CARE PROVIDERS

100,000 patient suffered injuries due to incompetence
13,000 patient died due to incompetence
estimated 80,000 die each year due to incompetence
estimated 1.2 million negative outcomes iatrogenic illness/death each year.

Source: Harvard Risk Management Foundation Study, 1990 *New England Journal of Medicine.*

Competencies should be directed toward essential mandatory aspects of performance, should have measurable clinical behaviors, should include evaluation mechanisms, and should test cognitive performance criteria.

Three-Part Competency Model

All registered nurses are accountable and responsible for all parts of the tasks associated with I.V. therapy and for tasks that are delegated to the licensed practical nurse or technician for care rendered to the patient while under care (Dugger, 1993). The three-part competency model is an effective tool for ensuring competent practice. A competency-based educational model requires developing the three major parts of the model: the competency statement, the performance criteria, and the evaluation and learning options. The model in Table 2–6 will be used as the framework for assessing the competency of the I.V. practitioner throughout this book.

Occupational Risks

There are two types of occupational hazards associated with I.V. therapy: physical hazards and hazardous materials. In the past, we relied on health care workers to voluntarily report accidental occupational injuries resulting in exposure to blood or body fluid. Up to 90% of theses injuries are never reported.

Physical Hazards

Physical hazards associated with I.V. therapy include, but are not limited to, accidents, abrasions, contusions, and chemical exposure.

Needle-Stick Injuries

An important risk to the health care worker is exposure to bloodborne pathogens. Needle-stick injuries are associated with recapping the needle, improper discarding of needle in container, and accidental needle sticks while performing tasks and carelessness. Accidental needle-stick injuries can lead to exposure to human immunodeficiency virus (HIV), hepatitis B, hepatitis C, and cytomegalovirus (Hibberd, 1995). Needle-stick injuries account for approximately 80% of all accidental exposures to blood, with 20% before or during use of needles and up to 70% after use and before disposal. Prevention of these injuries is imperative (Jagger, Hunt, & Brand-Elnagger, 1988). In April 1992, the FDA issued a Safety Alert urging hospitals to use a needleless or recessed needle system to access I.V. lines (FDA, 1992).

Tokars and colleagues (1992) found that needle-stick injuries occurred in 7% of 1382 observed surgical procedures. Risk factors for injury include (1) the type of procedures (more injuries were seen during gynecologic procedures), (2) prolonged operative time, and (3) use of fingers rather than a surgical instrument to hold tissue that was being sutured. The risk of injury for staff on medical wards may be 6 to 12 times lower than that for surgical personnel. On average, nurses are exposed to one percutaneous injury per year (Roberts & Bell, 1994).

Abrasions and Contusions

Abrasions and contusions can be caused by needle sticks and contact with broken glass, sharp edges of containers, or any jagged-edged item. Small or undetected skin abrasions can be potential portals for microorganisms or viruses such as *Staphylococcus aureus*, herpes simplex, and HIV. Use caution when assembling and manipulating I.V. equipment. Excellent hand-washing practices and use of barrier precaution prevent the invasion of microorganisms.

TABLE 2–6. EDUCATIONAL THREE-PART COMPETENCY PROGRAM MODEL

Part	Definition	Examples
Competency statement	Critical behaviors required for satisfactory performance; clearly articulated and written; consist of 5 parts: Description of a general category of behavior Oriented to the learner Description of measurable behavior Free of performance conditions and criteria Validated by experts	Correct procedure to initiate a peripheral venous access device
Performance criteria	A set of criteria that allow a preceptor or determine whether performance is satisfactory; can be a checklist	Steps to perform insertion of a venous access device: Prepare patient. Assemble all equipment. Prepare skin using appropriate aseptic technique. Insert over-the-needle cannula without contamination. Establish accurate flow rate. Apply dressing. Label dressing.
Evaluation and learning options	Tool to assist in evaluating clinical performance; can be developed directly from criteria established for each competency Skills certification and mastery set at a level higher than cognitive process 100% Mastery required for safe delivery of I.V. infusions (McGregor, 1990) Further study, review, and retest needed if mastery is not achieved Appropriate self-directed learning tools: audiotaped programs, videos, and selected readings	Review of credentials: Education Licensure Experience Written examination Skills demonstration Clinical observation Competency-based orientation

Chemical Exposure

OSHA published guidelines for the management of cytotoxic (antineoplastic) drugs in the workplace in 1986. Since that time, surveys indicated further clarification was needed in management of exposure to chemicals. OSHA revised its recommendations for hazardous drug handling in 1995. In order to provide recommendations

30

consistent with current scientific knowledge, the information was expanded to cover hazardous drugs, in addition to the cytotoxic (see Appendix D for list). The recommendations apply to all settings where employees are occupationally exposed to hazardous drugs (HD) (OSHA, 1995).

Hazardous drugs have demonstrated the ability to cause chromosome breakage in circulating lymphocytes and mutagenic activity in urine, along with causing skin necrosis after surface contacts with abraded skin or damage to normal skin. It is recommended that nurses preparing HDs wear surgical latex gloves (double gloves if they do not interfere with techniques) and wear a protective disposable gown made of lint-free, low-permeability fabrics with closed front, long sleeves, and elastic or knit-closed cuffs when indicated. Because surgical masks do not protect against the breathing of aerosols, a biologic safety cabinet or an air-purifying respirator should be used when preparing HDs. A plastic face shield or splash goggles should be worn if a biologic safety cabinet is not used. Refer to Chapter 14, Antineoplastic Agents, and Appendix D for further information on these guidelines.

Latex Allergy

Both latex and vinyl gloves protect the wearer from contact with blood and body fluids. Latex is a natural material, more flexible than vinyl. Latex molds to the wearer's hand, allowing freedom of movement. Its network of lattices that allows it to reseal tiny punctures automatically is an extremely valuable feature. Gloves made of polyvinyl chloride, the synthetic rubber known as vinyl, cannot reseal and are less flexible and durable than latex (Korniewicz, Kirwin, & Larson, 1991).

Numerous studies and case reports document hypersensitivity to natural rubber latex (Nutter, 1979; Nguyen, Burns, & Shapiro, 1991; Sussman, Tarlo, & Dolovich, 1991). Latex antigens can precipitate skin, mucous membrane, or respiratory reactions. There are three different types of reactions to natural rubber latex: (1) irritation, (2) delayed hypersensitivity (contact dermatitis), and (3) immediate hypersensitivity (anaphylactic symptoms).

Immediate latex hypersensitivity reactions include itching eyes, swelling of lips or tongue, dyspnea, dizziness, abdominal pain, nausea, hypotension, shock, and potentially death.

Persons most at risk for a latex allergy include:

- Those who work in the medical and dental profession who have daily exposure to latex products
- Those with a history of allergies and asthma
- Those with a history of reactions to latex (balloons, condoms, gloves)
- Those who are female
- Those who are allergic to bananas, avocados, tropical fruits, kiwi, and chestnuts
- Those with poinsettia plants that contain latex-producing lacticifers, which have been know to cause contact urticaria (Jackson, 1995)

To reduce the risk of an allergic response, avoid using hand lotions or lubricants that contain mineral oil, petroleum salves, and other hydrocarbon-based gels or lotions to prevent the breakdown of the glove material and maintain barrier protection. Do not reuse disposable examination gloves because disinfecting agents can damage barrier properties of gloves. Hand washing is recommended after gloves are removed and before a new pair is applied. Gloves should not be stored where they will be subjected to excessive heat, direct ultraviolet or fluorescent light, or ozone.

In 1991, the FDA issued a medical alert regarding allergic reactions to latex-containing medical devices and advised health care professionals to identify their latex-sensitive patients and to prepare to treat allergic reactions promptly.

> Call FDA Problem Reporting Program (800 638-6725) to report incidents of adverse reactions to latex or other materials used in medical devices.

Biologic Hazards

I.V. therapy nurses are constantly exposed to patient's secretions and excretions. Biologic agents such as bacteria and viruses are living organisms which are capable of causing infectious disease (Baldwin, 1992). The CDC has estimated that approximately 500 to 600 health care workers are hospitalized annually with hepatitis B virus-related diseases (US Department of Health and Human Services, 1989). Nurses should follow standards established by OSHA regarding gloving and hand-washing practices. All body secretions, and therefore fluids from patients, can be potentially infectious. Strict guidelines must be adhered to by all personnel having contact with patients.

OSHA's Rules for Occupational Exposure to Bloodborne Pathogens

OSHA has stiffened the rules by enforcing new regulations regarding universal precautions. OSHA's new standard makes universal precautions fully enforceable for the first time and spells out what inspectors will look for. Health care workers should be aware of how the rules are observed in each agency.

Health care employees face a significant risk as the result of occupational exposure to materials that may contain bloodborne pathogens, including hepatitis B virus (HBV), which causes hepatitis B (a serious liver disease) and HIV, which causes AIDS. The exposure can be minimized or eliminated using a combination of engineering and work practice controls, personal protective clothing and equipment, training, medical surveillance, hepatitis B vaccination, signs and labels, and other provisions (OSHA, 1991).

The following list is a summary of some of the rules to be observed in the workplace.

Hepatitis B Vaccine. The vaccine must be offered at no charge to the employee "at a reasonable time and place" and "within 10 working days of initial assignment."

Universal Precautions. It is now a legal requirement to observe this concept, in which "all human blood and certain human body fluids are treated as if known to be infection for HIV, HBV and other bloodborne pathogens."

Sharps and Waste Disposal. Reusable, contaminated sharps have to be placed in puncture, resistant, leak-proof, and labeled or color-coded containers that are "easily accessible . . . maintained upright, and placed routinely."

Protective Equipment. The whole range of equipment must be available wherever blood or other infectious materials might reach an employee's clothes, skin, eyes, mouth, or other mucous membranes.

Gloves. Gloves must be worn when hand contact with infectious materials can be reasonably anticipated. Utility gloves must be discarded if cracked, peeling, torn, or punctured. Hypoallergenic gloves must be provided to those allergic to other gloves.

Laundry. Contaminated laundry has to be handled "with a minimum of agitation" and moved in labeled or color-coded bags or containers. Wet laundry requires leak-proof containers. Laundry workers must wear gloves.

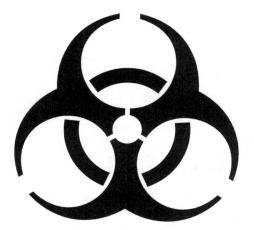

Figure 2–1. Universal symbol for biohazards.

Communicating Hazards. Orange-red or fluorescent orange warning labels must be affixed to containers of "regulated" waste, refrigerators and freezers containing infectious materials, and containers used to transport them. Labels must include the official BIOHAZARD legend (Fig. 2–1).

QUALITY PATIENT MANAGEMENT

Risk management handles "errors," whereas quality assurance (QA) seeks "perfection." Both are mutually compatible and interdependent. QA works at preventing malpractice claims and promotes better patient outcomes. All hospital departments are involved in both QA and risk management activities (Fiesta, 1991).

Risk management + quality assurance = quality management

Quality management is a systematic process to ensure desired patient outcomes. A quality management program includes both risk management and quality assurance and is established to objectively identify, evaluate, and solve problems associated with I.V. patient treatment modalities.

QA requirements have always been a part of the JCAHO's accreditation process, but introduction of the Agenda for Change in 1986 shifted the emphasis from problem-solving endeavors to continuous improvement of quality (Roberts, Coale, & Redman, 1989). With this shift, JCAHO initiated the transition from QA to continuous quality improvement (CQI). The goal was to create outcome monitoring and evaluation processes to assist organizations in improving the quality of care. QA is frequently focused solely on the clinical aspects of care rather than the interrelated managerial, governance, support, and clinical processes that affect patient care outcomes. Quality cannot be assured; it can only be assessed, managed, or improved. Dennis O'Leary, JCAHO president, has admitted that in retrospect quality assurance was an "unfortunate semantic selection because it does not accurately reflect JCAHO's vision of quality" (O'Leary, 1991).

Beginning in the 1980s, health care consumers, third-party payers, and health care providers, began looking at *positive patient outcomes* as a measure of quality. JCAHO was the driving force in this movement, along with peer review organizations (PROs), Medicare/Medicaid reimbursement regulations, federal and state laws, and court interpretations of liability and private health insurers' standards (Cassidy

33

& Friesen, 1990). In the early 1980s, guidelines initiated by JCAHO, were formed to provide a nursing quality assurance (NQA) committee. This committee recognized that QA had to be ongoing to ensure high-quality patient care. The committee in each facility should include management, chief nursing officers, and members of staff (O'Brien, 1988). NQA focuses on two endeavors: checking achievement of standards and solving patient care problems.

JCAHO (1995) has changed the wording of continuous quality improvement to performance improvement. The goal of improving organization performance is to continuously improve patient health outcomes.

Approaches to Quality Management

Assessing the achievement of nursing care standards involves measuring the quality of care provided. This is part of the nursing process: observing care delivered, assessing patient satisfaction, documentation of care received, and evaluation of outcomes based on short- and long-term goals. Involving staff in quality assessments can increase their awareness of standards, as well as enhancing their assessment skills (New & New, 1989).

Performance Improvement

Performance is what is done and how well it is done to provide health care. Dimensions of performance include:

Doing the right thing

Example
The efficacy of the procedure or treatment in relation to the patient's condition; the appropriateness of a specific test, procedure, or service to meet the patient's needs.

Doing the right thing well

Example
The availability of a needed test, procedure, treatment, or service to the patient who needs it; the timeliness with which the service is provided to the patient and the effectiveness with which the care was provided; the continuity of services with respect to other services, practitioners, and providers over time; the safety of the patient to whom the services are provided; the respect and caring with which the services are provided.

Continuous Quality Improvement

Continuous quality improvement (CQI) is an approach to quality management that builds on the traditional QA models. This approach was first introduced in 1992 as an effective way to improve the quality of health care. In 1992, JCAHO first introduced standards that mandated CQI methodology from hospitals receiving accreditation surveys (LaRochelle & Shahinpour, 1995). CQI broadens the focus to all facets of the organization that affect patient outcomes, not just to clinical aspects of care. An essential characteristic of CQI is that it is continuous process; outcomes are never optimized but may be constantly improved. A distinctive feature of CQI is that it emphasizes improvement in the interdisciplinary processes involved in patient care delivery. CQI incorporates leadership principles from total quality management and has become the central theme or standard in health care.

Total quality management (TQM) is an outgrowth of several health care organizations, which have adopted a management system that fosters continuous im-

TABLE 2–7. JCAHO 10-STEP MONITORING AND EVALUATION PROCESS

1. Assign responsibility.
2. Delineate the scope of care and service.
3. Identify important aspects of care and service.
4. Identify indicators.
5. Establish thresholds for evaluation.
6. Perform data collection.
7. Evaluate.
8. Take action.
9. Assess actions and document improvement.
10. Communicate relevant information.

Source: From the Joint Commission on the Accreditation of Healthcare Organizations (1992). *Accreditation manual for hospitals, 1992.* JCAHO.

provement at all levels and for all function by focusing on maximizing customer satisfaction. TQM and CQI share many characteristics; however, unlike CQI, TQM is not unique to health care. It requires that those in top management be committed to the program and provide clear vision for the organization; employees must participate actively in the quality improvement process. TQM contributes to a positive work environment, fosters collaboration, promotes teamwork to enhance interdepartmental communication (Milakovich, 1991).

In health care, the most widely used and accepted format for assessing quality is the 10-step monitoring and evaluation process outline by JCAHO (JCAHO, 1987). These standards emphasize the importance of planned, systematic, and ongoing monitoring and evaluation activities. (Table 2–7).

Types of Standards

I.V. therapy CQI includes compliance with policy and procedure manuals, documentation of I.V. therapy-related complications, equipment evaluation, and chart documentation. The quality improvement process may be performed by lengthy studies, short-term sampling, or problem solving with documentation and reporting (Weinstein, 1993). Three categories are used to create a model for quality management. Each category is linked as a measurement of quality patient care. The three components are:

- Structure
- Process
- Outcome

Structure

Structure refers to the conditions and mechanisms that provide support for the actual provision of care. This is defined as evaluation of resources: material and human. Material resources are classified as facilities, equipment, mission, philosophy, goals of organization, or financial resources. Human resources include the number and qualifications of nurses performing I.V.-related procedures.

35

STRUCTURE RESOURCES

Material Resources	Human Resources
1. Facilities 2. Equipment 3. Financial budget 4. Philosophy, goals, mission of organization	1. Number of nurses 2. Qualification of nurses performing I.V.-related nursing duties.

Process

Process denotes what is actually done in giving and receiving care. Process is a goal-directed, interrelated series of actions, events, mechanisms, or steps. It includes the patient's activities in seeking care and the practitioner's activities in making a nursing diagnosis, along with evaluation of actual performance of procedures. This link sets the standards by which evaluation can take place. Process standards focus on job descriptions, performance standards, procedures, and protocols.

PROCESS BASED ON STANDARDS OF PRACTICE

Patient Activities	Nurse Activities
1. Patient knowledge	1. Standards of care 2. Interventions and establishment of short- and long-term goals 3. Written procedures

Outcome

Outcome denotes the effect of care on the health status of patients. The result of the performance (or nonperformance) of a function or process is the outcome. Improvements in the patient's knowledge and changes in patient health status are components of outcome criteria. The assessment of outcomes is a method by which quality of care is established. Outcome in the practice of I.V. therapy should reflect final results of the therapy including patient recovery and rates of complications.

OUTCOME CRITERIA

Patient Knowledge	Evaluation of Care
1. Patient participation in care and verbal understanding of health status.	1. Evaluation of nursing compliance to institutional policy. 2. Evaluation that standards of care are met. 3. Patient is free of complications.

Table 2–8 gives an example of a quality management model for catheter-related sepsis.

Helpful guidelines for evaluation of CQI include the following:

1. Centers for Disease Control (CDC), *Guidelines for Prevention of Intravascular Infections*
2. Intravenous Nurses Society (INS), *Standards of Practice.*
3. Joint Commission on Accreditation of Healthcare Organizations (JCAHO) Performance Standards for I.V. Therapy
4. American Association of Blood Banking (AABB)

TABLE 2–8. **QUALITY MANAGEMENT MODEL: CATHETER-RELATED SEPSIS**

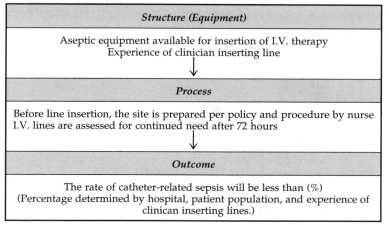

Structure (Equipment)
Aseptic equipment available for insertion of I.V. therapy Experience of clinician inserting line ↓
Process
Before line insertion, the site is prepared per policy and procedure by nurse I.V. lines are assessed for continued need after 72 hours ↓
Outcome
The rate of catheter-related sepsis will be less than (%) (Percentage determined by hospital, patient population, and experience of clinican inserting lines.)

In summary the goals of continuous quality improvement are to (1) prevent complications, (2) decrease morbidity and mortality, (3) decrease cost, (4) shorten hospital stay, (5) increase patient comfort, and (6) increase patient knowledge.

Intravenous Therapy Nursing Teams

A team involves a group of nursing personnel working together to meet patient needs. According to INS (S17), "Intravenous teams provide clinical expertise, cost effective care and decrease the risk of complications related to intravenous therapy. Intravenous nursing teams provide desired patient outcomes and decrease morbidity and mortality associated with this therapy."

The responsibilities of the I.V. team should be set by policy and procedure of the institution. These responsibilities include but are not limited to:

1. Inserting I.V. cannulas
2. Administering prescribed I.V. solutions, medications, and blood products
3. Monitoring and maintaining I.V. sites and systems
4. Evaluating the patient's response to prescribed therapy
5. Providing patient and family teaching and evaluating their comprehension
6. Documenting pertinent information of the patient's record
7. Compiling statistics to qualify and quantify I.V. services

I.V. nurses should also be active on committees relevant to the specialty practice of I.V. nursing, such as:

Pharmacy and therapeutics
Infection control
Nutritional support
Transfusion therapy
Quality assurance and risk management

KEY POINTS

RISK MANAGEMENT AND QUALITY PATIENT MANAGEMENT

Risk management
 Categories of risk management include:
  1. Patterns of risk through internal audits and "tracking"
  2. Reporting individual risk-related incidents
  3. Developing and participating in product evaluation system
  4. Monitoring patient care
  5. Preventing events most likely to lead to liability
 Strategies for risk management include:
  1. Understanding laws that govern practice
  2. Establishment of nursing standards of practice
  3. Use of incident reports
  4. Informed consent
  5. Developing and participating in product evaluation
  6. Developing nursing competency standards
  7. Documentation
  8. Identification of occupational risks
  9. Quality patient management
 Sources of laws
  Primary sources of law in the United States:
   Constitution
   Statutes
   Administrative law
   Common law
  Legal terms are:
   Criminal law
   Civil law
   Tort
   Malpractice
   Rule of personal liability
    Common torts in the nursing practice of I.V. therapy:
     Assault and battery
      Coercion of a rational adult patient to place an I.V. cannula device constitutes assault and battery.

Standards of care
 National level: standards of nursing practice established by the ANA and JCAHO
 State level: Nurse Practice Act
 Local level: hospital/agency policy and procedure manuals
 Breach of duty
  Breach of duty related to I.V. therapy includes:
  1. Delay in administration of medication
  2. Unfamiliarity with the drug
  3. Inappropriate route of administration
  4. Failure to qualify orders
  5. Negligence in patient teaching

Unusual occurrence reports
Unusual occurrence reports should be filed every time there is an unusual occurrence. Incident reports are simply a record of an event.
Informed consent
For a consent to be valid, three conditions must be met:
1. Patients must be capable of giving consent
2. Patients must receive the necessary information to make an intelligent decision
3. Consent must not be coerced

   The consent form is actually a risk management tool designed to avoid charges of malpractice.
Documentation
All charting should accurately describe the care rendered the patient, and it should be objective. Charting must be timely, complete, and accurate to help the patient secure a better quality of care and to help protect nurses, physicians, and hospitals.
Competency standards
Competency-based educational programs establish goals, accountability, and behaviors for practitioners. The framework for developing staff competencies includes:
1. Development of standards
2. Development of skill lists
3. Assessment of learning needs
4. Planning educational programs
5. Presentation of educational programs
6. Evaluation of learning outcomes

Three-part model

Step 1: Critical behavior are identified and competency statements are written.

Step 2: Steps of performance criteria are made.

Step 3: Evaluation and remediation take place.
Occupation risks
Physical hazards

Needle-stick injuries

Abrasions and contusions

Chemical exposure

Latex allergy

Biological hazards

Quality patient management
Quality management works at preventing malpractice claims and promotes better patient outcomes.

Approaches to quality patient management include:

Performance improvement

Continuous quality improvement (CQI)

Total quality management (TQM)

JCAHO 10-step monitoring and evaluation process

Goals of quality assessment
Prevent complications.

Decrease morbidity and mortality.

Decrease cost.

Shorten hospital stays.

Increase patient comfort.

Increase patient knowledge.

REFERENCES

Abbey, J. (1993). *FDA positions on regulation, education, and monitoring of infusion devices in relation to adverse events, in adverse events during infusion therapy.* Newport Beach: Communicore symposium 23–25.

Baldwin, D.R. (1992). Management of intravenous hazardous materials and hazardous wastes in the work environment. *Journal of Intravenous Nursing*, 15(2), 90–99.

Baker, D.L. (1990). Measuring outcome criteria. *Journal of Intravenous Nursing*, 13(4), 253–258.

Bernzweig, E.P. (1981). *Nurse's liability for malpractice* (3rd ed). New York: McGraw-Hill, 68.

Cassidy, D.A., & Friesen, M.A. (1990). QA: Applying JCAHO's generic model. *Nursing Management*, 21(6), 22–27.

Creighton, H. (1987). Legal significance of charting. Part II. *Nursing Management*, 18(10), 14–15.

Creighton, H. (1987). Legal importance of policy and procedures. Part I. *Nursing Management*, 18(4), 14–15.

Creighton, H. (1987). Legal importance of policy and procedures. Part II. *Nursing Management*, 18(5), 22–28.

Delaney, C.W., & Lauer, M.L. (1988). *Intravenous therapy: A guide to quality care.* Philadelphia: J.B. Lippincott.

Fiesta, J. (1991). Nurse's role as an expert witness. *Nursing Management*, 22(3), 28–29.

Fiesta, J. (1991). QA and risk management reducing liability exposure. *Nursing Management*, 22(2), 14–15.

Fiesta, J. (1988). *The law and liability: A guide for nurses* (2nd ed). New York: Wiley Medical Publications, 3–5, 51–79.

Gardner, C. (1987). Risk management of medication errors. *National Intravenous Therapy Association*, 10(1), 266–278.

Goldman, T.A. (1991). Risk management concepts and strategies. *Journal of Intravenous Nursing*, 14(3), 199–204.

Hibberd, P.L. (1995). Patients, needles and health care workers. *Journal of Intravenous Nursing*, 18(2), 65–76.

Hogue, E. (1986). What you should know about informed consent. *Nursing 86*, 6, 47–48.

Hughes, F.Y. (1987). Quality assurance in home care services. *Nursing Management*, 18(12), 33–36.

Jagger, J., Hunt, E., & Brand-Elnagger, J. (1988). Rates of needle-stick injury caused by various devices in a university hospital. *New England Journal of Medicine*, 319, 284.

Joint Commission of the Accreditation of Healthcare Organizations. (1995). *1996 Comprehensive Accreditation Manual for Hospitals.* Chicago, JCAHO, 239–273, 397–404.

Joint Commission on the Accreditation of Healthcare Organizations. (1992). *Accreditation manual for hospitals, 1992.* Chicago: JCAHO.

Korniewicz, D.M., Kirwin, M., & Larson, E. (1991). Do your gloves fit the task? *American Journal of Nursing*, 91(6), 38–39.

LaRochelle, D.R., & Shahinpour, N. (1995). Total quality management guest editorial. *Nursing Clinics of North America*, 30(1).

Lumsden, D.J. (1990). Legal risks in a changing practice environment. *Journal of Intravenous Nursing*, 13(1), 59–67.

Macklin, D.C. (1990). The evolution of standards. *Journal of Intravenous Nursing*, 13(4), 249–252.

Markey, J. (1994). Latex allergy implications for healthcare personnel and infusion therapy patients. *Journal of Intravenous Nursing*, 17(1), 35–39.

Masoorli, S. (1995). Infusion therapy lawsuits. *Journal of Intravenous Nursing*, 18(2), 88–91.

McCray, E. (1986). Occupational risk of acquired immunodeficiency syndrome among health care workers. *New England Journal of Medicine*, 314(17), 1127.

McGregor, R.J. (1990). A framework for developing staff competencies. *Journal of Nursing Staff Development*, (2), 79–83.

Meisenheimer, C.G. (1992). *Improving quality: A guide to effective programs.* Gaithersburg, MD: Aspen Publications, 53.

Micheletti, J.A., & Shlala, T.J. (1990). Evolving QA initiative in home healthcare. *Nursing Management*, 20(8), 24–28.

Milakovich, M.E. (1991). Creating a total quality health care environment. *Health Care Management Review*, 7, 126–128.

New, N.A., & New, J.R. (1989). QA that works. *Nursing Management*, 20(6), 21–24.

Nyugen, D., Burns, M., & Shaprio, G. (1991). Intraoperative cardiovascular collapse secondary to latex allergy. *Journal of Urology, 146*, 571–574.

Nutter, A.F. (1979). Contact urticaria to rubber. *Journal of Dermatology, 101*, 597–598.

O'Brien, B. (1988). QA: A commitment to excellence. *Nursing Management, 19*(11), 33–40.

OSHA (1986). OSHA work-practice for personnel dealing with cytotoxic (antineoplastic) drugs. *American Journal of Hospital Pharmacy, 43*, 1193.

Pierce, C. (1995). Intravenous nursing as a specialty. In *Intravenous Therapy Clinical Principles and Practices*. Philadelphia: W.B. Saunders.

Porter, A.L. (1988). Assuring quality through staff nurse performance. *Nursing Clinics of North America, 23*(3), 649–655.

Roberts, J.S., Bell, D.M., & Culver, D. (1994). HIV transmission in the health-care setting. *Infectious Disease Clinics of North America, 8*, 319–329.

Roberts, J.S., Coale, J.G., & Redman, R.R. (1989). A history of the joint commission on accreditation of hospitals. *JAMA, 238*, 936–940.

Schroeder, P. (1988). Directions and dilemmas in nursing QA. *Nursing Clinics of North America, 23*(3), 657–664.

Scott, W.L. (1990). Medical-device complications: Reporting a quality assurance mechanism. *Journal of Intravenous Nursing, 13*(3), 178–182.

Scrima, D.A. (1987). Assessing staff competency. *Journal of Nursing Administration, 17*(2), 41–45.

Sussman, G.L., Tarlo, S., & Dolovich, J.D. (1991). The spectrum of IgE-mediated responses to latex. *JAMA, 5*, 13.

Tan, M.W. (1990). Occurrence screens: A risk and quality control tool for I.V. nursing. *Journal of Intravenous Nursing, 13*(5), 308–311.

Tokars, J., Bell, D., & Culver, D. (1992). Percutaneous injuries during surgical procedures. *JAMA, 267*, 2899.

Wecht, C.H. (1979). Medical expert testimony. Every doctor's concern. *Legal Aspects of Medical Practice, 2*.

Weinstein, S. (1993). *Plumer's principles and practices of intravenous therapy* (5th ed). Philadelphia: J.B. Lippincott.

Weinstein, S. (1996). Legal implications/risk management. *Journal of Intravenous Nursing Supplement. 19* (3S) S16–S18.

Wilkinson, R., & Moore, B.T. (1990). *Quality assurance in ambulatory care* (2nd ed). Chicago: Joint Commission on the Accreditation of Healthcare Organizations.

Williams, H.F. (1995). Integrating the occupational safety and health administration mandates on bloodborne pathogens in the practice setting. *Journal of Intravenous Nursing (Suppl), 6S*(18), S9–S16.

UNIT TWO

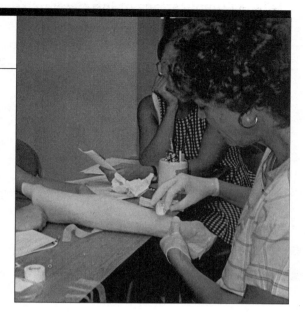

THE BASICS: FOUNDATION FOR PRACTICE

CHAPTER 3
Fundamentals of Fluid Balance

CHAPTER 4
Fundamentals of Electrolyte Balance

CHAPTER 5
Parenteral Solutions

CHAPTER 6
Infection Control

CHAPTER 7
Equipment

CHAPTER 8
Techniques for Peripheral Intravenous Therapy

CHAPTER 9
Complications of Intravenous Therapy

CHAPTER 10
Intravenous Therapy: Special Problems

Fundamentals of Fluid Balance

CHAPTER CONTENTS

GLOSSARY
LEARNING OBJECTIVES
PRE-TEST, CHAPTER 3
BODY FLUID COMPOSITION
FLUID DISTRIBUTION
FLUID FUNCTION
Fluid Transport
HOMEOSTATIC MECHANISMS
Kidneys
Heart and Blood Vessels
Lungs
Glands
PHYSICAL ASSESSMENT
Neurologic
Cardiovascular
Respiratory
Integumentary
Special Senses
Body Weight

FLUID VOLUME IMBALANCES
Fluid Volume Deficit
Fluid Volume Excess
NURSING PLAN OF CARE: FLUID VOLUME
  DEFICIT
PATIENT EDUCATION
HOME CARE ISSUES
NURSING PLAN OF CARE: FLUID VOLUME
  EXCESS
PATIENT EDUCATION
HOME CARE ISSUE
COMPETENCY CRITERIA: FLUID BALANCE
KEY POINTS
POST-TEST, CHAPTER 3
CRITICAL THINKING ACTIVITY
ANSWERS TO CHAPTER 3
Pre-Test
Post-Test
REFERENCES
BIBLIOGRAPHY

GLOSSARY

Active transport   The passage of a substance across a cell membrane by an energy-consuming process that permits diffusion to take place
Antidiuretic hormone (ADH)   A hormone secreted from the pituitary mechanism that causes the kidney to conserve water; sometimes referred to as the "water-conserving hormone"
Body fluid   Body water in which electrolytes are dissolved
Diffusion   The passage of molecules of one substance between the molecules of another to form a mixture of the two substances
Extracellular fluid (ECF)   Body fluid located outside the cells
Filtration   The process of passing of fluid through a filter using pressure
Fingerprinting   A condition in which imprints are made on the hands, sternum, or forehead when pressed firmly by the fingers
Homeostasis   The ability to restore equilibrium under stress

Hypertonic Having an osmotic pressure greater than that of the solution with which it is compared

Hypotonic Having an osmotic pressure less than that of the solution with which it is compared

Insensible loss Output that is difficult to measure, such as perspiration

Isotonic Having an osmotic pressure equal to that of blood; equivalent osmotic pressure

Interstitial fluid Body fluid between the cells

Intracellular fluid (ICF) Body fluid inside the cells

Intravascular fluid The fluid portion of blood plasma

Oncotic pressure The osmotic pressure exerted by colloids (proteins), as when albumin exerts oncotic pressure within the blood vessels and helps to hold the water content of the blood in the intravascular compartment

Osmolarity A measure of solute concentration. The concentration of a solution in terms of osmoles of solutes per liter of solution

Osmosis The movement of water from a lower concentration to a higher concentration across a semipermeable membrane

Syndrome of inappropriate antidiuretic hormone (SIADH) secretion A condition in which excessive ADH is secreted, resulting in hyponatremia

Sensible loss Output that is measurable

Solute The substance that is dissolved in a liquid to form a solution

LEARNING OBJECTIVES

Upon completion of this chapter, the reader will be able to:

- Define terminology related to fluids and electrolytes.
- Identify the three fluid compartments within the body.
- Identify the mechanisms of daily intake and daily output.
- State the functions of body fluid.
- Differentiate between active and passive transport.
- Define the concept of osmosis and delineate examples of this concept.
- State the average insensible loss for 24 hours.
- Recall the homeostatic organs.
- Compare and contrast the movement of water in hypotonic, hypertonic, and isotonic solutions.
- Summarize the major fluid balance disorders.
- List the six major body systems assessed for fluid balance disturbances.
- Identify the patient with fluid volume deficit and fluid volume excess, using the nurses' quick assessment guide.
- Determine the nursing diagnosis appropriate for care of the patient experiencing fluid balance disturbances.

PRE-TEST, CHAPTER 3

Match the term in column I to the definition in column II.

Column I

1. __B__ extracellular
2. __D__ intravascular
3. __E__ intracellular
4. __C__ osmolarity
5. __A__ homeostasis

Column II

A. Ability to restore equilibrium
B. Fluid outside the cell
C. A measure of solute concentration
D. The fluid portion of blood plasma
E. Fluid inside the cells

6. What are the three fluid compartments related to body fluid distribution?
   A. Intracellular, interstitial, intravascular
   B. Interstitial, extravascular, intravascular
   C. Extracellular, extravascular, interstitial

7. What are the functions of body fluid?
   A. Maintain blood volume
   B. Transport material to and from cells
   C. Assist digestion of food through hydrolysis
   D. Regulate body temperature
   E. All of the above

8. How is fluid primarily passively transported within the body?
   A. Osmosis
   B. Adenosine triphosphate (ATP) in cell membrane
   C. Diffusion
   D. The sodium-potassium pump

9. Which of the following is the range of milliosmoles (mOsm/liter) for an isotonic solution?
   A. 150–250   C. 320–460
   B. 250–375   D. 350–500

10. Which of the following may be signs and symptoms of fluid volume deficit?
    A. Bounding pulse, decreased blood pressure, and moist crackles
    B. Increased respiratory rate, warm moist skin, and decreased temperature
    C. Decreased pulse, decreased blood pressure, and poor skin turgor
    D. Dyspnea, jugular vein distention, and sternum fingerprinting

11. A patient has the following signs and symptoms: moist rales, increased respiratory rate, dyspnea, and 3+ edema of the ankles. What is the appropriate nursing diagnosis?
    A. Fluid volume deficit
    B. Fluid volume excess
    C. Tissue integrity impaired
    D. Tissue perfusion altered, renal

12. What is the average insensible loss in an adult?
    A. 200–400 mL per day
    B. 400–600 mL per day
    C. 500–1000 mL per day
    D. 800–1200 mL per day

13. Diffusion is a passive process in which molecules move from:
    A. An area of low concentration to one of high concentration
    B. An area of high concentration to one of low concentration
    C. A region of low pressure to one of high pressure, using hydrostatic pressure

True-False

14. T F Hypertonic solutions have a range of 250 to 300 mOsm/liter.

15. T F The area that can be used to assess for skin turgor in an adult is the sternum.

Chinese say that water is the most powerful element, because it is perfectly nonresistant. It can wear away rock and sweep all before it.

FLORENCE SCOVEL SHINN

BODY FLUID COMPOSITION

Body fluid refers to body water in which electrolytes are dissolved. Water is the largest single constituent of the body. Body water, the medium in which cellular reactions take place, constitutes approximately 60% of total body weight (TBW) in young male adults and 50% to 55% in female adults. See Table 3–1 for values of total body fluids in relation to age and sex. Fat tissue contains little water, and the percentage of total body water will vary considerably, based on the amount of body fat present. In addition, total body water progressively decreases with age, making up about 50% of body weight in the elderly (Metheny, 1996). See Figure 3–1 for values of total body fluids in relation to age and sex.

FLUID DISTRIBUTION

Total body water is distributed both within the cell and outside the cell. The body water within the cells is referred to as intracellular fluid (ICF); fluid outside the cells is referred to as extracellular fluid (ECF) and consists of two compartments: interstitial and intravascular. Approximately 40% (two thirds) of the TBW is composed of the fluid inside the cell (ICF). The other 20% is outside the cell (ECF) and is divided between interstitial and intravascular spaces, with 15% in the tissue (interstitial) space and only 5% represented in the plasma (intravascular) space. The interstitial fluid lies outside of the blood vessels in the interstitial spaces between the body cells. See Figure 3–2 for a diagrammatic representation of body water distribution.

✎ **NOTE:** Lymph and cerebrospinal fluids, although highly specialized, are usually regarded as interstitial fluid.

An exchange of fluid continuously occurs among the intracellular, plasma, and interstitial compartments. Of these three spaces, only the plasma is directly influenced by the intake or elimination of fluid from the body. Changes in the intracellular and

TABLE 3–1. **PERCENTAGES OF TOTAL BODY FLUID IN RELATION TO AGE AND SEX**

Age	% of Water = Body Weight
Full-term newborn	70–80
1-year-old	64
Puberty to 39 years	Men: 60
	Women: 55
40–60 years	Men: 55
	Women: 47
Over 60 years	Men: 52
	Women: 46

Source: From *Fluid and electrolyte balance: Nursing considerations* (2nd ed) by N.M. Metheny, 1992, Philadelphia: J.B. Lippincott. Copyright 1992 by J.B. Lippincott Company. Reprinted by permission.

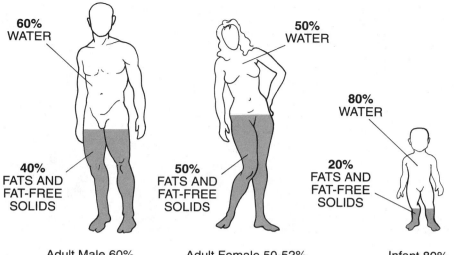

60% WATER	50% WATER	
		80% WATER
40% FATS AND FAT-FREE SOLIDS	50% FATS AND FAT-FREE SOLIDS	20% FATS AND FAT-FREE SOLIDS
Adult Male 60%	Adult Female 50-52%	Infant 80%

Figure 3–1. Percentages of body water.

interstitial fluid compartments occur in response to changes in the volume or concentration of the plasma.

The internal environment needs to remain in homeostasis; therefore, the intake and output of fluid must be relatively equal, as in healthy individuals. In illness this balance is frequently upset, and intake of fluid may become diminished or even cease. Output may vary with the influences of increased temperature, increased respirations, draining wounds, or gastric suction.

Normal sources of water per day include liquids, water-containing foods, and metabolic activity. In healthy adults, the intake of fluids varies from 1000 to 3000 mL/day, and 200 to 300 mL is produced from oxidation (O'Shea, 1993).

The elimination of fluid is considered sensible (measurable) loss and insensible

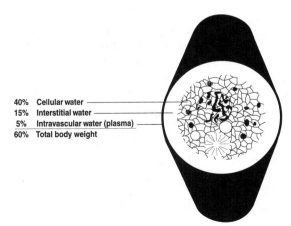

40% Cellular water
15% Interstitial water
5% Intravascular water (plasma)
60% Total body weight

Figure 3–2. Percentages of total body fluid.

49

TABLE 3–2. **WATER BALANCE: INTAKE AND OUTPUT**

Intake (mL)		Output (mL)	
Liquids	1200	Breathing	500
Food intake	1000	Perspiration	500
Oxidation	300	Urine	1400
Total	2500	Feces	100
		Total	2500

(not measurable) loss. Water is eliminated from the body by the skin, kidneys, bowels, and lungs. Approximately 300 to 500 mL is eliminated via the lungs every 24 hours, and approximately 500 mL/day of water is eliminated by the skin as perspiration. The amount of insensible loss in an adult is considered to be 500 to 1000 mL/day. Losses via the gastrointestinal tract are only about 100 to 200 mL per day because of the reabsorption of most of the fluid in the small intestines (Table 3–2). Increased losses of gastrointestinal fluids can occur from diarrhea or intestinal fistulas (Metheny, 1996).

✎ **NOTE:** Significant sweat losses occur if the patient's body temperature exceeds 101°F (38.3°C) or if room temperature exceeds 90°F. Insensible loss is also increased if respirations are increased to more than 20 per minute.

FLUID FUNCTION

Fluids within the body have several important functions. The ECF transports nutrients to the cells and carries waste products away from the cells by means of the capillary bed. Body fluids are in constant motion, maintaining living conditions for body cells (Metheny, 1996). The fluid within the body also has the following functions:

1. Maintains blood volume
2. Regulates body temperature
3. Transports material to and from cells
4. Serves as aqueous medium for cellular metabolism
5. Assists digestion of food through hydrolysis
6. Acts as solvent in which solutes are available for cell function
7. Serves as medium for the excretion of waste

Fluid Transport

Movement of particles through the cell membrane occurs via four transport mechanisms: diffusion, osmosis, filtration, and active transport. Materials are transported between the ICF and the extracellular compartment by these four mechanisms (Table 3–3).

Passive Transport

Passive transport includes diffusion, filtration, and osmosis

50

TABLE 3–3.
MECHANISMS OF TRANSPORT

Passive Transport
Diffusion
Filtration
Osmosis

Active Transport
ATP by cell membrane
Sodium-potassium pump

Diffusion

Diffusion is the passive movement of molecules or ions from a region of high concentration to an area of low concentration. Diffusion occurs through semipermeable membranes by either passing through pores, if small enough, or dissolving in the lipid matrix of the membrane wall. If there is no force opposing diffusion, particles will distribute themselves evenly. Many substances can diffuse through the cell membrane, and these substances diffuse in both directions. Influencing factors in the diffusion process are concentration differences, electrical potential, and pressure differences across the pores. The greater the concentration, the greater the rate of diffusion. Increase in the pressure on one side of the membrane increases the molecular forces striking the pores, thus creating a pressure gradient. Other factors that increase diffusion include:

Increased temperature
Increased concentration of particles
Decreased size or molecular weight of particle
Increased surface area available for diffusion
Decreased distance across which the particle mass must diffuse

Osmosis

Osmosis is the passage of water from an area of lower concentration of particles toward a higher concentration of particles across a semipermeable membrane. This process tends to equalize the concentration of two solutions.

Osmotic pressure develops as solute particles collide against each other. The concentration of a solution containing more solute particles increases the collisions creating a greater osmotic pressure. Osmotic pressure is measured in milliosmoles (mOsm). Osmolality refers to the total number of osmotically active particles per liter of solution, whereas osmolarity refers to the concentration of a solute in a volume of solution. The two terms are very similar and are often used interchangeably. The term osmolarity will be used within this text. The normal osmolarity of body fluids is between 280 and 295 mOsm/liter, and the osmolarity of ICF and ECF is always equal. The terms tonicity and osmolarity are used interchangeably (Chenevey, 1987). Tonicity reflects the concept and effects of hypotonic, hypertonic, and isotonic solutions on body cells. Figure 3–3 is a diagrammatic representation of the movement of water by osmosis in hypotonic, isotonic, and hypertonic solutions.

51

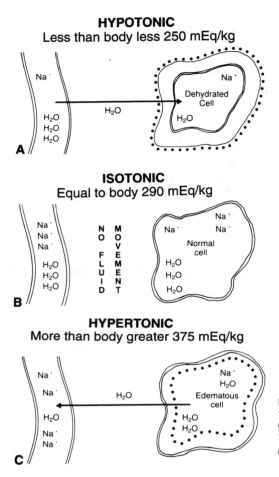

Figure 3–3. Effects of fluids shifts in isotonic, hypertonic, and hypotonic states. (From Mathewson-Kuhn, M., *Pharmacotherapeutics: A Nursing Process Approach*, 3rd ed. F.A. Davis, Philadelphia, 1994, p. 175, with permission.)

Isotonic solutions, such as 0.9% sodium chloride (NaCl), and 5% dextrose in water have the same osmolarity as that of normal body fluids. Solutions that have an osmolarity of 250 to 375 mOsm/liter are considered isotonic solutions and will have no effect on the volume of fluid within the cell; the solution will remain within the ECF space. Isotonic solutions are used to expand the ECF compartment.

Hypotonic solutions contain less salt than the intracellular space, and when infused, have an osmolarity below 250 mOsm/liter, and move water into the cell causing the cell to swell and possibly burst. By lowering the serum osmolarity the body fluids shift out of the blood vessels into the interstitial tissue and cells. Hypotonic solutions hydrate cells and can deplete the circulatory system. An examples of a hypotonic solution is 2.5% dextrose in water.

Hypertonic solutions, conversely, cause the water from within the cell to move to the ECF compartment where the concentration of salt is greater, causing the cell to shrink. Hypertonic solutions have an osmolarity of 375 mOsm/liter and above. These solutions are used to replace electrolytes. When hypertonic dextrose solutions are used alone, they also are used to shift ECF from interstitial tissue to plasma.

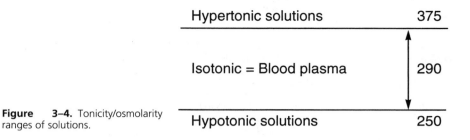

Hypertonic solutions	375
Isotonic = Blood plasma	290
Hypotonic solutions	250

Figure 3–4. Tonicity/osmolarity ranges of solutions.

Examples of hypertonic solutions are 5% dextrose, 0.9% NaCl, 5% dextrose, and Normosol M. Figure 3–4 is a chart of tonicity (osmolarity) ranges.

The osmotic pressure exerted by plasma colloids (or solutes) is called the colloid osmotic pressure or oncotic pressure. For example, albumin, a plasma protein, exerts oncotic pressure within the blood vessels and helps to hold the water content of the blood in the intravascular space. Proteinates are concentrated in the intracellular (55 mEq/L) and intravascular spaces (16 mEq/L).

Filtration

Filtration is the transfer of water and dissolved substance from a region of high pressure to a region of low pressure; the force behind it is hydrostatic pressure (the pressure on water at rest). The pumping heart provides hydrostatic pressure in the movement of water and electrolytes from the arterial capillary bed to the interstitial fluid. The plasma compartment contains more protein than the other compartments. Plasma protein, composed of albumin, globulin, and fibrinogen, creates an osmotic pressure at the capillary membrane, preventing fluid from the plasma from leaking into the interstitial spaces. Osmotic pressure created within the plasma by the presence of protein (mainly albumin) keeps the water in the vascular system (Chenevy, 1987).

Active Transport

Active transport is similar to the diffusion except that it acts against a concentration gradient. Active transport occurs when it is necessary for ions (electrolytes) to move from an area of low concentration to an area of high concentration. By definition, active transport implies that energy expenditure must take place for the movement to occur against a concentration gradient. Adenosine triphosphate (ATP) is released from the cell to enable certain substances to acquire the energy needed to pass through the cell membrane. For example, sodium concentration is greater in ECF; therefore, sodium tends to enter by diffusion into the intracellular compartment. This tendency is offset by the sodium-potassium pump, which is located on the cell membrane. In the presence of ATP, the sodium-potassium pump actively moves sodium from the cell into the ECF. Active transport is vital for maintaining the unique composition of both the extracellular and intracellular compartments.

HOMEOSTATIC MECHANISMS

Several homeostatic mechanisms are responsible for the balance of fluid and electrolytes within the body. These mechanisms involve organs that keep the composition and volume of body fluid within limits of normal: kidneys, lungs, heart, blood vessels, adrenal, parathyroid, and pituitary glands.

Kidneys

The kidneys are vital to control fluid and electrolyte balance. They normally filter 170 liters of plasma per day in the adult, while excreting only 1.5 liters of urine. They act in response to bloodborne messengers such as aldosterone and antidiuretic hormone (ADH). Functions of the kidneys in fluid balance are:

- Regulation of fluid volume and osmolarity by selective retention and excretion of body fluids
- Regulation of electrolyte levels by selective retention of needed substances and excretion of unneeded substances
- Regulation of pH of ECF by excretion or retention of hydrogen (H+) ions
- Excretion of metabolic wastes (primarily acids) and toxic substances (Metheny, 1992)

✎ NOTE: Renal failure can result in multiple fluid and electrolyte imbalances.

Heart and Blood Vessels

The pumping action of the heart provides circulation of blood through the kidneys under pressure, which allows urine to form; renal perfusion makes renal function possible. Blood vessels provide plasma to reach the kidneys in sufficient volume (20% of circulating blood volume) to permit regulation of water and electrolytes. Baroreceptors located in the carotid sinus and aortic arch respond to the degree of stretch of the vessel wall generated reacting to hypovolemia by stimulating fluid retention.

Lungs

The lungs are vital for maintaining homeostasis and constitute one of the main regulatory organs of fluid and acid-base balance. The lungs regulate acid-base balance by regulation of the H^+ ion concentration. Alveolar ventilation is responsible for the daily elimination of approximately 13,000 mEq of H^+ ions. The kidneys excrete only 40 to 80 mEq of hydrogen daily. Under influence from the medulla, the lungs act promptly to correct metabolic acid-base disturbances by regulating the level of carbon dioxide (a potential acid) in the ECF. Functions of the lungs in body fluid balance are:

- Regulation of metabolic alkalosis by compensatory hypoventilation, resulting in carbon dioxide (CO_2) retention and increased acidity of the ECF
- Regulation of metabolic acidosis by causing compensatory hyperventilation, resulting in CO_2 excretion and thus decreased acidity of the ECF
- Removal of 300 to 500 mL of water daily through exhalation (insensible water loss)

Glands

The glands responsible for aiding in homeostasis are the adrenal, pituitary, and parathyroid glands. The adrenal cortex is important in fluid and electrolyte homeostasis. The primary adrenocortical hormone influencing the balance of fluid is aldosterone. Aldosterone is responsible for the renal reabsorption of sodium, which results in the retention of chloride and water and the excretion of potassium. Aldosterone also regulates blood volume by regulating sodium retention.

Epinephrine, another adrenal hormone, increases blood pressure, enhances pulmonary ventilation, dilates blood vessels needed for emergencies, and constricts unnecessary vessels.

The adrenocortical hormone, cortisol, when produced in large quantities can produce sodium and fluid retention and potassium deficit.

The parathyroid gland is embedded in the corners of the thyroid gland and regulates calcium and phosphate balance. The parathyroid gland influences fluid and electrolytes, increases serum calcium levels, and lowers serum phosphate levels. A reciprocal relationship exists between extracellular calcium and phosphate levels. A decrease in parathyroid hormone (PTH) lowers serum calcium levels and increases serum phosphate levels. Another hormone that regulates calcium is calcitonin, a substance secreted by the thyroid gland. Calcitonin's action on calcium is opposite to that of PTH; calcitonin reduces plasma calcium concentrations.

The pituitary hormone influencing water balance is the antidiuretic hormone (ADH). This hormone, which affects renal reabsorption of water, is also referred to as the "water-conserving" hormone. Functions of ADH are to maintain osmotic pressure of the cells by controlling renal water retention or excretion and control of blood volume. Excessive secretion of ADH results in syndrome of inappropriate antidiuretic hormone secretion (SIADH).

PHYSICAL ASSESSMENT

A body systems approach is the best method for assessing fluid and electrolyte imbalances related to I.V. therapy. Begin by assessing vital signs, infusion rate of any I.V. infusions, and intake and output. Follow with assessing body systems at the beginning of each shift and as needed to monitor the patient's reactions to infusions.

Neurologic

There is a progressive loss of central nervous system (CNS) cells with advancing age, along with decrease in sense of smell and tactile sense. The thirst mechanism in the aged may be diminished and is a poor guide for fluid needs in the aged patient. An ill patient may not be able to verbalize thirst or to reach for a glass of water. Sensation of thirst depends on excitation of the cortical centers of consciousness. The use of antianxiety agents, sedatives, or hypnotics can lead to confusion and disorientation, causing the patient to forget to drink fluid. Changes in orientation can also be an indicator of fluid volume deficit.

Fluid volume changes, along with serum sodium levels affect the CNS cells, resulting in confusion, stupor, seizures, or coma. CNS cells shrink in sodium excess and expand when serum sodium levels decrease. Assessment of neuromuscular irritability is particularly important when imbalances in calcium, magnesium, and sodium are suspected.

Cardiovascular

The quality and rate of the pulse are indicators of how the patient is tolerating ECF volume. The peripheral veins in the extremities provide a way of evaluating plasma volume. Examination of hand veins can evaluate the plasma volume. Peripheral veins

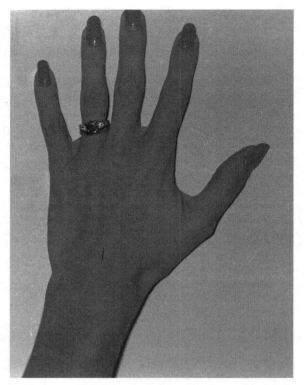

Figure 3–5. Hand vein assessment. Peripheral vein filling takes longer than 3 to 5 seconds in patients with sodium depletion and dehydration. Slow emptying of hand veins indicates overhydration and excessive blood volume.

empty in 3 to 5 seconds when the hand is elevated and fill in the same amount of time when lowered to a dependent position. Peripheral vein filling takes longer than 3 to 5 seconds in patients with sodium depletion and extracellular dehydration (Metheny, 1996). Slow emptying of the peripheral veins indicates overhydration and excessive blood volume (Fig. 3–5).

A 10-mm Hg fall in systolic blood pressure when shifting from the lying to the standing position usually indicates fluid volume deficit. The jugular vein provides a built-in manometer for evaluation of central venous pressure (CVP). Changes in fluid volume are reflected by changes in neck vein filling.

The external jugular veins, with the patient supine, fill to the anterior border of the sternocleidomastoid muscle. Flat neck veins in the supine position indicate a decreased plasma volume. When the patient is in a 45-degree position, the external jugular distends no higher than 2 cm above the sternal angle. Elevated venous pressure is indicated by neck veins distending from the top portion of the sternum to the angle of the jaw (Fig. 3–6).

Edema indicates expansion of interstitial volume. Edema can be localized (usually caused by inflammation) or generalized (usually related to capillary hemodynamics). Edema should be assessed over bony surfaces of the tibia or sacrum and

56

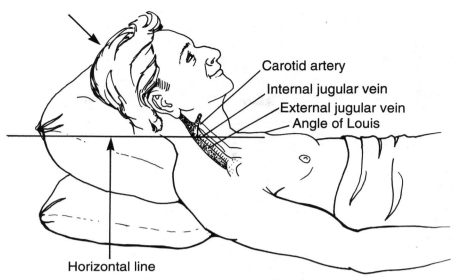

Figure 3–6. Jugular venous distention.

rated according to severity 1+ to 4+ (Horne & Swearingen, 1993; Fig. 3–7). The presence of periorbital edema suggests significant fluid retention.

Respiratory

A key to assessment of circulatory overload can be made by assessing the lung fields. Changes in respiratory rate and depth may be a compensatory mechanism for acid-base imbalance. Moist crackles, in the absence of cardiopulmonary disease, indicate fluid volume excess. Shallow, slow breathing could indicate metabolic alkalosis or respiratory acidosis. Deep rapid breathing could indicate respiratory alkalosis or metabolic acidosis. See Chapter 4 for further information on acid-base imbalances.

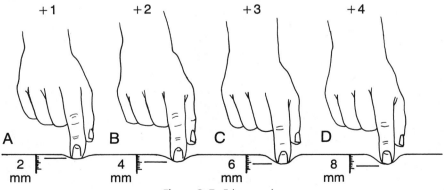

Figure 3–7. Edema scale.

Integumentary

The temperature and skin surface assessment are key in determining fluid volume changes. Turgor of the skin should be assessed by pinching the area over the hand, sternum, or forehead. In a normal person, the pinched skin immediately falls back to its normal position when released. This elastic property, referred to as turgor, is partially dependent on interstitial fluid volume. In a person with a fluid volume deficit, the skin may remain slightly elevated for many seconds. In persons over age 55, skin turgor is generally reduced because of loss of elasticity, particularly in areas that have been exposed to the sun. A more accurate assessment can be made on the skin over the sternum. A condition in which placement of fingers firmly on the patient's skin leaves finger imprints is called fingerprinting and is associated with fluid volume excess. Fingerprint edema is demonstrated by pressing a finger firmly over the sternum or other body surface for a period of 15 to 30 seconds. Upon removal of the finger, a positive sign is a visible fingerprint, similar to that seen when a fingerprint is made on paper with ink (Vanatta & Fogelman, 1988).

✎ **NOTE:** An increase in temperature can indicate a sodium excess, and flushing of the skin surfaces can indicate a magnesium deficit. See Chapter 4 for a detailed discussion of electrolyte imbalances.

Special Senses

The eyes, mouth, lips, and tongue are also key indicators of fluid volume imbalances. The absence of tearing and salivation in a child is a sign of fluid volume deficit. In a healthy person, the tongue has one longitudinal furrow. In the person with fluid volume deficit, the tongue has additional longitudinal furrows and is smaller because of fluid loss (Metheny, 1996).

Mucous membranes are often the first sign of dehydration; as fluid volume decreases, the mouth becomes dry and sticky and the lips dry and cracked. In fluid volume deficit, eyes tend to appear sunken; in significant fluid volume excess, periorbital edema is present.

✎ **NOTE:** Good oral hygiene is imperative with mouth-breathing patients. Also, if you are giving good oral care and the crusted, dry, furrowed tongue is not improving, fluid volume deficit must be restored to aid in solving this problem.

Body Weight

Taking daily weights of patients with potential fluid imbalances is an important clinical tool. Accurate body weight measurement is a better indicator of gains or losses than intake and output records. A loss or gain of 1 kg (2.2 lb) reflects a loss or gain of 1 liter of body fluid. Generally, fluid volume excess is considered severe when body weight is more than 15% higher than the person's normal body weight. Severe fluid volume deficit occurs when body weight is more than 15% less than the person's normal body weight. See Table 3–4 for a summary of assessment findings that indicate altered fluid status.

TABLE 3–4. **QUICK ASSESSMENT GUIDE FOR FLUID IMBALANCE**

System Assessed	Fluid Volume	
	Fluid Volume Excess	Deficit
Neurologic		Change in orientation Confusion
Cardiovascular	Bounding pulse Increased pulse rate Jugular distention Overdistended hand veins that are slow to empty (>3 s)	Decreased pulse rate Decreased blood pressure Narrow pulse pressure Slow hand vein filing (>3 s)
Respiratory	Moist crackles Respiratory rate >20 Dyspnea Pulmonary edema	Lungs clear
Integument	Warm, moist skin Fingerprinting over sternum	Decreased turgor over sternum and forehead Decreased skin temperature
Eyes	Periorbital edema (suggests significant fluid retention)	Dry conjunctiva Sunken eyes Decreased tearing
Mouth		Sticky, dry mucous membranes
Lips		Dry, cracked
Tongue		Extralongitudinal furrows
Body weight	Mild: <5% over normal Moderate: 5–10% over normal Severe: >15% over normal	Mild: <5% less than normal Moderate: 5–10% less than normal Severe: >15% less than normal

FLUID VOLUME IMBALANCES

Fluid volume imbalances may reflect an increase or a decrease in total body fluid or an altered distribution of body fluids. There are two major alterations in ECF balance: fluid volume deficit and fluid volume excess.

Fluid Volume Deficit

Extracellular fluid volume deficit reflects a contracted vascular compartment due either to a significant ECF loss or to an accumulation of fluid in the interstitial space. Gastrointestinal dysfunction is the most common cause of ECF deficit. Fluid volume deficit occurs when there is either an excessive loss of body water or an inadequate compensatory intake. The ECF consists predominantly of the electrolytes, sodium

59

and chloride, both of which tend to attract water; loss of these electrolytes also leads to loss of water. Other causes are listed in Table 3–5.

Clinically, ECF deficit is characterized by acute weight loss, altered cardiovascular function that reflects the underlying ECF volume deficit, and complaints of nausea and vomiting. Symptomatology reflects a dehydrated state with sunken eyeballs, poor skin turgor, and oliguria.

Laboratory findings in fluid volume deficit reflects hemoconcentration; the serum hemoglobin, hematocrit, and proteins are increased. Blood urea nitrogen is elevated above 20 mg/100 mL. The urine specific gravity reflects high solute concentration of more than 1.030.

Treatment for ECF volume deficit entails fluid replacement (orally or intravenously) until the oliguria is relieved and the cardiovascular and neurologic systems stabilize. Isotonic electrolyte solutions such as 0.9% NaCl or lactated Ringer's solution are used to treat the hypotensive patient in fluid volume deficit. A hypotonic electrolyte solution (0.45% NaCl) often is used to provide electrolyte and free water for renal excretion of metabolic wastes (Metheny, 1996).

✎ **NOTE:** Extreme caution must be exercised in fluid replacement therapy to avoid fluid overload.

Fluid Volume Excess

Extracellular fluid volume excess causes an expansion of the ECF compartment. The primary cause of ECF excess is cardiovascular dysfunction. Fluid volume excess is always secondary to an increase in total body sodium content, which causes total body water increase. Normally, the posterior pituitary decreases secretion of the ADH when excess water moves into the cells. This causes the kidney to eliminate excess fluid. However, if the patient has an excessive secretion of ADH, the water will be retained, placing the patient at risk for fluid volume excess. Excessive secretion of ADH can be caused by fear, pain, postoperative reaction 12 to 24 hours after surgery, and acute infections. See Table 3–5 for additional causes of ECF volume excess.

Clinically, ECF volume excess has distinct signs and symptoms, the most prominent being weight gain. Edema is usually not apparent until 2 to 4 kg of fluid have

TABLE 3–5. **EXTRACELLULAR FLUID DISORDERS: DEFICIT AND EXCESS**

	Fluid Volume Deficit	**Fluid Volume Excess**
Definition (Causes)	Hypovolemia	Hypervolemia
	Fever with diaphoresis	*Cardiovascular* dysfunction
	GI dysfunction (most common)	CHF, pulmonary edema
	Fluid and electrolyte loss	Too rapid administration of
	Diarrhea	saline I.V.
	Overdose of cathartics	*Renal* dysfunction
	Renal dysfunction	Serum protein depletion and
	Neurologic dysfunction	hyponatremia
	Lethargy and coma	Cirrhosis with ascites and
	Endocrine dysfunction	portal hypertension
	Diabetes insipidus	*Endocrine* dysfunction
		Hyperaldosteronism

TABLE 3–5. **EXTRACELLULAR FLUID DISORDERS: DEFICIT AND EXCESS**
(*Continued*)

	Fluid Volume Deficit	Fluid Volume Excess
Clinical Picture	Acute weight loss *Neurologic:* Change in mental status, disorientation, lethargy, convulsions *Cardiovascular:* Postural hypotension, dizziness Syncope, vertigo, pulse weak Absence of neck vein distention Decreased CVP, decreased cardiac output *GI:* Nausea, vomiting, anorexia *Fluid intake versus output:* Increased thirst, decreased urine output, poor skin turgor over sternum and forehead Dry skin and mucous membranes Sunken eyeballs; hyperthermia	Acute weight gain *Neurologic:* Changes in mental status and level of consciousness, seizures *Cardiovascular:* Hypertension, tachycardia bounding pulse Increased CVP, neck vein distention *Edema:* True pitting edema, taut and shiny skin *Respiratory:* SOB, tachypnea, dyspnea, cough, rales, pulmonary edema *Renal:* Urine output disproportionately less than fluid intake
Laboratory Data	Electrolyte parameter (by itself) indicative of fluid deficit *Serum* Hematocrit: Increased Hemoglobin: Increased Proteins: Increased Osmolarity: Normal BUN: > 20 mg/100 mL *Urine* Sodium: < 50 mEq/liter Osmolarity: > 500 mOsm/liter Specific gravity: 1.030	Electrolyte parameter (by itself) indicative of fluid excess *Serum* Hematocrit: Normal to low Hemoglobin: Normal to low Proteins: Normal to low Osmolarity: Normal BUN: Normal to low *Urine* Sodium: Reduced Osmolarity: < 500 mOsm/liter Specific gravity: < 1.010
Treatment	1. Restore fluid and electrolyte balance using I.V. isotonic saline. 2. Treat underlying cause.	1. Reduce fluid retention by salt and fluid restriction. 2. Diuretics to increase fluid excretion. 3. Treat underlying cause.

GI = Gastrointestinal; CHF = congestive heart failure; CVP = central venous pressure; SOB = shortness of breath; BUN = blood urea nitrogen.
Source: Adapted from Dolan, J. (1991). *Critical Care Nursing: Clinical Management Through the Nursing Process.* Philadelphia: F.A. Davis. Reprinted by permission.

FLUID VOLUME DEFICIT

Focus Criteria for Assessment

Subjective	*Objective*
History of contributing factors and cause, such as diabetes mellitus, cardiac disease, or gastrointestinal disorder	Present weight
	Changes in mentation
	Dry skin and mucous membranes
Recent weight loss	Poor skin turgor
History of laxative, enema, or diuretic overuse	Decreased pulse rate
	Decreased blood pressure
Fluid intake (amount and type)	Slow vein filling
	Decreased urine output
	Decreased urine specific gravity

Nursing Diagnoses

Fluid volume deficit related to failure or regulatory mechanisms
Fluid volume deficit related to loss of body fluid and inadequate fluid intake
Fluid volume deficit related to high-solute tube feedings

Nursing Diagnoses

Risk of injury related to confusion
Altered oral mucous membrane related to dehydration
Altered tissue perfusion: cardiopulmonary, renal, and peripheral related to hypovolemia

Outcome Criteria

The patient will:
Increase fluid intake to a minimum of 2000 mL/day, unless contraindicated.
Relate the need for increased fluid intake during stress or heat.
Maintain a urine specific gravity within normal range.
Demonstrate no signs and symptoms of dehydration.

Nursing Management: Critical Activities

Monitor fluid status, including intake and output.
Monitor specific gravity.
Monitor trends of daily weights.
Monitor hemodynamic status (central venous pressure when appropriate).
Observe for indicators of dehydration (e.g., poor skin turgor, delayed capillary refill, weak or thready pulse, severe thirst, dry mucous membranes, decreased urine output, and hypotension).
Monitor fluid loss (e.g., bleeding, vomiting, diarrhea, and perspiration tachypnea).
Administer isotonic solutions for extracellular rehydration, if appropriate.
Administer hypotonic solutions for intracellular rehydration, if appropriate.
Monitor hemoglobin and hematocrit.
Monitor serum sodium levels.
Encourage oral fluid intake.
Promote skin integrity (monitor areas at risk for breakdown).
Provide frequent oral hygiene.

Source: Carpenito, 1995; Poyss, 1987.

been retained. Alterations in respiratory and cardiovascular function are present and include hypertension and tachycardia.

In fluid volume excess, the hematocrit may be decreased because of hemodilution. The serum sodium and serum osmolarity will be decreased if hypervolemia occurs as a result of excessive retention of water.

Treatment of ECF volume excess is directed toward sodium and fluid restriction, administration of diuretics and the treatment of the underlying cause (Dolan, 1995).

PATIENT EDUCATION

Assess patient's understanding of the type of fluid loss being experienced.

Give verbal and written instructions for fluid replacement (drink at least 3 quarts of liquid).

Teach to increase the fluid intake during hot days, in the presence of fever or infection and to decrease activity during extreme weather.

Teach how to observe for dehydration (especially in infants).

Instruct to seek medical consultation for continued dehydration.

Teach appropriate use of laxatives, enemas, and diuretics.

HOME CARE ISSUES

Consider home care visit to follow up patients with diabetes mellitus, cardiovascular disorders, and severe gastrointestinal disorders.

Follow up with home care for patients on drug therapy for edema (diuretics).

Nursing Plan of Care

FLUID VOLUME EXCESS

Focus Criteria for Assessment

Subjective	*Objective*
History of symptoms, shortness of breath, or signs of fluid overload	Weight gain
Recent weight loss	Bounding pulse
History of contributing factors and cause, such as family or personal history of diabetes mellitus or cardiac or renal diseases	Increased respiratory rate
	Moist crackles in lungs
	Increased blood pressure
	Slow vein filling
	Peripheral edema
Alcoholism	Neck vein distention
Steroid therapy	
Excessive salt intake	
Excessive parenteral fluid replacement	

Nursing Diagnoses

Fluid volume excess related to infusion of sodium chloride solution

Fluid volume excess related to compromised regulatory function secondary to renal failure—acute or chronic

Fluid volume excess related to dependent venous pooling or venostasis

Impaired skin integrity related to altered circulation, edema

Continued on following page

Source: Carpenito, 1995; Poyss, 1987.

PATIENT EDUCATION

Inform to notify physician for excessive edema or weight gain (> 2 lb/day) or increased shortness of breath.
Provide literature concerning low-salt diets; consult with dietitian if necessary.
Write instructions for diet.
Have patient demonstrate use of Ace bandages or stockings.

HOME CARE ISSUE

Consider home care visit to follow up on diet and instructions on use of stockings.

COMPETENCY CRITERIA: Fluid Balance

Competency Statement: The competent intravenous therapy nurse will be able to monitor the patient for signs and symptoms of fluid volume disturbances.

COGNITIVE CRITERIA

	Skilled	Needs Education
1. Able to identify patients at risk for fluid volume disorders:		
Cardiac disorders		
CHF		
Renal		
Diuretic therapy		
Renal failure		
Gastrointestinal disorders		
Diarrhea		
Surgical		
N/G tube to suction		
Postoperative complications		
Neurologic		
Diabetis insipidus		

SUGGESTED EVALUATION CRITERIA

Written test

PERFORMANCE CRITERIA

	Skilled	Needs Education
1. Able to perform assessment directed at identifying fluid volume disorders:		
Accurate vital signs		
Accurate weight		
Accurate intake and output		
Specific gravity		
Cardiac		
Pulse		
Edema scale		
Blood pressure		
Jugular vein distention		

Hand vein filling

Pulmonary

Lung sounds

Rate

Integumentary

Skin turgor

Skin surfaces

Fontanel's (pediatric)

Special senses

Eyes:

Dry conjunctiva

Decreased tearing

Mouth:

Sticky, dry mucous membrane

Tongue: extra longitudinal furrow

Laboratory data

Hemaglobin and hematocrit

Proteins

Cretinine and BUN

SUGGESTED EVALUATION CRITERIA

Written test

Clinical case studies

Assessment skills performance at bedside or in simulated laboratory

KEY POINTS

Fundamentals fluid balance

Fluid is distributed in three compartments:

Intracellular	15%
Intravascular	5%
Interstitial	40%
TBW in water	60%

Fluid balance intake and output

Intake—liquids, food, and oxidation (2500 mL in 24 hours)

Output—Insensible loss: Sweat, respirations (500 to 1000 mL in 24 hours)

Sensible loss: Urine, feces (1500 mL in 24 hours)

Fluid transported passively by: filtration, diffusion and osmosis
  Electrolytes are actively transported by: ATP on cell membrane and the sodium-potassium pump
  Definition of osmosis: Movement of water from a lower concentration to a higher concentration across a semipermeable membrane.

Tonicity
  Isotonic solution: 250 to 375 mOsm/liter
  Hypotonic solutions: less than 250 mOsm/liter
  Hypertonic solutions: more than 375 mOsm/liter

Homeostatic organs
  Kidneys
  Heart and blood vessels
  Lungs
  Glands: adrenal, parathyroid, pituitary

Physical assessment includes:
  Neurologic
  Cardiovascular
  Respiratory
  Integumentary
  Special senses
  Body weight

Fluid volume imbalance
  ECF volume deficit
      Contracted vascular compartment
      Acute weight loss, altered cardiovascular function
      Laboratory findings: Hemoconcentration; increased serum hemoglobin, hematocrit, proteins; elevated BUN; urine specific gravity greater than 1.030
      Treatment: Replace fluids
      Isotonic multiple electrolyte solution for hypertensive patient.
      Hypotonic electrolyte solutions to provide electrolytes and free water for renal excretion of wastes
  ECF volume excess
      Expanded ECF compartment
      Usually secondary to increased sodium
      Acute weight gain, altered cardiovascular function, hypertension, tachycardia, and respiratory function alteration
      Laboratory findings: Hematocrit decreased because of hemodilution
      Treatment: Restrict sodium and fluids; administer diuretics; treat underlying cause

POST-TEST, CHAPTER 3

Match the term in column I with the definition in column II.

Column I

1. __C__ isotonic
2. __F__ hypertonic
3. __I__ hypotonic
4. __J__ osmolarity
5. __D__ homeostasis
6. __B__ ADH
7. __E__ intravascular fluid
8. __H__ intracellular fluid
9. __G__ interstitial fluid
10. __A__ insensible loss

Column II

A. Output that is difficult to measure, such as perspiration

B. Hormone secreted from the pituitary that causes kidneys to conserve water

C. Having an osmotic pressure equal to blood

D. Ability to restore equilibrium under stress

E. Fluid portion of the blood

F. Having an osmotic pressure higher than 375 mOsm/liter

G. Fluid between the cells

H. Fluid inside the cells

I. Having an osmotic pressure of less than 250 mOsm/liter

J. A measure of solute concentration

11. A physician orders 5% dextrose and 0.9% NaCl (mOsm 559). Fluid will move from the _____ space to the _____ space.
    A. Intracellular to vascular
    B. Vascular to interstitial
    C. Interstitial to the cellular

12. A physician orders 0.45% NaCl (mOsm 154). Fluid will move from the _____ space to the _____ space.
    A. Intracellular to vascular
    B. Vascular to intracellular
    C. Interstitial to cellular

13. A physician orders lactated Ringer's solution (mOsm 273). Fluid will _____ .
    A. Move from the intracellular space to the vascular space
    B. Move from the vascular space to the cellular space
    C. Stay in the vascular space

14. List two functions of the body fluid.
    A. __Temperature control__
    B. __Transport Nutrient to Cells__

15. List three homeostatic organs.
    A. __Heart__
    B. __Lungs__
    C. __Glands__

16. Fluid is transported passively by the mechanism/s of:
    A. Diffusion
    B. Osmosis
    C. Filtration
    D. All of the above

17. Identify one nursing diagnosis for fluid volume deficit.

Fluid volume deficit R/T Loss of body fluid

18. You have just completed a physical assessment of Mr. Marx, age 68. You find:
He knows who he is but is unsure of where he is (previous orientation normal).
Eyes are sunken.
Mouth is coated with an extra longitudinal furrow.
Lips are cracked.
Hand vein filling take more than 5 seconds.
Tenting of the skin appears over the sternum.
Vital signs: BP 128/60, pulse 78, respiratory rate 16 (previously 150/78, 76, 16, respectively)

Your assessment would lead you to suspect _Dehydration_ .

CRITICAL THINKING ACTIVITY

1. Within your work environment, identify the patients at risk for fluid volume deficit or excess. Remember that even outpatient units see patients at risk.

2. Using the six body systems to assess for fluid volume excess or deficit, choose four patients on your unit to assess and check for fluid volume changes.

3. Check I.V. solutions infusing on your patients and identify whether the solutions are isotonic, hypotonic, or hypertonic.

ANSWERS TO CHAPTER 3

PRE-TEST

1. B	5. A	9. B	13. B
2. D	6. A	10. C	14. F
3. E	7. E	11. B	15. T
4. C	8. A	12. C	

POST-TEST

1. C
2. F
3. I
4. J
5. D
6. B
7. E
8. H
9. G
10. A
11. A
12. B
13. C

14. Maintains blood volume, regulates body temperature, transports material to and from cells; acts as aqueous medium for cellular metabolism, assists in digestion of food, serves as a solvent in which solutes are available for cell function and as a medium for excretion of waste.
15. Kidneys, heart, blood vessels, adrenal, parathyroid, and pituitary glands.
16. D
17. Fluid volume deficit related to failure of regulatory mechanism.
    Fluid volume deficit related to loss of body fluid and inadequate fluid intake.
18. Fluid volume deficit.

REFERENCES

Carpenito, L.J. (1995). *Nursing diagnosis application to clinical practice* (6th ed). Philadelphia: J.B. Lippincott.

Carson, R. (1961). *The sea around us.* New York: New American Library.

Chenevey, B. (1987). Overview of fluids and electrolytes. *Nursing Clinics of North America,* 22(4), 749–759.

Dolan, J.T. (1995). *Critical care nursing: Clinical management through the nursing process.* Philadelphia: F.A. Davis.

Goldberger, E. (1986). *A primer of water, electrolytes and acid-base syndromes*, (7th ed). Philadelphia: Lea & Febiger.

Mathewson-Kuhn, M. (1994). *Pharmacotherapeutics: A nursing process approach* (3rd ed). Philadelphia: F.A. Davis.

Metheny, N.M. (1996). *Fluids and electrolyte balance: Nursing considerations* (3rd ed). Philadelphia: J.B. Lippincott.

Poyss, A.S. (1987). Assessment and nursing diagnosis in fluid and electrolyte disorders. *Nursing Clinics of North America, 22*(4), 773–783.

Washington Manual (1993). *Manual of medical therapeutics* (27th ed). Boston: Little, Brown.

BIBLIOGRAPHY

Baldwin, K.M., Garza C.S., Martin, R.N., et al. (1995). *Davis's manual of critical care therapeutics.* Philadelphia: F.A. Davis.

Berger, E. (1984). Nutrition in hypodermoclysis. *Journal of the American Geriatric Society, 32,* 199.

Burgess, R.E. (1965). Fluids and electrolytes. *American Journal of Nursing, 65*(10).

Maxwell, M., & Kleeman, C. (1980). *Clinical disorders of fluid and electrolyte metabolism* (3rd ed). New York: McGraw-Hill.

Rolls, B.J., & Phillips P.A. (1990). Aging and disturbances of thirst and fluid balance. *Nutrition Reviews, 48*(3), 137–143.

Rutherford, C. (1989). Fluid and electrolyte therapy: Considerations for patient care. *Journal of Intravenous Therapy, 12*(3), 173–184.

CHAPTER 4

Fundamentals of Electrolyte Balance

CHAPTER CONTENTS

GLOSSARY
LEARNING OBJECTIVES
PRE-TEST, CHAPTER 4
BASIC PRINCIPLES OF ELECTROLYTE BALANCE
ELECTROLYTES: FUNCTION, DEFICIT, EXCESS, AND TREATMENT
Sodium
Potassium
Calcium
Magnesium
Phosphorus
Chloride
NURSING PLAN OF CARE: ELECTROLYTE IMBALANCE
PATIENT EDUCATION
HOME CARE ISSUES
SUMMARY WORKSHEET #1: ELECTROLYTES

ACID-BASE BALANCE
Chemical Buffer Systems
MAJOR ELECTROLYTE IMBALANCES
Metabolic Acid-Base Imbalance
Respiratory Acid-Base Imbalance
SUMMARY WORKSHEET #2: ACID-BASE BALANCE
COMPETENCY CRITERIA: ELECTROLYTE BALANCE
KEY POINTS
CRITICAL THINKING ACTIVITY
POST-TEST, CHAPTER 4
ANSWERS TO CHAPTER 4
Pre-Test
Post-Test
REFERENCES

GLOSSARY

Acidosis   Blood pH below normal (less than 7.35)
Alkalosis   Blood pH above normal (greater than 7.45)
Anion   Negatively charged electrolyte
Antidiuretic hormone (ADH)   A hormone secreted from the pituitary mechanism that causes the kidney to conserve water; sometimes referred to as the "water-conserving hormone"
Cation   Positively charged electrolyte
Chvostek's sign   A sign elicited by tapping the facial nerve about 2 cm anterior to the earlobe, just below the zygomatic process; the response is a spasm of the muscles supplied by the facial nerve
Extracellular fluid (ECF)   Body fluid located outside the cells
Hyperkalemia   An excess of potassium in the blood
Hypokalemia   A low potassium concentration in the blood
Intracellular fluid (ICF)   Body fluid located between the cells
pH   Hydrogen ion (H^+) concentration

LEARNING OBJECTIVES

Upon completion of this chapter, the reader will be able to:

- Define terminology related to electrolytes.
- State the seven major electrolytes within the body fluids.
- Differentiate between cations and anions.
- Contrast each of the seven electrolytes and their major roles in body fluids.
- Identify signs and symptoms of deficits of sodium, potassium, calcium, magnesium, chloride, and phosphate.
- Identify signs and symptoms of excesses of sodium, potassium, calcium, magnesium, chloride, and phosphate.
- Recognize patients at risk for electrolyte imbalance.
- State the normal pH range of body fluids.
- Compare clinical manifestations of metabolic acidosis and alkalosis.
- Identify regulatory organs of acid-base balance.
- Identify nursing diagnoses and interventions related to electrolyte balance.

PRE-TEST, CHAPTER 4

Match the term in column I to the definition in column II.

Column I	Column II
1. __F__ acidosis	A. Electrolyte
2. __C__ hyperkalemia	B. Hydrogen ion (H^+) concentration
3. __B__ pH	C. An excess of potassium in the blood
4. __E__ cation	D. Continuous tonic spasm of a muscle
5. __G__ ECF	E. Positively charged electrolyte
6. __H__ alkalosis	F. H^+ ion concentration increases
7. __A__ ion	G. Extracellular fluid
8. __I__ ICF	H. H^+ ion concentration decreases
9. __D__ tetany	I. Intracellular fluid
10. __J__ anion	J. Negatively charged electrolyte

True-False

11. (T) F The normal pH range for arterial blood is 7.35 to 7.45.
12. (T) F The major function of sodium is maintaining ECF volume.
13. (T) F Calcium and phosphorous have a reciprocal relationship.
14. (T) F Magnesium is a major intracellular electrolyte.
15. T (F) The kidneys and liver are the organs of regulation in acid-base balance.

16. Which of the following electrolytes are positively charged?
   A. Potassium, sodium, bicarbonate
   B. Potassium, sodium, calcium
   C. Bicarbonate, phosphate, chloride
   D. Chloride, magnesium, bicarbonate

17. Which of the following signs and symptoms indicate alkalosis (bicarbonate excess)?
   A. Kussmaul breathing, confusion, increased respiratory rate
   B. Tetany, soft tissue calcification
   C. Dizziness, tingling of fingers and toes, carpopedal spasm

Match the signs and symptoms of the deficit with the electrolyte imbalance.

Electrolyte Imbalance

18. __C__ hypokalemia
19. __D__ hypocalcemia
20. __A__ hypomagnesemia
21. __C__ hyponatremia

Signs and Symptoms

A. Anorexia, exhaustion, muscle cramps, ataxia

B. Irritability, diminished reflexes, anorexia, nausea, vomiting

C. Numbness of fingers, cramps, mental changes, Chvostek's sign

D. Neuromuscular and nervous system irritability, paraesthesia, cardiac dysrhythmias, disorientation

When they went ashore the animals that took up a land life carried with them

a part of the sea in their bodies, a heritage which they passed on to their

children and which even today links each land animal with its origin in the

ancient sea.

RACHEL CARSON, 1961

BASIC PRINCIPLES OF ELECTROLYTE BALANCE

Chemical compounds in solution behave in one of two ways—they either separate and combine with other compounds or remain intact. One group of compounds remains intact; these are called nonelectrolytes (e.g., urea, dextrose, and creatinine). These compounds do not separate from their complex form when added to a solution. The second group of compounds—electrolytes—dissociate or separate in solution. These compounds break up into separate particles known as ions in a process called ionization. The major electrolytes in the body fluid include sodium, potassium, calcium, magnesium, chloride, phosphorous, and bicarbonate.

Ions, which are the dissociated particles of an electrolyte, each carry an electrical charge, either positive or negative. Negative ions are called anions, and positive ions are called cations (Table 4–1).

Electrolytes are active chemicals that unite. The ions are expressed in terms of milliequivalents (mEq) per liter rather than milligrams (mg). A milliequivalent measures chemical activity or combining power rather than weight. For example, when a hostess creates a guest list for a party, she does not invite 1000 pounds of boys per 1000 pounds of girls; she invites the same number of boys and girls. The total cations and anions in a given compartment is equal. There are 154 mEq of anions and 154 mEq of cations in the plasma. Each water compartment of the body contains electrolytes. The concentration and composition of electrolytes vary from compartment to compartment. See Table 4–2 for a diagrammatic comparison of electrolyte composition in the fluid compartments.

The electrolyte content of intracellular fluid (ICF) differs from that of extracellular fluid (ECF). Usually only *ECF* plasma electrolytes are measured because of the special techniques required to measure the concentration of electrolytes in the ICF. The serum plasma levels of electrolytes are important in the assessment and management of patients with electrolyte imbalances.

ELECTROLYTES: FUNCTION, DEFICIT, EXCESS, AND TREATMENT

Sodium

Normal reference value: 135 to 145 mEq/liter

TABLE 4–1. **POSITIVE AND NEGATIVE IONS IN BODY FLUIDS**

Cations	Anions
Sodium (Na^+)	Chloride (Cl^-)
Potassium (K^+)	Phosphate (HPO_4^{--})
Calcium (Ca^{++})	Bicarbonate (HCO_3^-) (Also SO_4^{--}, proteinates, and
Magnesium (Mg^{++})	organic acids)

TABLE 4–2. COMPARISON OF ELECTROLYTE COMPOSITION IN FLUID COMPARTMENTS

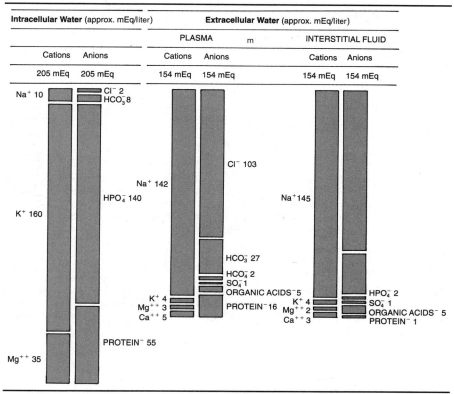

Intracellular Water (approx. mEq/liter)		Extracellular Water (approx. mEq/liter)			
		PLASMA	m	INTERSTITIAL FLUID	
Cations	Anions	Cations	Anions	Cations	Anions
205 mEq	205 mEq	154 mEq	154 mEq	154 mEq	154 mEq

Intracellular:
Na⁺ 10 — Cl⁻ 2, HCO₃⁻ 8
K⁺ 160 — HPO₄⁻ 140
Mg⁺⁺ 35 — PROTEIN⁻ 55

Plasma:
Na⁺ 142 — Cl⁻ 103, HCO₃⁻ 27, HCO₄⁻ 2, SO₄⁻ 1, ORGANIC ACIDS⁻ 5, PROTEIN⁻ 16
K⁺ 4, Mg⁺⁺ 3, Ca⁺⁺ 5

Interstitial Fluid:
Na⁺ 145 — HPO₄⁻ 2, SO₄⁻ 1, ORGANIC ACIDS⁻ 5, PROTEIN⁻ 1
K⁺ 4, Mg⁺⁺ 2, Ca⁺⁺ 3

Function

The major function of sodium is to maintain ECF volume. Extracellular sodium level has an effect on the cellular fluid volume based on the principle of osmosis. Sodium represents about 90% of all the extracellular cations. Sodium does not easily cross the cell wall membrane and is therefore the most abundant cation of ECF. The major roles of sodium include:

1. Maintenance of ECF volume
2. Transmission of impulses in nerve and muscle fibers
3. Regulation of acid-base when sodium combines with chloride or bicarbonate
4. Control of ICF volume

A low serum sodium level results in dilute ECF, therefore allowing water to be drawn into the cells (lower to higher concentration). Conversely if the serum sodium is high, water is drawn out of the cells leading to cellular dehydration. See Figure 4–1 for the relationship between sodium and cellular fluid. The normal daily requirement for sodium in adults is approximately 100 mEq.

77

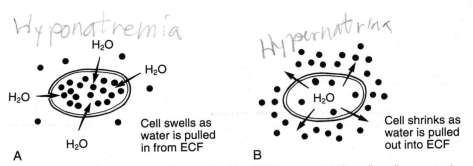

Hyponatremia

Hypernatremia

A

Cell swells as water is pulled in from ECF

B

Cell shrinks as water is pulled out into ECF

Figure 4–1. Sodium and cellular fluid relationship. (*A*) Hyponatremia. The cell swells as water is pulled in from the extracellular fluid (ECF). (*B*) Hypernatremia. The cell shrinks as water is pulled out into the ECF.

The kidneys are extremely important in the regulation of sodium. This regulation is primarily accomplished through the action of the hormone, aldosterone. Hyponatremia is a common complication of adrenal insufficiency because of aldosterone and cortisol deficiencies. The elderly have a slower rate of aldosterone secretion, which places them at risk for sodium imbalances.

Serum Sodium Deficit: Hyponatremia

Hyponatremia refers to a condition in which the sodium level is below normal—less than 135 mEq/liter. Low sodium can be the result of an excessive loss of sodium or an excessive gain of water; in either event, hyponatremia is due to a relatively greater concentration of water than of sodium.

Etiology

All gastrointestinal secretions contain sodium; therefore, any abnormal loss of gastrointestinal secretions can cause a sodium deficit. Excessive sweating, combined with excessive water consumption, use of thiazide diuretics (especially dangerous with low-salt diets), and adrenal insufficiency (aldosterone deficiency) also cause sodium loss.

Excessive use of I.V. dextrose and water solution, compulsive water drinking (psychogenic polydipsia), labor induction with oxytocin, and syndrome of inappropriate antidiuretic syndrome (SIADH) cause the amount of sodium per volume to be reduced, in turn causing a dilutional hyponatremia. Oxytocin has been shown to have an intrinsic antidiuretic hormone effect, acting to increase water reabsorption from the glomerular filtrate (Metheny, 1996).

✎ **NOTE:** "The syndrome of inappropriate SIADH has progressed from a rare occurrence to the most common cause of hyponatremia seen in a general hospital" (Anderson, Chung, & Kluge, 1985). SIADH occurs in patients with inflammatory disorders such as pneumonias, tuberculosis, abscess; oat cell cancer of the lung; and central nervous system (CNS) disorders such as meningitis, trauma, stroke, and degenerative disease (Metheny, 1996).

Chemical agents may also impair renal water excretion, therefore leading to sodium deficit. Pharmacologic agents that contribute to sodium deficit include: nicotine, diabinase, cytoxan, morphine, barbiturates, and acetaminophen.

78

Signs and Symptoms

Patients with chronic hyponatremia may experience impaired sensation of taste, anorexia, muscle cramps, feeling of exhaustion, apprehension: feeling of impending doom (with Na+ <115), and focal weaknesses: hemiparesis, ataxia.

✎ **NOTE:** Dehydration and chronic hyponatremia can lead to confusional states that interfere with fluid intake in the elderly. The elderly are very susceptible to dehydration (Rolls & Phillips, 1990).

Patients with acute hyponatremia due to water overload experience the same symptoms as well as fingerprint edema (sign of intracellular water excess) and specific gravity of 1.002 to 1.004.

Diagnostic Tests

Serum sodium—Less than 135 mEq/liter
Serum osmolarity—Less than 280 mOsm/liter
Urine specific gravity—Less than 1.004
Urine sodium—Decreased (usually less than 20 mEq/liter)

Treatment

Treatment of hyponatremia aims to provide sodium by the dietary, enteral, or parenteral route. Patients able to eat and drink can easily replace sodium by normal diet. Those unable to take sodium orally must take the electrolyte by the parenteral route. An isotonic saline or Ringer's solution may be ordered, such as 0.9% sodium chloride (NaCl), or lactated Ringer's solution.

✎ **NOTE:** When the primary problem is water retention, it is safer to restrict water than to administer sodium. An I.V. solution that can contribute to hyponatremia is excessive administration of 5% dextrose in water.

Generally, treatment guidelines for hyponatremia are:

1. Replace sodium and fluid losses through diet or parenteral fluids. (If serum sodium level is lower than 125 mEq/liter, it is important to quickly bring the level up to more than 125 mEq/liter, then gradually continue to return sodium to a normal level.)
2. Restore normal ECF volume.
3. Correct any other electrolyte losses such as potassium or bicarbonate.

Serum Sodium Excess: Hypernatremia

The serum level of sodium is elevated to above 145 mEq/liter in hypernatremia. This elevation can be caused by a gain of sodium without water or a loss of water without loss of sodium.

Etiology

Increased levels of serum sodium can occur with deprivation of water, occurring when a person cannot respond to thirst; during hypertonic tube feeding with inadequate water supplements; with excessive parenteral administration of sodium-containing solutions; and when drowning in sea water. Sodium is lost with watery diarrhea (a particular problem in infants), increased insensible loss; ingestion of sodium

79

in unusual amounts, profuse sweating; heatstroke, and diabetes insipidus when water intake is inadequate.

Signs and Symptoms

Patients with hypernatermia may experience thirst, elevated body temperature, swollen tongue and red, dry, sticky mucous membranes, severe hypernatremia, disorientation, irritability or hyperactivity when stimulated.

Diagnostic Tests

Serum sodium—Greater than 145 mEq/liter
Serum osmolarity—Greater than 295 mOsm/kg
Urine specific gravity—Greater than 1.015 (except for diabetes insipidus)
Dehydration test—Water is withheld for 16 to 18 hours. Serum and urine osmolarity are checked 1 hour after administration of antidiuretic hormone (ADH). This test is used to identify the cause of polyuric syndromes (central versus nephrogenic diabetes insipidus)

Treatment

The goal of treatment of hypernatremia is to *gradually* lower the serum sodium level, infusing a hypotonic electrolyte solution such as 0.45% normal saline or 5% dextrose in water. Gradual reduction is necessary to decrease the risk of cerebral edema. The sodium level should not be lowered more than 15 mEq/liter in an 8-hour period of time for adults (Weldy, 1996).

Generally, treatment guidelines for hypernatremia are:

1. Infusion of an isotonic solution (0.9% NaCl) or hypotonic electrolyte solution (0.45% NaCl or 5% dextrose in water).
2. Sodium levels can also be decreased by use of diuretics, which induce excretion of water and sodium.

✎ **NOTE:** Patients who are debilitated need to have fluids offered at regular intervals. The literature states that hypodermoclysis via infusion is a short-term method of aiding the elderly to reduce sodium levels (Berger, 1984).

Potassium

Normal reference value: 3.5 to 5.5 mEq/liter

Function

Potassium is an intracellular electrolyte with 98% in the ICF and 2% in the ECF. Potassium is a dynamic electrolyte. Cellular potassium will replace ECF potassium if it becomes depleted. Potassium is acquired through diet and must be ingested daily because the body has no effective method of storage. The daily requirement is 40 mEq. Potassium influences both skeletal and cardiac muscle activity. Alterations in the concentration of plasma potassium changes myocardial irritability and rhythm. Potassium moves easily into the intracellular space when glucose is being metabolized by the body. It moves out of the cells during strenuous exercise, when cellular metabolism is impaired or when the cell dies. Potassium, along with sodium, is responsible for transmission of nerve impulses. During nerve cell innervation, these ions exchange places, creating an electrical current (Metheny, 1996).

There is a relationship between acid-base imbalance and potassium balance. Hypokalemia can cause alkalosis, which in turn can further decrease serum potassium. Hyperkalemia can cause acidosis, which in turn can further increase serum potassium.

The regulation of potassium is related to several other processes, including:

- Sodium level—Enough sodium must be available for exchange with potassium.
- Hydrogen ion excretion—When there is an increase in hydrogen ion excretion, there is a decrease in potassium excretion.
- Aldosterone level—An increased level of aldosterone stimulates and increases excretion of potassium.

Serum Potassium Deficit: Hypokalemia

Hypokalemia refers to a serum potassium level below 3.5 mEq/liter. It usually reflects a real deficit in total potassium stores; however, it may occur in patients with normal potassium stores when alkalosis is present. Hypokalemia is a common disturbance; many factors are associated with this deficit, and many clinical conditions contribute to it.

Etiology

Many conditions can lead to potassium deficit including gastrointestinal and renal loss, increased use of increased perspiration, shifting of extracellular potassium into the cells, and poor dietary intake.

Gastrointestinal loss includes diarrhea or laxative overuse, prolonged gastric suction, and protracted vomiting.

Renal loss includes diuretic therapy, excessive use of glucocorticoids, ingestion of drugs such as sodium penicillin, carbenicillin, or amphotericin B, and excessive ingestion of European licorice.

Sweat loss includes heavy perspiration in persons acclimated to the heat.

Shifting into the cells can occur with total parenteral nutrition therapy without adequate potassium supplementation, alkalosis, and excessive administration of insulin.

Poor dietary intake can occur with anorexia nervosa, bulimia, and alcoholism.

Signs and Symptoms

Patients with hypokalemia may experience neuromuscular changes such as fatigue, muscle weakness, diminished deep tendon reflexes and flaccid paralysis (late). Other symptoms include anorexia, nausea, vomiting; irritability (early); increased sensitivity to digitalis; ECG changes; and death (in severe hypokalemia) due to cardiac arrest.

Diagnostic Tests

Serum potassium—less than 3.5 mEq/liter

Arterial blood gas (ABG)—May show metabolic alkalosis (increased pH and bicarbonate ion)

ECG—ST-segment depression, flattened T wave, presence of U wave, and ventricular dysrhythmias (Figure 4–2).

✎ **NOTE:** Clinical signs and symptoms rarely occur before the serum potassium level has fallen below 3 mEq/liter.

81

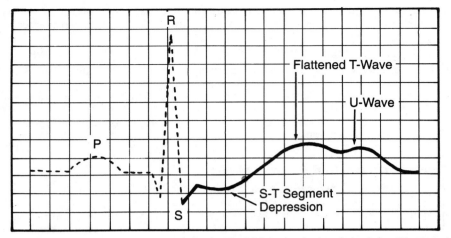

Figure 4–2. Sample ECG tracing: Hypokalemia. The ECG tracing for hypokalemia has ST-segment depression, flattened T wave, and the presence of a U wave.

Treatment

Replacement of potassium is the key concept in treatment of potassium deficit. General treatment guidelines include:

1. Mild hypokalemia is usually treated with dietary increases of potassium or oral supplements.
2. Salt substitutes contain potassium and can be used to supplement potassium intake (Morton Salt Substitute, Co-Salt, Adolph's Salt Substitute).
3. If the serum potassium is below 2 mEq/liter, monitor the patient's ECG and administer potassium by means of a secondary piggyback set in a volume of 100 mL (Metheny, 1996).

See Table 4–3 for critical guidelines for nursing in I.V. administration of potassium.

✎ **NOTE:** Potassium replacement must take place slowly to prevent hyperkalemia. Extreme caution should be used when potassium chloride replacement exceeds 120 mEq in 24 hours. The patient must be monitored for dysrhythmias.

Serum Potassium Excess: Hyperkalemia

Hyperkalemia occurs less frequently than hypokalemia, but it can be more dangerous for the patient. It seldom occurs in patients who have normal renal function. Hyperkalemia is defined as a serum plasma level of potassium above 5.5 mEq/liter. The main causes of hyperkalemia are (1) increased intake of potassium (oral or parenteral), (2) decreased urinary excretion of potassium, and (3) movement of potassium out of the cells and into the extracellular space.

Etiology

High levels of serum potassium can be caused by excessive administration of potassium parenterally or orally; severe renal failure resulting in reduced potassium excretion; release of potassium from damaged cells, such as with burns or crush

TABLE 4–3. **CRITICAL GUIDELINES FOR ADMINISTRATION OF POTASSIUM**

Guidelines for Administration of Potassium
1. **Never give a potassium I.V. push.**
2. Potassium chloride (KCl) should be added to a nondextrose solution such as isotonic saline to treat severe hypokalemia because administration of KCl in a dextrose solution may cause a small reduction in the serum potassium level.
3. Never administer concentrated potassium solutions without first diluting them as directed.
4. KCl concentrations greater than 60 mEq/liter **should not** be given in a peripheral vein. Concentrations greater than 8 mEq/100 mL can cause pain and irritation of peripheral veins and lead to postinfusion phlebitis (Rapp, 1987).
5. When adding KCl to infusion solutions, especially plastic systems, make sure the KCl mixes with the solution thoroughly. Invert and agitate the container to ensure mixing. *Do not add KCl to a hanging container!*
6. For patients with any degree of renal insufficiency or heart block, Zull (1989) recommends reducing the infusion by 50%. For example: 5 to 10 mEq/hr rather than 10 to 20 mEq/hr.
7. Administer potassium at a rate not to exceed 10 mEq/hr through peripheral veins. (Kokko, J., & Tannen R., 1990; Gahart, 1994).
8. For extreme hypokalemia, rates should be no more than 40 mEq/hr while constantly monitoring ECG (Kokko, J., & Tannen, 1990).
9. If KCl is administered into the subcutaneous tissue (infiltration), it is extremely irritating and can cause serious tissue loss. Use extravasation protocol in this situation.

injuries; and acidosis. Pseudohyperkalemia can occur with prolonged tourniquet application during blood withdrawal.

Signs and Symptoms

Patients with hyperkalemia may experience EEG changes, vague muscle weakness, flaccid paralysis, anxiety, nausea, cramping, and diarrhea.

Diagnostic Tests

Serum potassium—Greater than 5.5 mEq/liter
ABG values—Metabolic acidosis (decreased pH and bicarbonate ion)
ECG—Widened QRS, prolonged PR, and ventricular dysrhythmias (Fig. 4–3).

Treatment

The following are guidelines for the treatment of hyperkalemia:

1. Restrict dietary potassium in mild cases.
2. Discontinue supplements of potassium.
3. Administer I.V. calcium gluconate if necessary for cardiac symptoms.
4. Administer I.V. sodium bicarbonate, which alkalinizes the plasma and cause a temporary shift of potassium into the cells.
5. Administer regular insulin (10 to 25 U) and hypertonic dextrose (10%), which causes a shift of potassium into the cells.
6. Peritoneal dialysis or hemodialysis may be ordered.

See Table 4–4 for critical guidelines for nursing in treatment of potassium excess.

83

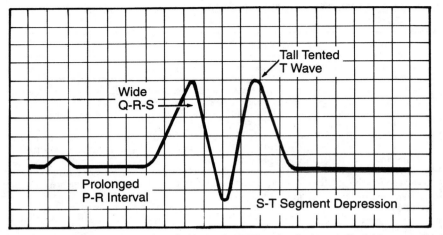

Figure 4–3. Sample ECG tracing: hyperkalemia. The ECG tracing for hyperkalemia shows progressive changes: tall, thin T waves; prolonged PR intervals; ST-segment depression; widened QRS; and loss of P wave. Eventually QRS becomes widened.

TABLE 4–4. **CRITICAL GUIDELINES FOR REMOVAL OF POTASSIUM**

Treatment Guidelines

1. **Sodium polystyrene sulfonate** is a cation exchange resin that removes potassium from the body by exchanging sodium for potassium in the intestinal tract. This method should not be the sole treatment for severe hyperkalemia because of its slow onset.
     Oral sodium polystyrene sulfonate (15–30 g): May repeat every 4–6 hours as needed; removes potassium in 1–2 hours.
     Rectal sodium polystyrene sulfonate (50 g) as retention enema: When administered, use an inflated rectal catheter to ensure retention of the dissolved resin for 30–60 minutes; removes potassium in 30–60 minutes. Each enema can lower the plasma potassium concentration by 0.5–1.0 mEq/liter (Rose, 1989).
2. **Dialysis** is used when more aggressive methods are needed. Peritoneal dialysis is not as effective as hemodialysis. Peritoneal dialysis can remove approximately 10–15 mEq/hr, whereas hemodialysis can remove 25–30 mEq/hr. (Kokko, & Tannen, 1990).
3. **Glucose and insulin**
     Insulin facilitates potassium movement into the cells, reducing the plasma potassium level. Glucose administration in nondiabetic patients may cause a marked increase in insulin release from the pancreas, producing desired plasma potassium-lowering effects (Rose, 1989).
     500 mL of 10% dextrose with 15–20 u of regular insulin over 1 hour; the potassium-lowering effects are delayed about 30 minutes, but are effective for 4–6 hours (Zull, 1989).
4. **Emergency measures**
     Calcium gluconate: 10 mL of 10% calcium gluconate administered slowly over 2–3 minutes. Administer only to patient who needs immediate myocardial protection against toxic effects of severe hyperkalemia. Protective effect begins within 1–2 minutes and lasts only 30–60 minutes. (Spital, 1989).
     Sodium bicarbonate: 45 mEq (1 ampule of 7.5% sodium bicarbonate) infused slowly over 5 minutes. This temporarily shifts potassium into the cells, and is helpful in patients with metabolic acidosis.

Calcium

Normal reference value: 8.5 to 10.5 mg/dL

Functions

The calcium ion is most abundant in the skeletal system, with 99% residing in the bone and teeth. Only 1% is available for rapid exchange in the circulating blood bound to protein. The parathyroid hormone (PTH) is responsible for transfer of calcium from the bone to plasma. PTH also augments the intestinal absorption of calcium and enhances net renal calcium reabsorption. Calcium is acquired through dietary intake. Adults require approximately 1 g of calcium daily, along with vitamin D and protein, which are required for absorption and utilization of this electrolyte.

Calcium is instrumental in activating enzymes and stimulating essential chemical reactions. It plays an important role in maintaining normal transmission of nerve impulses and has a sedative effect on nerve cells. Calcium plays its most important role in the conversion of prothrombin to thrombin, a necessary sequence in the formation of a clot.

Calcium and phosphate have a reciprocal relationship; that is, a rise in calcium level causes a drop in the serum phosphorus concentration, and a drop in calcium causes a rise in phosphorus.

Calcium is present in three different forms in the plasma: (1) ionized (50% of total calcium), (2) bound (less than 50% of total calcium), and (3) complexed (small percentage that combines with phosphate)

Only ionized calcium (calcium that is affected by plasma pH, phosphorus, and albumin levels) is physiologically important. A relationship between ionized calcium and plasma pH is reciprocal; an increase in pH decreases the percentage of calcium that is ionized. The relationship between plasma phosphorus and ionized calcium is also reciprocal. Albumin does not affect ionized calcium, but it does affect the amount of calcium bound to proteins.

Serum Calcium Deficit: Hypocalcemia

Hypocalcemia is caused by a reduction of total body calcium levels or a reduction of the percentage of ionized calcium.

Etiology

Total calcium levels may be decreased because of increased calcium loss, reduced intake secondary to altered intestinal absorption, and altered regulation, as in hypoparathyroidism.

The most common cause of hypocalcemia is inadequate secretion of PTH caused by primary hypoparathyroidism or surgically induced hypoparathyroidism. It can also result from calcium loss through diarrhea and wound exudate, acute pancreatitis, hyperphosphatemia usually associated with renal failure, inadequate intake of vitamin D or minimal sun exposure, prolonged nasogastric tube suctioning resulting in metabolic alkalosis, and infusion of citrated blood (citrate-phosphate-dextrose).

Patients on potent loop diuretics and digoxin are predisposed to hypocalcemia and hypermagnesemia.

Signs and Symptoms

Patients with hypocalcemia may experience neuromuscular symptoms such as numbness of the fingers, cramps in the muscles (especially the extremities), hyper-

85

active deep tendon reflexes, and a positive Trousseau's sign (see Fig. 4–4) and Chvostek's sign. (see Fig. 4–5)

Other symptoms include irritability, memory impairment, delusions, seizures (late), prolonged QT interval, and altered cardiovascular hemodynamics that may precipitate congestive heart failure. In patients with hypocalcemia due to citrated blood transfusion, the cardiac index, stroke volume, and left ventricular stroke work values have been found to be lower.

The most dangerous symptom associated with hypocalcemia is the development of laryngospasm and tetany-like contractions. A low magnesium level and a high potassium level potentiate the cardiac and neuromuscular irritability produced by a low calcium level. However, a low potassium level can protect the patient from hypocalcemic tetany (McFadden, Zaloga, & Chernow, 1983).

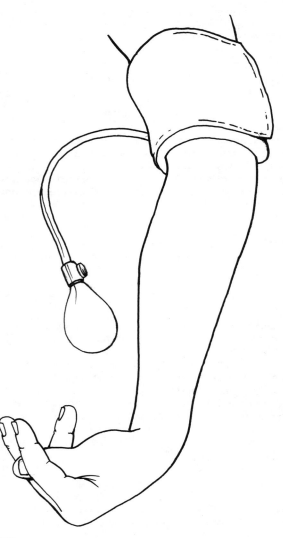

Figure 4–4. Positive Trousseau's sign. Carpopedal attitude of the hand when blood pressure cuff is placed on the arm and inflated above systolic pressure for 3 minutes. A positive reaction is the development of carpal spasm.

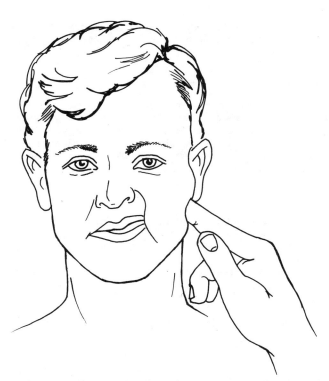

Figure 4–5. Positive Chvostek's sign, which occurs after tapping the facial nerve approximately 2 cm anterior to the earlobe. Unilateral twitching of the facial muscle occurs in some patients with hypocalcemia or hypomagnesemia.

Treatment

Treatment of hypocalcemia consists of administration of calcium gluconate, either orally (preferred) with calcium supplements, 1000 mg/day, to raise the total serum calcium level by 1 mg/dL (Clutter, 1993), or intravenously, 10 to 20 mL of a 10% solution in 5% dextrose in water over 20 minutes (Clutter, 1993).

Serum Calcium Excess: Hypercalcemia

Hypercalcemia can be very dangerous, with a 50% mortality rate, if untreated. Patients with hypercalcemia have one of the following three conditions: malignancy, hyperparathyroidism, or thiazide-diuretic use (Olinger, 1989).

Etiology

Most symptoms of hypercalcemia are present only when serum calcium is greater than 12 mg/dL and tend to be more severe if hypercalcemia develops quickly (Clutter, 1993). Causes of hypercalcemia include hyperparathyroidism, Paget's disease, multiple fractures, thiazide diuretics, and overuse of calcium-containing antacids. Patients with solid tumors that have metastasis, such as breast, prostate, and malignant melanomas, and hematologic tumors, such as lymphomas, acute leukemia,

87

and myelomas, are also at risk for developing hypercalcemia. Hypercalcemia is associated with use of certain chemotherapeutic regimens such as androgens and estrogens.

Signs and Symptoms

Patients with hypercalcemia may experience neuromuscular symptoms such as muscle weakness, incoordination, lethargy, deep bony pain, flank pain, pathologic fractures (due to bone weakening). Other symptoms include constipation, anorexia, nausea, vomiting, polyuria or polydipsia, leading to uremia if not treated, and renal colic caused by stone formation. Patients receiving digitalis must receive calcium with extreme care because it can precipitate severe dysrhythmias.

Diagnostic Tests

Total serum calcium—May be more than 10.5 mg/dL
Serum ionized calcium—5.5 mg/dL
Serum parathyroid hormone—Increased levels in primary or secondary hyperparathryoidism
X-rays—may reveal osteoporosis, bone cavitation, or urinary calculi

Treatment

Hypercalcemia should be treated according to the following guidelines:

1. Treat the underlying disease.
2. Saline diuresis: Fluids should be forced to help eliminate the source of the hypercalcemia. A solution of 0.45% NaCl or 0.9% NaCl I.V. dilutes the serum calcium level. Rehydration is important to dilute the Ca^+ ion and promote renal excretion.
3. Inorganic phosphate salts can be given orally (Neutra-Phos) or rectally (Fleet Enema).
4. Hemodialysis or peritoneal dialysis should be carried out to reduce serum calcium levels in life-threatening situations.
5. Furosemide, 20 to 40 mg every 2 hours, may be used to prevent volume overloading during saline administration.
6. Calcitonin, 4 to 8 U/kg intramuscularly or subcutaneous every 6 to 12 hours, will temporarily lower the serum calcium level by 1 to 3 mg/100 mL.
7. Biphosphonates inhibit bone resorption: Pamidronate is effective, 60 to 90 mg in 1 liter of 0.9% NaCl or 5% dextrose in water is infused over 24 hours.
8. Plicamycin (Mithramycin) inhibits bone resorption and reliably lowers serum calcium. It is used only in malignant hypercalcemia because of its toxicity. A single dose of 25 μg/kg in 500 mL of 5% dextrose in water is infused intravenously over 4 to 6 hours (Clutter 1993).

Magnesium

Normal reference value: 1.5 to 2.5 mEq/liter

Function

Magnesium is a major intracellular electrolyte. The normal diet supplies approximately 25 mEq of magnesium. Approximately one third of serum magnesium is bound to protein; the remaining two thirds exists as free cations. The same factors that regulate calcium balance have an influence on magnesium balance. Magnesium balance is also affected by many of the same agents that decrease or influence potassium balance.

Magnesium acts directly on the myoneural junction and affects neuromuscular irritability and contractility, possibly exerting a sedative effect. Magnesium acts as an activator for many enzymes and plays a role in both carbohydrate and protein metabolism. Magnesium affects the cardiovascular system, acting peripherally to produce vasodilation. Imbalances in magnesium predispose the heart to ventricular dysrhythmias (Metheny, 1996).

Serum Magnesium Deficit: Hypomagnesemia

Hypomagnesemia is an often overlooked problem in critically ill patients. This imbalance is considered to be one of the most underdiagnosed electrolyte deficiencies (Metheny, 1996). Symptoms of hypomagnesemia tend to occur when the serum level drops below 1 mEq/liter.

Etiology

Hypomagnesemia can result from chronic alcoholism; malabsorption syndrome, especially if the small bowel is affected; prolonged malnutrition or starvation; prolonged diarrhea; acute pancreatitis; administration of magnesium-free solutions for longer than 1 week; and prolonged nasogastric tube suctioning. Use of certain drugs, such as aminogylosides, diuretics, and cisplatin, and infusion of collected blood preserved with citrate can also cause hypomagnesemia (McFadden, Zaloga, & Chernow, 1983).

Signs and Symptoms

Patients with hypomagnesemia often experience neuromuscular symptoms such as hyperactive reflexes, coarse tremors, muscle cramps, positive Chvostek's and Trousseau's signs (see Figs. 4–4 and 4–5), seizures, paresthesia of the feet and legs, and painfully cold hands and feet. Other symptoms include disorientation, dysrhythmias, tachycardia, and increased potential for digitalis toxicity.

Diagnostic Tests

Serum magnesium—< 1.5 mEq/liter
Urine magnesium—Helps to identify renal causes of magnesium depletion.
Serum albumin—A decrease may cause a decreased magnesium level resulting from the reduction in protein-bound magnesium.
Serum potassium—Decreased because of failure of the cellular sodium-potassium pump to move potassium into the cell and because of the accompanying loss of potassium in the urine.
Serum calcium—May be reduced because of a reduction in the release and action of PTH.
ECG—Findings of tachydysrhythmias, prolonged PR and QT intervals, widening of the QRS, ST-segment depression, and flattened T waves. A form of ventricular tachycardia (torsades de pointes) associated with all three electrolyte imbalances (magnesium, calcium, and potassium) may develop.

TABLE 4–5. CRITICAL GUIDELINES FOR ADMINISTRATION OF MAGNESIUM

1. Double check the order for magnesium administration to ensure that it stipulates the concentration of the solution to be used. Do not accept orders for "amps" or "vials" without further clarification.
2. Use caution in patients with impaired renal function; watch urine output.
3. Reduce other CNS depressants when given concurrently with magnesium preparations.
4. Therapeutic doses of magnesium can produce flushing and sweating and occur most often if the administration rate is too fast.
5. Closely assess the patient receiving magnesium.

Treatment

Treatment of hypomagnesemia can include:

1. Administer oral magnesium salts.
2. Administer 40 mEq (5 g) magnesium sulfate added intravenously to 1 liter of 5% dextrose in water or 5% dextrose/NaCl.
3. Administer 1 to 2 g of 10% solution of magnesium sulfate by direct I.V. push at a rate of 1.5 mL/min (Phillips & Kuhn, 1996).

See Table 4–5 for critical guidelines for nurses administering magnesium.

✎ **NOTE:** Be aware that other CNS depressants could cause further depressed sensorium when magnesium sulfate is being administered. Therefore, be prepared to deal with respiratory arrest if hypermagnesemia inadvertently occurs during administration of magnesium sulfate.

Serum Magnesium Excess: Hypermagnesemia

Hypermagnesemia occurs when a person's serum level is greater than 2.5 mEq/liter. The most common cause of hypermagnesemia is renal failure in patients who have an increased intake of magnesium.

Etiology

Hypermagnesemia can result from renal failure, Addison's disease, hyperparathyroidism, and hyperthyroidism. Excessive magnesium administration during treatment of eclampsia, hemodialysis with excessively hard water with a dialysate inadvertently high in magnesium or ingestion of medications high in magnesium, such as antacids and laxatives, are iatrogenic causes of hypermagnesemia.

Signs and Symptoms

Patients with hypermagnesemia may experience neuromuscular symptoms such as flushing and sense of skin warmth, lethargy, sedation, hypoactive deep tendon reflexes, depressed respirations, and weak or absent cry in newborn. Other symptoms include hypotension, sinus bradycardia, heart block, and cardiac arrest (diastole serum level > 15 mEq/liter) at increased susceptibility to digitalis toxicity, nausea, vomiting, and seizures.

Diagnostic Tests

Serum magnesium—Greater than 2.5 mEq/liter
ECG—Findings of QT interval and atrioventricular block may occur (at levels greater than 12 mEq/liter) (Horne & Swearingen, 1993).

Treatment

Guidelines for treatment of hypermagnesemia are:

1. Decrease oral magnesium intake.
2. Administer calcium gluconate to antagonize the action of magnesium.
3. Support respiratory function.
4. Order peritoneal or hemodialysis in severe cases of hypermagnesemia.

Phosphorus

Normal reference value: 3.0 to 4.5 mg/dL

Function

Approximately 80% of phosphorus in the body is contained in the bones and teeth, and 20% is abundant in the ICF. The PTH plays a major role in homeostasis of phosphate because of its ability to vary phosphate reabsorption in the proximal tubule of the kidney. PTH also allows for the shift of phosphate from bone to plasma.

Phosphorus plays an important role in delivery of oxygen to tissues by regulating the level of 2,3-diphosphoglycerate (2,3-DPG), a substance in red cells that decreases the affinity of hemoglobin for oxygen.

Because phosphorus and calcium have a reciprocal relationship, an increase in the phosphorus level frequently causes hypocalcemia.

Serum Phosphate Deficit: Hypophosphatemia

Phosphorus is a critical constituent of all the body's tissues. Hypophosphatemia occurs when the serum level is below the lower limit of normal (less than 2.5 mg/dL). This imbalance may occur in the presence of total body phosphate deficit or may merely reflect a temporary shift of phosphorus into the cells.

Etiology

Hypophosphatemia can result from total parenteral nutrition administered without adequate phosphorus, malabsorption syndromes, alcohol withdrawal, prolonged respiratory alkalosis, and hyperparathyroidism. Treatment of diabetic ketoacidosis and overuse of phosphate-binding antacid gels, such as Amphojel and Basaljel, can also precipitate hypophosphatemia.

Signs and Symptoms

Hypophosphatemia can affect the CNS, the neuromuscular and cardiac status, and the blood. The patient may experience disorientation, confusion, seizures, paresthesia (early), profound muscle weakness, tremor, ataxia, incoordination, dysarthria, dysphagia and congestive cardiomyopathy. Hypophosphatemia affects all blood cells, especially red cells. It causes a decline in 2,3-DPG levels in erythrocytes. 2,3-DPG in red cells normally interacts with hemoglobin to promote the release of oxygen. With reduced 2,3-DPG, oxygen delivery to peripheral tissues is impaired.

Diagnostic Tests

Serum phosphorus—Less than 2.5 mg/dL (1.7 mEq/liter)
Serum PTH—Elevated

91

Serum magnesium—Decreased because of increased urinary excretion of magnesium

Serum alkaline phosphate—Increased with increased osteoblastic activity

X-rays—Skeletal changes of osteomalacia or rickets

Treatment

Treatment should include the folowing regimen:

1. For mild to moderate deficiency, oral phosphate supplements, such as Neutra-Phos or Phospho-Soda, can be administered.
2. For severe hypophosphatemia, administer I.V. phosphorus solutions in severe deficiency.

✎ **NOTE:** In treating be aware that calcium levels should be monitored closely (Horne & Swearingen, 1993).

Serum Phosphate Excess: Hyperphosphatemia

A variety of conditions can lead to hyperphosphatemia, but the major disorder is renal disease.

Etiology

Hyperphosphatemia can result from renal insufficiency, hypoparathyroidism, or increased catabolism. It is also seen in cancer states such as myelogenous leukemia and lymphoma.

Signs and Symptoms

Patients with hyperphosphatemia may experience many symptoms including hypocalcemia, tetany (short-term); soft tissue calcification (long-term); mental changes such as apprehension, confusion, coma; and increased 2,3-DPG in red blood cells.

Diagnostic Tests

Serum phosphorus—Greater than 4.5 mg/dL (2.6 mEq/liter)

Serum calcium—Useful in assessing potential consequences of treatment

Serum PTH—Decreased in hypoparathyroidism

Blood urea nitrogen—Assess renal function

X-rays—Skeletal changes of osteodystrophy

Treatment

Treatment should include the following regimen.

1. Identify the underlying cause of hyperphosphatemia.
2. Restrict dietary intake.
3. Administer phosphate-binding gels (e.g., Amphojel, Basaljel, or Dialume).

Chloride

Normal reference value: 95 to 108 mEq/liter

Functions

Chloride (Cl^-) is the major anion in the ECF. Changes in serum Cl^- concentration are usually secondary to changes in one or more of the other electrolytes. Cl^- has a reciprocal relationship with bicarbonate (HCO_3^-). For example, a drop in HCO_3^- concentrations results in a reciprocal rise in Cl^-; when Cl^- decreases, HCO_3^- will increase in compensation. Cl^- exists primarily combined as sodium chloride (NaCl) or hydrochloric acid (HCl). Measurement of serum Cl^- is most frequently done for its inferential value.

Reabsorption of Cl^- by the renal tubules is one of the major regulatory functions of the kidneys. As NaCl is reabsorbed, water follows through osmosis. It is through this function that vascular blood volume is maintained.

Cl^- plays its most important role in acid-base balance. Its role in the pH balance of the ECF is referred to as the "chloride shift". The Cl^- shift is an ionic exchange that occurs within red blood cells. This shift preserves the electrical neutrality of the red blood cells and maintains a $1:20$ ratio of carbonic acid and HCO_3^- that is essential for pH balance of the plasma.

Serum Chloride Deficit: Hypochloremia

Loss of Cl^- ions occurs mainly through gastrointestinal losses and significantly alters acid-base balance because of the reciprocal relationship with HCO_3^-.

Etiology

Hypochloremia results primarily from severe vomiting and diarrhea, pyloric obstruction, acute infection, and use of chlorothiazide diuretics.

Signs and Symptoms

Patients with hypochloremia may experience neuromuscular symptoms such as tetany, and hypertonic reflexes. Other symptoms include depressed respiration and excessive loss of Cl^- resulting in alkalosis owing to an increase in HCO_3.

✎ **NOTE:** A deficiency in chloride reflects a deficiency in potassium. When replacing potassium, use potassium chloride solution.

Diagnostic Tests

Serum chloride—Less than 96 mEq/liter
ABG values—Consistent with alkalosis
ECG—May show dysrhythmias related to associated hyperkalemia

Treatment

The principles of treating patients with hypochloremia are twofold: (1) treat the underlying cause (alkalosis) and (2) administer NaCl solutions.

Serum Chloride Excess: Hyperchloremia

Excessive Cl^- ions result from any condition that causes a decrease in HCO_3^- and can also influence acid-base balance.

Signs and Symptoms

Patients with hyperchloremia may experience symptoms related to acidosis such as drowsiness, lethargy, headache, weakness, tremors, dyspnea, tachypnea, Kussmaul's respirations (with pH less than 7.20), hyperventilation, and dysrhythmias.

Diagnostic Tests

Serum chloride—Greater than 106 mEq/liter
Serum carbon dioxide—Less than 22 mEq/liter when associated with acidosis
Serum pH—Less than 7.35 when associated with metabolic acidosis
ECG—Presence of dysrhythmias

Treatment

Hyperchloremia is treated by (1) treating the underlying cause of acidosis and (2) administering solutions free of NaCl.

Nursing Plan of Care

ELECTROLYTE IMBALANCE

Focus Criteria for Assessment (Table 4–6)

Subjective	*Objective*
History of precipitating illness or disorder	Serum laboratory values consistent with specific electrolyte imbalance
Complaints of weakness, lethargy, and fatigue	Urine specific gravity, pH, and osmolarity consistent with specific electrolyte imbalance
Use of drugs that may cause problem	Neuromuscular, cardiovascular, and neurologic assessment findings consistent with specific electrolyte imbalance

Nursing Diagnoses

Sensory-perceptual alterations secondary to hyponatremia
Altered health maintenance related to poor dietary habits or perceptual or cognitive impairment
Constipation related to weakened peristalsis
Fluid volume deficit related to failure of the regulatory mechanism
Impaired physical mobility related to activity intolerance, decreased strength and endurance, pain, discomfort, neuromuscular impairment, or musculoskeletal impairment related to electrolyte imbalance
Ineffective breathing pattern related to biochemical imbalances
Altered comfort related to injuring agent (e.g., stones associated with excessive calcium)
Risk for injury related to confusion, altered thought processes resulting from electrolyte imbalance, tetany and seizures resulting from severe hypocalcemia, or sensory changes resulting from hypercalcemia
Decreased cardiac output related to electrical disturbances resulting from severe hypokalemia, hypocalcemia, or hypophosphatemia
Impaired gas exchange related to altered oxygen resulting from laryngeal spasm in severe hypokalemia, hyperkalemia, hypocalcemia, or hypophosphatemia
Altered urinary elimination pattern related to changes in renal function resulting from hypercalcemia

Continued on following page

Nursing Diagnoses (continued)

Risk for impaired verbal communication related to confusion, lethargy, or electrolyte imbalance

Outcome Criteria

Patient will:

Be mobile without evidence of weakness, pain, or fractures

Have an adequate cardiac output, blood pressure with normal range, absence of clinical signs of heart failure or cardiac dysrhythmias

Exhibit voiding pattern and urine characteristics with normal range

Have no injury caused by neuromuscular or sensory alterations

Have an effective breathing pattern with normal depth and rate

Nursing Management: Critical Activities

Consult with physician if signs and symptoms of fluid or electrolyte imbalance persist or clinically worsen.

Monitor for abnormalities in serum electrolytes, as indicated.

Monitor ECG for dysrhythmias.

Monitor patient response to electrolyte replacement therapy.

Administer supplemental electrolytes, as indicated.

Monitor for loss of electrolyte-rich body fluids, such as nasogastric suctioning, ileostomy drainage, diarrhea, wound drainage, or diaphoresis.

Closely monitor serum potassium levels in patients taking diuretics with digoxin.

Monitor for side effects of prescribed electrolyte supplements.

Obtain ordered specimens for laboratory analysis of serum and urine electrolytes and ABGs, as indicated.

Maintain I.V. solution containing electrolytes at a constant flow rate.

Provide a safe environment for the patient with neurologic and neuromuscular manifestations of electrolyte imbalances.

Maintain accurate intake and output.

Maintain patent I.V. line.

PATIENT EDUCATION

Provide written material and verbal instructions regarding any medications.

Review indicators of digitalis toxicity, if appropriate.

Provide information on dietary sources of electrolytes in deficit situations when appropriate.

Provide information on over-the-counter medications (e.g., magnesium or aluminum hydroxide, antacids and/or phosphorus-binding antacids, laxatives, multivitamin and mineral supplements) when appropriate.

HOME CARE ISSUES

Patients that might require home electrolyte replacement:

Cardiopulmonary disorders: education regarding potassium replacement. Multiple electrolyte replacement or observation for development of imbalance with fistulas, gastrointestinal disorders, intractable diarrhea, hyperemesis gravidarum, and chemotherapy (before and after therapy).

Therapies last from 1 to 7 days and usually are administered via an indwelling venous access device unless long-term access device is available.

Assess for compliance because patients often discontinue therapy when they feel better.

TABLE 4–6. SUMMARY OF ELECTROLYTE IMBALANCE

Patients at Risk for Electrolyte Imbalance		
Patient Care Units	**Conditions that Can Lead to Imbalance**	**Potential Electrolyte Imbalances**
Geriatric	Prolonged diarrhea Proloned malnutrition Diuretic therapy	FVD Hypernatremia Hypokalemia
Medical	Anorexia nervosa Profuse sweating Overuse of antacids Gastroenteritis Hyperparathyroidism Diabetic ketoacidosis Alcoholism Renal failure SIADH	FVD Hyponatremia Hypomagnesemia Hypocalcemia Hyperkalemia Hypermangesemia Hypokalemia

Surgical	Infections
	Surgical hypoparathyroidism
	Nasogastric suction due to
	   alkalosis
	Postoperative complications
	Pharmacology agents: morphine,
	   penicillin and carbenicillen
	Ileus
		FVD or FVE
		Hypokalemia
		Hypomagnesemia
		Hypocalcemia
		Hypochloremia

Oncology	Myelogenous leukemia Lymphoma Cytoxan Hypertonic tube feeding Neoplastic disease Solid tumors: breast and prostate Malignant melanoma	Hyponatremia Hypercalcemia Hypernatremia Hypermagnesemia
Critical Care	Crushing injuries TPN administration Hypertonic tube feeding Burns Drowning in sea water Head injuries	Hypomagnesemia Hypercalcemia Hypernatremia Hyponatremia Hypophosphatemia Hyperkalemia

FVD = Fluid volume deficit; FVE = fluid volume excess; SIADH = syndrome of inappropriate antidiuretic hormone; TPN = total parenteral nutrition.

SUMMARY WORKSHEET 1: Electrolytes

CATIONS

SODIUM (Na⁺)   **Normal Lab:**

Key Points:

Deficit:

    Etiology   *Signs and Symptoms*

Excess

    Etiology   *Signs and Symptoms*

POTASSIUM (K⁺)   **Normal Lab:**

Key Points:

Deficit:

    Etiology   *Signs and Symptoms*

Excess:

    Etiology   *Signs and Symptoms*

CALCIUM (Ca⁺⁺)   **Normal Lab:**

Key Points:

Deficit:

    Etiology   *Signs and Symptoms*

Excess:

    Etiology   *Signs and Symptoms*

MAGNESIUM (Mg^{++})   **Normal Lab:**

Key Points:

Deficit:

    Etiology   *Signs and Symptoms*

Excess:

    Etiology   *Signs and Symptoms*

ANIONS

CHLORIDE (Cl$^-$)   **Normal Lab:**

Key Points:

Deficit:

    Etiology   *Signs and Symptoms*

Excess:

    Etiology   *Signs and Symptoms*

PHOSPHATE (HPO$_4^-$)   **Normal Lab:**

Key Points:

Deficit:

    Etiology   *Signs and Symptoms*

Excess:

    Etiology   *Signs and Symptoms*

ACID-BASE BALANCE

The regulation of the hydrogen ion concentration of body fluids is actually the key component of acid-base balance. The pH of a fluid reflects the hydrogen ion concentration of that fluid. The normal pH of arterial blood ranges from 7.35 to 7.45.

The inverse proportion of the pH to the concentration of hydrogen ions is reflected in the concept that the higher the pH value the lower the hydrogen ion concentration. Conversely, the lower the pH value, the higher the hydrogen ion concentration. Therefore, a pH below 7.35 reflects an acidotic state. A pH greater than 7.45 indicates alkalosis and a lower hydrogen ion concentration. A variation from 7.35 to 7.45 of 0.4 in either direction can be fatal. See Figure 4–6 for the pH scale.

Three mechanisms operate to maintain the appropriate pH of the blood:

1. Chemical buffer systems in the ECF and within the cells
2. Removal of carbon dioxide by the lungs
3. Renal regulation of the hydrogen ion concentration

Chemical Buffer Systems

Chemical buffer systems act like a sponge to combine with any acid or alkali to prevent excessive change in the hydrogen ion concentration. The bicarbonate buffer system is just one.

The pH of the plasma is determined by the ratio of sodium bicarbonate ($NaHCO_3$) to carbonic acid (H_2CO_3), which is the main buffer pair. Because the body has a strong tendency toward acidity, the body requires a more basic over an acidic buffering system. The ratio of HCO_3^-, a base, to H_2CO_3, is normally 20:1. The $NaHCO_3/H_2CO_3$ buffer system is responsible for approximately 45% of all hydrogen ion buffering.

Two other buffer systems in the body are the phosphate buffer system and the protein buffer system. Both act in a manner identical with that of the bicarbonate buffer system (Chenevey, 1987).

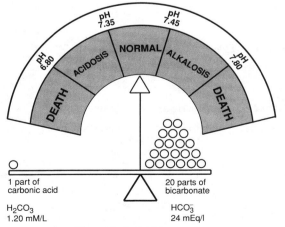

Figure 4–6. Acid-base scale.

99

Respiratory Regulation

When carbon dioxide combines with water, H_2CO_3 is formed. Therefore, an increase in the acid carbon dioxide lowers the pH of blood creating an acidotic state; a decrease in the carbon dioxide level increases the pH, causing the blood to become more alkaline. After H_2CO_3 is formed, it dissociates into carbon dioxide and water. The carbon dioxide is transferred to the lungs, where it diffuses into the alveoli and is eliminated via exhalation. Therefore, the rate of respiration affects the hydrogen ion concentration. An increase in respiratory rate will cause carbon dioxide to be blown off by the lungs, resulting in an increase in pH. Conversely, a decrease in respiratory rate will cause retention of carbon dioxide and thus a decrease in pH.

Renal Regulation

The kidneys regulate the hydrogen ion concentration by increasing or decreasing the HCO_3 ion concentration in the body fluid by a series of complex chemical reactions that occur in the renal tubules. The regulation of acid-base balance by the kidney occurs chiefly by increasing or decreasing the HCO_3 ion concentration in body fluids. Hydrogen is secreted into the tubules of the kidney, where it is eliminated in the urine. At the same time, sodium is reabsorbed from the tubular fluid into the ECF in exchange for hydrogen and combines with HCO_3 ions to form the buffer, $NaHCO_3$.

The kidneys help to regulate the extracellular concentration of HCO_3. Two buffer systems help the kidney to eliminate excess hydrogen in the urine: the phosphate buffer system and the ammonia buffer system. With each of these, an excess of hydrogen is secreted and HCO_3 ions are formed; sodium is reabsorbed, thus forming $NaHCO_3$.

The time it takes for a change to occur in the acid-base balance can range from a fraction of a second to more than 24 hours. Although the kidneys are the most powerful regulating mechanism, they are slow to make major changes in the acid-base balance (Chenevey, 1987).

MAJOR ELECTROLYTE IMBALANCES

There are two types of major electrolyte imbalances: (1) metabolic (base bicarbonate deficit and excess) acidosis and alkalosis and (2) respiratory (carbonic acid deficit and excess) acidosis and alkalosis.

Metabolic Acid-Base Imbalance

Normal reference value: 22 to 26 mEq/liter

Base Bicarbonate Deficit: Metabolic Acidosis

Metabolic acidosis (HCO_3^- deficit) is a clinical disturbance characterized by a low pH and a low plasma HCO_3 level. This condition can occur by a gain of hydrogen ($H+$) ion or a loss of HCO_3^-.

Etiology

Metabolic acidosis occurs with loss of HCO_3 from diarrhea, draining fistulas, and administration of TPN. Diabetes mellitus, alcoholism, and starvation cause ketoacidosis. Respiratory or circulatory failure, ingestion of certain drugs or toxins, some hereditary disorders, and septic shock cause lactic acidosis. It can also result

100

when renal failure results in excessive retention of hydrogen ions and with excessive ingestion of aspirin, ethylene alcohol, and ammonium chloride.

✎ **NOTE:** Hyperkalemia is usually present in clinical cases of acidosis (Metheny, 1996).

Signs and Symptoms

Patients with metabolic acidosis may experience CNS-related symptoms such as headache, confusion, drowsiness, increased respiratory rate, and kussmaul breathing. Other symptoms include nausea, vomiting, decreased cardiac output, and bradycardia (when serum pH is less than 7.0).

Diagnostic Tests

ABG values
   pH less than 7.35
   HCO_3^- less than 22 mEq/liter
   $Paco_2$ less than 38 mm Hg
Serum HCO_3—Less than 22 mEq/liter
Serum electrolytes—Elevated potassium possible, because of exchange of intracellular potassium for hydrogen ions in the body's attempt to normalize acid-base environment.
ECG—Dysrhythmias caused by hyperkalemia (Horne & Swearingen, 1993)

Treatment

Metabolic acidosis is treated by (1) reversing the underlying cause (diabetic ketoacidosis, alcholism related to ketoacidosis, diarrhea, acute renal failure, renal tubular acidosis, poisoning, lactic acidosis); (2) eliminating the source (if cause is due to excessive administration of NaCl); and (3) administering $NaHCO_3$ (7.5% 44.4 mEq/50 mL or 8.4% 50 mEq/50 mL I.V. when pH is equal to or less than 7.2. Concentration depends on severity of acidosis and presence of any serum sodium disorders

✎ **NOTE:** Give $NaHCO_3$ cautiously to avoid metabolic alkalosis and pulmonary edema secondary to sodium overload.

Potassium replacement: hyperkalemia is usually present but potassium deficit can occur. If deficit of less than 3.5 mEq/liter is present the potassium deficit must be corrected before $NaHCO_3$ is administered because when the acidosis is correct, the potassium shifts back into the ICF (Horne & Swearingen, 1993).

Base Bicarbonate Excess: Metabolic Alkalosis

Metabolic alkalosis (HCO_3^- excess) is a clinical disturbance characterized by a high pH and a high plasma HCO_3^- concentration. It can be produced by a gain of HCO_3^- or a loss of hydrogen ion.

Etiology

Metabolic alkalosis occurs with gastrointestinal loss of hydrogen ions from gastric suctioning and vomiting. Renal loss of hydrogen ions occurs from potassium-losing diuretics, excess of mineralocorticoid, and hypercalcemia and hypoparathyroidism. In hypokalemia and carbohydrate refeeding after starvation, hydrogen ions shift from ECF into the cells depleting serum levels. This also occurs when excessive ingestion of alkalis, such as antacids and Alka-Seltzer, parenteral administration of

$NaHCO_3$ during cardiopulmonary resuscitation and massive blood transfusions increase serum levels of HCO_3^-.

Signs and Symptoms

Patients with metabolic alkaloses may experience dizziness and depressed respirations in addition to impaired mentation, tingling of fingers and toes, circumoral paresthesia, and hypertonic reflexes. Other symptoms include hypotension, cardiac dyrhythmias, hyperventilation, hypokalemia, and decreased ionized calcium (carpopedal spasm).

Diagnostic Tests

ABG values
   pH greater than 7.45
   HCO_3^- greater than 26 mEq/liter
   Pa_{CO_2} greater than 42 mm Hg
Serum HCO_3—Greater than 26 mEq/liter
Serum electrolytes—Low serum potassium (less than 4 mEq/liter) and low serum
   chloride
ECG—Assess for dysrhythmias (Horne & Swearingen, 1993)

✎ **NOTE:** Hypokalemia is often present in alkalosis.

Treatment

Metabolic alkalosis is treated by (1) reversing the underlying cause; (2) administering sufficient chloride for the kidney to excrete the excess HCO_3; and (3) replacing potassium if a chloride deficit is also present (Horne & Swearingen, 1993).

Respiratory Acid-Base Imbalance

Normal reference value: Partial pressure of carbon dioxide (Pa_{CO_2})—38–42 mm Hg.

Carbonic Acid Excess: Respiratory Acidosis

Respiratory acidosis is due to inadequate excretion of carbon dioxide and inadequate ventilation resulting in an increase of serum levels or carbon dioxide and H_2CO_3. Acute respiratory acidosis is usually associated with emergency situations.

Etiology

Acute respiratory acidosis can result from pulmonary, neurologic, and cardiac causes such as: pulmonary edema, aspiration of a foreign body, pneumothorax, severe pneumonia, and severe, prolonged exacerbation of acute asthma, overdose of sedatives, cardiac arrest, and massive pulmonary embolism.

Chronic respiratory acidosis results from emphysema, bronchial asthma, bronchiectasis, postoperative pain, obesity, and tight abdominal binders.

Signs and Symptoms

Acute signs and symptoms include tachypnea, dyspnea, dizziness, seizures, warm, flushed skin, and ventricular fibrillation. Chronic signs and symptoms occur if Pa_{CO_2} exceeds the body's ability to compensate, which include respiratory symptoms.

Diagnostic Tests

Acute
  ABG values
    pH less than 7.35
    Paco greater than 42 mm Hg
    HCO_3^- greater than 26 mEq/liter
Chronic
  pH less than 7.35
  $Paco_2$ greater than 42 mm Hg
  HCO_3^- normal or slight increase
Serum HCO_3—Reflects acid-base balance; initial values normal unless mixed disorder is present
Serum electrolytes—Usually not altered
Chest x-ray—Determines the presence of underlying pulmonary disease
Drug screen—Determines the quantity of drug if patient is suspected of taking an overdose (Horne & Swearingen, 1993)

Treatment

Respiratory acidosis is treated by carrying out the following:

1. Improve ventilation.
2. Administer bronchodilators or antibiotics for respiratory infections, as indicated.
3. Administer oxygen, as indicated.
4. Administer adequate fluids (2 to 3 liters/day) to keep mucous membranes moist and help to remove secretions.

Carbonic Acid Deficit: Respiratory Alkalosis

Respiratory alkalosis is usually due to hyperventilation, which causes "blowing off" of carbon dioxide and a decrease in H_2CO_3 content. Respiratory alkalosis can be acute or chronic (Table 4–7).

Etiology

Acute respiratory acidosis results from pulmonary disorders that produce hypoxemia or stimulation of the respiratory centers. Underlying causes of hypoxemia include: high fever, pneumonia, congestive heart failure, pulmonary emboli, hypotension, asthma, and inhalation of irritants. Causes of stimulation of respiratory centers include anxiety (most common), excessive mechanical ventilation, CNS lesions involving the respiratory center, and salicylate overdose (an early sign).

Signs and Symptoms

Respiratory alkalosis causes light-headedness; inability to concentrate; numbness and tingling of extremities (circumoral paresthesia); and tinnitus, palpitations, epigastic pain, blurred vision, precordial pain (tightness), sweating, dry mouth, tremulousness, seizures and loss of consciousness.

Diagnostic Tests

ABG values
  pH greater than 7.45
  $Paco_2$ less than 38 mm Hg
  HCO_3^- less than 22 mEq/liter

Serum electrolytes—Presence of metabolic acid-base disorders
Serum phosphate—May fall to less than 0.5 mg/dL
ECG—Determines cardiac dysrhythmias (Horne & Swearingen, 1993)

Treatment

Treatment of respiratory alkalosis consists of (1) treating the source of anxiety (instruct patient to breathe slowly into a paper bag); (2) administering a sedative, as indicated; and (3) treating the underlying cause (Metheny, 1996).

TABLE 4–7. SUMMARY OF ACUTE ACID-BASE IMBALANCES

Acid-Base Imbalance	pH	Paco$_2$	HCO$_3^-$	Signs and Symptoms	Causes
Acute metabolic acidosis	↓	↓	↓ *	Tachypena-Kussmaul respirations, hypotension, cold, clammy skin, coma, dysrhythmias	Shock, arrest, ketoacidosis, starvation, acute renal failure, ingestion of acids, diarrhea
Metabolic alkalosis	↑	↑	↑ *	Muscular weakness hyporeflexia, dysrhythmia, apathy, confusion, stupor	Volume depletion gastric drainage, vomiting, diuretic usage, aldosteronism, severe potassium depletion, excessive alkali intake
Respiratory acidosis	↓	↑	No change	Tachycardia, tachypnea diaphoresis, headache, restlessness, coma, cyanosis, dysrhythmias, hypotension	Acute respiratory failure, drug overdose, chest wall trauma, asphyxiation, CNS trauma, cardiopulmonary disorders, impaired muscle of respiration
Respiratory alkalosis	↑	↓	No change	Paresthesia (fingers) dizziness, lethargy, confusion	Hyperventilation, salicylate poison, hypoxia with pneumonia, pulmonary edema, gram-negative sepsis, CNS lesion, inappropriate mechanical ventilation

*Compensatory response.

SUMMARY WORKSHEET 2: Acid-Base Balance

METABOLIC ACID-BASE IMBALANCE: BASE BICARBONATE DEFICIT AND EXCESS

Bicarbonate (HCO_2):   **Normal Lab:**

Key Points:

Deficit: Acidosis

    Etiology   *Signs and Symptoms*

Excess: Alkalosis

    Etiology   *Signs and Symptoms*

RESPIRATORY ACID-BASE IMBALANCE: CARBONIC ACID EXCESS AND DEFICIT

Carbonic Acid (H_2CO_3)   **Normal Lab:**

Key Points:

Excess: Respiratory Acidosis

    Etiology   *Signs and Symptoms*

Deficit: Respiratory Alkalosis

    Etiology   *Signs and Symptoms*

COMPETENCY CRITERIA: Electrolyte Balance

Competency Statement: The competent I.V. therapy nurse will be able to: Identify the patient with signs and symptoms of electrolyte imbalance and acid-base imbalance.

COGNITIVE CRITERIA

	Skilled	*Needs Education*
1. Ability to identify patients at risk for electrolyte imbalances:		
Sodium		
Potassium		
Magnesium		
Calcium		
Phosphorus		
2. Ability to identify patients at risk for metabolic acid-base imbalances:		
Acidosis		
Alkalosis		

PERFORMANCE CRITERIA

	Skilled	*Needs Education*
3. Ability to perform specific assessments related to electrolyte imbalances:		
Sodium		
Skin turgor		
Mentation		
Potassium		
Monitor		
ECG tracing		
Calcium		
Trousseau's sign		
Chvostek's sign		
Review of laboratory data specific for electrolyte imbalances		
Serum electrolytes		
ABGs		
Urine		

SUGGESTED EVALUATION CRITERIA

Written test—Cognitive

Physical assessment of patient

Assessment skills performance in simulated lab

Clinical case studies

Review of clients on unit or in home care setting and choosing those at risk for electrolyte imbalances

KEY POINTS

FUNDAMENTALS OF ELECTROLYTES

The 7 major electrolytes and their symbols are:

Cations	Anions
Sodium (Na^+)	Chloride (Cl^-)
Potassium (K^+)	Phosphate (HPO_4^-)
Calcium (Ca^{++})	Bicarbonate (HCO_3^-)
Magnesium (Mg^{++})	

The prefix hypo = deficit in an electrolyte

The prefix hyper = excess in an electrolyte

Sodium: 135–145 mEq/liter

Function: Maintenance of extracellular fluid volume

Transmission of impulses in nerve and muscle fibers

Regulation of acid-base when sodium combines with chloride ore bicarbonate control of intracellular fluid volume

Hyponatremia: Gastrointestinal losses, use of thiazide diuretics, adrenal insufficiency, excessive infusion of 5%D/W, SIADH

S&S: anorexia, muscle cramps, exhaustion, apprehension, ataxia

Treatment: Replace sodium

Hypernatremia: Excessive IV administration of sodium chloride solutions, profuse sweating

S&S: Thirst! elevated body temperature, disorientation

Treatment: Gradually lower serum sodium level using hypotonic electrolyte solution or isotonic solutions

Potassium: 3.5–5.5 mEq/liter

Function: Responsible for transmission of nerve impulses

Hypokalemia: Main cause gastrointestinal losses

S&S: Irritability, fatigue, muscle weakness, diminished deep tendon reflexes, ECG changes, flaccid paralysis

Treatment: Replace potassium

Hyperkalemia: Excessive administration of potassium, renal failure, crushing injury, acidosis

S&S: ECG changes, vague muscle weakness, nausea, diarrhea

Calcium: 8.5 to 10.5 mg/dL
Function: Activation of enzymes and stimulating essential chemical reactions
Role in maintaining normal transmission of nerve impulses
Sedative effect on nerve cells
Conversion of prothrombin to thrombin
Calcium and phosphate have a reciprocal relationship
Hypocalcemia: Increased calcium loss, reduced intake related to altered intestinal absorption, altered regulation
S&S: Neuromuscular changes: numbness of fingers, cramps, hyperactive deep tendon reflexes, positive Trousseau's sign and Chvostek's sign
CNS: Irritability
CV: altered cardiovascular hemodynamics, prolonged QT interval
Treatment: Replace calcium with calcium gluconate (10 mL to 20 mL of a 10% solution in 5% dextrose in water over 20 minutes)
Hypercalcemia: malignancy, hyperparathyroidism, thiazide-diuretic use
S&S: Neuromuscular: muscle weakness, lethargy, deep bony pain, pathologic fractures
GI: anorexia, nausea, vomiting, constipation
Renal: polyuria renal colic stones
Cardiac: Note: Patient receiving digitalis must receive calcium with extreme care because it can precipitate severe dysrhythmias

Magnesium: 1.5 to 2.5 mEq/liter
Function: Acts directly on myoneural junction and affects neuromuscular irritability and contractility. Activator for many enzymes, role in carbohydrate and protein metabolism
Hypomagnesemia: chronic alcoholism, malabsorption syndromes, prolonged malnutrition or starvation. Drugs such as gentamicin, diuretics, cisplatin, prolonged gastric suctioning
S&S: Neuromuscular: hyperactive reflexes, coarse tremors, muscle cramps, positive Chvostek's and Trousseau's signs, convulsions. CV: dysrhythmias, tachycardia
Treatment: Administer 40 mEq (5 Gm) magnesium sulfate IV to 1 liter of 5%D/W or 5%D/NACL or 1–2 GM of 10% solution direct IV push at rate of 1.5 mL/minute
Hypermagnesemia: renal failure, excessive administration of magnesium via IV, hyperparathyroidism
S&S: Neuromuscular: flushing and sense of skin warmth, lethargy, sedation, hypoactive deep tendon reflexes CV: hypotension, sinus bradycardia, heart block, cardiac arrest
GI: nausea and vomiting
Treatment: Administer calcium gluconate, support respiratory function, hemodialysis

Phosphorus: 3.0–4.5 mg/dL
Function: Role in delivery of oxygen to tissues regulating level of 2,3-diphosphoglycerate (2,3DPG)
Hypophosphatemia: Hyperalimentation (inadequate amounts of phosphorus), malabsorption syndromes, alcohol withdrawal, treatment of diabetic ketoacidosis, prolonged respiratory alkalosis
S&S: Neuromuscular: paresthesia, muscle weakness, tremors, dysarthria, dysphagia
Central: disorientation, convulsions. Hematological: affects all blood cells—red cells primarily
Treatment: IV phosphate solutions

Hyperphosphatemia: Renal disease
S&S: Neuromuscular changes: hypocalcemia, tetany Central: mental changes, apprehension. Hematologic: Increased red blood cell 2,3-DPG levels
Treatment: Treat underlying cause, restrict dietary intake, administer phosphate binding gels

Chloride: 95–108 mEq/liter

Function: Acid-base balance. Preserves electrical neutrality of red blood cells and maintains of 1:20 ratio of carbonic acid and bicarbonate
Hypochloremia: severe vomiting, diarrhea, pyloric obstruction
S&S: tetany, hypertonic reflexes, depressed respirations

✎ **NOTE:** Excessive loss of chloride results in alkalosis due to increase in bicarbonate ion.

Treatment: treat underlying cause, administer sodium chloride solutions

Hyperchloremia: Any condition that decreases bicarbonate ions: acidosis
S&S: deep rapid breathing, stupor, weakness, signs and symptoms of acidosis
Treatment: Treat underlying cause of acidosis, administer solutions free of sodium chloride

Acid-base balance

Three mechanisms control the pH of body fluids
1. Chemical buffer systems
2. Lungs
3. Kidneys

The H^+ ion concentration is reflected in the pH. The normal pH of body fluids is 7.35–7.45, a variation in 0.4 in either direction can be fatal
Deficit in base bicarbonate = Acidosis. Excess of base bicarbonate = Alkalosis Lab values of importance in screening for acid/base poroblems are: pH, HCO_3- and $PaCO_2$

CRITICAL THINKING ACTIVITY

1. In your work environment, list the types of patients that are at risk for potassium deficit.

2. If you have a patient who is receiving total parenteral nutrition, read the I.V. solution container and write down the contents. Is this patient receiving phosphorus and magnesium?

3. Review the chemistry laboratory report on one patient. Write down the patient's chemistry values and compare these values with normal lab values. Did you pick up any deficits or excesses?

4. Conduct a conference on your unit on the relationship between nasogastric tubes and the effects on electrolyte imbalances. What was the response of the nurses? How many nurses knew there was such a risk with nasogastric tubes?

5. Why are patients who have nasogastric tubes at risk for alkalosis?

POST-TEST, CHAPTER 4

Match the term in column I with the definition in column II.

Column I

1. _____ acidosis
2. _____ SIADH
3. _____ ion
4. _____ anion
5. _____ alkalosis
6. _____ cation
7. _____ Trousseau's sign
8. _____ pH
9. _____ Chvostek's sign
10. _____ intravascular fluid

Column II

A. Electrolyte
B. H^+ ion concentration decreases, pH greater than 7.45
C. Positively charged ion
D. Syndrome of inappropriate antidiuretic hormone
E. H^+ ion concentration increases, pH less than 7.35
F. Negatively charged ion
G. H^+ concentration
H. Fluid in the plasma
I. Spasm of muscle supplying facial nerve
J. Spasm of hand elicited when blood supply to hand is decreased

11. List the four cations in the body fluid.
    A. _____
    B. _____
    C. _____
    D. _____

12. You assess your patient and find the following signs and symptoms: fatigued muscles, complaints of nausea and anorexia, irritability and diminished deep tendon reflexes. You check serum electrolytes and find: chloride 92 mEq/liter, potassium 3.1 mEq/liter and sodium 135 mEq/liter. What would you suspect?
    A. Hyponatremia
    B. Hyperchloremia
    C. Hypokalemia
    D. Hypernatremia

13. Your patient has a nasogastric tube to continuous suction. What electrolytes are at risk for deficit with this type of patient?
    A. Sodium
    B. Potassium
    C. Chloride
    D. All of the above

True-False

14. **T F** The normal pH of body fluid is 7.35 to 7.45.

15. **T F** The major electrolytes in the intracellular compartment are sodium and chloride.

16. **T F** Potassium influences skeletal and cardiac muscle activity.

17. **T F** Normal potassium level is 3.5 to 5.0 mEq/liter.

111

18. List as many nursing diagnoses (nursing problems) as could occur for electrolyte
    imbalances _____

    _____

    _____

19. Which are the regulatory organs in acid-base balance.
    A. Lungs and liver
    B. Lungs and kidneys
    C. Pituitary glands and adrenal glands

20. In the medical-surgical setting, identify one type of patient at risk for electrolyte
    imbalance and explain why?

21. On the oncology unit, identify one type of patient at risk for electrolyte imbalance and
    explain why?

22. A patient presents with the following signs and symptoms: confusion, respirations 30,
    blood pressure 100/70 mm Hg, prior admission for renal failure. ABG values are: pH
    7.32, HCO_3^- 20 mEq/liter, $Paco_2$ 34 mm Hg. What would you suspect?
    A. Metabolic acidosis
    B. Metabolic alkalosis
    C. Respiratory acidosis

23. The most common cause of hypermagnesemia is:
    A. Nasogastric tubes to suction
    B. Renal failure
    C. Overzealous administration of I.V. potassium chloride
    D. Respirators

24. In critical care units, patients are at risk for the following electrolyte imbalances:
    A. Hypomagnesemia, hypercalcemia, and hypophosphatemia
    B. Hyperkalemia, hypernatremia, and hyperchloremia
    C. Hyponatremia, hypernatremia, and hyperkalemia

ANSWERS TO CHAPTER 4

PRE-TEST

1. F	7. A	12. T	17. B
2. C	8. I	13. T	18. C
3. B	9. D	14. T	19. D
4. E	10. J	15. F	20. A
5. G	11. T	16. B	21. C
6. H			

POST-TEST

1. E	6. C	11. Magnesium Mg^+	13. D
2. D	7. J	Sodium Na^+	14. T
3. A	8. G	Potassium K^+	15. F
4. F	9. I	Calcium Ca^{++}	16. T
5. B	10. H	12. C	17. T

18. Sensory-perceptual alterations secondary to hyponatremia

Altered health maintenance related to poor dietary habits, perceptual/cognitive impairment

Constipation related to weakened peristalsis

Fluid volume deficit related to failure of regulatory mechanism

Impaired physical mobility related to activity intolerance; decreased strength and endurance; pain, discomfort; neuromuscular impairment; musculoskeletal impairment resulting from electrolyte imbalance

Ineffective breathing pattern related to biochemical imbalances

Altered comfort, pain, related to injuring agent (e.g., stones associated with calcium, excess)

Risk of injury related to confusion; altered thought process related to electrolyte imbalance; tetany and seizures secondary to severe hypocalcemia; sensory changes with hypercalcemia

Decreased cardiac output related to electrical factors (risk of ventricular dysrhythmias) secondary to severe hypokalemia, hyperkalemia, hypocalcemia, or hypophoshatemia

Impaired gas exchange related to altered oxygen supply secondary to laryngeal spasm occurring with severe hypocalcemia; decreased strength of respiratory muscles, and decreased 2,3-DPG in hypophosphatemia

Altered pattern of urinary elimination related to changes in renal function occurring with hypercalcemia

High risk for impaired verbal communication related to confusion, lethargy, and electrolyte balance

19. B
20. Patient with nasogastric tube to suction
21. Patient with myelogenous leukemia, lymphoma
22. A
23. B
24. A

REFERENCES

Anderson, R.J., Chung, H., & Kluge, R. (1985). Hyponatremia: A prospective analysis of its epidemiology and the pathogenetic role of vasopressin. *Annals of Internal Medicine, 102*, 164–168.

Berger, E. (1984). Nutrition in hypodermoclysis. *Journal of American Geriatric Society, 32*, 199.

Burgess, R.E. (1965). Fluids and electrolytes. *American Journal of Nursing, 65*(10).

Calloway, C. (1987). When the problem involves magnesium, calcium or phosphate. *RN, 5*, 30–35.

Carson, R. (1961). *The sea around us.* New York: New American Library.

Chenevey, B. (1987). Overview of fluids and electrolytes. *Nursing Clinics of North America, 22*(4), 749–759.

Clutter, W.E. (1993). Mineral and metabolic bone disease. In: Woodley, M., & Whelan A. (eds) *Manual of medical therapeutics,* (27th ed). Boston: Little, Brown.

Gahart, B.L. (1994). *Intravenous medications: A handbook for nurses and other allied health personnel* (10th ed). St. Louis: C.V. Mosby.

Goldberger, E. (1986). *A primer of water, electrolytes and acid-base syndromes* (7th ed). Philadelphia: Lea & Febiger.

Horne, M.M., & Swearingen, P.L. (1993). *Pocket guide to fluids, electrolytes and acid-base balance.* St. Louis: Mosby-Year Book.

Kokko, J., & Tannen R. (1990). *Fluids and electrolytes* (2nd ed). Philadelphia: W.B. Saunders.

Lamb, C. (1986). SIADH: Why is the serum sodium low? Interviews with Culpepper, M., Porter, G.A., & Roddam, R. *Patient Care,* 94–110.

McFadden, E., & Zaloga, G.P. (1983). Calcium regulation. *Critical Care Quarterly, 12*, 12–21.

McFadden, E., Zaloga, G., & Chernow, B. (1983). Hypocalcemia: A medical emergency, *American Journal of Nursing, 80*, 226–230.

Metheny, N.M. (1990). Why worry about IV fluids? *American Journal of Nursing* (6), 50–55.

Metheny, N.M. (1996). *Fluids and electrolyte balance: Nursing considerations* (3rd ed). Philadelphia: J.B. Lippincott.

Olinger, M. (1989). Disorders of calcium and magnesium. *Emergency Medical Clinics of North America, 7*(4), 769.

O'Shea, M.H. (1992). Fluid and electrolyte management. In: Woodley, M., & Whelan, A. (eds). *Manual of medical therapeutics* (27th ed). Boston: Little, Brown.

Poyss, A.S. (1987). Assessment and nursing diagnosis in fluid and electrolyte disorders. *Nursing Clinics of North America, 22*(4), 773–783.

Rapp, R. (1987). Use of lidocaine to reduce pain associated with potassium chloride. *Clinical Pharmacy, 6*, 98.

Rolls, B.J., & Phillips, P.A. (1990). Aging and disturbances of thirst and fluid balance. *Nutrition Reviews, 48*(3), 137–143.

Rose, B. (1984). *Clinical physiology of acid-base and electrolyte disorders* (2nd ed). New York: McGraw-Hill.

Rutherford, C. (1989). Fluid and electrolyte therapy: Considerations for patient care. *Jounral of Intravenous Therapy, 12*(3), 173–184.

Shrier, R. (1986). *Renal and electrolyte disorders* (3rd ed). Boston: Little, Brown.

Spital, A. (1989). Bicarbonate in the treatment of severe hyperkalemia. *American Journal of Medicine, 85*, 51.

Vanatta, J., & Fogelman, M. (1988). *Moyers fluid balance* (3rd ed) Chicago: Year Book Medical Publishers.

Weldy, N.J. (1996). *Body fluids and electrolytes. A programmed presentation* (7th ed). St. Louis: Mosby, pp. 83–119, 127.

Zaloga, G., & Chernow, B. (1983). Magnesium metabolism in critical illness. *Critical Care Quarterly 4*, 22–27. (1989). Hyperkalemia—silent and deadly. *Lancet*, 1240.

Zull, D. (1989). Disorders of potassium metabolism. *Emergency Medical Clinics of North America, 7*(4), 771.

CHAPTER 5

Parenteral Solutions

CHAPTER CONTENTS

GLOSSARY
LEARNING OBJECTIVES
PRE-TEST, CHAPTER 5
RATIONALES AND OBJECTIVES OF
  PARENTERAL THERAPY
Maintenance Therapy
Replacement Therapy
Restoration Therapy
SUMMARY WORKSHEET #1: OBJECTIVES OF
  I.V. THERAPY
KEY ELEMENTS IN PARENTERAL SOLUTIONS
Water
Carbohydrates (Glucose)
Protein
Vitamins
Electrolytes
pH
HYPOTONIC, ISOTONIC, AND HYPERTONIC
  SOLUTIONS
Hypotonic Fluids

Isotonic Fluids
Hypertonic Fluids
TYPES OF PARENTERAL SOLUTIONS
Crystalloid Solutions
SUMMARY WORKSHEET #2: PARENTERAL
  CRYSTALLOID SOLUTIONS
Colloid Solutions
SUMMARY WORKSHEET #3: PARENTERAL
  COLLOID SOLUTIONS
NURSING PLAN OF CARE: ADMINISTRATION
  OF PARENTERAL FLUIDS
COMPETENCY CRITERIA: ADMINISTRATION OF
  PARENTERAL FLUIDS
KEY POINTS
CRITICAL THINKING ACTIVITY
POST-TEST, CHAPTER 5
ANSWERS TO CHAPTER 5
Pre-Test
Post-Text
REFERENCES

GLOSSARY

Balanced solution Parenteral solution that contains portions of electrolytes similar to plasma; also contains bicarbonate or acetate ion
Catabolism The breakdown of chemical compounds by the body; an energy-producing metabolic process
Colloid A substance that does not dissolve into a true solution and is not capable of passing through a semipermeable membrane (e.g., blood, plasma, albumin, dextran)
Crystalloid A substance that forms a true solution and is capable of passing through a semipermeable membrane (e.g., lactated Ringer's solution, isotonic saline)
Dehydration A deficit of body water; can involve one fluid compartment or all three
Hydrating fluids A solution of water, carbohydrate, Na^+, and Cl^-, used to determine adequacy of renal function
Maintenance therapy Fluids that provide all nutrients necessary to meet daily patient requirements
Normal saline Solution of salt (0.9% sodium chloride)
Oliguria Diminished amount of urine
Plasma substitute A solution of a synthetic substance such as dextran used as a substitute for plasma

Replacement therapy Replenishment of losses when maintenance cannot be met and when patient is in a deficit state

Restoration therapy Reconstruction of fluid and electrolyte needs on a continuing basis until homeostasis returns

LEARNING OBJECTIVES

Upon completion of this chapter, the reader will be able to:

- Define terminology related to parenteral solutions.
- Identify the three objectives of parenteral therapy.
- List the key elements in intravenous (I.V.) solutions.
- List the uses of maintenance fluids.
- List the four functions of glucose as a necessary nutrient when administered parenterally.
- Explain the roles of vitamin C and vitamin B complex in maintenance therapy.
- Describe the uses of hypotonic, isotonic, and hypertonic fluids.
- Identify the major groupings of I.V. solutions.
- Compare the advantages and disadvantages of dextrose, sodium chloride, hydrating fluids, and multiple electrolyte fluids.
- Identify the main role of hydrating fluids.
- Compare the properties of a crystalloid with those of a colloid solution.
- Identify the use of alkalinizing and acidifying fluids.
- State the most commonly used hypotonic multiple electrolyte solution.
- State the most commonly used isotonic multiple electrolyte fluid.
- State the use of albumin, hetastarch, and dextran.

PRE-TEST, CHAPTER 5

Match the term in column I with the definition in column II.

Column I

1. _____ maintenance therapy
2. _____ replacement therapy
3. _____ restoration therapy

Column II

A. Objective required to meet daily needs; usually includes water, carbohydrates, and electrolytes

B. Objective for continuing (ongoing) losses; reassess every 4 hours

C. Objective for meeting previous losses

4. List four key components of I.V. solution.

A. _____

B. _____

C. _____

D. _____

Match the term in column I to the definition in column II.

Column I

5. _____ sodium chloride solution

6. _____ oliguria

7. _____ hydrating solution

8. _____ colloid

9. _____ crystalloid

Column II

A. A substance that does not dissolve into a true solution

B. Solution of salt (0.9% sodium chloride)

C. Diminished amount of urine

D. A substance that forms a true solution

E. Solution of water, carbohydrates, sodium, and chlorine used to determine adequacy of renal function

10. Hypotonic solutions are used to
    A. Hydrate cells
    B. Increase vascular space
    C. Supply sodium and chloride in deficit states

11. Hypertonic solutions are used to
    A. Shift extracellular fluid (ECF) from intracellular space to plasma
    B. Hydrate cells
    C. Supply free water to vascular space

12. What is/are the function(s) of glucose parenterally?
    A. Improve hepatic function
    B. Supply necessary calories for energy
    C. Spare body protein
    D. Minimize ketosis
    E. All of the above

13. What is the role of vitamin C in parenteral therapy?
    A. To increase the tensile strength of collagen
    B. To protect cells against oxidation
    C. To promote wound healing
    D. To help with metabolism of carbohydrates

14. What is the *main* role of a hydrating solution?
    A. To check kidney function
    B. To expand the ECF compartment
    C. To hydrate the cells
    D. To supply sodium and chloride in deficit states

15. What is the most commonly used multiple electrolyte solution?
    A. 5% dextrose in water
    B. 0.9% sodium chloride
    C. Lactated Ringer's solution
    D. 5% dextrose and sodium chloride

16. What is the most common complication of dextran administration?
    A. Fluid overload
    B. Hypersensitivity reactions
    C. Hyponatremia
    D. Hyperkalemia

17. What is the purpose of a colloid solution?
    A. To expand the interstitial compartment
    B. To replace electrolytes
    C. To expand the intravascular compartment
    D. To correct acidosis

Let the patient's taste decide. You will say that, in cases of great thirst, the patient's craving decides that it will drink a great deal of tea, and that you cannot help it. But in these cases be sure that the patient requires diluents for quite other purposes than quenching the thirst; he wants a great deal of some drink, not only of tea, and the doctor will order what he is to have, barley water or lemonade, or soda water and milk, as the case may be.

FLORENCE NIGHTINGALE, 1859

In the mid-1950s less than 20% of hospital patients received intravenous (I.V.) therapy. I.V. solutions at that time were used primarily during surgery and for treatment of dehydration. Solutions for the surgical patients were infused over 3- to 4-hour periods and discontinued at night. The only solutions available were 5% dextrose in water and 5% dextrose and 0.9% sodium chloride. Today, more than 90% of hospitalized patients receive I.V. therapy with over 200 different types of parenteral solutions.

RATIONALES AND OBJECTIVES OF PARENTERAL THERAPY

To understand the use of parenteral solutions the nurse must understand two important concepts: (1) the rationale for the physician's order of I.V. therapy, and (2) the type of solution ordered and the composition and clinical use of that solution.

Objectives or rationales for administration of I.V. therapy fall into three broad categories: maintenance therapy for daily body fluid requirements, replacement therapy for present losses, and restoration therapy for concurrent or continuing losses.

These three objectives differ in the time necessary to complete the therapy, the purpose of the I.V. fluid, and the type of patient who is to receive the I.V. solution. Factors affecting the choice of objective in prescribing parenteral fluid and the rate of administration by the physician are the patient's:

Renal function
Daily maintenance requirements
Existing fluid and electrolyte imbalance
Clinical status
Disturbances in homeostasis as a result of parenteral therapy (Metheny, 1996)

Maintenance Therapy

In maintenance therapy, water has priority. The body needs water to replace insensible loss, which can occur as perspiration from the skin and moisture from respirations. The average adult loses 500 to 1000 mL of water over 24 hours through insensible loss. Water is also an important dilutor for waste products excreted by the kidney. Approximately 30 mL of fluid is needed per kilogram of body weight (15 mL/kg) for maintenance needs (Metheny, 1992). Also, an individual's fluid requirements are based on age, height, weight, and amount of body fat.

Maintenance therapy provides nutrients that meet the daily needs of a patient for water, electrolytes, and dextrose. Water has priority. The typical patient profile for maintenance therapy is one who is allowed nothing by mouth (NPO) or has

118

restricted oral intake for any reason (O'Shea, 1993). Remember that insensible loss is approximately 500 to 1000 mL per 24 hours. Maintenance therapy should be 1500 mL per square meter (m^2) of body surface over 24 hours (Metheny, 1996).

Example
A male weighing 85 kg (187 lb) has a body surface area of 2 (m^2).

1500 mL $\times$ 2 = 3000 mL for maintenance therapy.

(See Appendix for nomogram of body surface areas).

Balanced solutions for maintenance therapy include water, daily needs of sodium and potassium, and glucose. Glucose, a necessary component in maintenance therapy, is converted to glycogen by the liver. It has four main uses in parenteral therapy:

1. Improves hepatic function
2. Supplies necessary calories for energy
3. Spares body protein
4. Minimizes ketosis

✎ **NOTE:** The basic caloric requirement for an adult is 1600 calories/day for a 70-kg adult at rest. Approximately 100 to 150 g of carbohydrates are needed daily to minimize protein catabolism and prevent starvation. In 1 liter of 5% dextrose in water, there are 50 g of dextrose (Metheny, 1996).

Hospitalized patients receiving additional saline or glucose infusions are prone to develop potassium deficiency. Hospitalized patients are usually under stress. Excretion of potassium in urine can rise to 60 to 120 mEq/day even with limited intake. Tissue injury significantly increases the loss of potassium. Normal dietary intake of potassium is 80 to 200 mEq/day.

Vitamins are necessary for utilization of other nutrients. Vitamin C and vitamin B complex are used frequently in parenteral therapy, especially in postoperative patients. Vitamin C promotes wound healing, and vitamin B complex has a role in metabolism of carbohydrates and maintenance of gastrointestinal function (Weinstein, 1993).

Replacement Therapy

Replacement therapy is necessary to meet the fluid, electrolyte, or blood product deficits of patients in acute distress and are supplied within 48 hours. Examples of conditions of patients needing replacement infusion therapy (and their replacement requirements) are:

Hemorrhage (replacement of cells and plasma)
Low platelets (replacement of clotting factors)
Vomiting and diarrhea (replacement of losses of electrolytes and water)
Starvation (replacement of loss of water and electrolytes)

When maintenance of body requirements cannot be met, replacement therapy is instituted by the physician. The physician must figure the losses and calculate replacement over a 48-hour period. *The very first thing to check before replacement therapy can begin is kidney function.* Patients requiring replacement therapy, except those in shock, require potassium. Patients under stress from tissue injury, wound infection, or gastric or bowel surgery also require potassium. Potassium, 20 mEq/liter, achieves adequate replacement (Metheny, 1996).

119

✎ **NOTE:** Never give over 120 mEq of potassium in 24 hours, unless cardiac status is monitored continuously, because it can create a life-threatening situation.

Carefully monitor balanced solutions with potassium for the following patients:

1. Those with dysfunction of:
   Renal system
   Cardiovascular system
   Adrenal glands
   Pituitary gland
   Parathyroid gland
2. Those with deficits of:
   Sodium
   Calcium
   Base bicarbonate deficit or excess
   Blood volume (hypovolemic)

3. Those with excess of:
   Extracellular potassium
   Extracellular calcium

✎ **NOTE:** *Key nursing assessment*: Check kidney function before administration of potassium in replacement therapy.

Restoration Therapy

Restoration therapy for concurrent losses is achieved on an ongoing daily basis. Critical evaluation of concurrent losses of fluid and electrolyte therapy is done at least every 24 hours. Of extreme importance in this type of management of fluid and electrolyte therapy is accurate documentation of intake and output. Restoration of homeostasis depends on the nursing assessment of intake of I.V. fluids, as well as on the documentation of all body fluid losses. The types of clinical patients who require 24-hour evaluation are those with draining fistulas, abscesses, nasogastric tubes, burns, and abdominal wounds.

The fluid and electrolyte management of these patients cannot be completed in 48 hours. Therefore, maintenance therapy and replacement therapy do not meet these patients' needs. A day-by-day restoration of vital fluids and electrolytes is necessary. With these types of patients you will see frequent changes in the types of solution ordered, in the amount of electrolytes ordered based on laboratory values ordered, and in the rate of infusion.

The type of restoration fluid ordered depends on the type of fluid being lost. For example, excessive loss of gastric fluid must be replaced by solutions resembling that fluid; with nasogastric suctioning, chloride, potassium, and sodium are lost continually. Restoration of electrolyte imbalance is imperative for proper homeostatic management therapy. Rather than waiting to make daily rounds to evaluate the 24-hour totals and change infusion orders, physicians are ordering multiple electrolyte solutions to be used as a replacement solution via the main infusion system on an ongoing basis. This replacement need is reevaluated every 1 to 8 hours.

Example
The physician orders 1000 mL of 5% dextrose/0.45% sodium chloride every 8 hours as a primary solution. A multiple electrolyte solution, such as lactated Ringer's solution, is ordered in addition to the primary solution to replace nasogastric output mL for mL over 4 hours. The primary I.V. solution is continuously infused at 125 mL/hour. If the nasogastric suction container is emptied for 400 mL of gastric secretions, the nurse will need

TABLE 5–1. **SAMPLE SCHEDULE FOR RESTORATION THERAPY FOR NASOGASTRIC SUCTIONING**

Time	8:00 AM	9:00 AM	10:00 AM	11:00 AM	12:00 PM	1:00 PM
Gastric Suction Fluids	**(400 ml)**				**(300 ml)**	
Primary (5% Dextrose and NaCl)	125	125	125	125	125	125
Restoration (Lactated Ringers Solution)	100	100	100	100	75	75
TOTAL	**225**	**225**	**225**	**250**	**200**	**200**

to infuse 400 mL of lactated Ringer's solution over the next 4 hours, or 100 mL/hour. The primary solution (5% dextrose/0.5% sodium chloride) will infuse at 125 mL, and the lactated Ringer's solution will infuse at 100 mL/hour for a total of 225 mL/hour. The nurse will then empty the nasogastric suction container 4 hours later and recalculate the replacement solution (Table 5–1).

This type of restoration of fluids and electrolytes is challenging for nurses. One must be on time and accurate so as not to overload the patient or get behind in fluid therapy.

SUMMARY WORKSHEET 1: Objectives of I.V. Therapy

1. MAINTENANCE THERAPY FOR DAILY BODY FLUID REQUIREMENTS

Time: Purpose: Patient Profile:

2. REPLACEMENT THERAPY FOR PREVIOUS LOSSES

Time: Purpose: Patient Profile:

Key nursing assessment 1: _____

3. RESTORATION THERAPY FOR CONCURRENT OR CONTINUING LOSSES

Time: Purpose: Patient Profile:

KEY ELEMENTS IN PARENTERAL SOLUTIONS

The key elements that make up parenteral fluids include water, carbohydrates (glucose), protein, vitamins, electrolytes, and pH.

Water

Normal maintenance requirements for water in an adult are roughly 1000 mL/day. These water needs are increased in patients with sensible water losses such as respirations above 20, fever, diaphoresis, and in low humidity; in patients with decreased renal concentration ability; and in the elderly. The average adult loses 500 to 1000 mL in the form of insensible water per 24 hours. Water must be provided for adequate kidney function.

✎ NOTE: High humidity, such as that in an incubator, minimizes insensible water loss (Metheny, 1996).

Carbohydrates (Glucose)

Glucose, a nutrient included in maintenance, restoration, and replacement therapies, is converted into glycogen by the liver, improving hepatic function. By supplying calories for energy, it spares body protein. Sources of carbohydrates include dextrose (glucose) and fructose. When glucose is supplied by infusion, all the parenteral glucose is bioavailable.

✎ NOTE: The addition of 100 g of glucose per day minimizes starvation. Every 2 liters of 5% dextrose in water contains 100 g of glucose (Weinstein, 1993).

Protein

Protein is the body-building nutrient whose major function is contributing to tissue growth and repair; replacement of body cells; healing of wounds and synthesis of vitamins and enzymes. Amino acids are the basic units of protein. Current parenteral proteins are elemental, provided as synthetic crystalline amino acids. These proteins are available in concentrations of 3% to 11.4% and are used in total parenteral nutrition (TPN) centrally or peripherally. When administered by infusion, protein bypasses the gastrointestinal and portal circulation (Metheny, 1996).

✎ NOTE: The usual daily requirement is 1 g protein/kg of body weight. For example, a 54-kg woman needs 54 g protein.

Vitamins

Vitamins are added to restorative and replacement therapies. Certain vitamins are necessary for growth and act as catalysts for metabolic processes. These are fat-soluble A, D, E, and K and water-soluble B and C. Some disease conditions alter vitamin requirements (Metheny, 1996). Vitamins B and C are the most frequently used in parenteral therapy. Vitamin B complex is important in metabolism of carbohydrates and maintaining gastrointestinal function, which is especially important in postoperative patients. Vitamin C promotes wound healing.

Electrolytes

The major additive to replacement and restorative therapies are electrolytes. The correction of electrolyte imbalances is important in prevention of serious complications associated with excess or deficit of electrolytes. There are seven major electrolytes contained in normal body fluids and seven major elements supplied in manufactured I.V. solutions (see Chapter 4 for a review of electrolyte functions). The electrolytes of major importance in parenteral therapy are potassium, sodium, chloride, magnesium, phosphorus, calcium, and bicarbonate or acetate ion (important for acid-base balance).

pH

The pH reflects the degree of acidity or alkalinity of a solution. For routine parenteral therapy, blood pH is not a significant problem. Normal kidneys can achieve an acid-base balance as long as enough water is supplied. The USP standards require that solution pH must be slightly acidic, between a pH of 3.5 and 6.2. Many solutions have a pH of 5. The acidity of solutions allows them to have a longer shelf life (Weinstein, 1993).

✎ NOTE: As the acidity of a solution increases, irritation to the vein wall increases.

HYPOTONIC, ISOTONIC, AND HYPERTONIC SOLUTIONS

The choice of I.V. solution depends on the amount of solutes in the solution and the osmolarity of the infusate. The effect of I.V. fluid on the body fluid compartments depends on how its osmolarity compares with the patient's serum osmolarity. I.V. fluids can change the fluid compartment in one of three ways: (1) they can expand the intravascular compartment; (2) they can expand the intravascular compartment and deplete the intracellular and interstitial compartments; or (3) they can expand the intracellular compartment and deplete the intravascular compartment. I.V. fluids are hypotonic, isotonic, or hypertonic, depending on the amount of solutes in the solution.

Hypotonic Fluids

Hypotonic fluids have an osmolarity below 250 mOsm/liter. By lowering serum osmolarity, the body fluids shift out of blood vessels into cells and interstitial spaces. Hypotonic solutions hydrate cells and can deplete the circulatory system.

> Example: 0.45% sodium chloride, mOsm/liter = 154.
> Uses: To hydrate cells and lower serum sodium levels.
> Caution: Hypotonic fluids cause depletion of the circulatory system.

Water moves from the vascular space to the intracellular space when hypotonic fluids are infused.

✎ NOTE: Do not give hypotonic solutions to patients with low blood pressure because it will further a hypotensive state.

Isotonic Fluids

Isotonic solutions have an osmolarity of 250 to 375 mOsm/liter. They are used to expand the extracellular fluid (ECF) compartment. Many isotonic solutions are available; the most common are:

> Examples: 0.9% sodium chloride, 5% dextrose in water, lactated Ringer's solution
> Use: To expand the intravascular compartment.
> Caution: The danger with the use of isotonic solutions is circulatory overload. These solutions do not cause fluid shifts into other compartments. The problem with overexpanding the vascular compartment is that the fluid dilutes the concentration of hemoglobin and lowers hematocrit.

Hypertonic Fluids

Hypertonic fluids have an osmolarity of 375 mOsm/liter or higher. These fluids are used to replace electrolytes. When hypertonic dextrose solutions are used alone, they also are used to shift ECF from interstitial fluid to plasma.

> Common hypertonic solutions available are:

> Examples: 5% dextrose and 0.9% sodium chloride, 5% dextrose and lactated Ringer's solution, 10% dextrose in water, 20% dextrose in water (Keithley & Fraulini, 1982).
> Uses: To replace electrolytes and to shift fluid from interstitial space to plasma.
> Caution: Hypertonic fluids are irritating to vein walls and may cause hypertonic circulatory overload.

✎ **NOTE:** Give hypertonic solutions slowly to prevent circulatory overload (Kuhn, 1994).

TYPES OF PARENTERAL SOLUTIONS

Crystalloid Solutions

Crystalloid solutions form a true solution and are capable of passing through semipermeable membranes; they can be hypotonic, isotonic, or hypertonic. The vascular fluid is 25% of the ECF, and 25% of any crystalloid administered will remain in the vascular space. Crystalloids must be given in three to four times the volume to expand the vascular space equal to a **colloid** solution. Types of crystalloid solutions include dextrose solutions, sodium chloride solutions, multiple electrolyte solutions, and alkalizing and acidifying solutions.

Dextrose in Water

Carbohydrates can be administered by parenteral route as dextrose, fructose, or invert sugar. Dextrose is the most commonly administered carbohydrate. Approximately 1600 calories are needed daily for an adult at bedrest; this is a basal figure and does not allow for fever or other causes of increased metabolism (Metheny, 1996). When carbohydrate needs are inadequate, the body will use its own fat to supply calories. Dextrose fluids are used to provide calories for energy, reduce catabolism of protein, and reduce protein breakdown of glucose to help prevent a negative nitrogen balance (Weinstein, 1993). See Table 5–2 for the types of available dextrose solutions.

125

TABLE 5–2. CONTENTS OF AVAILABLE INTRAVENOUS FLUIDS

Solution	Osmolarity	Dextrose	pH	Cal/100 mL	Na	Cl	K	Ca	Mg	Acete	Lactate
Dextrose in Water (D/W)											
2.5%D/W	Hypotonic	2.5		8							
5% D/W	Isotonic	5	4.8	17							
10% D/W	Hypertonic	10	4.7	34							
20% D/W	Hypertonic	20	2.8	68							
50% D/W	Hypertonic	50	4.6	170							
70% D/W	Hypertonic	70		237							
Sodium Chloride (NaCl)											
0.2% NaCl (1/4 strength)	Hypotonic				34	34					
0.45% NaCl (1/2 strength)	Hypotonic		5.9		77	77					
0.9% NaCl (full strength)	Isotonic		6.0		154	154					
3% NaCl	Hypertonic		6.0		513	513					
5% NaCl	Hypertonic				855	855					
Dextrose and Sodium Chloride (D/NaCl)											
0.2% D and 0.9% NaCl	Isotonic										
5% D and 0.2% NaCl	Isotonic	5	4.6	17	34	34					
5% D and 0.45% NaCl	Hypertonic	5	4.6	17	77	77					
5% D and 0.9% NaCl	Hypertonic	5	4.4	17	154	154					
2.5% D and 0.45% NaCl	Hypotonic										
5% D and 0.45% NaCl	Hypertonic										
Multiple Electrolyte Solutions											
Lactated Ringer's	Isotonic		6.5		130	109	4	3			28
Ringer's injection	Isotonic		6.0		147	156	4	4			
Normosol-R	Isotonic		6.4	18	140	98	5		3	27	
Plasmalyte-A	Isotonic		7.4		140	98	5		3	27	
Isolyte E	Isotonic		6.0		140	103	10		3	49	
Specialty Solutions											
1/6M Sodium lactate	Hypertonic		6.5		167						167
10% Mannitol	Hypertonic		5.7								
20% Mannitol	Hypertonic		5.7								
NaHCO$_3$	Hypertonic		8.0		595						595
6% Dextran and 0.9% NaCl	Isotonic		4.5		154	154					
10% Dextran and 0.9% NaCl	Isotonic		4.5		154	154					

Ca = Calcium; Cal = calories; Cl = chloride; K = potassium; Mg = magnesium.

It is difficult to administer enough calories by I.V. infusion, especially with 5% dextrose in water, which provides only 170 calories/liter. One would have to administer 9 liters to meet calorie requirements and most patients cannot tolerate 9000 mL of fluid in 24 hours. Concentrated solutions of carbohydrates in 20% to 70% dextrose are useful for supplying calories. The solutions containing high percentages of dextrose must be administered slowly for adequate absorption and utilization by the cells (Metheny, 1992).

Dextrose is a nonelectrolyte, and the total number of particles in a dextrose solution does not depend on ionization. Dextrose is thought to be the closest to the ideal carbohydrate available because it is well metabolized by all tissue. The tonicity of dextrose solutions depends on the particles of sugar in the solution. Dextrose 5% is rapidly metabolized and has no osmotically active particle once in the plasma. The osmolarity of a dextrose solution is determined differently from that of an electrolyte solution. Dextrose is distributed inside and outside the cells, with 8% remaining in the circulation to increase blood volume. The USP pH requirements for dextrose is 3.5 to 6.5 (Weinstein, 1993).

✎ **NOTE:** Hypotonic solutions hydrate the intracellular compartment more than they hydrate the intravascular space.

The other two types of carbohydrates used for infusions, fructose and invert sugar, have their own specific uses. Fructose is similar to glucose but less irritating to veins. The important point about fructose is that it can be metabolized by adipose tissue independent of insulin. However, fructose cannot be used if the patient is in acidosis. Invert sugar contains the same equimolar quantities of glucose and fructose, but less invert sugar is lost in the urine (Metheny, 1996).

ADVANTAGES
- Acts as a vehicle for administration of medications
- Provides nutrition
- Can be used as treatment for hyperkalemia (using high concentrations of dextrose)
- Can be used in treatment of dehydration
- Provides free water

✎ **NOTE:** Before any medication is added to a dextrose solution, compatibility information should be checked. Dextrose may also affect the stability of admixtures (e.g., ampicillin sodium) (Terry & Hedrick, 1995).

DISADVANTAGES
- Solutions of 20% to 70% dextrose, if infused rapidly, act as an osmotic diuretic and pull interstitial fluid into plasma, causing severe cellular dehydration. Any solution of dextrose infused rapidly can place the patient at risk for dehydration. To prevent this adverse reaction, infuse the dextrose solution at the prescribed rate.

✎ **NOTE:** Do not play "catch up" if the solution infusion is behind schedule. Make sure the I.V. solution does not "run away" and infuse rapidly into the patient.

If 20% to 70% dextrose is infused too rapidly, it can irritate the vein wall. Rapid infusion of 20% to 70% dextrose can also lead to transient hyperinsulin reaction, in which the pancreas secretes extra insulin to metabolize the infused dextrose. Sudden discontinuation of any hypertonic dextrose solution may leave a temporary excess of insulin. To prevent hyperinsulinism, infuse an isotonic dextrose solution (5% to

127

10%) to wean patient off hypertonic dextrose. The infusion rate should be gradually decreased over 48 hours. When administering dextrose solutions, remember that they do not provide any electrolytes. Dextrose solutions cannot replace or correct electrolyte deficits, and continuous infusion of 5% dextrose in water places the patient at risk for deficits in sodium, potassium, and chloride. Also, dextrose cannot be mixed with blood components because it causes hemolysis (agglomeration) of the cells.

Sodium Chloride

Sodium chloride injection (0.9%) is an isotonic solution. It is isotonic owing to the higher than normal sodium (Na^+) and chloride (Cl^-) ions. Sodium chloride 0.9% solution has 154 mEq of both sodium and chloride or about 9% higher than normal plasma levels of sodium and chloride ions without other plasma electrolytes. See Table 5–2 for the type of available sodium chloride solutions.

ADVANTAGES
- Provides ECF replacement when chloride loss is greater than or equal to sodium losses (e.g., a patient on nasogastric suctioning)
- Treats metabolic alkalosis in the presence of fluid loss (the 154 mEq of chloride will help compensate for the increase in bicarbonate ions)
- Treats sodium depletion
- Initiates or terminates a blood transfusion (the saline solutions are the *only* solutions to be used with any blood product)

DISADVANTAGES
- Provides more sodium and chloride than a patient needs, causing hypernatremia. The adult dietary sodium requirements are 90 to 250 mEq daily. (Three liters of sodium chloride [0.9%] will provide the patient with 462 mEq of sodium, a level that exceeds normal tolerance.) To prevent this overload of electrolytes, assess for signs and symptoms of sodium retention.

✎ NOTE: During stress, the body retains sodium, adding to hypernatremia.

- Can cause acidosis in patients receiving continuous infusions of 0.9% sodium chloride because sodium chloride provides one third more chloride than is present in ECF. The excess chloride leads to loss of bicarbonate ions, leading to an imbalance of acid.
- May cause low potassium levels (hypokalemia), because of the lack of the other important electrolytes over a period of time.
- Can lead to circulatory overload. Isotonic fluids expand the ECF compartment, which can lead to overload of the cardiovascular compartments.

✎ NOTE: Hypotonic saline (0.45%) can be used to supply normal daily salt and water requirements safely. Hypertonic saline solution (3% to 5%) is used only to correct severe sodium depletion and water overload (Keithley & Fraulini, 1982).
Be aware of the increased dangers in administering saline solutions to elderly patients, patients with severe dehydration, and patients with chronic glomerulonephritis.

Dextrose and Sodium Chloride

When sodium chloride is infused, the addition of 100 g dextrose prevents formation of ketone bodies. Dextrose prevents catabolism and consequently the loss of potassium and intracellular water (Weinstein, 1993).

128

Carbohydrates and sodium chloride fluid combinations are best used when there has been an excessive loss of fluid through sweating, vomiting, or gastric suctioning (Kuhn, 1994). See Table 5–2 for types of available dextrose and sodium chloride solutions.

ADVANTAGES
- Temporarily treats circulatory insufficiency and shock due to hypovolemia in the immediate absence of a plasma expander
- Provides early treatment of burns, along with plasma or albumin
- Replaces nutrient and electrolytes
- Acts as a hydrating solution to check kidney function before replacement of potassium

DISADVANTAGES
- Same as for sodium chloride solutions (see earlier section): hypernatremia, acidosis, and circulatory overload

Hydrating Fluids

Solutions that contain dextrose and hypotonic saline provide more water than is required for excretion of salt and useful as hydrating fluids. Hydrating fluids are used to assess the status of the kidneys. The administration of a hydrating solution at a rate of 8 mL/m^2 of body surface per minute for 45 minutes is called a *fluid challenge*. When urinary flow is established, it indicates that the kidneys have begun to function; the hydrating solution may then be replaced with a specific electrolyte solution. If after 45 minutes the urinary flow is not restored, the rate of infusion should be reduced and monitoring of the patient should continue without electrolyte additives (especially potassium) (Metheny, 1996). Carbohydrates in hydrating solutions reduce depletion of nitrogen and liver glycogen and are also useful in rehydrating cells. See Table 5–2 for types of hydrating fluids.

ADVANTAGES
- Assesses the status of the kidneys before replacement therapy is started
- Hydrates patients in dehydrated states
- Promotes diuresis in dehydrated patients (Weinstein, 1993)

DISADVANTAGES
- Requires cautious administration in edematous patients (e.g., patients with cardiac, renal, or liver disease)

✎ NOTE: Do not give potassium to any patient unless kidney function has been established. Use hydrating fluid to check kidney function.

Multiple Electrolyte Fluids

A variety of balanced electrolyte fluids are available commercially. Balanced fluids are available as hypotonic or isotonic maintenance and replacement solutions. Maintenance fluids approximate normal body electrolyte needs; replacement fluids contain one or more electrolytes in amounts over those found in normal body fluids. Balanced fluids also may contain lactate or acetate (yielding bicarbonate), which helps to combat acidosis and provide a truly "balanced solution." See Table 5–2 for types of multiple electrolyte solution.

129

Multiple electrolyte fluids are recommended for use in patients with trauma, alimentary tract fluid losses, dehydration, sodium depletion, acidosis, and burns (Keithley & Faundini, 1982).

✎ **NOTE:** Dextrose (5%) is usually added to balanced multiple electrolyte solutions.

Balanced Hypotonic Fluids (Maintenance Fluids)

Hypotonic balanced multiple electrolyte fluids are used for maintaining body homeostasis. These solutions contain 5% dextrose for its protein-sparing effect. Dextrose increases tonicity of these solutions. The balancing of hypotonic electrolytes (lower than within normal body levels) is ideal for maintaining body homeostasis. Balanced solutions contain sodium, potassium, calcium, magnesium, chloride, and lactate. Potassium is usually not added to maintenance multiple electrolyte fluids.

Hypotonic multiple electrolyte fluids are used for (1) routine maintenance, (2) conditions that increase fluid losses through urine, stool, or expired air, and (3) stress leading to inappropriate release of antidiuretic hormone.

ADVANTAGES
- Useful for maintaining water: Water maintenance equals 1600 mL/m^2 body surface area per day (Drug and Therapeutic Information, 1970). Because of the hypotonicity of these multiple electrolyte fluids, water should be provided for urinary and metabolic needs to take advantage of the body's homeostatic mechanisms (Weinstein, 1993).

DISADVANTAGES
- Hyperkalemia
- Water intoxication

Balanced Isotonic Fluids

Balanced isotonic multiple electrolyte fluids do not contain dextrose.

Balanced Isotonic and Hypertonic Fluids (Replacement Fluids)

Many types of replacement fluids are available. Special fluids are available by each manufacturer for gastric replacement, which provide the typical electrolytes lost by vomiting or gastric suction. These isotonic fluids usually contain ammonium ions, which are metabolized in the liver to hydrogen ions and urea, replacing hydrogen ions lost in gastric juices. Lactated Ringer's injection is considered an isotonic multiple electrolyte solution.

Hypertonic multiple electrolyte solutions are also used as replacement fluids and usually have the addition of 5% dextrose, which raises the osmolarity of the solution.

✎ **NOTE:** Do not use gastric replacement fluid in patients with hepatic insufficiency or renal failure.

ADVANTAGES
- Isotonic multiple electrolyte solutions are balanced and have an ionic composition similar to that of plasma.

DISADVANTAGES
- May cause hypernatremia (3 liters of isotonic multiple electrolyte fluid can provide up to 390 mEq of sodium).

130

Lactate Fluids

The Ringer's solutions (Ringer's injection and lactated Ringer's injection) are classified as balanced or isotonic solutions because their fluid and electrolyte content is similar to that of plasma. They are used to replace electrolytes at physiologic levels in the ECF compartment. Ringer's injection is a fluid and electrolyte replenisher, which is used over 0.9% sodium chloride for treatment of dehydration after reduced water intake or water loss. Lactated Ringer's injection is the most commonly prescribed solution. Ringer's injection and lactated Ringer's fluids are used for the following:

- Treatment of any type of dehydration
- Restoration of fluid balance before and after surgery
- Replacement of fluids lost in burns
- Peritoneal irrigation
- Treatment of metabolic acidosis that occurs with mild renal insufficiency
- Treatment of infant diarrhea
- Treatment of diabetic ketoacidosis
- Treatment of salicylate overdose

Ringer's Injection

Ringer's solution (injection) is similar to normal saline with the substitution of potassium and calcium for some of the sodium ions in concentrations equal to the plasma. Ringer's injection, however, is superior to 0.9% sodium chloride as a fluid and electrolyte replenisher and it is preferred to normal saline for treatment of dehydration after drastically reduced water intake or water loss (e.g., with vomiting, diarrhea, or fistula drainage).

Ringer's injection does not contain enough potassium or calcium to be used as a maintenance fluid or to correct a deficit of these electrolytes (Remington, in Griffith, 1986).

Lactated Ringer's Injection

ADVANTAGES
- Contains less sodium, calcium, and chloride than the Ringer's injection but contains the bicarbonate precursor to assist in acidosis.
- Most similar to the body's extracellular electrolyte content.

DISADVANTAGES
- Lactated Ringer's solution should not be used in patients with impaired lactate metabolism, such as patients with:
- Liver disease
- Addison's disease
- Severe metabolic acidosis or alkalosis
- Profound hypovolemia
- Profound shock or cardiac failure

In these patients, serum lactate levels may already be elevated (Griffith, 1986).

Alkalizing Fluids and Acidifying Infusions Fluids

Alkalizing

Metabolic acidosis can occur in clinical situations in which dehydration, shock, liver disease, starvation, or diabetes causes retention of chlorides, ketone bodies, or organic salts or when excessive bicarbonate is lost. Treatment consists of infusion of

131

an alkalizing fluid. Two I.V. fluids are available when excessive bicarbonate is lost and metabolic acidosis occurs: 1/6 molar isotonic sodium lactate and 5% sodium bicarbonate injection. The lactate ion must be oxidized in the body to carbon dioxide before it can affect acid-base balance. Sodium lactate to bicarbonate requires 1 to 2 hours. Oxygen is needed to increase bicarbonate concentrations.

Alkalizing fluids are used for vomiting, starvation, uncontrolled diabetes mellitus, acute infections, renal failure, and severe acidosis with severe hyperpnea (sodium bicarbonate injection).

The 1/6 molar sodium lactate solution is useful whenever acidosis has resulted from sodium deficiency. The isotonic solution sodium bicarbonate injection provides bicarbonate ions in clinical situations in which excessive bicarbonate is lost.

✎ **NOTE:** The reason sodium bicarbonate injection is used to relieve dyspnea and hyperpnea is that the bicarbonate ion is released in the form of carbon dioxide through the lungs, leaving behind an excess of sodium.

The 1/6 molar sodium lactate fluid is *contraindicated* in patients suffering from lack of oxygen or in patients with liver disease. Patients receiving this fluid should be watched for signs of hypocalcemic tetany (Weinstein, 1993).

Acidifying

Metabolic alkalosis is a condition associated with an excess of bicarbonate and deficit of chloride. Isotonic sodium chloride (0.9%) provides conservative treatment of metabolic alkalosis. Ammonium chloride is the solution used to treat metabolic alkalosis. Acidifying fluids are used for severe metabolic alkalosis due to loss of gastric secretions or pyloric stenosis.

An advantage is that the ammonium ion is converted by the liver to hydrogen ion and to ammonia, which is excreted as urea. However, a disadvantage is that ammonium chloride must be infused at a slow rate to enable the liver to metabolize the ammonium ion. In fact, rapid infusion can result in toxicity, causing irregular breathing and bradycardia.

✎ **NOTE:** This I.V. fluid must be used with caution in patients with severe hepatic disease or renal failure and is contraindicated in any condition with a high ammonium level.

Potassium Chloride

Several premixed solutions of potassium chloride (KCl) are available from the manufacturer. Potassium, 20 mEq or 40 mEq, is added to 5% dextrose in water or 5% dextrose and 0.45% sodium chloride. Follow special nursing considerations in administration of I.V. KCl. See Table 4–4 for critical guidelines for the administration of potassium chloride fluids. Note that the electrolyte is clearly marked in red to distinguish it from I.V. solutions without additives.

SUMMARY WORKSHEET 2: Parenteral Crystalloid Solutions

DEXTROSE
Uses:

Advantages:
1.
2.
3.
4.

Disadvantages:
1.
2.
3.
4.

SODIUM CHLORIDE
Uses:

Advantages:
1.
2.
3.
4.

Disadvantages:
1.
2.
3.
4.

DEXTROSE AND SODIUM CHLORIDE
Uses:

Advantages:
1.
2.
3.
4.

Disadvantages:
1.
2.
3.

MULTIPLE ELECTROLYTE FLUIDS
Uses:

Advantages: Disadvantages:

   Ringer's Injection   *Ringer's Injection*

   Lactated Ringer's   *Lactated Ringer's*

ALKALIZING AND ACIDIFYING FLUIDS
Uses:

Advantages: Disadvantages:

   Alkalizing Fluids   *Alkalizing Fluids*

   Acidifying Fluids   *Acidifying Fluids*

134

Colloid Solutions

Patients with fluid and electrolyte disturbances occasionally require treatment with colloids. Colloid solutions contain protein or starch molecules which remain distributed in the extracellular space and do not form a "true" solution. When colloid molecules are administered, they remain in the vascular space for several days in patients with normal capillary endothelium. These fluids increase the osmotic pressure within the plasma space, drawing fluid to increase intravascular volume.

Colloid solutions do not dissolve and do not flow freely between fluid compartments. Infusion of a colloid solution increases intravascular colloid osmotic pressure (pressure of plasma proteins). Colloid solutions are further discussed in the chapter.

Dextran

Dextran fluids are polysaccharides that behave as colloids. They are available as low molecular weight dextran (Dextran 40) and high molecular weight dextran (Dextran 70). Dextran 70 is more effective than dextran 40 as a substitute for plasma expansion. It is important to monitor pulse, blood pressure, and urine output every 5 to 15 minutes for the first hour of administration of dextran and then every hour. Dextran should be administered at a rate of 20 mL/kg of body weight over 24 hours to prevent hypersensitivity reactions and decrease risk of bleeding (Phillips & Kuhn, 1996).

Dextran fluids are used for plasma substitute or expansion. An advantage of dextran use is that the intravascular space is expanded in excess of the volume infused. Disadvantages are hypersensitivity reactions (anaphylaxis) and an increased risk of bleeding.

✎ **NOTE:** Dextran is contraindicated in patients with severe bleeding disorder, congestive heart failure, and renal failure. It is important to draw blood for typing and cross-matching prior to administration of dextran.

Albumin

Albumin is a natural plasma protein prepared from donor plasma. This colloid is available as a 5% or 25% solution. Five percent albumin is osmotically and oncotically equivalent to plasma. The 25% solution is equivalent to 500 mL of plasma or 2 U of whole blood (Phillips & Kuhn, 1996).

Albumin is used for maintenance of blood volume, emergency treatment of shock due to acute blood loss, hypovolemic shock caused by plasma rather than whole blood loss, hypoproteinemic conditions and treatment of erythroblastosis fetalis (25% solution).

ADVANTAGES
- These products are subject to an extended heating period during preparation and therefore do not transmit viral disease.

DISADVANTAGES
- May precipitate allergic reactions (urticaria, flushing, chills, fever, or headache)
- May cause circulatory overload (greatest risk with 25% albumin)
- May cause pulmonary edema
- May alter laboratory findings

✎ **NOTE:** Albumin is not a source of nutrition (Phillips & Kuhn, 1996).

Mannitol

Mannitol is a sugar alcohol substance that is available in concentrations from 5% to 25%. It is used to promote diuresis in oliguric acute renal failure, promote excretion of toxic substances in the body, reduce excess cerebrospinal fluid, reduce intraocular pressure, and treat intracranial pressure and cerebral edema.

ADVANTAGES
- May reduce excess cerebrospinal fluid within 15 minutes

DISADVANTAGES
- May cause fluid and electrolyte imbalances
- May cause cell dehydration or fluid overload by drawing fluid from cells into the vascular system
- Requires cautious use for patients with impaired cardiac or renal system
- May lead to skin irritation and tissue necrosis because of extravasation of mannitol (Terry & Hedrick, 1995)

Hetastarch

Hetastarch (hydroxyethyl glucose) is a synthetic colloid made from starch. It is available under the name Hespan as a 6% or 10% solution, diluted in isotonic sodium chloride in a 500-mL container. These starches are not derived from donor plasma and are therefore less toxic and less expensive. Hetastarch is equal in plasma volume expansion properties to 5% human albumin.

ADVANTAGES
- Hetastarch does not interfere with blood typing and cross-matching, as do other colloidal solutions.

DISADVANTAGES
- The possibility of allergic reaction
- Hetastarch may alter the coagulation mechanism, that is, with transient prolongation of the prothrombin, partial thromboplastin, and clotting times.

Thus, this solution is contraindicated in patients with severe bleeding disorders, severe congestive heart failure, and anuric renal failure (Terry & Hedrick, 1995).

✎ **NOTE:** Use cautiously in patients whose conditions predispose them to fluid retention.

See Table 5–3 for a summary of common I.V. fluids—their composition, uses, advantages, and disadvantages.

TABLE 5-3. QUICK-GLANCE CHART OF COMMON I.V. FLUIDS

Product	Uses	Advantages	Side Effects/Precautions
Carbohydrate Solutions 5% Dextrose 10% Dextrose 20% Dextroe 50% Dextrose	• Provides calories • Provides free water • Acts as a diluent for I.V. drugs • Treats dehydration • Treats hyperkalemia	Spares body protein; provides nutrition	Possible compromise of glucose tolerance by stress, sepsis, hepatic and renal failure, corticosteroids, and diuretics; does not provide any electrolytes; may cause vein irritation, water intoxication, and possible agglomeration **Note** Hypertonic fluids may cause hyperglycemia, osmotic diuresis, hyperosomolar coma, or hyperinsulinism
Sodium Chloride (NaCl) Solutions 0.2% NaCl 0.45% NaCl 0.9% NaCl	• Replaces sodium and chloride • Treats hyperosmolar diabetes • Acts as a diluent for I.V. drug administration • Used for initiation and discontinuation of blood products	Replaces ECF, electrolytes	Hyponatremia (excessive use of 0.25 or 0.45% NaCl); calorie depletion; hypernatremia or hyperchloremia; circulatory overload; deficit of other electrolyte
3% and 5%	• Replaces severe sodium and chloride deficit • Helps to correct water overload	Same as NaCl fluids	Same as NaCl fluids

(continued)

PARENTERAL SOLUTIONS

TABLE 5–3. QUICK-GLANCE CHART OF COMMON I.V. FLUIDS (*Continued*)

Product	Uses	Advantages	Side Effects/Precautions
Combination Dextrose and NaCl Solutions			
5% Dextrose/0.2% NaCl 5% Dextrose/0.45% NaCl 5% Dextrose/0.9% NaCl	• For temporary treatment of circulatory insufficiency hydrating fluids • Replaces nutrients and electrolytes	Assesses kidney function; hydrates cells; promotes diuresis	Cautious use in edematous patients, patients with cardiac, renal or liver disease
Note: 5% and 0.2% NaCl and 5% D/0.45% NaCl are hydration solutions.			
Multiple Electrolyte Solutions Maintenance: Normosol-M Plasmalyte-A	• Provides routine maintenance • Relieves stress leading to inappropriate release of the antidiuretic hormone • Provides free water	Provides calories; provides electrolytes	Hyperkalemia; water intoxication
Replacement: Normosol-R Isolyte E Plasmalyte-R Lactated Ringer's Ringer's injection	• Replaces fluid for severe vomiting, diarrhea, or diuresis • Corrects metabolic alkalosis loss • Replaces fluid loss from trauma or burns • Replaces fluid losses for alimentary tract losses and in hyponatremia	Ionic composition similar to plasma	Hypernatremia; contraindicated in metabolic acidosis **Note:** Lactated Ringer's solution is contraindicated in liver disease, Addison's disease, severe metabolic acidosis and alkalosis, and profound hypovolemia. Ringer's injection does not provide enough potassium or calcium to be used as a maintenance fluid.

Specialty Fluids

Alkalizing:		
Sodium bicarbonate 1/6 molar sodium lactate	• Corrects metabolic acidosis • Reduces severe hyperkalemia • Treats uncontrolled diabetes mellitus, acute infections, and renal failure	Treats metabolic acidosis; relieves dyspnea and hyperpnea	1/6 Molar contraindicated in patients suffering from lack of oxygen or in those with liver disease; hypcalcemic tetany
Plasma expanders:		
6% and 10% Dextran	• Counteracts shock/anticipated shock related to trauma, surgery, burns, or hemorrhage • Prevents venous thrombosis and pulmonary embolism prophylactically during surgery • Promotes diuresis and excretion of toxic substances • Increases granulocyte yield during leukapheresis	Provides plasma expansion	Hypersensitivity reactions; increased risk of bleeding; hypervolemia preexisting conditions should be considered (e.g., renal or cardiac disease)
10% and 20% Mannitol		Reduces intraocular pressure; decreases intracranial pressure, reducing cerebral edema	Hypervolemia, extravasation, skin irritation, and tissue necrosis; interferes with laboratory testing **Note:** Preexisting conditions should be considered with caution owing to possible crystal formation.
5% and 25% Albumin	• Counteracts shock/impending shock due to hypovolemia • Provides protein (for hypoproteinemia) • Treats hyperbilirubinemia and erythroblastosis fetalis	Extensive heating period during preparation prevents transmission of viral disease	Allergic reactions; circulatory overload; alteration of laboratory tests
6% or 10% Hetastarch	• Provides volume expansion • Leukapheresis	Does not interfere with blood typing and cross-matching	May alter coagulation mechanism; allergic reactions; hypervolemia

SUMMARY WORKSHEET 3: Parenteral Colloid Solutions

Dextran

Uses:

Advantages: Disadvantages:

Albumin

Uses:

Advantages: Disadvantages:

Mannitol

Uses:

Advantages: Disadvantages:

Hetastarch

Uses:

Advantages: Disadvantages:

Nursing Plan of Care

ADMINISTRATION OF PARENTERAL FLUIDS

Focus Criteria for Assessment

Subjective

History of present illness of fluid loss

Objective

Observe ability to ingest and retain fluids.
Monitor vital signs.
Monitor weight.
Assess symptoms of fluid disturbance.
Assess for complications associated with infusion therapy (phlebitis, erratic flow rates, infiltration)

Nursing Diagnoses

Anxiety (mild, moderate, severe) related to threat to or change in health status; misconceptions regarding therapy
Altered nutrition less than body requirements related to inability to ingest or digest food or absorb nutrients; inadequate nutrient replacement
Decreased cardiac output related to reaction to parenteral solution, contamination
Fluid volume excess related to infusion of I.V. fluid
Knowledge deficit related to new procedure and maintaining I.V. therapy
Fluid volume deficit related to deviations affecting intake and absorption of fluids; factors influencing fluid needs (e.g., hypermetabolic state)
Impaired tissue integrity related to irritating fluids
Risk for infection related to broken skin or traumatized tissue
Risk for sleep pattern disturbance related to external sensory stimuli (e.g., I.V. fluid and tubing)

Patient Outcome Criteria

The patient will:
Demonstrate improved fluid balance as evidenced by urine output of 30 mL/hour with normal specific gravity, stable vital signs, moist mucous membranes, good skin turgor and capillary refill of less than 3 seconds.
Verbalize understanding of condition and treat.

Nursing Management: Critical Activities

Administer I.V. fluids at room temperature.
Administer I.V. medications at prescribed rate and monitor for results.
Monitor I.V. site during infusion.
Monitor for fluid overload and physical reactions.
Monitor for I.V. patency prior to administration of I.V. medications.
Replace I.V. cannula, apparatus every 48–72 hours.
Replace fluid containers at least every 24 hours.
Flush I.V. lines between administration of incompatible solutions.
Record intake and output.
Monitor urine output and specific gravity.
Provide information outlining current I.V. therapy.
Maintain universal precautions.
(McCloskey & Bulechek, 1992)

PATIENT EDUCATION

Instruct on reason for therapy (e.g., replacement fluid, vitamins, nutrition, volume replacement)

Instruct to report signs and symptoms of complications (e.g., burning at infusion site, redness, any discomfort).

HOME CARE ISSUES

Most infusion therapies in the home are used for delivery of specific treatment such as antibiotics, chemotherapy, total parenteral nutrition, growth hormones, blood products, and hydration therapy.

Home care for hydration therapy is used for dehydration and fluid and electrolyte imbalance resulting from:

Cardiopulmonary disorders
Fistulas
Hyperemesis gravidarum
Intractable diarrhea
Chemotherapy (before and after)
Radiation enteritis
Short-bowel syndrome

Short-term therapy lasts from 1 to 7 days and is usually administered via a peripheral lock or long-term access device. Be sure to educate hydration patients about the need for therapy, aseptic technique, set-up and administration of specific solution, and possible complications. Monitor home care patients' weight, hydration status, and laboratory tests (Grace & Tomaselli, 1995).

COMPETENCY CRITERIA: Administration of Parenteral Fluids

Competency Statement: The competent I.V. therapy nurse will be able to deliver parenteral therapy safely following policy and standardized procedures.

COGNITIVE CRITERIA

	Skilled	Needs Education
1. Identifies composition, uses, advantages, and disadvantages of solutions:		
Carbohydrate fluids		
Sodium chloride fluids		
Alkalinizing fluids		
Acidifying fluids		
Multiple electrolyte fluids		

PERFORMANCE CRITERIA

	Skilled	Needs Education
1. Verify appropriate fluid type, rate, and volume of delivery.		
2. Inspects fluids for abnormalities and defects.		
3. Describe I.V. tubing and dressing maintenance policies.		
4. Document appropriately according to institutional policy.		
5. Educate patient and family concerning I.V. therapy.		

SUGGESTED EVALUATION CRITERIA

1. Observation of nurse administering I.V. therapy

2. Written test on composition of I.V. fluids

143

KEY POINTS

Parenteral solutions
Three main objectives of I.V. therapy:
    Maintain daily requirements
    Replace previous losses
    Restore concurrent losses

Key elements in parenteral therapy
    Water
    Carbohydrates
    Protein
    Vitamins
    Electrolytes
The pH is important in acidity of the solution and its stability.

Hypotonic, Isotonic, and Hypertonic Solutions
    Hypotonic
        250 mOsm/liter or below
    Isotonic
        Range between 250 mOsm/liter and 375 mOsm/liter
    Hypertonic
        Above 375 mOsm/liter

Types of parenteral fluids
    Crystalloid solutions
        Dextrose in water
        Sodium chloride
        Dextrose and sodium chloride
        Hydrating fluids
        Multiple electrolyte fluids
        Alkalizing fluids and acidifying infusions
        Potassium chloride
    Colloid solutions
        Dextran
        Albumin
        Mannitol
        Hetastarch

CRITICAL THINKING ACTIVITY

1. Describe a situation in which you observed a solution administered too rapidly.

2. Become familiar with the solutions available in your work environment. Are they primarily solutions without additives? If they are multiple electrolyte solutions, are they arranged on the shelf so as not to be mistaken for each other?

3. The solutions with red lettering on top are usually solutions with additives such as lidocaine and aminophylline. How are these solutions dispensed at your facility? Are they in such a place that they could be "grabbed" by mistake and hung in an emergency?

4. You discover that a solution has been rapidly infused into a patient. Can this potentially harm the patient? What would you do to remedy this situation?

POST-TEST, CHAPTER 5

Match the term in column I with the definition in column II.

Column I

1. _____ crystalloid
2. _____ hydrating solution
3. __B__ homeostasis
4. _____ colloid
5. _____ catabolism

Column II

A. Substance does not dissolve, does not pass through a semipermeable membrane

B. Ability to restore equilibrium

C. Solution of water, carbohydrate, sodium chloride used to check kidney function

D. Breakdown of chemical compounds by the body energy producing metabolic process

E. A substance that forms a true solution

6. The three objectives of I.V. therapy are:
   A. Maintenance, peristaltic, and replacement therapy
   B. Replacement, expansion, and restoration therapy
   C. Maintenance, replacement, and restoration therapy
   D. Restoration, hydration, and dehydration therapy

7. The functions of glucose in parenteral therapy include all of the following except:
   A. Provides calories for energy
   B. Helps to prevent negative nitrogen balance
   C. Reduces catabolism of protein
   D. Serves as vehicle for blood transfusions

8. Maintenance solutions are used for patients who are:
   A. Having nothing by mouth for a short period of time.
   B. Experiencing hemorrhage
   C. Dehydrated from gastrointestinal losses
   D. Experiencing draining fistulas

Match the term in column I with the definition in column II

Column I

9. _____ hypotonic
10. _____ isotonic
11. _____ hypertonic

Column II

A. Osmolarity of 375 mOsm/liter and higher. Replaces electrolytes

B. Equal to blood plasma

C. Used for cellular dehydration; osmolarity below 250 mOsm/liter

12. The average adult insensible loss is between _____ and _____ mL/day.

13. The main role of a hydrating solution is to_____

_____ .

14. Identify two uses of lactated solutions.

_____

_____

15. The most commonly used multiple electrolyte solution is _____ .

16. List one advantage and one disadvantage of the following three groups of fluids.

Dextrose Fluids

Advantage: Disadvantage:

Sodium Chloride Fluids

Advantage: Disadvantage:

Multiple Electrolyte Fluids

Advantage: Disadvantage:

17. Dr. Jacob orders 1000 mL of 5% dextrose/0.45% sodium chloride to infuse every 8 hours for Mrs. Black. Mrs. Black has a nasogastric tube to suction. Dr. Jacob additionally orders lactated Ringer's injection as a replacement for gastric losses mL for mL every 4 hours. How many mL/hour total will you be giving Mrs. Black if you empty the nasogastric tube as 8 AM and have a 500-mL output of gastric contents.
    _____ mL/hour of primary solution
    _____ mL/hour of nasogastric replacement solution
    _____ Total mL/hour

ANSWERS TO CHAPTER 5

PRE-TEST

1. A
2. C
3. B
4. Free water, carbohydrates, electrolytes, protein, vitamins, and pH
5. B
6. C
7. E
8. A
9. D
10. A
11. A
12. E
13. C
14. A
15. C
16. B
17. C

POST-TEST

1. E
2. C
3. B
4. A
5. D
6. C
7. D
8. A
9. C
10. B
11. A
12. 500 to 1000 mL/day
13. Check kidney function before administration of potassium.
14. To treat dehydration
    To restore fluid balance before and after surgery
    To restore fluid loss in infant diarrhea
    To treat diabetic ketoacidosis
    To provide short-term replacement for blood
15. Lactated Ringer's injection

16. Dextrose fluids
    Advantages:
       Vehicle for administration of
         medication
       Provide nutrition
       Treat hyperkalemia
       Treat dehydration
    Sodium chloride fluids
    Advantages:
       Replace extracellular fluid
       Treat metabolic alkalosis
       Treat sodium depletion
       Initiate blood transfusion
    Multiple electrolyte fluids
    Advantages:
       Treat acidosis
       Replace fluids and electrolytes

    Disadvantage:
       Acts as osmotic diuretic if infused too
         rapidly

    Disadvantages:
       Hypernatremia
       Overload of sodium and chloride
       Circulatory overload

    Disadvantage:
       Circulatory overload

17. 125 mL/hour of primary solution
    125 mL/hour of replacement solution
    250 mL/hour total

REFERENCES

Drug and Therapeutic Information, Inc. (1970). Parenteral water and electrolyte solutions. *Medical Letter on Drugs and Therapeutics, 12*(19), 77.

Gasparis, L., Murray, E.B., & Ursomanno, P. (1989). I.V. Solutions—Which one's right for your patient? *Nursing 89, 4,* 62–64.

Grace, L.A., & Tomaselli, B.J. (1995). Intravenous therapy in the home. In Terry, J., Baranowski, L., Lonsway, R. & Hedrick, C. (eds.): *Intravenous therapy: Clinical principles and practice.* Philadelphia: W.B. Saunders, p. 513.

Griffith, C.A. (1986). The family of Ringer's solutions. *Journal of Intravenous Therapy Association, 9,* 480–483.

Keithley, J.K. & Fraulini, K.E. (1982). What's behind that I.V. line? *Nursing 82,* 34–42.

Kuhn, M. (1994). *Pharmacotherapeutics: A nursing process approach* (3rd ed). Philadelphia: F.A. Davis, 173–193.

McCloskey, J.C., & Bulechek, G.M. (1992). *Iowa intervention project: Nursing interventions classification (NIC).* St. Louis: Mosby-Year Book, p. 320.

Metheny, N.M. (1996). *Fluid and electrolyte balance: Nursing considerations* (3rd ed). Philadelphia: J.B. Lippincott, pp. 169–171.

Moore, V.B. (1973). I.V. fluids. *Nursing 73, 6,* 32–38.

O'Shea, M.H. (1993). Fluid and electrolyte management. In Woodley, M. & Whelan, A. (eds.): *Manual of medical therapeutics* (27th ed). Boston: Little, Brown, p. 42.

Phillips, L.D., & Kuhn, M. (1996). *Manual of I.V. Drugs.* Boston: Little, Brown.

Sommers, M. (1990). Rapid fluid resuscitation. *Nursing 90, 1,* 52–59.

Terry, J., & Hedrick, C. (1995). Parenteral fluids. In Terry, J., Baranowski, L., Lonsway, R., & Hedrick, C. (eds.): *Intravenous therapy: Clinical principles and practices.* Philadelphia, W.B. Saunders, pp. 151–164.

Weinstein, S. (1993). *Principles and practices of I.V. therapy* (5th ed.). Boston: Little, Brown, p. 304.

CHAPTER 6

Infection Control

CHAPTER CONTENTS

GLOSSARY
LEARNING OBJECTIVES
PRE-TEST, CHAPTER 6
IMMUNE SYSTEM FUNCTION
Organs
Mechanisms of Defense
Impaired Host Resistance
BASIC PRINCIPLES OF EPIDEMIOLOGY
Colonization
Dissemination
Nosocomial Infections
Chain of Infection
STRATEGIES FOR PREVENTION OF INFECTION
I.V.-RELATED INFECTIONS
Infusion Phlebitis
Septicemia/Fungemia

Cannula-Related Infections
Infusate-Related Infections
NURSING PLAN OF CARE: INFECTION
  CONTROL
PATIENT EDUCATION
HOME CARE ISSUES
TECHNOLOGIC ADVANCES
COMPETENCY CRITERIA: INFECTION CONTROL
KEY POINTS
CRITICAL THINKING ACTIVITY
POST-TEST, CHAPTER 6
ANSWERS TO CHAPTER 6
Pre-Test
Post-Test
REFERENCES

GLOSSARY

Active acquired immunity Immunity that comes from direct contact with antigens by disease

Antigens Microbic invaders that bombard the body and trigger immune response

Asepsis Freedom from infection or infectious material, absence of viable pathogenic organisms

Bloodborne pathogen Microorganisms that is transmitted via the blood

Colonization Growth of microorganisms in a host without overt clinical symptoms or detected immune reaction

Contamination Microorganisms present on a body surface without tissue invasion or physiologic reaction

Dissemination Movement of microorganisms from an individual into the immediate environment, or movement of microorganisms from a confined site (e.g., skin, kidney) to the bloodstream to other parts of the body

Endogenous Produced within or caused by factors within the organism

Epidemiology Branch of science concerned with the study of the factors determining and influencing the frequency and distribution of disease, injury, and other health-related events and their causes in a defined human population for the purpose of establishing programs to prevent and control their development and spread

Exogenous Developed or originating outside the organism

Extrinsic contamination Of external origin

Hematogenous Produced by or derived from the blood; disseminated through the bloodstream or by the circulation

Host The organism from which a microorganism obtains its nourishment

Immunosuppression   Inhibition of the formation of antibodies to antigens that may be present

Intrinsic contamination   Contamination during manufacture

Leukocytes   Reduction of the number of leukocytes in the blood to a count being 5000 or less

Nosocomial infection   Hospital-acquired infection, which was not present or incubating at the time of admission

Passive acquired immunity   Transient immunity that develops from a person-to-person passage of immune cells or from gamma-globulin infusion

Pathogens   Any disease-producing agent or microorganism

Phlebitis   Inflammation of a vein

Reservoir   The place where the organism maintains its presence, metabolizes, and replicates

Sepsis   The presence of pathogenic microorganisms or their toxins in the blood or other tissues; the condition associated with such presence

Transmission   The movement of an organism from the source to the host

Virulence   Relative power and degree of pathogenicity possessed by organisms to produce disease

LEARNING OBJECTIVES

Upon completion of this chapter, the reader will be able to:

- State the definitions of the glossary terms.
- Discuss the function of the immune system.
- Identify the organs involved in the immune system.
- Identify the factors important for maintaining the well-being of the host.
- State the four clinical symptoms of an impaired host.
- State the causes of secondary immune deficiencies.
- Identify the three carrier states.
- Discuss the links in the chain of infection.
- Identify strategies to prevent infection.
- State the factors that influence formation of infusion phlebitis.
- State the Intravenous Nurses Standards of Practice for prevention of infection.
- Discuss sources of intravenous (I.V.) cannula-related infections.
- State the most prevalent microorganisms found in I.V.-related infections.
- Relate the critical nursing interventions for infection control.

PRE-TEST, CHAPTER 6

Match the term in column I to the definition in column II.

Column I

1. _____ colonization
2. _____ endogenous
3. _____ exogenous
4. _____ intrinsic contamination
5. _____ pathogen
6. _____ virulence

Column II

A. Relative power and degree of pathogenicity to produce disease

B. Growth of microorganisms in a host without over clinical symptoms

C. Contamination during manufacture

D. Produced within or caused by factors within the organism

E. Any disease-producing agent

F. Originating outside the organism

7. The purpose of the immune system is to provide:
   A. the body with a way to recognize and destroy invading antigens
   B. the body with antigens
   C. a way to inhibit the formation of antibodies to antigens
   D. a way for the movement of an organism from the source to the host

8. All of the following are organs of the immune system *except*:
   A. Thymus
   B. Bone marrow
   C. Heart
   D. Lungs

9. An immunosuppressed host has all of the following characteristics *except*:
   A. Frequent infections
   B. Infections are more severe than usual
   C. Incomplete response to treatment
   D. Leukocyte count of 5000 to 10,000

10. Identify the links in the chain of infection.

_____

_____   _____

11. All of the following strategies are to prevent infection *except*:
    A. Handwashing
    B. Isolation guidelines
    C. Epidemiologist
    D. Know what is clean, disinfected and sterile

12. Which of the following cutaneous antiseptics are used for prevention of I.V. device–related septicemias?
    A. Providone-iodine
    B. Hexachlorophene
    C. Acetone
    D. Polyantibiotic ointment

13. Which of the following is the *most* prevalent microorganism found in I.V.-related infections?
    A. *Staphylococcus*
    B. Tribe Klebsielleae
    C. *Pseudomonas*
    D. *Yersinia* spp

14. All of the following are factors that can contribute to the contamination of infusion equipment *except*:
    A. Faulty handling of equipment
    B. Injection ports
    C. Antibiotics
    D. Three-way stopcocks

15. Which of the following is a critical nursing intervention when caring for a patient with an infusion-related infection?
    A. Monitoring for signs and symptoms of sepsis
    B. Monitoring for dysrhythmias
    C. Use of full barrier protection
    D. Educating the patient on good handwashing techniques.

It may seem a strange principle to enunciate as the very first requirement in a Hospital that it should do the sick no harm. It is quite necessary to lay down such a principle

FLORENCE NIGHTINGALE, 1859

IMMUNE SYSTEM FUNCTION

The immune system provides the body with a way of distinguishing itself from foreign invaders. These invaders constantly bombard the body and trigger immune response. They are termed antigens and can include microbes such as viruses, bacteria, and parasites (Gurka, 1989). Appropriate immune response occurs when the immune system recognizes and destroys invading antigens.

The immune system also acts as a "clean-up crew" disposing of used, mutant, or damaged cells that result from catabolism, growth, and injury (Grady, 1988).

Organs

The organs and cells involved in the immune system form a complex when antigens and immune system cells are constantly moving via the lymph system, blood circulation, and lymphatic organs. The primary organs of the immune system are the thymus and bone marrow. Secondary organs include lymph nodes, spleen, liver, Peyer's patches, appendix, tonsils and adenoids, and lungs (Frey, 1991). See Table 6–1 for location and function of these organs.

Mechanisms of Defense

A mutual compatibility exists between a healthy host (human) and environmental microbes. The factors most important in maintaining the well-being of the host are nonspecific responses and specific immune response. The natural immune response consists of nonspecific defenses present at birth. These mechanisms function without prior exposure to an antigen. Nonspecific mechanisms include:

FIRST LINE
Physical
    Skin
    Mucous membranes
    Epiglottis
    Respiratory tract cilia
    Sphincters
Chemical
    Tears
    Vaginal secretions
    Gastric acidity
Mechanical
    Lacrimation
    Intestinal peristalsis
    Urinary flow

SECOND LINE
Phagocytosis
Complement cascade

153

TABLE 6–1. ORGANS OF THE IMMUNE SYSTEM

Organs	Location	Function
Primary		
Thymus	Mediastinal cavity	Provides immune function in early years; T-cell development
Bone marrow	Ribs, sternum, long bones	Produces stem cells, which are precursors to leukocytes and lymphocytes
Secondary		
Lymph nodes	Interconnected system of vessels and nodes; chains of pathway of lymph drainage	Stores T cells, B cells, macrophages; circulates leukocytes; drains and filters waste products (cellular debris)
Spleen	Left upper abdominal quadrant beneath diaphragm	Stores red cells, leukocytes, platelets, lymphocytes; serves as hematopoietic organ; filters out antigens
Liver	Right upper abdominal quadrant	Kupffer's cells filter out antigens
Peyer's patches, appendix	Small intestine Right lower abdominal quadrant	Areas of lymphoid tissue that contain B cells and T cells
Tonsils and adenoids	Pharynx	Unknown
Lungs	Thoracic cavity	Filter antigenic material and cellular debris

Source: From Frey, A.M. (1991). The immune system and intravenous administration of immune globulin. Part I. *Journal of Intravenous Nursing, 14*(5), 316, with permission.

Nonspecific Immune Response

Physical nonspecific mechanisms of defense against infections include intact skin and mucosal barriers. The skin forms the first barrier against infection; it is a physical barrier and contains secretions that have an antibacterial action. This tight network of cells provides an impenetrable physical barrier against invasion by microbes that reside on the external or internal environment (Brachman, 1992).

Chemical barriers inhibit growth and invasion by environmental microbes, such as occurs with acid secretion by mucus, with urine acidity, and with a variety of lipids secreted in the skin. There are also physiologic mechanisms. The large airway of the lungs secretes mucus that traps inspired particles; the inspired debris is removed by epithelium and expectorated.

Through mechanical action, peristalsis in the gastrointestinal tract and urinary tract expel organisms from the internal environment of the host (Hudak & Gallo, 1994).

Age influences nonspecific factors and is associated with decreased resistance at either end of the age spectrum—the very young and the very old. Factors such as surgery and the presence of chronic disease such as diabetes, blood disorders, certain lymphomas and collagen diseases alter host resistance, which influences nonspecific factors (Massanari, 1989).

154

Specific Immune Response

Acquired or specific host defense mechanisms function most efficiently when there has been prior exposure to invading antigens. Passive acquired immunity is transient and develops by passage of immune cells from one person to another or by gamma-globulin infusion. Active acquired immunity develops from direct contact with antigens by disease. The key players in specific immune response are leukocytes, T-cell lymphocytes, B lymphocytes, immunoglobulin, and complement cascade.

Leukocytes make up one of the most important components of the immune system. A differential white blood cell (WBC) count provides specific information related to infections and disease. Leukopenia is defined as a reduction of the number of leukocytes in the blood to a count less than $5,000/mm^3$. Normal WBC count ranges from 5000 to 10,000/mL (Corbett, 1992). Another component of the immune system are the B and T lymphocytes, which form the specific immune response system. Lymphocytes have specific antigen recognition and can neutralize toxin and phagocytize invading bacteria and viruses (DiJulio, 1991). Lymphocytes recognize an antigen because of genes known as human leukocyte antigen (HLA) genes.

Immunoglobulin circulates through the body, aiding in destruction of microorganisms and neutralizing toxin. Immunoglobulins are divided into five major classes: IgA, IgD, IgE, IgG, and IgM. The absence of one or more of these substances has been linked to infection or disease processes (Frey, 1991).

The phagocytic cells provide a first line of defense against invasion by bacteria and selected fungi. These cells circulate in the bloodstream until summoned by chemical mediators to sites of infections. The immune system provides a surveillance network that enables the host to monitor and identify foreign material and generate specific protection against invading pathogens. Immunologic responses are mediated through the production of antibodies that circulate in the plasma.

The complement system consists of a complex of about 17 different proteins that are responsible for several steps in the inflammatory process, including summoning phagocytic cells to the site of infection. Complement also attaches to the infectious agent and promotes ingestion by the phagocyte. The complement proteins are numbered C1 through C9 and act in a cascade fashion to initiate action of the next protein. These proteins are part of the nonspecific and specific response system. As a nonspecific immune response, C3 and C5 increase vascular permeability and chemically attract granulocytes (Grady, 1988). As part of the specific response, the normally inactive proteins are activated by specific antibodies in two pathways. The classic pathway requires interaction of C1 with antigen-antibody complex, or the alternative pathway occurs with the absence of a specific antibody (Frey, 1991).

Impaired Host Resistance

Many factors can result in impaired host defense. Persons who acquire an infection because of a deficiency in any of their multifaceted host defenses are referred to as compromised hosts. Persons with major defects related to specific immune responses are referred to as immunosuppressed hosts. These two terms often are used interchangeably.

The following is a general clinical picture of immune dysfunction:

- Infections occur frequently.
- Infections are more severe than usual.
- Unusual infecting agents or infections with opportunistic organisms.

- There is an incomplete response to treatment without complete elimination of the infecting agent.

Primary immunodeficiency disorders are congenital or inherited. B-cell immunodeficiencies account for about 50% of primary immunodeficiences; T-cell immunodeficiencies account for about 40% (Frey, 1991a).

Secondary immunodeficiencies arise from disease processes or therapies that decrease immune system organ or cell function. These deficiencies are acquired. Causes of secondary immune deficiency are age, stress, trauma, poor nutritional status, and drug therapy. Often, this type of immunodeficiency is transient and responds well to antibody therapy with IgG or removal of cause (Gurka, 1989).

BASIC PRINCIPLES OF EPIDEMIOLOGY

Epidemiology is the "study of things that happen to people." Historically, it involves the study of epidemics. Epidemiology is the study of determinants, occurrence, and distribution of health and disease in a population (Patterson & Hierholzer, 1992).

Colonization

Infection is the replication of organisms in the tissue of a host; development of clinical signs and symptoms. Colonization is the presence of a microorganism in or on a host, with growth and multiplication of the microorganisms with no clinical symptoms or detected immune reaction at the time of isolation.

A carrier (or colonized person) is an individual colonized with a specific microorganism and from whom the organism can be recovered but who shows no signs and symptoms of presence of the microorganism. A carrier may have a history of previous disease. The carrier state may be transient (short-term), intermediate (on occasion), or chronic (long-term, permanent, or persistent).

Dissemination

Dissemination is the shedding of microorganisms from a person carrying them into the immediate environment. Cultures of air samples, surfaces, and objects reveal dissemination or shedding of microorganisms. Nurses can disseminate *Staphylococcus* from their skin by shedding stratum corneum epidermial cells, which leads to the transmission of *Staphylococcus* to patients.

Nosocomial Infections

More than 50% of all epidemics of nosocomial bacteremia or candidemia reported in the world literature between 1965 and 1991 were derived from some kind of vascular access devices (Maki, 1990). Nosocomial infections develop within a hospital or are produced by organisms acquired during hospitalization (Brachman, 1992). These infections may involve anyone in contact with the hospital environment including staff, volunteers, visitors, and workers. Nosocomial infections are preventable, and their sources can be endogenous or exogenous.

Endogenous infections are caused by a person's own flora. Exogenous infections are from sources outside a person's body.

156

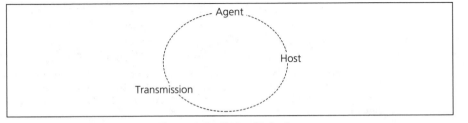

Figure 6–1. Chain of infection.

Chain of Infection

Infections result from interaction between infectious agents and susceptible hosts. This interaction is called transmission. The chain of infection refers to agent, transmission, and host; the links interrelate (Fig. 6–1).

✎ **NOTE:** To control nosocomial infection, the chain of infection must be attacked at its weakest link.

Agent

The first link in the chain of infection is the microbial agent, which may be a bacterium, fungus, virus, or parasite. Most nosocomial infections are caused by bacteria and viruses (Brachman, 1992). The ability of the organisms to induce disease is called its virulence or invasiveness.

All organisms have a reservoir and a source; these may be the same or different, and it is important to distinguish between these. The reservoir is the place where the organism maintains its presence, metabolizes, and replicates. Viruses survive better in human reservoirs; the reservoir of gram-positive bacteria is usually a human, whereas gram-negative bacteria may have either a human or animal reservoir or an inanimate reservoir. The source is the place from which the infectious agent passes to the host, either by direct contact or by indirect contact through a vehicle as the means of transmission. Sources can be animate or inanimate (Brachman, 1992).

The exit site is important in transmission of infection. Organisms from humans usually have a single portal of exit. The major portals of exit are the respiratory and gastrointestinal tracts, as well as the skin (e.g., in wounds). In addition, blood may be a portal of exit and is a concern for infusion nurses.

Transmission

The second link in the chain of infection involves the movement of organisms from source to host, that is, the mechanisms of transmission. There are four different routes of transmission: contact, common vehicle, airborne, and vectorborne. An organism may have a single route of transmission or two or more routes.

Contact

In contact transmission, the host has contact with the source, which occurs directly, indirectly, or by droplets. *Direct* contact transmission is spread by physical person-to-person contact between source and host. *Indirect* contact transmission involves participation of an intermediate object (usually inanimate) that is passively involved in transmission of the infectious agent from source to host. The intermediate object may become contaminated from an animate or inanimate source. An example

157

of an indirectly transmitted infection is one that is caused by the use of a tourniquet on an infected person and reuse of the same tourniquet on another person.

✎ **NOTE:** Intact skin is the best defense against infection; for verticle spread in this manner you must have a portal of exit and re-entry with nonintact skin.

Droplet transmission refers to the brief passage of the infectious agent through the air when the source and host are relatively near each other (usually within several feet). The transmission generally occurs by talking or sneezing. Examples of droplet-spread infections are measles and streptococcal pharyngitis.

Common Vehicle

In common vehicle transmission of infection, a contaminated inanimate vehicle serves as the vector for transmission to many people. The hosts become infected after contact with the common vehicle. The organisms replicate while in the vehicle, as *Salmonella* replicates in food, or is passively carried by a vehicle such as hepatitis A in food.

Airborne

Airborne transmission involves organisms that have an airborne phase in their route of dissemination, which is usually a distance of more than several feet between source and host. The droplets are 5 μm or smaller and may remain suspended in the air for a prolonged period of time. Dust particles that have settled on surfaces may become suspended by physical action and may also remain airborne for a prolonged period. Skin squamae may become airborne and provide a mechanism for the airborne transmission of organisms such as staphylococci. Studies have shown that the tubercle bacilli and nosocomial staphylococcal disease can be transmitted by the airborne route (Riley, 1959; Waller, Buntsin & Brubaker, 1963).

Vectorborne

Vectorborne transmission of infection includes external and internal vector transmission. *External* vectorborne transmission is the mechanical transfer of microorganisms on the body or appendages of the vector (e.g., shigellae and salmonellae are transferred by flies). *Internal* vectorborne transmission includes harborage and biologic transmission. In transmission by harborage, there is no biologic action between vector and agent. In biologic transmission, the agent goes through biologic changes within the vector, as when malaria parasites change within the mosquito.

Host

The third link in the chain of infection is the host. Note that disease does not always follow the transmission of infectious agents to a host. This may be due to certain host factors that influence the development of infections, such as the site of deposition of the agent and the host's defense mechanism.

Breaking the Chain of Infection

Available methods in which to break the chain of infection include the following:

1. New microbiologic methods. New laboratory methods can determine strains of bacterial organisms at the molecular level. In the 1990s, standard nosocomial outbreak investigations often involve some type of molecular analysis.
2. Advancement of epidemiologic methods. At one time epidemiologic methodology was descriptive and analytical; now sophisticated methods include relative risk, risk ratios, regression analysis, and correlation coefficients to

study nosocomial infections. Computerization of infection control surveillance has expanded epidemiology databases.

3. Continuous quality improvement (CQI) programs. The linking of hospital reimbursement to quality of care and assessment has been a strong incentive to expand the model and methods of hospital epidemiology to CQI surveillance. Quality assessment of noninfectious risks requires risk and outcome definitions.

4. Risk management. Formal programs have been established to deal with poor outcome evaluation and control in patients with liability-centered and malpractice-related risk management programs.

5. Antibiotic use. The Joint Commission on Accreditation of Healthcare Organizations (JCAHO) requires the medical staff to develop a systematic process for evaluating empiric, therapeutic, and prophylactic use of drugs; this includes programs for review of antibiotic use. Each hospital should provide support for a group concerned with appropriate use of antibiotics. This team should be headed by an infectious disease physician. Strategies to improve antibiotics use include education, ordering policies, drug utilization review, restriction policies, control of laboratory susceptibility testing, and limitation of contact time between physician and pharmaceutical representatives (Patterson & Hierholzer, 1992) (Table 6–2).

TABLE 6–2. **STRATEGIES TO IMPROVE ANTIBIOTIC USE**

Strategy	Advantages	Disadvantages
Education	Palatable; does not encroach the practice of medicine	Requires reinforcement; effectiveness difficult to document
Hospital formulary	Immediate impact; enables generic and therapeutic equivalency substitutions	Requires strong Pharmacy and Therapeutics Committee; perception that patient care is being compromised
Ordering policies	Special order sheets shown to be effective; automatic stop orders also useful	Extra paperwork; physicians may be resentful; automatic stop orders may at times compromise patient care
Drug utilization review	Provides feedback to physicians; ongoing, comprehensive review enables intervention	Labor-intensive; requires contact time between reviewers and physician
Restriction policies	Enables tight control, especially of the newer, more expensive agents	Limits freedom of physicians; may arouse resentment against the "antibiotic police"
Control of laboratory susceptibility testing	Easily accomplished; can influence prescribing habits	May hinder appropriate use, especially of the newer agents
Limitation of contact time between physicians and pharmaceutical representatives	Probably effective in the teaching setting; minimizes confusion among residents	Probably ineffective in the private practice setting

Source: From Bryan, C.S. (1989). Strategies to improve antibiotic use. *Infectious Disease Clinics of North America*, 1:723. Reprinted with permission.

TABLE 6–3. **ANTIMICROBIAL AGENTS EFFECTIVE AGAINST CERTAIN NOSOCOMIAL PATHOGENS**

Organism	Antimicrobial Agents
Gram-Positive	
Staphylococci (methicillin-sensitive)	First-generation cephalosporin, nafcillin
Staphylococci (methicillin-resistant)	Vancomycin
Enterococci	Ampicillin or vancomycin with or without aminoglycoside
Clostridium difficile (diarrhea, colitis)	Oral vancomycin, oral metroidazole
Gram-Negative	
Klebsiella spp	Cephalosporin, quinolone
Escherichia coli	
Enteric bacilli (*Enterobacter, Citrobacter, Serratia*) *Pseudomonas aeruginosa*	Imipenem or third-generation cephalosporin with or without aminoglycoside Ceftazidime, aztreonam, or extended-spectrum penicillin with or without aminoglycoside, ciprofloxacin
Acinetobacter spp	Imipenem, ciprofloxacin
Legionella spp	Erythromycin with or without rifampin
Other	
Candida	Amphotericin B, fluconazole, ketoconazole
Aspergillus spp	Amphotericin B, itraconazole
Anaerobes	Clindamycin, metronidazole, ticarcillin/clavulanate, ampicillin/sublactam

Source: From Perucca, R., Hedrick, C., Terry, J., & Johnson, J. (1995). Infection control. In Terry, J., Baranowski, L., Lonsway, R., & Hedrick C. (eds.): *Intravenous therapy: Clinical principles and practices*. Philadelphia: JB Lippincott, p. 145. Reprinted with permission.

To break the chain of infection, antimicrobial therapy is used in three stages. Stage 1 therapy is used when an infection is diagnosed or suspected and broad-spectrum therapy by I.V. route is initiated. Stage 1 is guided by a report of sample microscopy (e.g., morphology or Gram's stain). Usually, stage 1 patients are unstable from the standpoint of the infection process. The causative organisms should be cultured prior to initiation of antibiotics. See Table 6–3 for a list of antibiotics and their effectiveness against certain pathogens at this stage. Stage 2 is adjusted to antimicrobials active against the isolated organism. Results of antibiotic sensitivity testing are used to guide therapy. Antimicrobials with a narrower spectrum of activity are often used. A third and final stage is reached when the patient shows signs of successful treatment and is converted to oral therapy prior to discharge.

6. Pharmacoepidemiology (study of effects of drugs, beneficial and adverse). JCAHO requires that hospitals have the capacity to document and evaluate adverse drug reactions in their patients. The link between antibiotic use issues and adverse drug reactions has involved epidemiologists in pharmacoepidemiology.

7. Emporiatics (study of disease in travelers). The physician involved in infection control is often asked for travel advice. It is relevant for the hospital epidemiologist to stay apprised of current infectious disease events worldwide.

STRATEGIES FOR PREVENTION OF INFECTION

Nurses involved in maintenance of vascular access devices must have the knowledge base and competency to initiate infusion-related protocols to prevent infection. The principles of infection control provide the foundation for the delivery of I.V. therapy. Prevention begins with knowledge regarding the techniques to prevent infection. These techniques include (1) follow **handwashing** procedure; (2) know what is clean, disinfected, and sterile; (3) know what is dirty (contaminated); (4) correct contamination immediately; and (5) follow isolation guidelines.

Follow Handwashing Procedure

Vigorous handwashing, ideally with antiseptic-containing preparations, must always precede the insertion of a peripheral I.V. cannula and should also precede later handling of the device or the administration set. Handwashing reduces the nurse's and patient's risk of infection. A vigorous 15- to 20-second scrub with antiseptic soap using friction removes most microbes. Gloves do not replace handwashing and do not provide complete protection (Crow, 1989).

✎ **NOTE:** The combination of wearing gloves and washing hands after their removal markedly reduces the risk of contamination. Handwashing is the single most important means of preventing spread of infection. Sterile gloves are recommended for inserting peripheral I.V. cannulas in high-risk patients, such as those with leukemia (Maki, 1989).

KEY POINTS
- Wash hands before and after touching patients or patient care items, especially before and after handling patients' body fluids.
- Wash hands after touching any area of a patient's body.
- Wash all areas of hands including wrists between care of different patients for at least 10 seconds (Garner, 1992).

There is some degree of noncompliance among nursing staff regarding this simple and inexpensive technique to prevent infections. The following reasons have been suggested to account for this low level of compliance:

1. Lack of priority over other required procedures
2. Insufficient time to accomplish handwashing
3. Inconvenient placement of sinks or other handwashing tools
4. Allergy or intolerance to the handwashing solutions
5. Lack of leadership
6. Lack of personnel commitment to the routine of handwashing (Garner, 1992)

Know What Is Clean, Disinfected, and Sterile

Items are considered *clean* when they have been thoroughly washed and dried. Cleaning should be done by appropriately attired personnel in a controlled area. The use of an instrument cleaner is recommended. Items that are cleaned, dried, and soaked in disinfectant solution such as glutaraldehyde are considered *disinfected*. An item is *sterile* when it has been cleaned, dried, packaged, and sterilized in steam or gas. Steam or gas sterilization provides high levels of disinfection, killing all microbes except resistant bacterial spores (Crow, 1989).

✎ **NOTE:** Disinfectants used for cleaning equipment can be toxic to personnel.

Know What Is Dirty

The words "dirty" and "contaminated" tend to be synonymous in relation to infection control. Any instrument used to invade a patient's body is considered contaminated. It is important to clean and process items contaminated from patient's excreta immediately after use. Items that do not enter the body, such as sphymomanometers, may be used from patient to patient unless contaminated. (Disposable sphymomanometers are being used more frequently.)

✎ NOTE: Contaminated items should be stored separately from clean equipment.

Correct Contamination Immediately

If contamination has occurred, immediate action must be taken. Nurses are patient advocates and must speak up at the moment a break in technique is noticed. Too often the incident is reported to the infection control department or reported by means of an unusual occurrence report only to delay corrective action and possibly jeopardize a positive patient outcome.

Follow Isolation Guidelines

Universal Precautions

An approach to preventing the transmission of bloodborne pathogens is the concept of "Universal Precautions," which was recommended by Centers for Disease Control and Prevention (CDC) and supported by the Occupational Safety and Health Administration (OSHA) in its final rule in 1991. The lastest guidelines from CDC were available September 1995. Universal precautions should be used in the care of all patients, especially those in emergency care settings in which the risk of blood exposure is increased and the infection status is usually unknown. See appendices and Chapter 2 for specific guidelines.

Alternative Isolation System Body Substance Isolation

Body substance isolation was recommended by the CDC in 1987 and is composed of two part. The first and primary part focuses on the isolation of moist body substances through the use of barrier precautions, primarily gloves; this part is used for all patients, regardless of the diagnosis. A single universal reminder sign that defines body substances and describes the barrier precautions to be taken is placed in each single patient room or at the bedside. The second part of body substance isolation is a diagnosis-driven component that is used for patients who have some of the diseases that are transmitted exclusively or in part by airborne transmission. Body substance isolation includes the following:

Barrier precautions: gloves
Handwashing
Use of gowns, aprons, masks, or goggles
Disposal of soiled reusable items
Disposal of needles
Private room

In addition, personnel should be immune to or immunized against infectious agents transmitted by airborne or droplet routes (measles, mumps, rubella, and varicella).

CDC System for Isolation Precautions

The CDC recommends that hospitals use either category-specific or disease-specific isolation precautions. Since 1970, CDC-recommended, category-specific isolation precautions group diseases for which similar isolation precautions are indicated. Disease-specific isolation precautions recommended by the CDC in 1983 consider each infectious disease individually so that only those precautions indicated to interrupt transmission of that disease are recommended (Bennett & Brachman, 1993).

Six isolation categories recommended for category-specific isolation precautions:

1. Strict isolation
2. Contact isolation
3. Respiratory isolation
4. Tuberculosis (AFB) isolation
5. Enteric precautions
6. Drainage/secretion precautions

✎ **NOTE:** The previous category of blood and body fluid precautions was superseded by universal precautions in 1987.

Government Regulations

Government agencies such as the Health Care Financing Administration (HCFA) and the CDC issue regulations and guidelines for health care. Private organizations such as the JCAHO also issue standards and recommendations. In its chapter on infection control the JCAHO (1995) lists the following standards:

Standard 1: There is an effective hospital-wide program for the surveillance, prevention, and control of infection.

Standard 2: A multidisciplinary committee oversees the program for surveillance, prevention, and control of infection.

Standard 3: Responsibility for the management of infection surveillance, prevention, and control is assigned to a qualified person.

Standard 4: There were written policies and procedures for infection surveillance, prevention, and control for all patient care departments and services.

Standard 5: Patient care support departments and services, such as central services, housekeeping services, and linen and laundry services, are available to assist in the prevention and control of infections and are provided with adequate direction, staffing, and facilities to perform all required infection surveillance, prevention, and control functions.

I.V.-RELATED INFECTIONS

Each year in the United States, approximately 150 million intravascular devices are purchased by hospitals and clinics. Most are peripheral venous catheters; however, 5 million central venous devices of various types are sold in the United States annually (Maki, 1992). More than 50% of all epidemics of nosocomial bacteremia or candidemia reported in the world literature between 1965 and 1991 were derived from vascular access in some form (Maki, 1990).

Infusion Phlebitis

Infusion phlebitis is a common cause of pain and discomfort to the millions of patients who receive infusion therapy through peripheral cannulas. Infusion phlebitis is primarily a physiochemical phenomenon, and studies have shown that the following influence phlebitis formation:

- Cannula material
- Length and bore size

- Operator skill on insertion
- Anatomic site of cannulation
- Duration of cannulation
- Frequency of dressing changes
- Character of the infusate
- Host factors such as patient age, race, and gender and the presence of underlying disease significantly influence the risk of infusion phlebitis.

In a study by Maki and associates (1991), the risk for phlebitis exceeded 50% by the fourth day after cannula placement. According to Maki and associates (1991), the factors influencing the development of infusion phlebitis include I.V. antibiotics, female gender, catheterization for longer than 48 hours, and catheter material. See Table 6–4 for a complete list of risk factors for infusion phlebitis.

The three major types of phlebitis are mechanical, chemical, and bacterial—all of which are described in Chapter 9. Bacterial phlebitis (septic phlebitis) occurs when the I.V. infusate becomes contaminated, allowing bacteria to enter and proliferate, which in turn leads to septicemia. Bacterial phlebitis can occur because of compromised aseptic technique during admixture of fluids, inadequate skin preparation, failure to inspect containers for cracks or leaks, and improper cleansing of injection sites prior to administration of medications.

TABLE 6–4. **RISK FACTORS FOR INFUSION PHLEBITIS IN PERIPHERAL I.V. THERAPY**

Catheter Material	**Infusate**
Polypropylene > Teflon	Low pH
Silicone elastomer > polyurethane	Potassium chloride
Teflon > polyurethane*	Hypertonic glucose, amino acids lipid
Teflon > steel needles	**Antibiotics** (especially beta-lactams, vancomycin, metronidazole)
Catheter size	High flow of intravenous fluid (>90 mL/hr)
Large bore > smaller bore	
Insertion in emergency room > inpatient units	Daily intravenous dressing change every 48 hr
Increasing duration of catheter placement	Host factors
	"Poor quality" peripheral veins
	Insertion site: upperarm, wrist > hand
	Age
	Children: older > younger
	Adults: younger > older
	Sex: Female > male
	Race: white > black
	Individual biologic vulnerability

* Factors found to be significant predictors of risk in a recent prospective study of 1054 peripheral I.V. catheters in the University of Wisconsin Hospital and Clinics are indicated by italic type

NOTE: The > symbol denotes a significantly greater risk of phlebitis. Factors found to be significant predictors of risk in this study are denoted in boldface type.

Source: From Maki, D.G., & Ringer, M. (1991). Risk factors for infusion-related phlebitis with small peripheral venous catheters: A randomized controlled study. *Annals of Internal Medicine, 114,* 845.

Septicemia/Fungemia

Infusates are parenteral fluids, blood products, or I.V. medications administered through an intravascular device. Infusion-related septicemia and fungemia are more likely than cannula-related infections to culminate in frank shock and are often unrecognized. Fortunately there is a low incidence of bloodstream infection (less than 1%) (Maki, 1992). Of 30 million patients in the United States receiving infusions each year, this translates to 50,000 to 100,000 cases of septicemia (Maki, 1990).

Most infusion-related septicemia is by gram-negative bacilli introduced by intrinsic contamination (i.e., by manufacturer) or by extrinsic contamination (i.e., during its preparation and administration). See Table 6–5 for microorganisms most frequently encountered in various forms of intravascular-related infections. Intravascular device–related sepsis is preventable. To prevent this type of sepsis, the nurse must know the reservoirs of nosocomial pathogens, modes of transmission to patient's infusion, and rational and effect guidelines for prevention.

The two major sources of bloodstream infections associated with any intravascular device are infection of cannula wound and contamination of infusate.

TABLE 6–5. **MICROORGANISMS MOST FREQUENTLY FOUND IN I.V.-RELATED INFECTIONS**

Source	Pathogen
Peripheral I.V. catheters	*Staphylococcus aureus*
	Coagulase-negative staphylococci
	Candida spp
Central venous catheters	Coagulase-negative staphylococci
	Staphylococcus aureus
	Candida spp.
	Corynebacterium spp.
	Klebsiella and *Enterobacter* spp.
	Mycobacterium spp.
	Trichophyton beiglii
	Fusarium spp.
	Malassezia furfur
Contaminated I.V. infusate	Tribe Klebsielleae
	Enterobacter cloacae
	Enterobacter agglomerans
	Serratia marcescens
	Klebsiella spp
	Pseudomonas cepacia
	Citrobacter freundii
	Flavobacterium spp
	Candida tropicalis
Contaminated blood products	*Enterobacter cloacae*
	Achromobacter spp
	Flavobacterium spp
	Pseudomonas spp
	Salmonella spp
	Yersinia spp

Source: Maki, D.G. (1992). In J.V. Bennett & P.S. Brachman, *Hospital Infections* (3rd ed). Boston: Little, Brown, p. 856, with permission.

In a study (Beck-Sague, Jarvis, & National Nosocomial Infections Surveillance System, 1993) nosocomial fungemia were more than three times as likely in patients with central intravascular catheters compared to those who did not have a central intravascular catheter. Patients with bloodstream infections receiving total parenteral nutrition or in intensive care units were more likely to have fungemia compared to those not receiving total parenteral nutrition or not in intensive care units.

Factors that contribute to contamination and infection include:

1. *Faulty handling.* Glass containers can become cracked or damaged and plastic bags punctured. Bacteria and fungi may invade a hairline crack in an I.V. container.

✎ **NOTE:** Before use, containers of fluid should be examined against a light and dark background for cracks, defects, turbidity, and particulate matter. Any glass container lacking a vacuum when opened should be considered contaminated.

2. *Admixtures.* The risk of contamination when admixtures are prepared is decreased when trained personnel prepare mixtures under laminar flow hoods. The use of strict aseptic technique is vital.

3. *Manipulation of in-use I.V. equipment.* Faulty technique in handling equipment can lead to contamination. When an administration set is inserted into the container and the container is inverted, the fluid tends to leak from the vent onto the unsterile surface of the container. Regurgitation of the contaminated fluid can occur.

✎ **NOTE:** Squeezing the drip chamber of the administration set before inserting it into the container and releasing it when the container is inverted will prevent regurgitation of fluid and minimize the risk of contamination.

4. *Injection ports.* Aseptic technique must be maintained when injection ports are used for "piggyback" or secondary infusions. The injection port located at the distal end of the tubing can expose the patient to excreta and drainage.

✎ **NOTE:** The injection port must be scrubbed at least 1 minute with an accepted antiseptic (e.g., 70% isopropyl alcohol) or 30 seconds with an antiseptic microbial (e.g., providone-iodine) solution. Securely taping the needle, needle protector system, or needleless system firmly in the port will prevent the in-and-out motion of the needle from introducing bacteria into the infusion.

5. *Three-way stopcocks.* These adjunct devices are potential sources of transmission of bacteria because their ports, unprotected by sterile covering, are open to moisture and contaminants. These devices are usually connected to central venous catheters and arterial lines and are frequently used for drawing blood. Aseptic technique is vital.

✎ **NOTE:** Whenever fluid is noted to be leaking at injection sites, connections, or vents, the I.V. set should be replaced.

Cannula-Related Infections

Peripheral intravascular device–related sepsis is the least recognized nosocomial infection. Over the past two decades there has been a change in the number of gram-positive, rather than gram-negative, species reported as the cause of bloodstream infections (BSI). The majority of intravascular catheter-related bloodstream infections are caused by four pathogens: coagulase-negative staphylococci, candida, enterococci, and *Staphylococcus aureus* (Banerjee et al, 1991).

Staphylococcus epidermidis (coagulase-negative staphylococci) has become the most frequently isolated pathogen and accounts for 28% of all nosocomial BSIs reported during 1986 to 1989 (Schaberg, Culver, & Gaynes, 1991). *Staphylococcus aureus* now accounts for 16% of reported nosocomial BSIs, while before 1986 it was the leading cause. Approximately 8% of infections are caused by Enterococci. However, more alarming is the emergence of the vancomycin-resistant enterococci (VRE). From 1989 to 1993, 3.8% of the blood isolates from BSIs reported to CDC were vancomycin resistant (CDC, 1993). Fungal pathogens represented an increasing proportion of nosocomial infections during 1980–1990. Candida albicans accounted for more than 75% of all nosocomial fungal infections reported (Voss et al, 1994).

Sources of Cannula-Related Infections

The major sources of cannula-related infections are the skin flora, contamination of the catheter hub, contamination of infusate, and hematogenous colonization of the device (Figure 6–2).

Use of short-term devices like the steel needle or Teflon or polyurethane catheters indicate the lowest rate of infection, while the polyvinyl chloride or polyethylene catheter has been associated with bloodsteam infections (Maki & Ringer, 1991). Percutaneous-inserted noncuffed central venous catheters used for hemodialysis have been associated with the highest rates of bacteremia, a range of 10% (Cheesbrough, Finch, & Burden, 1986). Barrier precautions during catheter insertion provide adequate protection against infection. CDC and INS guidelines for changing catheters, administration sets, and catheter site care are shown in Table 6–6.

Recent studies note that peripherally inserted central catheters (PICC) pose a subsequently lower risk of catheter-related bloodstream infections (Dietrich, & Lobos 1988; Graham et al., 1991). However, further studies are needed to adequately determine how long PICCs can be safely left in place. CDC (1995) recommends change at least every 6 weeks with no recommendation for frequency of change when the duration of therapy is expected to exceed 6 weeks.

The central venous catheter in all its forms poses the greatest risk of septicemia today (Wey et al., 1989; Trilla et al., 1991). The lowest rate of infection with central

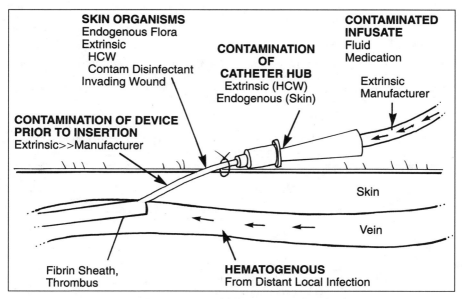

Figure 6–2. Sources of I.V. cannula-related infections. HCW = health care worker.

TABLE 6–6. NURSING PROCEDURE: STEPS IN CATHETER CULTURING

Equipment Sterile scissors Sterile gloves 70% Alcohol swab Sterile specimen container Label
Steps Explain procedure to patient. Remove dressing over I.V. site. Wash hands and put on sterile gloves. Wipe skin around puncture site with 70% alcohol to cleanse area of any blood or antimicrobial ointment. Withdraw catheter carefully. Be sure to direct the removed portion of the catheter upward to keep it away from patient's skin. Hold catheter over specimen container, and with sterile scissors cut half the length of the catheter and drop it into the container. Close container and label.

venous catheters (CVC) has been with surgically implanted Hickman or Broviac catheters that incorporate a Dacron cuff. The totally implantable intravascular devices have the lowest reported rates of catheter-related blood septicemias, possibly because they are located beneath the skin with no orifice for ingress of microorganisms (Groeger, Lucas, & Thaler et al., 1993). Strategies for prevention of catheter-related infections are shown in Table 6–7. In their current recommendations CDC states, "because insertion and maintenance of intravascular catheters by inexperienced staff may increase the risk of catheter colonization and catheter related bloodstream infections, many institutions have established infusion therapy teams. Available data suggest that trained personnel designated with the responsibility for insertion and maintenance of intravascular devices provide a service that effectively reduced catheter related infections and overall costs" (CDC, 1995).

Culturing Techniques

If the I.V. catheter is in any way compromised, it should be cultured. The recommended method for culturing a catheter, is the semiquantitative culture technique (Table 6–6). The semiquantitative culture technique involves thoroughly cleaning the area around the insertion site with 70% alcohol and permitting the area to air-dry.

TABLE 6–7. THREE CUTANEOUS ANTISEPTICS USED FOR PREVENTION OF I.V. DEVICE-RELATED SEPTICEMIA

Source of Septicemia	10% Providone-Iodine (n=227)	70% Alcohol (n=227)	2% Chlorhexidine (n=214)
Catheter-related	6	3	1
Contaminated infusate	—	3	—
Contaminated hub	1	—	—
All sources	7	6	1

Source: Maki, D.G., Alvarado, C.J., & Ringer, M. (1991). A prospective, randomized trial of providone-iodine, alcohol and chlorhexidine for prevention of infection with central venous and arterial catheters. *Lancet, 3389,* 339.

Alcohol is recommended because the residual antimicrobial activity of iodine-containing solutions may kill organisms on the catheter when it is removed. After the catheter is withdrawn, at least 5 cm of the tip and the catheter segment, beginning 1 to 2 mm inside the skin-catheter junction point, is clipped off with sterile scissors and dropped into a sterile specimen tube or cup. Purulent drainage at the site should be cultured prior to cleaning the site.

✎ **NOTE:** A positive, semiquantitative culture of 15 or more colony-forming units (CFUs) confirms a local cannula infection (Maki, 1992).

Disadvantages of this semiquantitative method are that (1) this method may fail to detect bacteremia of the internal lumen of the catheter tips and (2) the catheter must be removed for culturing and may not be the source of infection.

✎ **NOTE:** Culture any purulent drainage from the site. If the I.V. solution is the suspected source of infection, send the fluid container and tubing to the laboratory for analysis (Castle, 1983).

Blood cultures drawn through a peripheral vein and through the I.V. cannula can be a helpful alternative to culturing the cannula. If the results of the catheter blood sample are five times the peripheral blood sample, a catheter-related infection is suspected and the catheter should be removed.

Infusate-Related Infections

The occurrence of epidemic gram-negative bacteremia across the United States in 1970 and 1971 brought awareness that fluids given in I.V. infusions also are vulnerable to contamination (Maki, 1976). From 1965 to 1978, 28 of the 30 epidemics of infusion-related bacteremia were traced to containers of infusates contaminated during manufacturing. Most epidemics of infusion-related septicemia have been traced to contamination of infusate by gram-negative bacilli, introduced during manufacture (intrinsic contamination) or during its preparation and administration in the hospital (extrinsic contamination) (Maki, 1990).

The proliferation of microbes in 5% dextrose in water is most commonly related to tribe Klebsielleae: *Pseudomonas cepacia, Acinetobacter*, and *Serratia*. In 0.9% sodium chloride fluids, most bacteria grow except *Candida*. *Candida* species flourish in synthetic amino acids and 25% dextrose solutions (Maki, 1992).

Mechanisms of Fluid Contamination

Parenteral fluids can become contaminated during administration owing to the duration of uninterrupted infusion through the same administration set and to the frequency with which the set is manipulated. Microorganisms gain access from air entering bottles, from entry points into administration set, from the I.V. device through the line or at the junction between the administration seen and the catheter hub.

Molds gain access into glass I.V. bottles through microscopic cracks long before the bottle is hung for use; visible cloudiness or filmy precipitates and "fungus balls" in an I.V. bottle are visible to the nurse.

Total parenteral nutrition fluids should be used as soon as possible after preparation and stored at 4°C for growth of *Candida albicans* to be suppressed.

KEY POINTS
- Inspect all infusates before administration.
- Observe stringent asepsis during preparation and compounding of admixtures in the central pharmacy or on individual patient care units.
- Follow good aseptic techniques when infusions are handled during use, such as during injection of medications or changing of bags or bottles of fluids.

169

- Replace the administration set at periodic intervals to prevent the buildup of dangerous introduced contaminants and to further reduce the risk of related septicemia (Maki, 1993).

Reporting

If intrinsic contamination of a commercially distributed product is identified or even strongly suspected, especially if clinical infections have occurred as a consequence, the local, state, and federal (e.g., CDC and the Food and Drug Administration) public health authorities must be contacted immediately. The unopened lot or lots should be quarantined and saved for analysis.

Cutaneous Antiseptic

Cutaneous antiseptics are important because many I.V. device-related infections result from cutaneous colonization at the insertion site. A study by Maki and associates (1991) used providone-iodine, alcohol, and aqueous chlorhexidine for disinfection of the site before insertion and for site care every other day (Table 6–7). Chlorhexidine was associated with the lowest incidence of catheter-related infection and catheter-related bacteremia.

✎ **NOTE:** Use of acetone to defat the skin was found to be of no benefit (although still practiced) and only added to the inflammation and discomfort of the patient (Maki & McCormick, 1987). Use of topical polyantibiotic ointments on peripheral venous catheter has shown only moderate or no benefit (Maki, 1981), and use of polyantibiotic ointments has been associated with an increased incidence of *Candida* infection (Maki & Band, 1981; Flowers et al., 1989).

Dressings

The purpose of an I.V. site dressing is to prevent trauma to the catheter wound and cannulated vessel and to prevent extrinsic contamination of the wound. Transparent dressings permit continuous inspection of the site, secure the device reliably, and generally are more comfortable than gauze and tape. Transparent dressings permit patients to bathe and shower without saturating the dressing. Factors that affect cutaneous floral growth beneath the dressings include differences in physical properties such as moisture, vapor transmission rate, oxygen transmission, and cutaneous adherence. Transparent polyurethane dressings are more expensive than gauze and tape.

Technologic Advances

Innovations in the design or construction of the infusion apparatus are being developed, which deny access of microorganisms into the system or prevent organisms that might gain access from proliferating to high concentrations. Some technologic advances under development are:

- The incorporation of an antiseptic (providone-iodone) into a transparent catheter dressing to suppress subcutaneous colonization under the dressing (at this time not effective).
- Chlorhexidine over providone-iodine for cutaneous disinfection of vascular catheter sites (incorporating chlorhexidine into dressing's adhesive (possibly more effective than providone-iodine alone).
- A catheter hub engineered to reduce the risk of central venous catheter hub contamination. Strotter and associates (1982) showed that the device reduces significantly the rate of central venous catheter–related septicemia. (A non-

170

toxic, biodegradable, or easily metabolized antiseptic to I.V. fluid or I.V. admixtures might eliminate the hazard of fluid contamination altogether and reduce the risk of hub contamination.)

✎ **NOTE:** Pediatric infection control practices will be covered in Chapter 10; infection control issues related to blood products will be covered in Chapter 11; central venous catheter infections will be discussed in Chapter 13; and issues of infection control related to parenteral nutrition will be covered in Chapter 15.

Presently in use are the following:

- An interface barrier (Vita-Cuff, Vitafore Corporation, San Carlos, CA), to incorporate the aspect of technology of Hickman and Broviac catheters. This device consists of detachable cuff made of biodegradable collagen to which silver ion is chelated. The silver ion provides an additional chemical barrier against contamination (Maki, 1988).
- A catheter material resistant to colonization, which binds a nontoxic antiseptic or antimicrobial to the catheter surface, is being developed by Kamal and associates (1991).

Nursing Plan of Care:

INFECTION CONTROL

Focus Criteria for Assessment

Subjective
History of risk factors: fever, diarrhea

Objective
Baseline immunologic studies: T-cell count, white blood cell count (WBC), differential
Vital signs, especially temperature
Redness, inflammation, purulent drainage, tenderness, and warmth of insertion site

Nursing Diagnosis
Risk for infection related to immunodeficiency and malnutrition
Risk for impaired gas exchange related to alveolar-capillary membrane changes with infection
Risk for altered thought processes related to HIV or opportunistic infection of central nervous system
Risk for knowledge deficit related to illness and impact on patient's future
Risk for infection transmission

Patient Outcome Criteria
Patient will:
Be free from nosocomial infection.
Maintain adequate oxygenation.
Verbalize understanding of precautions for catheter care.
Report any need for additional dressing changes.
Not contaminate health care team, other patient, or family.

Nursing Management: Critical Activities
Use universal precautions.
Use aseptic technique and follow appropriate protocols when changing catheter dressing, I.V. tubing, and solutions.
Use sterile technique when inserting and removing catheter and when maintaining system.
Continued on following page

PATIENT EDUCATION

Instruct on management of I.V. access devices.
Instruct on handwashing, aseptic technique, and concept of dirty, clean, and sterile.
Provide information on dressing changes.
Instruct on site assessment and the key signs and symptoms to report to the home care agency, hospital health care worker, or physician.

HOME CARE ISSUES

It is generally believed that at-home risk factors for developing a catheter-related infection should be somewhat reduced from risk factors in a hospital setting. Research and study are needed to describe infection risks in the home setting.

The Environmental Protection Agency (EPA) has developed many advisory committees regarding infectious waste disposal in the home care setting. The Medical Waste Tracking Act of 1988 mandated to the EPA the investigation and development of guidelines for handling home-generated medical waste. The home care provider should establish policies and procedures for handling waste (Weinstein, 1993). Pre-packaged kits are available from a number of manufacturers and include Sharp's disposal systems and the CHemBLOC spill kit.

TECHNOLOGIC ADVANCES

Innovations in the design and construction of infusion equipment are being developed which deny access of microorganisms into the system or prevent organisms which might gain access from proliferating to high concentrations. Technology currently under development include:

- The incorporation of an antiseptic (povidone-iodine) into a transparent catheter dressing to suppress subcutaneous colonization under the dressing (at this time not been ineffective)
- Chlorhexidine over providone-iodine for cutaneous disinfection of vascular catheter sites incorporating chlorhexidine into the dressing's adhesive (possibly more effective than providone-iodine alone)
- An interface barrier (Vita-Cuff, Vitafore Corporation, San Carlos, CA) to incorporate the aspect of technology of Hickman and Broviac catheters.

This device consists of detachable cuff made of biodegradable collagen to which silver ions are chelated. The silver ions provide an additional chemical barrier against contamination (Maki, 1988)

- A catheter material resistant to colonization, which binds a nontoxic antiseptic or antimicrobial to the catheter surface (Kamal, Pfaller, Rempe, & Jebson, 1991).
- A catheter hub engineered to reduce the risk of central venous catheter hub contamination. Strotter and associates (1982) showed that the device reduces significantly the rate of central venous catheter-related septicemia. (A nontoxic, biodegradable or easily metabolized antiseptic to I.V. fluid or I.V. admixtures might eliminate the hazard of fluid contamination altogether and reduce the risk of hub contamination.)

COMPETENCY CRITERIA: Infection Control

Competency Statement: The competent I.V. therapy nurse will be able to use CDC guideliness for infection control practices in management of peripheral and central intravenous catheters.

COGNITIVE CRITERIA

	Skilled	Needs Education
1. States principles of cross-contamination.		
2. States mechanisms of transmission of bloodborne disease.		

PERFORMANCE CRITERIA

	Skilled	Needs Education
1. Demonstrates good handwashing techniques:		
15–20-second scrub with antimicrobial soap		
2. Uses Universal Precautions:		
Gloving		
Use of goggles, gowns, extra protective gear		
Use of biohazard waste bags		
3. Uses appropriate CDC isolation categories:		
Strict		
Contact		
Respiratory		
Tuberculosis (AFB)		
Enteric		
Drainage/secretion		
Neutropenic precautions		
4. Uses sterile technique:		
Central lines		
Dressing management		

SUGGESTED EVALUATION CRITERIA

1. Observation of Universal Precautions and sterile technique
2. Written test
3. Demonstration of dressing management using sterile technique

KEY POINTS

Infection control
Immune system function
    Purpose of immune system—to recognize and destroy invading antigens
    Organs
        Primary
            Thymus
            Bone marrow
        Secondary
            Lymph nodes
            Spleen
            Liver
            Peyer's patches
            Appendix
            Tonsils and adenoids
            Lungs
    Factors in maintaining the well-being of the host
        Nonspecific
            Physical
            Chemical
            Mechanical
            Phagocytosis
            Complement cascade
        Specific
            T and B lymphocytes
            Immunoglobulin
            Complement cascade
    Impaired host resistance
        B-cell immunodeficiencies (50% of primary immunodeficiencies)
        T-cell immunodeficiencies (40% of primary immunodeficiencies)

Basic principles of epidemiology
    Colonization—Presence of microorganism in or on a host
    Dissemination—Shedding of microorganisms from the person carrying them into the immediate environment
    Nosocomial infection—Infections that develop within a hospital or are produced by organisms acquired during hospitalization
    Endogenous infections—Infections caused by a patient's own flora
    Exogenous infections—Infections from sources other than patient
    Chain of infection
        Agent
        Transmission
        Host

Strategies for prevention of infection
Follow handwashing procedures.
Know what is clean, disinfected, and sterile.
Know what is dirty.
Correct contamination immediately.
Follow isolation guidelines.
Culturing Techniques

I.V.-related infections
Phlebitis
Factors affecting infusion phlebitis
Teflon higher risk than polyurethane material
Insertion in the emergency room higher risk than inpatient unit
Duration of cannulation
Placement in upper arm, wrist rather than hand
Individual biologic vulnerability
Infusate: antibiotics
Gender: female higher risk than male
Septicemia
Factors contributing to contamination
Faulty handling
Admixtures
Manipulation of in-use I.V. equipment
Injection ports
Three-way stopcocks
Cannula related infections
Staphylococcus aureus
Coagulase-negative staphylococci
Candida spp
Risk factors for infection
Percutaneously inserted noncuffed central venous catheters used for hemodialysis—highest risk
Peripherally inserted central venous catheters—lower risk
Surgically implanted central venous catheters—lowest risk

NOTE: Central venous catheters in all forms pose greatest risk of septicemia. Skin *insertion* site is the most common source of organism colonization.

Infusate-related infections
Tribe Klebsielleae
Pseudomonas cepacia
Candida spp.
Key Points
Inspect all infusates.
Observe stringent asepsis during preparation and compounding.
Follow good aseptic technique when infusion is handled during use.
Replace administration set at periodic intervals.
Dressings
Purpose
Prevent extrinsic contamination of wound.
Permits continuous inspection of site (transparent dressing)

CRITICAL THINKING ACTIVITY

1. During a given shift, note how many times nurses on your unit wash their hands.

2. Do you know where to locate the isolation policies and procedures for your agency? List the location.

3. Does your agency have a policy regarding reporting of contaminated infusates or I.V. equipment? Is that information accessible to you?

4. Describe a situation in which you cared for a patient with a suspected nosocomial infection. Was it catheter-related or infusate-related?

POST-TEST, CHAPTER 6

Match the term in column I to the definition in column II

Column I

1. _____ immunosuppression
2. _____ epidemiology
3. _____ nosocomial
4. _____ transmission
5. _____ reservoir

Column II

A. Place where the organism maintains its presence, metabolizes, and replicates

B. Inhibition of the formation of antibiotics to antigens that may be present

C. Movement of organism from source to the host.

D. Hospital-acquired infection

E. Concerned with the study of the factors determining and influencing frequency and distribution of disease

6. Which of the following constitute the first line of nonspecific defense mechanisms?
   A. Phagocytosis, complement cascade
   B. Leukocytes, proteins
   C. Physical and chemical barriers
   D. Immune system and phagocytes

7. The complement system consists of 17 different
   A. Glucose molecules
   B. Proteins
   C. Fatty acids
   D. Immune responses

8. The most common immunodeficiency disorders are
   A. B-cell immunodeficiencies
   B. T-cell immunodeficiencies
   C. Induced by drug therapy
   D. Due to poor nutritional status

9. All of the following are carrier states *except*:
   A. Transient
   B. Intermediate
   C. Chronic
   D. Acute

10. Which of the following describes dissemination?
    A. Shedding of microorganisms from a person carrying them into the environment
    B. Infections that develop within a hospital or are produced by organisms during hospitalization
    C. Infections caused by a patient's own flora
    D. The first link in the chain of infections

11. All of the following describe the movement of organisms from source to host *except*:
    A. Contact spread
    B. Airborne
    C. Dissemination
    D. Vectorborne

12. List four strategies to improve antibiotic usage.

    A. _____

    B. _____

178

C. _____

D. _____

13. Factors that influence formation of phlebitis include all of the following *except*:
    A. Cannual material
    B. Frequency of dressing changes
    C. Character of the infusate
    D. Low flow rates of I.V. solutions

14. Microorganisms frequently found in contaminated blood products include all of the following *except*:
    A. *Pseudomonas* species
    B. *Salmonella* species
    C. *Enterobacter cloacae*
    D. *Staphylococcus aureus*

15. List four factors that contribute to contamination and lead to sepsis.

    A. _____

    B. _____

    C. _____

    D. _____

ANSWERS TO CHAPTER 6

PRE-TEST

1. B
2. D
3. F
4. C
5. E
6. A
7. A
8. C
9. D
10. Agent–transmission–host
11. C
12. A
13. A
14. C
15. A

POST-TEST

1. B
2. E
3. D
4. C
5. A
6. C
7. B
8. A
9. D
10. A
11. C
12. Education
    Hospital formulary
    Ordering policies
    Drug utilization review
    Restriction policies
    Control of laboratory susceptibility
    testing
    Limitation of contact time between
    physicians and pharmaceutical
    representatives
13. D
14. D
15. Faulty handling
    Admixtures
    Manipulation of in-use I.V. equipment
    Injection ports
    Three-way stopcocks

REFERENCES

Banerjee, S.M., et al. (1991). Secular trends in nosocomial primary bloodstream infections in the United States. *American Journal of Medicine, 91*(Suppl 3B), 86S.

Beck-Sague, C.M., Jarvis, W.R. (993). Secular trends in the epidemiology of nosocomial fungal infections in the United States, 1980–1990. *Journal of Infectious Diseases* 167, 1247–1251.

Brachman, P.S. (1992). Epidemiology of nosocomial infections. In Bennett, J.V., & Brachman, P.S. (eds.): *Hospital infections* (3rd ed.). Boston: Little, Brown.

Bryan, C.S. (1989). Strategies to improve antibiotic use. *Infectious Disease Clinic of North America,* 3, 723.

Castle, M. (1983). Intravenous catheter cultures. In *Procedures: Nurse's reference library.* Springhouse, PA: Intermed Communications.

Cheesbrough, J.S., Finch, R.G., & Burden, R.P. (1986). A prospective study of the mechanisms of infection associated with hemodialysis catheters. *Journal of Infectious Disease, 154,* 579.

Corbett, J. (1992). *Laboratory tests and diagnostic procedures with nursing diagnoses.* Norwalk, CT: Appleton & Lange.

Crow, S. (1989). Asepsis: An indispensable part of the patient's care plan. *Critical Care Nursing Quarterly, 11*(4), 11–16.

Department of Health and Human Service (1995). Intravascular Device-Related Infections Prevention guideline availability; Notice. Federal Register. *Centers for Disease Control.* Georgia: Atlanta, 49993-49996.

Dietrich, K.A., & Lobos, J.G. (1988). Use of a single Silastic IV catheter for cystic fibrosis pulmonary exacerbations. *Pediatric Pulmonology, 4,* 181.

DiJulio, J. (1991). Hematopoiesis: An overview. *Oncology Nursing Forum, 18*(3), 6.

Flowers, R.H. III, et al. (1989). Efficacy of an attachable subcutaneous cuff for the prevention of intravascular catheter-related infection. *JAMA, 261,* 878.

Frey, A.M. (1991). The immune system and intravenous administration of immune globulin. Part I. The immune system. *Journal of Intravenous Nursing, 14*(5), 315–329.

Garner, J.S. (1992). Universal Precautions. In Bennett, J.V., & Brachman, P.S. (eds): *Hospital infections* (3rd ed). Boston: Little, Brown.

Grady, C. (1988). Host defense mechanisms: an overview. *Seminar Oncology Nursing, 4* (2), 86–94.

Graham, D.R., et al. (1991). Infectious complications among patients receiving home intravenous therapy with peripheral, central or peripherally placed central venous catheters. *American Journal of Medicine, 91*(Suppl 3B), 95S.

Groeger, J.S., Lucas, A.B., Thaler, H.T. et al. (1993). Infectious morbidity associated with long-term use of venous access device in patients with cancer. *Annals of Internal Medicine, 119,* 74.

Gurka, A.M. (1989). The immune system: Implications for critical care nursing. *Critical Care Nurse, 9*(7), 24–35.

Hudak, C.M., & Gallo, B.M. (1994). *Critical care nursing: A holistic approach.* Philadelphia: J.B. Lippincott.

Joint Commission on the Accreditation of Healthcare Organization's (1995). *1996 Comprehensive accreditation manual for hospitals.* Illinois: JCAHO.

Kamal, G.D., Pfaller, M.A., Rempe, L.E., & Jebson, P.J.R. (1991). Reduced intravascular catheter infection by antibiotic bonding. *Journal of the American Medical Association, 265*(18), 2364.

Maki, D.G., Rhame, F.S., Mackel, D.C. & Bennett, J.V. (1976). Nationwide epidemic of septicemia caused by contaminated intravenous products. *American Journal of Medicine, 60,* 471.

Maki, D.G., & Band J.D. (1981). A comparative study of polyantibiotic and iodophor ointments in prevention of catheter-related infection. *American Journal of Medicine, 70,* 739.

Maki, D.G., Botticelli, J.T., LeRoy, M.L., & Thielke, T.S. (1987). Prospective study of replacing administration sets for intravenous therapy at 48 vs 72 hour intervals. *JAMA, 258,* 1777.

Maki, D.G., & McCormick, R.D. (1987). Defatting catheter insertion sites in total parenteral nutrition is of no value as an infection control measure. *American Journal of Medicine, 83,* 833.

Maki, D.G., et al. (1988). An attachable silver-impregnated cuff for prevention of infection with central venous catheters: A prospective randomized multi-center trial. *American Journal of Medicine, 85,* 307.

Maki, D.G. (1989). The use of antiseptics for hand-washing by medical personnel. *Journal of Chemotherapy,* (Suppl 1), 3.

Maki, D.G. (1990). *The epidemiology and prevention of nosocomial bloodstream infection.* In Program and Abstracts of Third International Conference on Nosocomial Infection. Atlanta: Centers for Disease Control. The National Foundation for Infectious Diseases and American Society for Microbiology.

Maki, D.G., & Ringer, M. (1991). Risk factors for infusion-related phlebitis with small peripheral venous catheters. *Ann Intern Med, 114*(10), 845.

Maki, D.G. (1992). Infection due to infusion therapy. In Bennett, J.V., & Brachman, P.S. (eds.): *Hospital infections* (3rd ed.). Boston: Little, Brown.

Maki, D.G., Wheeler, S.J., Stolz, S.M., & Mermel, L.A. (1991). *Clinical trial of a novel antiseptic central venous catheter*. In Program and abstracts of the Thirty-First Interscience Conference on Antimicrobial Agents and Chemotherapy. Chicago: American Society for Microbiology.

Massanari, R.M. (1989). Nosocomial infections in critical care units: Causation and prevention. *Critical Care Nursing Quarterly, 11*(4), 45–47.

Mermel, L., McCormick, R., & Maki, D.G. (1991). Epidemiology and pathogenesis of infection with Swan-Ganz catheters: A prospective study using molecular epidemiology. *American Journal of Medicine, 91* (Suppl 3B), 197.

Patterson, J.E., & Hierholzer, W.J. (1992). The hospital epidemiologist. In Bennett, J.V., & Brachman, P.S. (eds.): *Hospital infections* (3rd ed.). Boston: Little, Brown.

Perruca, R., Hedrick, C., Terry, J., & Johnson, J. (1995). Infection control. In Terry, J., Baranowski, L., Lonsway, R., & Hedrick, C. (eds.): *Intravenous therapy: Clinical principles and practice*. Philadelphia: W.B. Saunders.

Riley, R.L. et al. (1959). Aerial dissemination of pulmonary tuberculosis: A two year study of contagion in a tuberculosis ward. *American Journal of Hygiene, 70*, 185.

Schalberg, D.R., Culver, D.H., & Gaynes, R.P. (1991). Major trends in the microbial etiology of nosocomial infections. *American Journal of Medicine* (suppl 3 B), B72S–75S.

Trilla, A., et al. (1991). Risk factors for nosocomial bacteremia in a large Spanish teaching hospital: A case-control study. *Infection Control Hospital Epidemiology, 12*, 150.

Tully, J.L., Friedland, G.H., Baldini, L.M., & Goldmann, D.A. (1981). Complications of intravenous therapy with steel needles and Teflon catheters: A comparative study. *American Journal of Medicine, 70*, 702.

Voss, A., Hollis, R.J., Pfaller, M.A., Wenzel, R.P., & Doebbeling, R.N. (1994). Investigation of the sequence of colonization and candidemia in nonneutropenic patients. *Journal of Clinical Microbiology, 32*, 975–980.

Waller, C.W., Kunstin, R.B., & Brubaker, M.M. (1963). The incidence of airborne wound infections during operation. *JAMA, 186*, 908.

Weinstein, S.W. (1993). *Plumer's principles & practices of intravenous therapy*. Philadelphia: J.B. Lippincott.

Wey, S.G., et al. (1989). Risk factors for hospital-acquired candidemia: A matched case-control study. *Archives of Internal Medicine, 149*, 2349.

CHAPTER 7

Equipment

CHAPTER CONTENTS

GLOSSARY
LEARNING OBJECTIVES
PRE-TEST, CHAPTER 7
INFUSION DELIVERY SYSTEMS
Glass System
Plastic System
ADMINISTRATION SETS
Primary
Secondary
Primary Y
Large Bore
PERIPHERAL INFUSION DEVICES
Scalp Vein Needles
Over-the-Needle Catheters
Inside-the-Needle Catheters
Midline Catheters
Dual-Lumen Peripheral Catheters
Central Infusion Devices
Percutaneous Catheters
Central Venous Tunneled Catheters
Peripherally Inserted Central Venous Catheters
Midclavicular
INLINE I.V. SOLUTION FILTERS
Depth
Membrane
I.V. Set Saver
BLOOD FILTERS
Standard Clot

Microaggregate
Leukocyte Depletion
ELECTRONIC INFUSION DEVICES (EIDs)
Controllers
Positive-Pressure Infusion Pumps
Mechanical Infusion Devices
Implantable Pumps
Programming Electronic Infusion Devices
ACCESSORY EQUIPMENT
Fluid Warmer
Latex Resealable Lock
Add-On Devices
Needle Protector Systems and Needleless
    Systems
NURSING PLAN OF CARE: PATIENTS RECEIVING
    PERIPHERAL I.V. THERAPY
PATIENT EDUCATION
HOME CARE ISSUES
COMPETENCY CRITERIA: EQUIPMENT
    MANAGEMENT
KEY POINTS
CRITICAL THINKING ACTIVITY
POST-TEST, CHAPTER 7
ANSWERS TO CHAPTER 7
Pre-Test
Post-Test
REFERENCES

GLOSSARY

Cannula A tube or sheath used for infusing fluids
Coring Visible, as well as microscopic, particles of rubber bung displaced by the spike during piercing of the glass container
Drip chamber Area of the intravenous (I.V.) tubing usually found under the spike where the solution drips and collects before running through the I.V. tubing
Filter A special porous device used to prevent the passage of undesired substances
Gauge Size of cannula opening
Groshong catheter Surgically implanted, long-term indwelling catheter; unique in that it has a two-way valve adjacent to the closed tip that prevents backflow of blood
Heparin lock Intermittent I.V. device used to maintain patent venous access

Hickman catheter   Long-term indwelling catheter inserted surgically via an incision in the deltopectoral groove through the superior vena cava, terminating near the right atrium

Hub   Female connection point of an I.V. cannula where the tubing or other equipment will attach

Infusate   I.V. solution

INS   Intravenous Nursing Society

Lumen   The space within an artery, vein, or catheter

Macrodrip   Drop factor of 10 to 20 drops equivalent to 1 mL based on manufacturer

Microaggregate   Microscopic collection of particles, such as platelets, leukocytes, and fibrin that can occur in stored blood

Microdrip   Drop factor of 60 drops/1 mL

Midclavicular catheter   Long (24–24 in) intravenous access device made of a soft flexible material inserted into one of the superficial veins of the peripheral vascular system and advanced to proximal axillary or subclavian veins

Midline   Peripherally inseted catheter with the tip terminating in the proximal portion of the extremity, usually 6 in in length

PCA   Patient-controlled analgesia

PICC   Long (20–24 in) intravenous access device made of a soft flexible material inserted into one of the superficial veins of the peripheral vascular system and advanced to the superior vena cava

Port   Point of entry

Radiopaque   Material used in I.V. catheter that can be identified by x-ray

Rubber bung   Stopper of glass container composed of numerous substances including rubber, chemical particles, and cellulose fibers

Stylet   Needle or guide that is found inside a catheter used for vein penetration

LEARNING OBJECTIVES

Upon completion of this chapter, the reader will be able to:

- Identify the terminology related to I.V. equipment.
- Identify types and characteristics of three infusate containers.
- Describe gravity flow systems.
- Compare vented and nonvented administration sets.
- Identify types and characteristics of peripheral and central infusion devices.
- State the major complications associated with over-the needle catheters and scalp vein needles.
- Identify the characteristics and uses of controllers and pumps to regulate infusions.
- Describe the use of filters in the infusion of solutions and blood products.
- Describe the use of miscellaneous adjuncts to aid in administration of safe infusions.
- Identify the Intravenous Nurses Society and the Centers for Disease Control and Prevention recommendations for standards of practice related to equipment safety and use.

PRE-TEST, CHAPTER 7

The pre-test is to review prior knowledge of equipment for safe delivery of infusions. Each question is based on the learning objectives of the chapter.

1. When using a closed-glass system, the administration set should be:
   A. Vented
   B. Nonvented

2. What are inline filters useful for?
   A. Filtering nonviable contaminants such as particles of metal, lint, and glass

B. Filtering viable contaminants such as bacteria and fungi
C. Filtering air from the administration set
D. All of the above

3. A major hazard of using Teflon over-the-needle catheters for peripheral infusion is:
A. The risk of phlebitis
B. The risk of infiltration
C. That they can be used for only 24 hours
D. The risk of septicemia

4. The infusate solution containers should be inspected for:
A. Clarity, expiration date, and air vents
B. Clarity, expiration date, and punctures or cracks
C. Puncture or cracks, presence of ports, and clarity

5. Volumetric pumps require:
A. A 170-micron filter
B. A 0.22-micron filter
C. Special cassette (cartridge) tubing
D. Microdrip tubing

True-False

6. **T F** Scalp vein needles have a higher rate of infiltration than do over-the-needle catheters.

7. **T F** According to the Intravenous Nursing Standards of Practice, primary tubing changes should coordinate with catheter changes at 48 hours.

8. **T F** Controllers eliminate the need for frequent monitoring of the patient by the nurse.

9. **T F** Controllers are gravity-dependent.

Match the term in column I with the definition in column II.

Column I

10. _____ port
11. _____ lumen
12. _____ radiopaque
13. _____ macrodrip
14. _____ filter

Column II

A. Porous device used to prevent passage of undesirable substances

B. Drop factor of 10 to 20 drops equivalent to 1 mL based on manufacturer

C. Space within an artery, vein, or catheter

D. Material used in catheters that can be identified by x-ray

E. Point of entry

All rituals and ceremonials which our modern worship of efficiency may devise, and all our elaborate scientific equipment will not save us if the intellectual and spiritual elements in our art are subordinated to the mechanical, and if the means come to be regarded as more important than ends.

STEWART, 1929

INFUSION DELIVERY SYSTEMS

Two infusion systems are available for delivery of intravenous (I.V.) fluids: the glass system and the plastic system. Sterile evacuated glass containers became available in 1929. The rigid glass containers contain a standard mix of materials, glass, metal, and rubber. The combination of materials is a disadvantage because of incompatibilities with other fluids and additives and breakdown of the materials during heat sterilization. In 1950, plastic containers became accessible for the storage and delivery of blood products. Today, the plastic system is used 90% to 95% of the time for administration of solutions and blood products (Ausman, 1984).

Glass System

The glass system has a partial vacuum and requires air vents (unlike the plastic system) (Fig. 7–1). In the open-glass system, air enters through a plastic tube in the container and collects in the air space in the bottle, allowing for displacement of the solution. In the closed-glass system, air is filtered into the container via vented tubing. The closed-glass system must use vented tubing to allow air into the container. For advantages and disadvantages of the glass system see Table 7–1.

✎ NOTE: In the open-glass system, the straw must extend above the fluid level to prevent bubbling of the air through the infusate (I.V. solution). Bubbling increases the risk of contamination. This system has been replaced by the use of closed-glass and plastic systems.

The glass system has a stopper, also called the rubber bung. During insertion of the administration set, coring can occur, which results in the introduction of fragments of the rubber core into the solution. Visible and microscopic particles of the rubber bung can be displaced by twisting the spike through the rubber bung (Delaney & Lauer, 1988).

Because of the combination of materials in the glass system, there have been some disadvantages to this system during heat sterilization procedures. Openings between the external environment and the internal container occur at peak heating and early cooling phases of sterilization. Recalls of endogenously contaminated fluids in the United States were caused by the expansion of metal, rubber, and glass during the sterilization procedure (Ausman, 1984).

Checking the Glass System for Clarity

To ensure safety in the administration of solutions, the nurse must check the solution's clarity and expiration date before connection to the administration set. To check the glass system, hold the glass bottle up to the light and check for flashes of light,

186

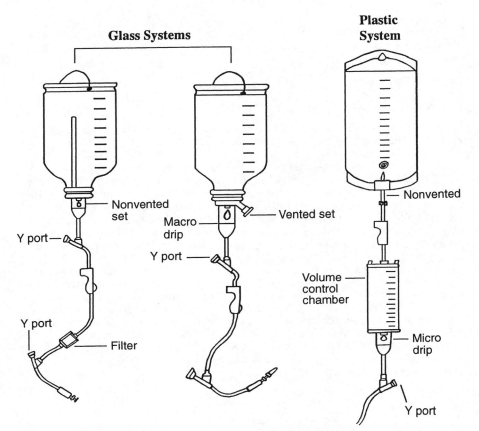

Figure 7–1. Comparison of infusate containers and administration sets. (Drawing by Timothy D. Mitas.)

TABLE 7–1. **ADVANTAGES AND DISADVANTAGES OF THE GLASS SYSTEM**

Advantages	Disadvantages
Crystal clear; allows for good visualization of contents	Breakage and shattering of glass
Fluid level easily read	Storage
Inert; has no plasticizers	Coring (due to rubber bung)
	Cumbersome disposal
	Rigidity
	Container constructed of mixed materials

floating particles, or discoloration. The glass system should be crystal clear; if not, mark the container contaminated and return it to central supply. Check the expiration date on the label.

Plastic System

Flexible and Rigid Plastic

Most I.V. fluids are packaged in plastic containers—either flexible or semirigid (Fig. 7–2). The flexible plastic container has several unique features. The entire structure that comes in contact with the fluid, including the closure, is made of the same material; it is all polyvinyl chloride (PVC) or other suitable material. There is no combination of metal, rubber, or glass as in the rigid glass system. The plastic system is a truly closed system. The introduction of PVC plastic solution containers has been accompanied by concerns of compatibility, specifically with the plasticizer diethylhexylphthalate (DEHP). These concerns have been addressed by the health care industry; however, solutions that remain a concern with regard to compatibility to plastic are insulin, nitroglycerin, fat emulsions, lorazepam, and others (Olin, 1991). For advantages and disadvantages of the plastic system, see Table 7–2.

The plastic system does not contain a vacuum; therefore, the containers must be flexible and collapsible (see Fig. 7–1). The plastic system does not need air to replace fluid flowing from the container. Either a vented or nonvented administration set is acceptable for delivery of the infusate. A membrane seals both the medication and the administration ports of the container, and there is no entry of air into this system. Because there is no rubber bung on the plastic system, spiking the system can be accomplished by means of a simple twisting motion (Fig. 7–3). Since the plastic can be easily perforated during use, careful attention should be paid to the integrity of this container during preparation and infusion delivery.

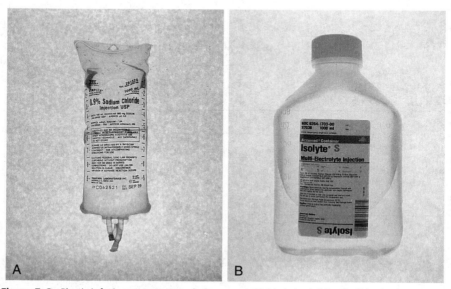

Figure 7–2. Plastic infusion system. I.V. solutions are available in both (A) a flexible plastic container and (B) a more rigid type of container. (Courtesy of D. Anderson, Chico, California.)

188

TABLE 7–2. **ADVANTAGES AND DISADVANTAGES OF THE PLASTIC SYSTEM**

Advantages	Disadvantages
Closed system	Punctures easily
Flexible	Fluid level difficult to determine
Lightweight	Composed of plasticizers
Container composed of one substance	Not completely inert (leaching)
Better storage	

The advantage of the semirigid, hard plastic unit is that it contains no plasticizers, and the the marks that indicate fluid levels are easier to read. This system is also impermeable to moisture. A disadvantage is that it does not completely collapse; therefore, the last 50 mL of the solution may be difficult to infuse.

The flexible and semirigid plastic systems, when used in a series with other similar containers, may promote movement of residual air into the I.V. line (Delaney & Lauer, 1988).

Checking the Plastic System for Clarity

The plastic container should be held up to the light and checked for clarity. If the plastic system is not crystal clear, any discoloration or floating particles in the solution

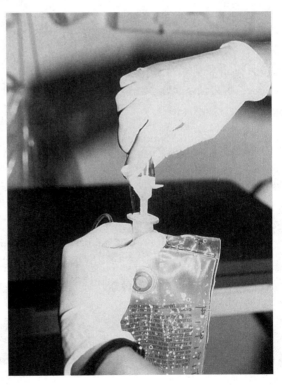

Figure 7–3. To spike the plastic container, insert the piercing pin of the I.V. tubing into the outlet port of the infusion bag using a twisting motion to ensure that the seal is pierced completely open.

189

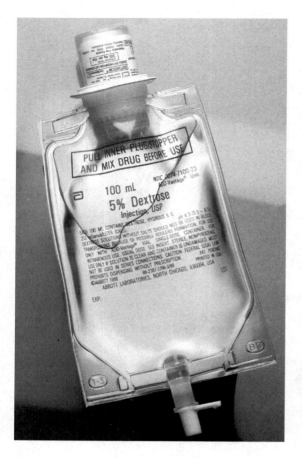

Figure 7–4. Use activated system. This Abbott ADD-Vantage™ system allows drugs to be quickly and safely reconstituted in an appropriate amount of diluent immediately before use. (Courtesy of Abbott Laboratories, North Chicago, IL. Used with permission.)

should be identified and labeled contaminated. The plastic system must be squeezed to check for pinholes. Check the expiration date on the label to ensure patient safety. The outer wrap of the plastic system should be free of pooled solution.

Use-Activated Containers

Use-activated containers are compartmentalized with premeasured ingredients that form an admixture when mixed. The containers are useful for high use infusions that have a short shelf-life after admixture. These systems are of benefit in the emergency department because they enable ease of use in acute situations (as in ambulances), in field use, and during transport. The ambulatory and home care settings can also benefit from use-activated systems (Fig. 7–4).

ADMINISTRATION SETS

Administration sets vary among manufacturers. These sets vary in drop factor, but all have the basic components (Fig. 7–5). The most frequently used administration sets include:

190

Primary (standard) sets
Secondary sets
    Piggyback
    Volume-controlled
Primary Y

BASIC COMPONENTS OF ADMINISTRATION SETS:

1. **Spike/piercing pin**: The spike/piercing pin is a sharply tipped plastic tube designed to be inserted into the infusate container. It is connected to the flange, drop orifice, and drip chamber.
2. **Flange**: The flange is a plastic guard that helps prevent touch contamination during insertion of the spike.
3. **Drop orifice**: The drop orifice is an opening that determines the size and shape of the fluid drop. The size of this drop orifice determines the drop factor.
4. **Drip chamber**: The drip chamber is a pliable, enlarged clear plastic tube that contains the drop orifice. It is connected to the tubing.
5. **Tubing**: The plastic tubing connects to the drip chamber. Depending on the manufacturer, the tubing may have a variety of clamps, ports, connectors, or filters built into the system. The average length of primary tubing is 66 to 100 in. The length of secondary administration sets averages from 32 to 42 in.
6. **Clamp**: The flow clamp control device operates on the principle of compres-

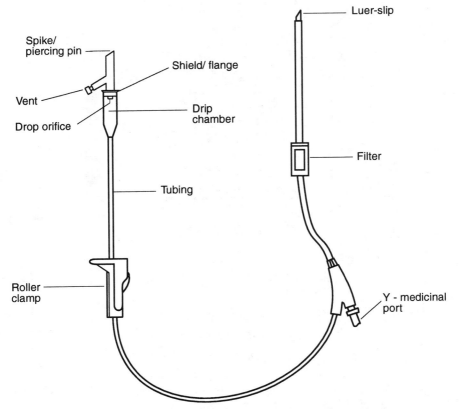

Figure 7–5. Basic administration set. (Drawing by Timothy D. Mitas.)

191

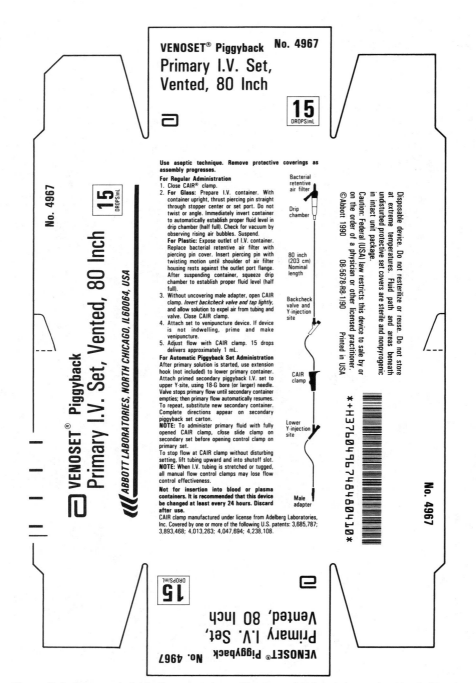

Figure 7–6. Primary administration set package. (Courtesy of Abbott Laboratories, Hospital Products Division, Abbott Park, IL.)

sion of the tubing wall. Each manufacturer supplies a clamp (roller, screw, or slide), and all operate on the principle of compression. The roller and screw clamps are equally reliable. The slide clamp is viewed as less reliable in controlling flow.

7. **Injection ports**: Injection ports serve as an access into the tubing and are located at various points along the administration set. Usually, the ports are used for administration of medication. Small needles should be used to access these ports (21- to 25-gauge) to ensure resealing.

8. **Final filter**: The final filter removes foreign particles from the infusate. It can be purchased as part of the administration set tubing, or filters can be added on.

Primary

Primary sets are referred to as standard sets and are available as vented or nonvented. Vented sets have an air filter attached to the spike pin that allows air to enter the container. Vented sets must be used on the closed-glass system. Nonvented sets have a straight spike pin without an air vent device. Nonvented sets can be used on any open-glass or plastic system. Primary sets are available in macrodrip form (10 to 20 drops/mL), or in microdrip form (60 drops/mL). The calibration is clearly specified on the box of each administration set, as well as in the accompanying literature. The microdrip set, also called a *minidrip* or *pediatric set*, is used when small amounts of fluid are required, such as in keep-vein-open rates (Fig. 7–6).

Secondary

Two types of secondary administration sets are available: the piggyback set and the volume-controlled set.

Piggyback Set

The piggyback set has short tubing (30 to 36 in) with a standard drop factor of 10 to 20 drops/mL. It is used to deliver 50 to 100 mL of infusate. In setting up the piggyback set, the primary infusion container is positioned lower than the secondary container, using the extension hook provided in the secondary line box. The secondary tubing connects to the primary line at the Y port.

Volume-Controlled Set

The volume-controlled set, also called metered-volume chamber set, is designed for intermittent administration of measured volumes of fluid with a calibrated chamber. These sets are calibrated in much smaller increments than other infusion devices, thus limiting the amount of solution available to the patient (usually for reasons of safety). Most chambers hold 100 to 150 mL of solution; neonatal chambers may hold only 10 to 50 mL. The volume-controlled set is most frequently used for pediatric patients and critically ill patients when small, well-controlled delivery of medication or solution is needed (Fig. 7–7).

Primary Y

The primary Y administration set is used for rapid infusion or for administration of more than one solution at a time. Each leg of the Y set is capable of being the primary

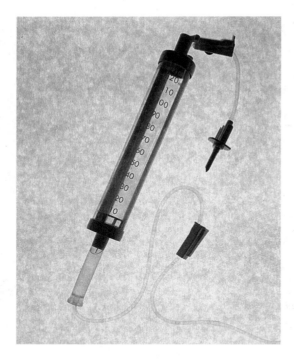

Figure 7–7. Volume chamber control set for intermittent infusion. (Courtesy of D. Anderson, Chico, CA.)

set. The Y set has two separate spikes with a separate drip chamber and short length of tubing with individual clamps. Primary Y sets are made up of large-bore tubing, because this tubing is meant to infuse large amounts of fluid in acute situations. Blood components can be administered through primary Y sets. A Y set allows for priming of the administration set before the blood is administered. Most blood administration Y sets contain inline filters with a pore size of 170 microns. Y sets have a drop factor of 10 to allow for the safe infusion of blood cells.

✎ **NOTE:** Primary Y sets are not provided as vented sets, so caution applies to bottles with venting straws or a venting apparatus added to the bottle. Collaps-

---

STANDARDS OF PRACTICE FOR ADMINISTRATION SETS

Centers for Disease Control and Prevention Standards of Practice Recommendations (1995)

Peripheral catheters: Change I.V. tubing, including piggyback tubing, no more frequently than every 72 hours.

Change tubing used to administer blood, blood products, or lipid emulsions within 24 hours of completing the infusion.

Midline catheters: Change I.V. tubing, including piggyback tubing, no more frequently than every 72 hours.

Central venous catheters: Change I.V. tubing, including piggyback, no more frequently than every 72 hours.

Peripherally inserted central venous catheters: Change I.V. tubing, including piggyback tubing, no more frequently than every 72 hours.

ible containers should be used with Y sets. Any air emboli associated with tubing of this inner lumen size are considered significant (Jensen, 1995).

Large Bore

Large-bore tubing sets are available for trauma care. These sets provide up to 514 mL/min for rapid flow rates, along with a 55% packed-cell flow rate faster than that of standard blood administration sets (Weinstein, 1993).

PERIPHERAL INFUSION DEVICES

Several types of peripheral infusion devices are commercially available; scalp vein needles, over-the-needle catheters, and inside-the-needle catheters, midline catheters, and dual-lumen catheters. The catheter-type devices usually have radiopaque material or stripping added to ensure radiographic visibility. Radiopacity aids in the identification of a catheter embolus, a rare complication. For a comparison of the types of peripheral infusion devices, see Table 7–3.

Scalp Vein Needles

The wing-tipped or butterfly needle are types of scalp vein needles. Scalp vein needles are made of stainless steel with odd-numbered gauges (17, 19, 21, 23, 25), and lengths of $\frac{1}{2}$ in to $1\frac{1}{4}$ in. The wings attached to the shaft are made of rubber or plastic,

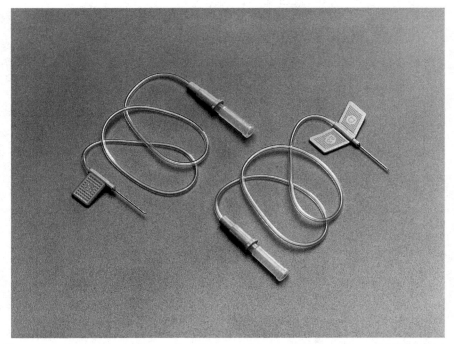

Figure 7–8. Types of scalp vein needles. (Courtesy of Becton-Dickinson, Deseret Division, Sandy, UT.)

TABLE 7-3. **COMPARISON OF PERIPHERAL INFUSION DEVICES**

Cannula	Advantages	Disadvantages	Uses
Scalp Vein Needle	Excellent for one-time I.V. medication, blood withdrawal, in patients allergic to nylon or Teflon Wings allow ease of insertions and secure taping Attached extension permits easy tubing change	Needle increases risk of infiltration Not recommended for use in flexor areas Needle not flexible Repuncture by contaminated needle possible	Infants and children Elderly and other adults with small veins Adults receiving short-term therapy
Over-the-Needle	Easy to insert Stays patent longer Catheter tip tapered to prevent peelback Radiopaque feature makes x-ray detection easy Infiltration rare Winged cannula easy to tape Stable: allows for greater patient mobility	Depending on the hub, sometimes difficult to secure with tape Long inflexible stylet increases risk of accidental puncture; pressure marks from hub Some catheters drag through the skin on insertion Increased risk of phlebitis	Long-term therapy Delivery of viscous liquids—blood and total parenteral nutrition Arterial monitoring
Inside-the-Needle	Permits insertion of catheter into superior vena cava Less likely to damage vein Stable Plastic sleeve reduces risk of touch contamination	Needle remains secured outside the skin; risk of catheter embolus Plastic catheter may support infection or trigger phlebitis in central veins	Long-term therapy Delivery of viscous liquid Delivery of drugs Central venous pressure monitoring Rarely used

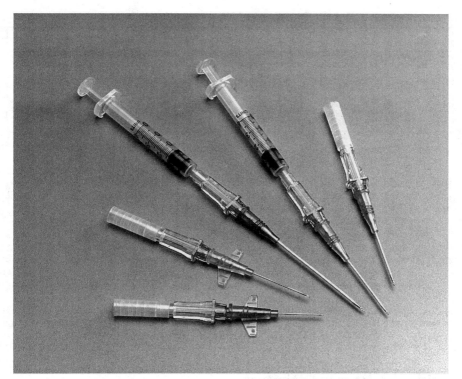

Figure 7–9. Types of over-the-needle catheters. (Courtesy of Becton-Dickinson, Deseret Division, Sandy, UT.)

and the flexible tubing extending behind the wings varies from 3 to 12 in long (Fig. 7–8). These needles are most frequently used for short-term therapy, usually in patients with expected indwelling catheter times of less than 24 hours, such as with single-dose therapy, I.V. push medication, or blood samples retrieval (Jensen, 1995). The steel needle is biocompatible and low rates of inflammation or phlebitis have been documented. The steel cannula does not flex or yield with resistance, therefore, the steel tip can easily puncture the vasculature after placement, increasing the risk of infiltration.

Over-the-Needle Catheters

The over-the-needle catheter (ONC) consists of a needle with a catheter sheath (Fig. 7–9). The cannula consists of a catheter with a length of $\frac{3}{4}$ in to 2 in and gauges of even numbers ranging from 12 to 24. (Table 7–4 is a guide regarding when to use the different sizes of gauge catheters.) The point of the needle extends beyond the tip of the catheter. After venipuncture, the needle (stylet) is withdrawn and discarded, leaving a flexible catheter within the vein.

Materials vary in ONCs, such as Teflon, Aquavene (which softens and expands), and vialon (which softens with body temperature). Teflon, a polyurethane material, has been shown to provide low cost, low rates of infiltration, and comparatively low rates of phlebitis. Teflon is a plastic-coated catheter material that is less thrombogenic

197

TABLE 7–4. GUIDE FOR OVER-THE-NEEDLE CATHETER USE

Gauge	
14–16	Multiple trauma, heart surgery, and transplantation procedures
18	Major trauma or surgery, blood administration
20	Minor trauma or surgery, blood administration
22	Pediatric, small veins, platelets, plasma
Note: Avoid use of 22-gauge catheter with packed red blood cells and whole blood, and antibiotic therapy in selected patients.)	

and less inflammatory than simple PVC or polyurethane (Altavela, Haas, & Nowak, 1993). Teflon ONCs tend to increase the risk of infusion-related phlebitis with small peripheral venous catheters (Maki & Ringer, 1991).

Aquavene is different from other venous access materials in that it changes physical properties after insertion. It softens in the vessel, expands 2 gauge sizes, and reduces thrombogenicity because of its biocompatibility. This catheter material is an elastomeric hydrogel, which undergoes predictable softening and dimension changes after contact with aqueous fluids.

Vialon, an elastomer of polyurethane, is a high-strength material that provides a smooth-surfaced catheter for easy insertion. Once inside the vein, vialon becomes soft and pliable, permitting the catheter to float in the vein rather than against the intima of the vein wall. Vialon is also designed to minimize local reactions under conditions of extended use (McKee et al., 1989).

Inside-the-Needle Catheters

The inside-the-needle catheter (INC) consists of a catheter between 14 and 19 gauge in diameter lying inside a needle. The needle may be from $1\frac{1}{2}$ to 2 in long, and the catheter may be 8 to 36 in long. The clear plastic sleeve over the catheter protects it from touch contamination during insertion. After the catheter is placed, the needle is withdrawn and secured outside the skin. Since the catheter is radiopaque, confirmation by x-ray can be done before administration of viscous solutions. These catheters have been largely replaced by the peripherally inserted central catheter (PICC).

✎ NOTE: With any catheter, use the shortest length and the smallest gauge to deliver the ordered therapy. Also, use a vein large enough to sustain sufficient blood flow, since this will decrease irritation to the vein wall.

Midline Catheters

Any catheter placed between the antecubital area and the head of the clavicle is called a midline catheter. The midline catheter is designed for intermediate-term therapies of two weeks or more. This catheter is 6 in long and is made of elastomeric hydrogel. Approximately 2 hours after insertion, it becomes 50 times softer, allowing it to increase two gauges in size and 2.5 cm in length (Meares, 1992). It is placed midline in the antecubital region in the basilic, cephalic, or median antecubital sites and is then advanced into the larger vessels of the upper arm for greater hemodilution. The arm should be measured from the proposed insertion site to the desired placement of the

198

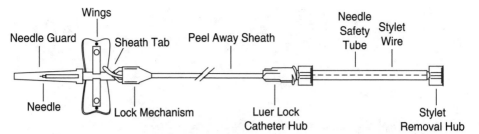

Figure 7–10. Midline catheter. This Landmark® Midline Catheter illustrates the features of this type of catheter. (Courtesy of Johnson & Johnson Medical Inc., Arlington, TX.)

catheter tip. In most adults this is about 5 to 6 in (Hadaway, 1990). X-ray verification for tip location is not necessary (See Fig. 7–10).

Dual-Lumen Peripheral Catheters

The dual-lumen peripheral catheter is available in a range of catheter gauges with corresponding lumen sizes. Two totally separate infusion channels exist, making it possible to infuse two solutions simultaneously. The catheters are available as 16-gauge catheters with 18-gauge and 20-gauge lumens or as 18-gauge catheters with 22-gauge and 20-gauge lumens (See Fig. 7–11).

✎ **NOTE:** Controversy still exists regarding simultaneous infusions of known incompatible solutions or medications through a dual-lumen peripheral catheter because of the limited hemodilution achievable in any peripheral vessel (Collins & Lutz, 1991).

Central Infusion Devices

Long-term I.V. therapy may require venous access over weeks, months, or even years. Special central venous catheters have been designed specifically for long-term access, patient comfort, and decreased complications associated with multiple therapies. There are three general types of placement of central venous lines: centrally placed percutaneous catheters and central venous tunneled catheters, both of which must be inserted by a physician, and the peripherally inserted central catheters, which can be inserted by a nurse.

    Percutaneous catheters
    Central venous tunneled catheters
        Hickman
        Broviac
        Groshong
        Implantable venous access port
    Peripherally inserted central catheter

Various types of central line catheters in use today will be discussed in detail in Chapter 13.

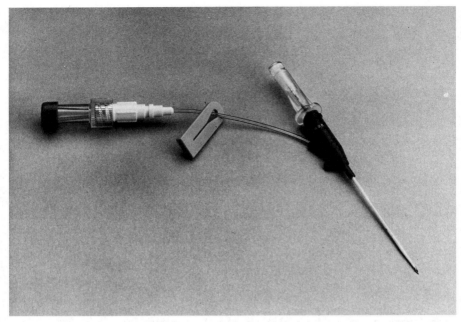

Figure 7–11. Dual-lumen peripheral catheter. This Twin-Cath® allows for two separate infusions through different ports by one access device. (Courtesy of Arrow International, Reading, PA. Used with permission.)

Percutaneous Catheters

In 1961, the first I.V. catheter for accessing the central circulation was introduced (Stewart & Sanislow, 1961). The percutaneous catheter is placed by an infraclavicular approach through the subclavian vein (or the jugular or femoral vein) and secured by suturing. It may remain in placed for a few days to several weeks. This type of catheter provides access to larger venous circulation for delivery of hypertonic solutions.

Central Venous Tunneled Catheters

Central venous tunneled catheters are made of silicone and are commercially available in many designs. These catheters are 20 to 30 in long and have a 22- to 17-gauge internal lumen diameter. The thickness of the silicone wall varies by manufacturer. Silicone catheters can be single, dual, or triple lumen (Fig. 7–12).

Hickman

The Hickman catheter is a 90-cm long, 1.6-mm diameter, long-term indwelling catheter equipped with one or two Dacron cuffs. It is made of silicone Silastic and is a modified Broviac catheter (see below) with a larger diameter. This central catheter allows for central drawing of blood samples.

The Hickman catheter is inserted surgically through an incision in the deltopectoral groove into the superior vena cava and terminates just before the right atrium.

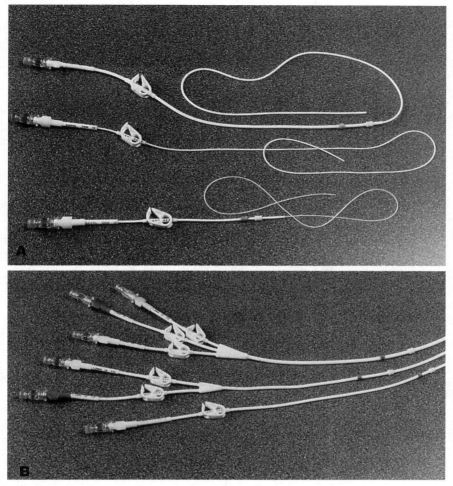

Figure 7–12. (*A*) Hickman (*top*) and Broviac (*bottom two*) catheters. (*B*) Triple-lumen (*top*), double-lumen (*middle*), and single-lumen (*bottom*) central venous tunneled catheters.

The catheter is tunneled subcutaneously and exits in an area that allows the patients to care for the site and port. The surgeon sutures the catheter in place via a Dacron polyester cuff that adheres to the tissues; this further secures the catheter and helps to prevent entrance of bacteria.

After the incision and exit sites heal, only the external catheter is visible. The patient or nurse can infuse medications, chemotherapeutic drugs, or blood through the Hickman catheter; blood specimens can be obtained also (see Fig. 7–12).

Broviac

The Broviac catheter is a 90-cm long, 1-mm diameter silicone Silastic long-term indwelling catheter equipped with cuffs. It allows for infusion of I.V. fluids including parenteral nutrition. Because of the Broviac's diameter, this catheter is used primarily in pediatric patients.

Groshong

The Groshong catheter is a thin-walled translucent silicone rubber catheter with an encapsulated barium sulfate radiopaque stripe and a patented two-way slit valve adjacent to a rounded, closed tip. A small Dacron cuff attached to the catheter promotes ingrowth of fibrous tissue, which helps to secure the catheter and reduces the potential for infection. Although similar to the Hickman catheter, its design allows for both fluid administration and blood sampling through the same lumen. The Groshong catheter is available in single- or triple-lumen style (Fig. 7–13).

Implantable Venous Access Ports

The implantable venous access port is a completely closed system composed of an implanted device with a drug reservoir, or port, with a self-sealing system connected to an outlet catheter. The device is surgically implanted into a convenient body site in a subcutaneous pocket. The self-sealing septum can withstand up to 2000 needle punctures. This device provides venous access for blood withdrawal, I.V. solution infusion, blood transfusion, and chemotherapy. The implanted port must be accessed with a Huber needle (noncoring) for safe and proper penetration of the septum of the port. Because these are noncoring needles, they contribute to the long lifetime of the port. The needles are sized from 19- to 24-gauge and range from $\frac{1}{2}$ to $2\frac{1}{2}$ in in length. The needles are available in 90-degree angle or straight-needle designs (Fig. 7–14).

Peripherally Inserted Central Venous Catheters

A PICC catheter is placed with tip location in the superior vena cava (SVC). A midclavicular catheter is placed so that the tip location is in the proximal axillary or subclavian vein. This catheter usually ranges from 16- to 25-gauge and 20 to 24 in in length. The peripheral catheter is inserted into a peripheral site and advanced into the superior vena cava. To reach the superior vena cava in the average adult a catheter at least 20 in long is required. The catheter is made of silicone, which has proven reliability and biocompatibility over the years in central venous catheter application

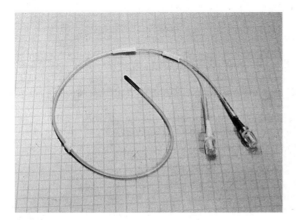

Figure 7–13. Groshong catheter. (Courtesy of Daval, Inc., a subsidiary of C.R. Bard, Inc., Specialty Access Products, Salt Lake City, UT.)

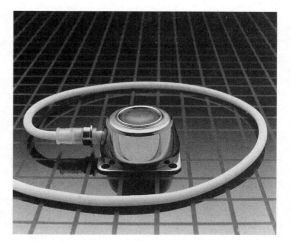

Figure 7–14. Implanted port. (Port-A-Cath, courtesy of Pharmacia Deltec Inc., St. Paul, MN.)

as well as a variety of implant uses. Silicone elastomer is soft, flexible, non-thrombogenic, and biocompatible (refer to Fig. 7–15). PICC may be used to deliver all types of therapy and is the appropriate choice for parenteral nutrition with dextrose content greater than 10%, continuous infusion of vesicant medications or medications with the ability to cause necrosis if they infiltrate, therapies with extreme variations in tonicity of pH, or anticipated extended I.V. therapy.

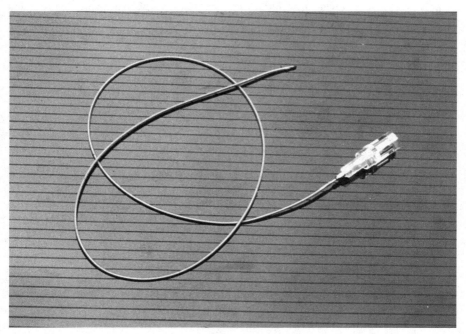

Figure 7–15. Peripherally inserted central catheter. (Courtesy of Daval, Inc., a subsidiary of C.R. Bard, Inc., Specialty Access Products, Salt Lake City, UT.)

203

Midclavicular

The midclavicular catheter has been referred to by several names including: longline, halfway, midline, PIC, and long-arm. The tip locations in this anatomical area is not considered a "midline" or a peripherally inserted central catheter (PICC). The intended tip location is the proximal axillary or subclavian vein. If a catheter is intended for the superior vena cava but falls short and ends up in the branchiocephalic (innominate) vein, it should be considered midclavicular. Midclavicular catheters may be the appropriate choice for I.V. fluid, electrolytes, and other medication commonly administered through peripheral veins, administration of isotonic solutions, and may be most appropriate if disease-produced or surgically created anomalies present tip location in SVC. Guidelines for PICC and midclavicular catheters are presented in Chapter 13.

INLINE I.V. SOLUTION FILTERS

Inline, or "final," filters are used in delivery of I.V. therapy to filter microorganisms, which, if alive, will multiply in the bloodstream or, if dead, will enter the tissue and cause a sterile abscess. There are two groups of particulate matter: nonviable contaminants such as particles of metal, lint, asbestos, rubber, cotton, dust, and glass; and viable contaminants, consisting of bacteria and fungi. Inline filters remove undissolved drug powders or crystals and precipitates from incompatible admixtures as well (Gurevich, 1986).

Inline filters are available in a variety of forms, sizes, and material. Two commonly used filters are the depth filter and the membrane filter.

The Food and Drug Administration (FDA, 1994) recommends the use of inline filter devices for removal of bacteria, fungi, particulates, air, and some endotoxins from intravenous-delivered fluids. The National Coordinating Committee on Large Volume Parenteral (NCCLVP) has established priorities for the use of filters, and recommends the use of filters with TPN admixtures, for immune-deficient or immunocompromised patients and for intravenous infusions containing additives, especially those that are heavily precipitated (Sevick, 1995).

Depth

The depth filter is composed of fibers or fragmented material that has been pressed or bonded to form a maze; the pore size is nonuniform. Fluid flows through a random path that absorbs and traps the particles. These filters can clog when large amounts of particles are retained. Depth filters prime easily and are capable of air elimination.

Membrane

Membrane filters are screen filters with uniformly sized pores. A 5-micron screen will retain on the flat portion of the membrane all particles greater than 5 microns. Filters of 0.2 micron are for bacteria, fungus, and air retention. The 0.22-micron air-venting filters automatically vent air through a nonwettable (hydrophobic) membrane and permit uniform high-gravity flow through large wettable (hydrophilic) membrane (Weinstein, 1993) (Fig. 7–16).

To be effective, an infusion filter must have the ability to:

- Maintain high flow rates
- Automatically vent air

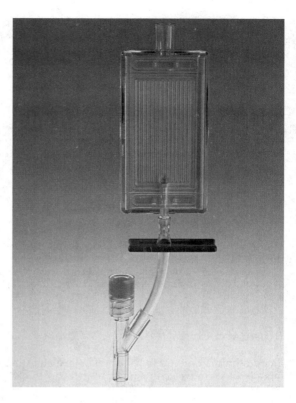

Figure 7–16. Inline solution filter. This Pall ELD-96™ filter removes inadvertent particulate matter, entrained air, microbial contaminants, and their associated endotoxins that may be present in I.V. solutions. The filter is effective for up to 96 hours. (Courtesy of Pall Corporation, Port Washington, NY. Used with permission.)

- Retain bacteria, fungi, particulate matter, and endotoxins
- Tolerate pressures generated by infusion pumps
- Act in a nonbinding fashion to drugs (Weinstein, 1993)

Filter are used under the following circumstances:

1. An additive has been combined with the solution.
2. The injection port on the tubing will be used.
3. The patient is susceptible to infusion phlebitis or infection.
4. The infusion is given centrally.

Filter sizes range from 5 microns (largest) to 0.22 micron (smallest). They allow liquids but not particles to pass through them. The finer the membrane, the more fully it will filter the liquid. See Table 7–5 for function of filters.

TABLE 7–5. **FUNCTION OF FILTERS**

Filter Size (Micron)	Function
5–1	Removes most particulate matter; does not remove fungi or bacteria
0.45	Removes fungi and most bacteria
0.22	Removes all fungi and bacteria but reduces flow rate; should be routinely used for the delivery of I.V. therapy (INS, 1996)

205

The drugs creating the greatest problem from incomplete dissolution of reconstituted mediations, recrystallization of drugs, and precipitates from incompatible mixtures are penicillin G, potassium, cephalothin sodium, ampicillin sodium, mannitol, and drugs manufactured by the "dry fill" process (Gurevich, 1986).

I.V. Set Saver

This inline set extends the set life and provides protection from inadvertent microbial, endotoxin, air, and particulate contamination for up to 96 hours. This filter can also be added to central lines because of its high flow rate and capacity. The I.V. set saver also is capable of retaining endotoxin molecules for up to 96 hours (Pall Biomedical Corporation, 1990).

BLOOD FILTERS

The American Association of Blood Banks states that blood must be transfused through a sterile, pyrogen-free transfusion set that has a filter capable of retaining particles that are potentially harmful to the recipient (Widman, 1991). Commercially available filters include the standard clot filter, the microaggregate filter, and the leukocyte depletion filter.

Standard Clot

Blood administration sets have a standard clot filter of 170- to 220-microns and are intended to remove coagulated products, microclots, and debris resulting from collection and storage. These filters do allow the passage of smaller particles called microaggregates, which are composed of nonviable leukocytes—primarily granulocytes, platelets, and fibrin strands. The microaggregates can cause pulmonary dysfunction (adult respiratory distress syndrome) when large quantities of stored bank blood are infused.

Microaggregate

A supplementary filter (transfusion filter) can be added to an in-use administration set, permitting infusion of blood, easy replacement of the filter, (if clogging occurs), and multiple infusion of blood units. The 20-micron microaggregate blood filters remove most debris from the transfusion product but can slow the administration of blood to an undesirable rate. The 40-micron filter allows blood to be transfused easily in the specified period of time; however, filtration is less refined. The 80-micron filter is the filter of choice in many institutions because of its safe level of filtration and high flow rate potential (Jensen, 1995). Microaggregate filters are added to blood administration sets for delivery of whole blood and packed red cells stored more than 4 days to eliminate microaggregates.

Leukocyte Depletion

The leukocyte depletion filter is used to remove leukocytes (including leukocyte-mediated viruses) from red blood cells and platelets. Leukocyte-poor filters are classified according to efficiency level, not micron size (Pall Biomedical Corporation,

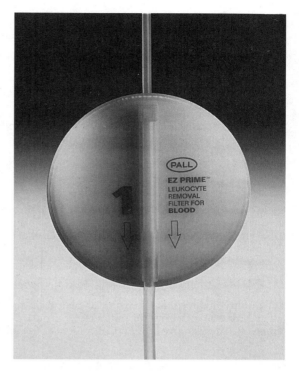

Figure 7–17. Leukocyte depletion filter. This Pall EZ Prime™ High Efficiency Leukocyte filter delivers low leukocyte residuals, averaging less than 2×10^5 white blood cells per transfusion and reducing the risk of leukocyte-related transfusion complications. It can be self-primed by gravity or primed rapidly by squeezing the blood bag. (Courtesy of Pall Corporation, Port Washington, NY. Used with permission.)

1990). These filters can be used to remove 95% to 99.9% of leukocytes from red blood cells and platelets (Pall, 1996). (Fig. 7–17).

ELECTRONIC INFUSION DEVICES (EIDs)

The use of flow control devices should be guided by the patient's age and condition, setting, and prescribed therapy. The nursing professional is responsible and accountable for the use of electronic infusion devices. To use these devices effectively, the nurse should know: (1) indications for their use, (2) their mechanical operation, (3) how to troubleshoot, (4) their psi rating, and (5) safe usage guidelines (Weinstein, 1993).

Infusion control devices have come a long way since their introduction in 1958. The very early models had serious accuracy and safety problems: air embolisms, fluid containers running dry, and clogged catheters were common. The pumps were large, hard to troubleshoot, and limited in their reliability and usability.

IVAC corporation introduced the concept of the rate controller in 1972; today there are many models and types on the market, including:

Controllers
Positive-pressure infusion pumps
    Volumetric
    Peristaltic
    Syringe

207

Ambulatory infusion
Multichannel and dual-channel
Patient-controlled analgesia
Mechanical infusion devices
Elastomere balloons

Recently, small portable units specifically designed for home use have been made available.

✎ **NOTE:** Because of the many controllers and volumetric and peristaltic pumps on the market, refer to the manufacturer's recommendations.

Controllers

Controllers operate strictly on gravity flow and do not exert positive pressure greater than the head height of the infusion bag, which is usually 2 pounds per square inch (psi) (Fig. 7–18). Some controllers can reach a psi of 5, but this pressure is uncommon. The maximum flow rate is affected by how high the I.V. container is hung above the I.V. site (Millam, 1990).

✎ **NOTE:** One psi and 50 mm Hg exert the same amount of pressure.

The gravity flow of fluid is regulated by a drop sensor and electric feedback mechanism. Controllers reduce the potential for rapid infusion of large amounts of solution (runaways) and empty bottles. Controllers assist the nurse in detecting infiltrations

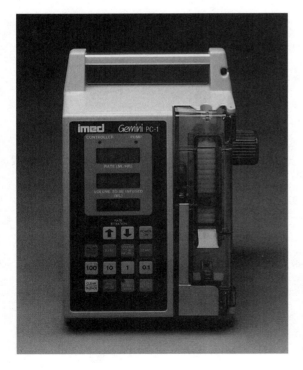

Figure 7–18. IMED Gemini PC-1® Controller. This single channel infusion device is designed to operate either as a controller or a volumtric infusion pump. (Courtesy of IMED Corporation. San Diego, CA. Used with permission.)

and maintaining accurate flow rates. It is estimated that 80% of I.V. fluid and drug administration can safely be regulated by the use of a controller.

The I.V. bag is usually hung 36 inches above a patient's head for adequate gravity pressure. When there is resistance to the flow, the controller's alarm will sound, signaling that it cannot maintain the preset rate. Resistance can occur when the patient is restless and frequently changing positions, if the catheter tip is at a flexion point, or if the patient lies on the tubing. Many of the newer controllers can deliver blood components safely.

Positive-Pressure Infusion Pumps

Positive-pressure infusion pumps average 10 psi, although newer technology has the psi set as low as 5 psi. Older pumps still in use may pump at dangerous pressures of 16 to 22 psi. Pressures greater than 10 to 20 psi should be used with extreme caution.

Positive-pressure infusion pumps are used for delivery of high volumes and for delivery of complex therapies in high-acuity situations. The pumps are more precise than controllers, deliver the fluid accurately as programmed, and have many features including the ability to keep track of fluid amounts and to sound alarms for various malfunctions. These pumps totally control the flow rate.

Volumetric

The volumetric pump calculates the volume delivered by measuring the volume displaced in a reservoir that is part of the disposable administration set. The pump calculates every fill and empty cycle of the reservoir. The reservoir is manipulated internally by a specific action of the pump. Industry standards for accuracy of electronic volumetric infusion pumps is plus or minus 5% (Jensen, 1995).

Pressure terminology includes the terms *fixed* and *variable*. With fixed infusion pressure, the pump is set internally to infuse up to a certain psi but not more (occlusion limit). Variable pressure pumps allow individual judgment about the psi needed to safely deliver therapy. A variable pressure pump can be adjusted by the nurse through programming. Variable pressure devices have a conservative upper limit (usually 10 psi) and a lower limit of 2 psi similar to that of a controller. A psi setting of 4 to 8 is common; pressures greater than 12 to 14 psi are rarely necessary.

Volumetric pumps have proved invaluable in neonatal, pediatric, and adult intensive care units, where critical infusions of small volumes of fluid or doses of high-potency drugs are indicated. These pumps have a cartridge that pumps the solution to be delivered; therefore, blood and red blood cells can be administered without damage to the blood cells.

Many pumps use microprocessor technology for a more compact unit and for easier troubleshooting. *All volumetric pumps require special tubing* (Fig. 7–19).

✎ NOTE: Reading the literature, becoming familiar with the pump, and observing all precautions are imperative measures to ensure safe, efficient operation.

Peristaltic

"Peristaltic" refers to the controlling mechanisms: a peristaltic device moves fluid by intermittently squeezing the I.V. tubing. The device may be rotary or linear. In a rotary peristaltic pump, a rotating disk or series of rollers compresses the tubing along a curved or semicircular chamber, propelling the fluid when pressure is re-

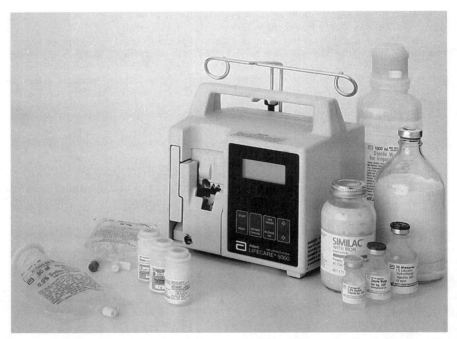

Figure 7–19. Lifecare 5000 Plum Pump. (Courtesy of Abbott Laboratories, Hospital Products Division, Abbott Park, IL.)

leased. In a linear device, one or more projections intermittently press the I.V. tubing. Peristaltic pumps are primarily used for infusion of enteral feedings.

Syringe

The syringe pump is a piston-driven infusion pump that provides precise infusion by controlling the rate by drive speed and syringe size, thus eliminating the variables of the drop rate. Syringe pumps are valuable for critical infusions of *small* doses of high-potency drugs. These pumps are used most frequently for delivery of antibiotic and small-volume parenteral therapy. Syringe pump technology was applied to patient-controlled analgesia (PCA) infusion devices. Syringe pumps are used frequently in the areas of anesthesia, oncology, and obstetrics.

The volume of the syringe pump is limited to the size of the syringe—usually a 60-mL syringe is used. However, the syringe can be as small as 5 mL. The tubing usually is a single, uninterrupted length of kink-resistant tubing with a notable lack of Y injection ports. Syringe pumps can use primary or secondary sets, depending on the intended use (Jensen, 1995).

Ambulatory

The ambulatory pump is a lightweight, compact infusion pump that has made a significant breakthrough in long-term care. This device allows the patient freedom to resume a normal life pattern. Ambulatory pumps range in size and weight—most being under 6 pounds and capable of delivering most infusion therapies. Features include medication delivery, delivery of several different dose sizes at different in-

210

tervals, memory of programs, and safety alarms. The main disadvantage of ambulatory pumps is limited power supply; they function on a battery system that requires frequent recharging (Fig. 7–20).

Multichannel and Dual-Channel

In the future, all multiple-drug delivery systems will be computer-generated, and many already use computer-generated technology. Dual-channel and multichannel pumps can deliver several medications and fluids simultaneously or intermittently from bags, bottles, or syringes (Weinstein, 1993). Multichannel pumps (usually three or four channels) require manifold-type sets to set up all channels—whether or not they are in use; each channel must be programmed independently. Programming a multichannel pump can be challenging.

The dual-channel pump offers a two-pump mechanism assembly, with a common control and programming panel. This type of pump uses one administration set for each channel.

Patient-Controlled Analgesia

Patient-controlled analgesia (PCA) pumps have been developed to assist the patient in controlling pain at home or in the hospital. These pumps are different from other infusion devices in that they have a remote bolus control in which the patient or

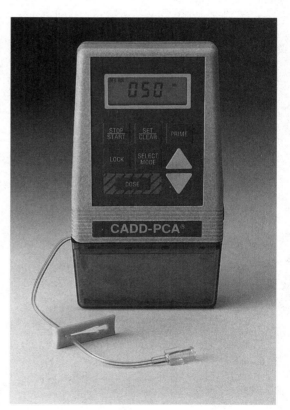

Figure 7–20. Portable infusion pump CADD-PCA. (Courtesy of Pharmacia Deltec Inc., St. Paul, MN.)

211

nurse can deliver a bolus of medication at set intervals. PCA pumps are available in ambulatory or pole-mounted models.

There are three types of PCA pumps: basal, continuous, and demand. All three afford some type of pain control with varying degree of patient interaction. The *continuous* mode of therapy is designed for the patient who needs maximum pain relief; it usually does not fluctuate from hour to hour and should completely relieve pain or achieve a constant effect. The *basal* mode is designed to achieve pain relief with minimal medication with intermittent dosing, thus allowing the patient to remain alert and active without sedation. The *demand* dose is delivered by intermittent infusion when a button attached to the pump is pushed. The demand dose can be used alone or with the basal type of infusion (Fig. 7–21).

✎ **NOTE:** The PCA pump must be programmed with parameters to prevent overmedication.

Mechanical Infusion Devices

Elastomere Balloons

The elastomere balloon system is a portable device with an elastomeric reservoir or balloon. The balloon, which is made of a soft rubberized material capable of being inflated to a predetermined volume, is safely encapsulated inside a rigid, transparent container. When the reservoir is filled, the balloon exerts positive pressure to administer the medication with an integrated flow restrictor that controls the flow rate. This system requires no batteries or electronic programming and is not reusable.

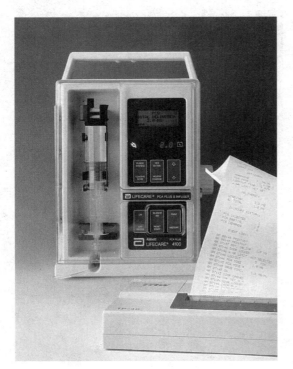

Figure 7–21. PCA Plus II infuser pump. (Courtesy of Abbott Laboratories, Hospital Products Division, Abbott Park, IL.)

✎ **NOTE:** Elastomere balloon devices are used primarily for delivery of antibiotics. The typical volume for these devices is 50 to 100 mL, but these balloons are available in sizes up to 250 mL (Fig. 7–22).

Implantable Pumps

Implantable infusion pumps have become popular because of their convenience and reliability. These pumps are now used to deliver morphine and other pain medications for patients with chronic pain.

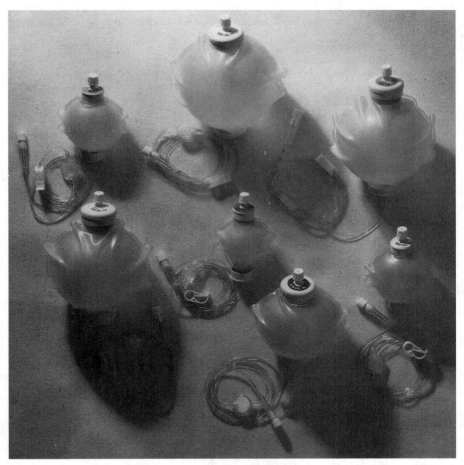

Figure 7–22. Home Pump Eclipse is a durable, portable, compact infusion system designed for the delivery of intermittent antibiotics. This disposable elastomeric infusion system offers volumes ranging from 50 mL to 500 mL. (Courtesy of Block Medical, Inc., Carlsbad, CA.)

Programming Electronic Infusion Devices

To be able to program any type electronic infusion device, one needs to be familiar with the terminology for delivering infusion and the device enhancements.

INFUSION TERMINOLOGY

Rate: Amount of time over which a specific volume of fluid infuses. Infusion pumps deliver in increments of mL/hr. The most common rate parameters for regular infusion pumps are 1 to 999 mL/hr. Many newer pumps are capable of setting rates that offer parameters of 0.1 mL in increments of 0.1 mL up to 99.9 mL, then in 1 mL increments up to 999 mL.

Volume infused: Measurement that tells how much of a given solution has been infused. This measurement is used to monitor the amount of fluid infused in a shift, or it can be used in home health to monitor the infusion periodically during the day or over several days. The "counter" must be returned to zero at the beginning of each shift.

Volume to be infused: Usually the amount of solution hanging in the solution container. A pump is designed to sound an alarm when the volume to be infused is reached.

ENHANCEMENT TERMINOLOGY

Drop sensors: Used with a controller to confirm the presence or absence of flow. The drop sensor is attached to the drop chamber of the administration set or can be located internally on the controller as the flow passes through a chamber.

✎ **NOTE:** The drop chamber must remain still to ensure that the counter senses or detects each drop as it falls. Splashing or multiple drops result in sudden rate changes.

ALARMS

Air-in-line: Designed to detect only visible bubbles or microscopic bubbles. This alarm is necessary for all positive-pressure pumps and infusion controllers. Volumetric pumps are usually equipped with air-in-line detectors.

Occlusion: Standard alarm for infusion pumps and controllers. Controllers may be able to indicate only "no flow." With an occlusion alarm, controllers are able to indicate upstream (between pump and container) or downstream (between patient and pump) occlusion by absence of flow. (Many newer pumps are able to differentiate between upstream and downstream occlusion.)

✎ **NOTE:** The pressure can be set as low as 2 to 5 psi for infusion of vesicants or routine fluids through veins. Occlusion alarms with low psi settings are common because the pumps are sensitive to even slight changes in pressure.

Infusion complete: Alarm triggered by a preset volume limit ("infusion complete"). These alarms are helpful in preventing the fluid container from running dry because they can be set to sound before the entire solution container is infused.

Low battery or low power: Gives the user ample warning of the pump's impending inability to function. A low-battery alarm means that the batteries need to be replaced or external power source needs to be connected. As a protective measure when low-battery and low-power alarms are continued over a preset number of minutes, the pumps usually convert to a "keep-vein-open" (KVO) rate. The preset KVO rate is usually between 0.1 and 5 mL.

Nonfunctional: Alarm that means the pump is operating outside parameters and the problem cannot be resolved. When this alarm sounds the pump should be disconnected from the patient and returned to biomedical engineering or to the manufacturer for evaluation. The nonfunctional alarm may be worded in many ways, depending on manufacturer.

Not infusing: Indicates that all of the pump infusion parameters are not set. This feature prevents tampering or setting changes from happening accidentally. The pump must be programmed or changed and then told to "start."

Parameters: Reminds the programmer that not all settings have been completed.

Tubing: Ensures that the correct tubing has been loaded into the pump. Also, if tubing incorrectly loaded, this alarm will sound.

Door: Indicates that the door that secures the tubing is not closed.

Free flow: Detects the rapid infusion of fluid, which can occur when the set is removed from the pump. Disengaging the tubing from the pump requires a deliberate act.

ADDITIONAL ENHANCEMENTS

Many other functions have been added to newer pumps:

Preprogrammed drug compatibility
Retrievable historical data
Infiltration or thrombus detection alarm
Central venous pressure monitor
Positive-pressure fill stroke
Modular self-diagnosing capability
Printer read-out

Nurse call system
Remote site programming
Syringe use for secondary infusion
Adjustable occlusion pressures
Opaque infusions (for blood, fat emulsions, iron dextran)
Secondary rate settings
Bar coding

ACCESSORY EQUIPMENT

Several types of accessory equipment are available to increase the efficiency and accuracy of delivering I.V. solutions.

Fluid Warmer

The fluid warmer is used primarily for the administration of blood to prevent stress of the cardiac system and to diminish hypothermia in multiple transfusions. Several companies have devised units consisting of blood-warming coils that are placed in warm water baths. Warming devices must undergo careful and continuing quality-control procedures. Standard blood tubing connected to the coils is usually needed (Weinstein, 1993). *Never put the blood tubing directly into warm water.*

Latex Resealable Lock

Also called a PRN device, this locking device is a capped resealable latex diaphragm that may have a Luer lock or Luer slip connection. This type of device can convert continuous I.V. infusion to an intermittent device when a resertable plug is inserted into the cannula hub. The latex resealable lock is used for saline or heparin flush. See Figure 7–23.

Since injection ports vary in their length from $\frac{1}{2}$ in to 2 in, a shorter lock is less bulky under dressing and allows less dead space during priming. A short injection port may allow needles to penetrate into the hub of the infusion catheter, which could compromise the catheter or tubing.

✎ NOTE: Large-bore needles or frequent needle punctures may remove a plug of rubber from the port, resulting in coring. The risk of coring is difficult to predict;

215

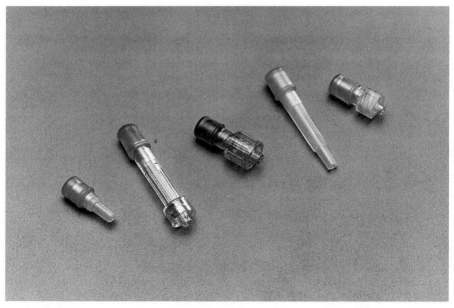

Figure 7–23. PRN adaptors. (Courtesy of Becton-Dicksinson, Deseret Division, Sandy, UT.)

therefore, latex injection caps should be routinely changed according to institutional protocol.

A disadvantage of the latex resealable lock is that it can separate at the hub or plug junction, allowing bacteria to enter the system because of inadequate flushing of blood cells from under the latex rubber. In addition, an occlusion or blood clot can occur within the locking device.

Add-On Devices

T-, J- or U-Shaped Port Devices

A J-, U-, or T-shaped port device may be used at the injection site. The T port is a common add-on device that is usually about 4 to 6 in long and made of standard or microbore tubing with a hard plastic T-shaped connector on one end. One leg of the T connector attaches to the I.V. device and the other is a resealable latex port.

The J loop or U connectors have the same purpose as the T connectors. Their rigid shape is maintained when connected to an I.V. site.

Disadvantages of I.V. loops are an increased cost and an additional site for bacteria to enter the system.

Microbore Extension Tubing

These are add-on sets that come in various lengths to add I.V. line for active patients. The extension sets aid in tubing changes without site manipulation. This tubing is frequently used as primary tubing for syringe pumps and ambulatory pumps. Disadvantages are an added cost and an additional site for bacteria to enter the system.

Needle Protector Systems and Needleless Systems

The use of protected needles or needleless equipment significantly decreases the risk of needle-stick injuries (Chiarello, Nagin, & Laufer, 1992). Three types of devices are available: I.V. delivery systems that are needleless or have recessed needles, shielded needles for percutaneous injection, and blunt needles.

The needle protection system covers the needle and protects against accidental needle sticks during blood sampling, I.V. push medications, intermittent I.V. medications, chemotherapy administration, and other catheter access procedures. The following recessed needles are available (Gurevich, 1994):

Centurion Keen-Needle (Tri-State)
LifeShield Connector (Abbott Laboratories)
NeedleLock Device (Baxter)
Protected Needle (McGaw)
Safety-Gard IV Needle (Becton-Dickinson)
Saf-T Floe (Ryan Medical)

IV catheter/stylet with protected needle:

Landmark (Johnson & Johnson)—Retractable needle
Protective IV Catheter (Critikon)—Plastic guard
SafeStick IV Catheter (Phase Medical)—Retractable needle
Saf-T Intima (Becton-Dickinson)—Safety shield

The needleless or needle-free I.V. systems have taken the place of 80% of needles used in I.V. therapy (Beason, Bourguignon, et al. 1992). The following needleless devices are available:

Clave (ICU Medical)—One piece needleless I.V. connection device
Interlink IV Access System (Baxter/Becton-Dickinson)—Blunt cannula
LifeShield (Abbott)—Blunt cannula, prepierced reseal injection site
Monject LifeShield (Sherwood Medical)—Blunt steel cannula
SafeLine (McGaw)—Blunt plastic cannula
Safesite (B. Braun Medical)—Reflux valve

The B. Braun Medical's Safesite is a two-way valve used in place of a male adaptor cap on a heparin-locked I.V. catheter. The valve is opened when accessed by a syringe or tubing. The Luer taper on the syringe or tubing opens the valve diaphragm and allows infusion or aspiration of fluids. The diaphragm closes when the syringe or tubing is removed (Fig. 7–24).

✎ NOTE: When choosing a product, evaluate its compatibility with other systems you use. An independent research agency, ECRI, issued test result data in September 1994 on safer needle devices.

To purchase a report on needle-stick prevention devices, write:

ECRI
5200 Butler Pike
Plymouth Meeting, PA 19462

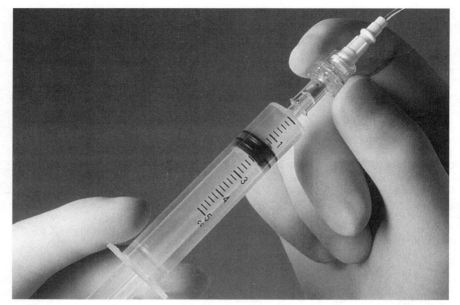

Figure 7–24. Safesite Needle-Free Access System. (Courtesy of Burron Medical, Inc., Bethlehem, PA.)

Nursing Plan of Care

PATIENTS RECEIVING PERIPHERAL I.V. THERAPY

Focus Assessment

Subjective

Knowledge of therapies and equipment used to deliver therapy

Objective

Suitable vascular access for choice of cannula

Adequate level of consciousness and compliance

Patient Outcome Criteria
The patient will be:
1. Free of complications associated with I.V. therapy
2. Free of injury

Nursing Diagnoses
Risk for injury related to environmental conditions, lack of knowledge regarding equipment
Knowledge deficit related to new procedure and maintaining I.V. therapy
Impaired physical mobility related to placement and maintenance of I.V. cannula
Anxiety (mild, moderate, or severe) related to new equipment technology

Continued on following page

Nursing Management: Critical Activities

Follow manufacturer's guidelines on setup and maintenance of specific electronic infusion devices.

Select and prepare infusion pump as indicated.

Correct malfunctioning equipment.

Plug equipment into electrical outlets connected to an emergency power source.

Have equipment periodically checked by bioengineering as appropriate.

Set alarm limits on equipment as appropriate.

Respond to equipment alarms appropriately.

Consult with other health care team members and recommend equipment and devices for patient use.

Compare machine-derived data with nurse's perception of patient's condition.

Explain potential risks and benefits of using equipment technology.

Follow INS Standards of Practice in rotation of I.V. sites, administration set changes, and dressing management to maintain integrity of site.

Use filters where appropriate.

Use appropriate administration set (vented or nonvented) with the appropriate fluid container.

Inspect fluid containers, administration sets, and cannulas for integrity prior to use.

PATIENT EDUCATION

Instruct patient by demonstration of preparation and administration of therapy.

Teach patient and family how to operate equipment as appropriate.

Advise patient regarding alarms of pump and advise to contact nurse if alarm is triggered.

Instruct on use of PCA pump for pain control.

Teach patient and family the expected patient outcomes and side effects associated with using the equipment.

HOME CARE ISSUES

Reimbursement is a challenge in the home care setting. Before any equipment is acquired the reimbursement status of the clientele served and the anticipated need should be thoroughly explored (Jensen, 1995).

Home care infusion devices are designed to allow the patient maximum portability and freedom of movement. The aim is for small, quiet, lightweight infusion pumps with pouches to enclose the infusion container. Equipment used at home must offer safety features because the caregiver in most situations is the patient or family.

Equipment used frequently in home care management include:

Medical teaching dolls (Legacy Products)—Facilitate visual, hands-on approach to educate patients of all ages and families about vascular access site, equipment, and procedures

Vascular access devices—Easy to administer medication by home-health care professional, patient, or family

Tubing, connectors, and filters—Include needle protector and needleless systems for use in home to prevent needle-stick injuries

Electronic infusion devices—Syringe pumps, elastomeric infusers, ambulatory pumps

Premixed medications

Transport storage pouch

219

COMPETENCY CRITERIA: Equipment Management

Competency Statement: The competent I.V. nurse will be able to demonstrate use of technical equipment and devices to deliver I.V. therapy.

PERFORMANCE CRITERIA:

	Skilled	Needs Education
1. Identifies types and indication for use:		
Scalp vein needles		
Over-the-needle catheters		
Midline catheters		
2. Chooses appropriate gauge and length cannula for patient.		
3. Demonstrates use of electronic infusion devices:		
Controller		
Pump		
Patient-controlled analgesia		
Ambulatory pump		
Elastomere pump		
4. Demonstrates use of inline filters:		
0.22 micron		
70 micron		
Leukocyte		
Microaggregate		
5. Inspects equipment for product integrity:		
Glass system		
Plastic system		
Administration sets		
6. Determines most appropriate accessory equipment and uses appropriately:		
Needleless/needle protector systems		
J, U, or T connectors		
Fluid warmers		
Resealable locks (PRN devices)		

220

SUGGESTED EVALUATION CRITERIA

1. Demonstrates setup and troubleshooting of equipment
2. Demonstrates appropriate choice of equipment in patient care setting

KEY POINTS

Equipment
Infusion delivery systems
  Glass
  Plastic
    Rigid
    Flexible

Administration sets
  Primary (standard) set
    Vented or nonvented
    Vented used for closed glass
  Secondary set
  Primary Y sets
  Volume control sets

Peripheral infusion devices
  Scalp vein needles—For short-term therapy
  Over-the-needle catheters (OMC)—For long-term peripheral therapy; made from Teflon, vialon or Aquavene
  Inside-the-needle catheter (INC)—Rarely used; catheter is threaded through a large-bore needle, peripherally inserted central venous catheters used instead of INC

Central infusion devices
  Percutaneous catheters
  Central venous tunneled catheters
    Hickman—Long-term indwelling catheter placed surgically (by a physician) and tunneled into place with a Dacron cuff
    Broviac—Long-term indwelling, small-diameter silicone catheter used for pediatric patients
    Groshong—Long-term indwelling catheter with a two-way valve at the end to prevent blood return; placed surgically and tunneled
    Implantable ports—closed system composed of implanted device with reservoir, port, and self-sealing system; requires use of a noncoring needle to access port
  Peripherally inserted central catheters (PICC)—Inserted peripherally and threaded to superior vena cava; can be placed by physicians, nurses, or nurse practitioners
  Midclavicular—Inserted peripherally and advanced to proximal axillary or subclavian vein

Inline I.V. solution filters
  Depth—Filters in which pore size is nonuniform
  Membrane (screen)—Air-venting, bacteria-retensive, 0.22-micron filter

221

Blood filters

Standard clot—170 to 220 microns; used on blood administration sets to remove coagulated products, microclots, and debris

Microaggregate—20, 40, and 80 microns; can be added to an in-use blood administration set, permitting infusion of blood, and easy replacement of the filter for delivery of multiple units

Leukocyte depletion—Used to remove 95% to 99.9% of leukocytes from red blood cells

Electronic infusion devices (EIDs)

Controller—Used in 80% of situations requiring rate control device; gravity-dependent; many are nonvolumetric, some volumetric controllers available with peristaltic action

Pumps

Volumetric—Calibrated in mL/hr; requires special cassette or cartridge to be used with the machine, very accurate, and used in delivery of high-potency drugs or when accuracy is imperative

Peristaltic—Calibrated in mL/hr; used primarily for delivery of enteral feedings; has a rotary disk or rollers to compress tubing

Syringe—Piston-driven pump that controls rate of infusion by drive speed and syringe size

Ambulatory infusion—Lightweight, compact infusion pumps

Multichannel and dual-channel—Computer-generated for delivery of multiple medications or fluids

Patient-controlled analgesia (PCA)—Can be used at home or in hospital to deliver pain medication

Mechanical infusion devices

Elastomere balloons—Portable device designed with an elastomeric reservoir for delivery of medication

Accessory equipment

Fluid warmers—Used for warming blood

Latex resealable locks (PRN device)—Attaches to hub of catheter and converts the cannula into an intermittent device

Add-on devices I.V. loop—J or U loop, connected to hub of catheter to turn tubing in a different direction

Microbore extension tubing—Add-on set to extend tubing

Needle protector and needleless system—Device to protect against needle sticks

CRITICAL THINKING ACTIVITY

1. You are asked to set up an I.V. piggyback of 150 mL of 5% dextrose in water and 20 mEq of potassium chloride. What type of rate regulation device would you use?

2. In setting up the regulation infusion device for the potassium piggyback, you find that the facility in which you are working uses a regulation pump that you have never used. What are your options for solving this problem?

3. You walk into a room at the beginning of your shift to check on a unit of packed cells. You find the packed cells being pumped via a volumetric pump and that the bag of packed cells is placed in a wash basin of warm water. Is the rate control device appropriate for the administration of blood? Is the warm water bath appropriate?

4. You are asked to add an inline filter (0.22 micron) to an I.V. line that is connected to an infusion pump. What do you have to do before adding the filter?

5. The extended-care facility in which you are working is using a closed-glass system for delivery of I.V. fluids. What type of administration set must you use?

POST-TEST, CHAPTER 7

Match the term in column I with the definition in column II.

Column I

1. _____ cannula
2. _____ drip chamber
3. _____ infusate
4. _____ lumen
5. _____ hub
6. _____ microdrip
7. _____ macrodrip
8. _____ port
9. _____ stylet
10. _____ gauge

Column II

A. A point of entry

B. Size of cannula opening

C. Needle guide that is found inside a catheter

D. A tube or sheath used for infusing fluids

E. Area of the I.V. tubing usually found under the spike where the solution drips and collects

F. I.V. solution

G. Space within an artery, vein, or catheter

H. Small drop factor—60 drops/mL

I. Standard drop factor—10 to 20 drops/mL

J. Female connection point of an I.V. cannula where the tubing or other equipment will attach

11. List the two types of infusate containers.

  A. _____

  B. _____

12. In using a flexible plastic system, which type of administration set should you choose:
  A. Vented
  B. Nonvented
  C. Vented or nonvented; both work with this system

13. Advantages of the ONC include all of the following *except*:
  A. Is patent longer than scalp vein needle
  B. Is radiopaque
  C. Has decreased infiltration risks
  D. Has low incidence of mechanical phlebitis

Match the venous access device in column I with the description in Column II

Column 1

14. _____ PICC
15. _____ Hickman
16. _____ Groshong
17. _____ implanted port

Column II

A. Long-term catheter inserted surgically via an incision in the deltopectoral groove terminating near the right atrium

B. Surgically implanted catheter; has two-way valve adjacent to the closed tip

C. Completely closed system, placed in a subcutaneous pocket with a self-sealing septum

D. Long-term peripheral catheter inserted in peripheral vein and threaded to the midclavicular or superior vena cava site

18. A 0.22-micron filter should be used when:
    A. An additive has been combined with the solution.
    B. The patient is susceptible to infusion phlebitis.
    C. Infusion is delivered by central route.
    D. All of the above.

19. The standard blood administration set has a cot filter of _____ microns.
    A. 170
    B. 40
    C. 20
    D. 0.22

20. Microaggregate filters are used for:
    A. Administration of protein solutions
    B. Administration of whole blood and packed cells stored more than 5 days
    C. Removal of bacteria for infusion
    D. Filtering of air from set

True-False

21. _____ Controllers are gravity-dependent.

22. _____ Volumetric pumps require special cassette tubing.

23. _____ Peristaltic pumps are primarily used for delivery of enteral feedings.

24. _____ Syringe pumps are useful in delivery of large volumes.

25. _____ According to INS standards of practice, intermittent administration sets should be changed every 24 hours.

26. Fluid warmers are used primarily for:
    A. Administration of total parenteral nutrition
    B. Administration of solutions to the pediatric patient
    C. Administration of blood
    D. Administration of solutions to the geriatric patient

27. Locking devices must be monitored every 4 hours and kept patent with:
    A. Saline flushes
    B. Heparin flushes
    C. Medication
    D. Saline or heparin based on hospital policy and physician preference

28. Needle protector systems are now being marketed to:
    A. Decrease risk of needle-stick injuries
    B. Protect the I.V. line's integrity
    C. Decrease tubing changes
    D. Enable quicker blood draws

29. Which of the following is a disadvantage of the glass system?
    A. Breakable and difficult to store
    B. Reacts with some solutions and medications
    C. May be difficult to read fluid levels
    D. May develop leaks

ANSWERS TO CHAPTER 7

PRE-TEST

1. A	5. C	9. T	12. D
2. D	6. T	10. E	13. B
3. A	7. T	11. C	14. A
4. B	8. F		

POST-TEST

1. D	9. C	17. C	24. F
2. E	10. B	18. D	25. T
3. F	11. Glass and plastic	19. A	26. C
4. G	12. C	20. B	27. D
5. J	13. C	21. T	28. A
6. H	14. D	22. T	29. A
7. I	15. A	23. T	
8. A	16. B		

REFERENCES

Altavela, J.L., Haas, C.E., & Nowak, D.R. (1993). Comparison of polyethylene and polyvinyl chloride sets for the administration of intravenous nitroglycerin to treat ischemic heart disease (abstract). Presented at the American College of Clinical Pharmacists Annual Meeting. Reno, NV.

Ausman, R.K. (1984). *Intravascular infusion systems: Principles and practices.* Boston: MTP Press Limited.

Centers for Disease Control and Prevention. (1995). *Guideline for prevention of intravenous therapy-related infections.* U.S. Department of Health and Human Services, Atlanta, GA.

Chiarello, L.A., Nagin, D., & Laufer, F. (1992). *Pilot study of needle stick prevention devices.* Albany: New York State Department of Health.

Collins, J.L., & Lutz, R.J. (1991). In vitro study of simultaneous infusion of incompatible drugs in multilument catheters. *Heart Lung 20,* 271–277.

Crocker, K.S., Devereaux, G.B., Ashmore, D.L., & Coker, M.H. (1990). Clinical evaluation of elastomeric hydrogel peripheral catheters during home infusion therapy. *Journal of Intravenous Nursing, 13*(2), 89–97.

Delaney, C.W., & Lauer, M.L. (1988). *Intravenous therapy: A guide to quality care.* Philadelphia: J.B. Lippincott.

Food and Drug Administration (1994). Safety alert: hazards of precipitation associated with parenteral nutrition. *American Journal of Hospital Pharmacy,* 51, 1427–1428.

Gurevich, I. (1986). Are I.V. in-line filters worth the price? *Nursing 86,* 42–43.

Gurevich, I. (1994). Preventing needlesticks: A market survey. *RN 11,* 4–8.

Hadaway, L.C. (1990). An overview of vascular access devices inserted via the antecubital area. *Journal of Intravenous Nursing,* 13(5), 297–306.

Jensen, B.L. (1995). Intravenous therapy equipment. In J. Terry, L. Baranowski, R. Lonsway, & C. Hedrick (eds.): *Intravenous therapy: Clinical principles and practice,* pp 303–338. Philadelphia: W.B. Saunders.

Maki, D.G., & Ringer, M. (1991). Risk factors for infusion-related phlebitis with small peripheral venous catheters: A randomized controlled study. *Annals of Internal Medicine,* 114, 945.

McKee, J.M., Shell, J.A., Warren, T.A., & Campbell, V.P. (1989). Complications of intravenous therapy: A randomized perspective study—Vialon vs Teflon. *Journal of Intravenous Therapy,* 12(5), 288.

Meares, C. (1992). P.I.C.C. & M.L.C. lines options worth exploring. *Nursing,* 92(10), 52–56.

Millam, D.A. (1990). Controlling the flow: Electronic infusion devices. *Nursing 90,* 65–68.

Moorhatch, P., & Chiou, W.L. (1974). Interactions between drugs and plastic intravenous fluid bags. *American Journal of Hospital Pharmacy,* 31, 149–152.

Olin, B.R. (1991). Intravenous nitroglycerin. In *Drug facts and comparisons,* p. 143a–4. Philadelphia: J.B. Lippincott.

Pall Biomedial Corporation. (1990). *Pall PC 50 and RC 100 leukocyte removal filters: Product brochure.* New York: Pall Biomedical Products Corporation.

Rasor, J. (1991). Landmark midline catheter performance: Analysis of an 830 catheter database. *MCP, 1*(3), 1–9.

Sevick, S (1995). Intravenous in-line filtration: choice or necessity? *Technical Report Gelman Sciences,* 1–3.

Stewart, R.D., & Sanislowk, G.A. (1961). Silastic intravenous catheters. *New England Journal of Medicine,* 265, 1238–1285.

Weinstein, S. (1993). *Plumer's principles and practices of intravenous therapy*. Philadelphia: J.B. Lippincott.

Weinstein, S.M. (1991). Electronic delivery in the 1990's and beyond: A nursing perspective. *Infusion Management Update, 1*(1), 1–2.

Widman, F.K. (1991). *Standards for blood banks and transfusion services* (14 ed.), p 39. Arlington, VA: American Association of Blood Banks.

Wolfrum, J. (1994). A follow-up evaluation to a needle-free I.V. system. *Nursing Management, 12*, 33–37.

CHAPTER 8

Techniques for Peripheral Intravenous Therapy

CHAPTER CONTENTS

GLOSSARY
LEARNING OBJECTIVES
PRE-TEST, CHAPTER 8
ANATOMY AND PHYSIOLOGY RELATED TO
  I.V. PRACTICE
Skin
Sensory Receptors
Venous System
SUMMARY WORKSHEET #1: SUPERFICIAL
  VEINS OF THE UPPER EXTREMITIES
APPROACHES TO VENIPUNCTURE
Precannulation
Cannulation
Postcannulation
SUMMARY OF STEPS IN INITIATING I.V.
  THERAPY
Precannula Insertion
Cannula Insertion
Postcannula Insertion
SUMMARY WORKSHEET #2: RATE
  CALCULATIONS
RECOMMENDATIONS FOR USE OF PERIPHERAL
  VENOUS CATHETERS
Centers for Disease Control and Prevention
  (1995)

DISCONTINUATION OF I.V. CANNULA
Procedure
LATEX RESEALABLE LOCKS (PRN DEVICES)
HEPARIN FLUSH VERSUS SALINE FLUSH
Heparin Lock Flush
Saline Lock Flush
CONTROVERSIAL PRACTICES
Lidocaine
Transdermal Analgesia
Topical Nitroglycerin
NURSING PLAN OF CARE: INITIATION OF
  VENIPUNCTURE
PATIENT EDUCATION
HOME CARE ISSUES
COMPETENCY CRITERIA: PERIPHERAL I.V.
  THERAPY
KEY POINTS
CRITICAL THINKING ACTIVITY
POST-TEST, CHAPTER 8
ANSWERS TO CHAPTER 8
Pre-Test
Post-Test
REFERENCES

GLOSSARY

Antimicrobial   An agent that destroys or prevents development of microorganisms
Bevel   Slanted edge on opening of a needle or cannula device
Cannula   A hollow plastic tube used for accessing the vascular system
Distal   Farther from the heart; farthest from point of attachment (below previous site of cannulation)
Endothelial lining   A thin layer of cells lining the blood vessels, and heart
Gauge   Size of a cannula (catheter) opening; gradual measurements of the outside diameter of a cannula
Microabrasion   Superficial break in skin integrity that may predispose the patient to infection
OSHA   Occupational Safety and Health Administration
Palpation   Examination by touch

229

Prime To fill the administration set with infusate for the first time
Proximal Nearest to the heart; closest point to attachment, (above previous site of cannulation)
Spike To insert the administration set into the infusate container

LEARNING OBJECTIVES

Upon completion of this chapter, the reader will be able to:
- Define the terminology related to peripheral veins.
- Recall the anatomy and physiology related to the venous system.
- Identify the five tissue structures that the therapist must penetrate for a successful venipuncture.
- Identify the peripheral veins appropriate for venipuncture.
- List the factors affecting site selection.
- Document the initiation of I.V. therapy.
- Demonstrate the Phillips 15-step approach for initiating I.V. therapy.
- List the sites appropriate for labeling.
- State the Intravenous Nursing Standards of Practice for site management.
- Recall the steps in performing a heparin or saline lock flush.
- Describe the advantages and disadvantages of latex resealable lock.
- Contrast the advantages and disadvantages of saline lock flush versus heparin lock flush.
- Identify use of lidocaine and topical creams in the initiation of I.V. therapy.
- Calculate drops per minute, using varied drop-factor tubing.
- Use the nursing process in techniques for initiation of I.V. therapy.

PRE-TEST, CHAPTER 8

1. The three layers of a vein are:
   A. Tunica center, tunica media, and facia
   B. Tunica intima, tunica media, and tunica adventitia
   C. Tunica intima, epidermis, and dermis

Match the definition in column II to the correct term in column I.

Column I	Column II
2. _____ cannula	A. Farthest from the heart
3. _____ bevel	B. Size of cannula opening
4. _____ gauge	C. Slanted edge on opening of a cannula device
5. _____ proximal	D. Nearest to the heart
6. _____ distal	E. Catheter

7. A physician's verbal order must be validated by a written order within _____ hours.
   A. 12
   B. 24
   C. 48
   D. 72

8. The first step in heparin flush of an intermittent infusion device is to:
   A. Flush with sodium chloride
   B. Check for patency of the catheter

230

C. Flush with heparin
D. Administer medication

9. According to the Centers for Disease Control, I.V. sites should be rotated every _____ hours.
A. 24 to 48
B. 36 to 48
C. 48 to 72
D. 72 to 96

10. What peripheral vein is appropriate for antibiotic therapy?
A. Cephalic vein
B. Dorsal metacarpal vein
C. Digital vein
D. Median antecubital vein

11. The calculation of the drop rate depends on:
A. Tubing length
B. Filter size
C. Drop factor of tubing
D. mL/hour

12. Labels should be applied to the:
A. Catheter site
B. Tubing
C. Solution container
D. All of the above

13. What factors affect site selection?
A. Type of solution
B. Condition of vein
C. Duration of therapy
D. Presence of disease, shunts, or grafts in the extremity
E. All of the above

14. The purpose of intermittent infusion devices is to:
A. Prevent phlebitis
B. Provide access to the vascular system without administration of solutions
C. Administer solutions at a more rapid rate
D. Prevent infiltration

Challenges make you discover things about yourself that you really never knew. They're what make the instrument stretch—what make you go beyond the norm.

CICELY TYSON, AMERICAN ACTRESS.

ANATOMY AND PHYSIOLOGY RELATED TO I.V. PRACTICE

To accurately perform I.V. therapy, the nurse must know the anatomy and physiology of the skin and venous system and be familiar with the physiologic response of a vein to heat, cold, and stress. It is also important to become familiar with the skin thickness and consistency at various sites.

Skin

The skin consists of two main layers—epidermis and dermis—overlying the superficial fascia. The epidermis, composed of squamous cells that are less sensitive than underlying structures, is the first line of defense against infections. The epidermis is the thickest on the palms of the hands and soles of the feet and is thinnest on the inner surfaces of the extremities. Thickness varies with age and exposure to the elements, such as wind and sun.

The dermis, a much thicker layer, is located directly below the epidermis. The dermis consists of blood vessels, hair follicles, sweat glands, sebaceous glands, small muscles, and nerves. As with the epidermis, the thickness of the dermis varies with age and physical condition. The skin is a special sense touch organ, and the dermis reacts quickly to painful stimuli, as well as to temperature changes and pressure

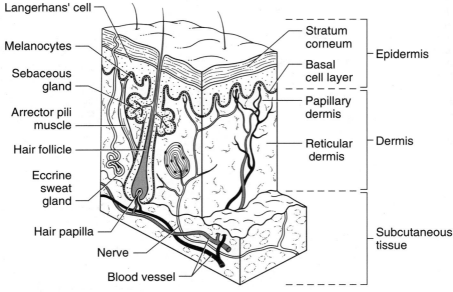

Figure 8–1. Anatomy of skin.

232

sensation. This is the most painful layer during venipuncture because of the large amount of blood vessels and the many nerves contained in this sheath.

The hypodermis, or fascia, lies below the epidermis and dermis and provides a covering for blood vessels. This connective tissue layer varies in thickness and is found over the entire body surface. Because any infection in the fascia, called superficial cellulitis, spreads easily throughout the body, it is essential to use strict aseptic technique when inserting infusion devices. This superficial tissue layer connects with deeper fascia (Fig. 8–1).

Sensory Receptors

There are five types of sensory receptors, four of which affect parenteral therapy. The sensory receptors transmit along afferent fibers. Many types of stimulation such as heat, light, cold, pressure, and sound are processed along the sensory receptors (Guyton, 1991). Sensory receptors related to parenteral therapy include:

1. Mechanoreceptors, which process skin tactile sensations, deep tissue sensation (palpation of veins)
2. Thermoreceptors, which process cold, warmth, and pain (application of heat or cold)
3. Nociceptors, which process pain (puncture of vein for insertion of cannula)
4. Chemoreceptors, which process osmotic changes in blood, decreased arterial pressure (decreased circulating blood volume)

✎ **NOTE:** To decrease pain during venipuncture, keep the skin taut by applying traction to it and move quickly through the skin layers and past the pain receptors.

Venous System

The body transport mechanism, the circulatory system, has two main subdivisions— the cardiopulmonary and the systemic systems. The systemic circulation, particularly the peripheral veins, is used in I.V. therapy. Veins function similarly to arteries, but are thinner and less muscular (Table 8–1). The wall of a vein is only 10% of the total diameter of the vessel, compared with 25% in the artery. Because the vein is thin and less muscular, it can distend easily allowing for storage of large volumes of blood under low pressure. Approximately 75% of the total blood volume is contained in the veins.

Some veins have valves, particularly those that transport blood against gravity as in the lower extremities. Valves, made up of endothelial leaflets, help prevent the distal reflux of blood. Valves occur at points of branching producing a noticeable bulge in the vessel (Smeltzer & Bare, 1992). Arteries and veins have three layers of tissue that form the wall, the tunica intima, tunica adventitia, and, tunica media. (Fig. 8–2).

TABLE 8–1. **COMPARISON OF ARTERY AND VEIN**

Artery*	Vein*
Thick-walled	Thin-walled
25% of arterial wall	10% of vein wall
Lacks valves	Greater distensibility
Pulsates	Valves present approximately every 3 in

*Has three tissue layers.

Tunica Adventitia

The outermost layer, called the tunica adventitia, consists of connective tissue that surrounds and supports a vessel. The blood supply of this layer, called the vasa vasorum, nourishes both the adventitia and media layers. Sometimes during venipuncture you can feel a "pop" as you enter the tunica adventitia.

Tunica Media

The middle layer, called the tunica media, is composed of muscular and elastic tissue with nerve fibers for vasoconstriction and vasodilation. The tunica media in a vein is not as strong and rigid as it is in an artery, so it tends to collapse or distend as pressure falls or rises. Stimulation by change in temperature or mechanical or chemical irritation can produce a response in this layer. For instance, cold blood or infusates can produce spasms that impede blood flow and cause pain. Application of heat promotes dilation, which can relieve a spasm or improve blood flow (Weinstein, 1993).

✎ NOTE: During venipuncture if the tip of the catheter has nicked the tunica adventitia or is placed in the tunica media layer, a small amount of blood will appear in the catheter; however, the catheter will not thread because it is trapped between layers. If you cannot get a steady backflow of blood the needle might be in this layer, so advance the stylet of the cannula slightly before advancing the catheter.

Tunica Intima

The innermost layer, called the tunica intima, has one thin layer of cells, referred to as the endothelial lining. The surface is smooth, allowing blood to flow through vessels easily. Any roughening of this bed of cells during venipuncture, while the

TABLE 8–2. SELECTING AN INSERTION SITE FOR THE SUPERFICIAL VEINS OF THE DORSUM OF THE HAND

Vein	Location	Insertion Device	Considerations
Digital	Lateral and dorsal portions of the fingers	Small-gauge cannula 20- to 22-gauge catheter 21- to 25-gauge steel needle	Use a padded tongue blade to splint the cannula. Use only solutions that are isotonic without additives because of the risk of infiltration.
Metacarpal	Dorsum of the hand formed by union of digital veins between the knuckles	20- to 22-gauge to $\frac{3}{4}$–1 in length over the needle catheter 21- to 25-gauge steel needle (short-term)	Good site to begin therapy Usually easily visualized Avoid if infusing antibiotics, potassium chloride, or chemotherapeutic agents

catheter is in place, or upon discontinuing the system fosters the process of thrombosis formation (see Chapter 9).

Veins of the Hands and Arms

Several veins can be used to infuse I.V. fluids, but the veins of the hands or arms are most commonly used (Figs. 8–3 and 8–4). When selecting the best site, many factors must be considered, such as ease of insertion and access, type of needle or catheter that can be used, and comfort and safety for the patient. See Tables 8–2 and 8–3 for identifying and selecting the most effective I.V. site for the clinical situation of the patient.

TABLE 8–3. **SELECTING AN INSERTION SITE FOR THE SUPERFICIAL VEINS OF THE ARM**

Vein	Location	Insertion Device	Considerations
Cephalic	Radial portion of the lower arm along the radial bone of the forearm	18- to 22-gauge cannulas, usually over-the-needle catheter	Large vein, easy to access First use most distal section and work upward for long-term therapy Useful for infusing blood and chemically irritating medications
Basilic	Ulnar aspect of the lower arm and runs up the ulnar bone	18- to 22-gauge, usually over-the-needle catheter	Difficult area to access Large vein, easily palpated, but moves easily; stabilize with traction during venipuncture Often available after other sites have been exhausted
Accessory cephalic	Branches off the cephalic vein along the radial bone	18- to 22-gauge, usually over-the-needle catheter	Medium to large size and easy to stabilize May be difficult to palpate in persons with large amounts of adipose tissue Valves at cephalic junction may prohibit cannula advancement Short length may prohibit cannula use
Upper cephalic	Radial aspect of upper arm above the elbow	16- to 20-gauge, usually over-the-needle catheter	Difficult to visualize Excellent site for confused patients (who tend to pull at their I.V. line)
Median antebrachial	Extends up the front of the forearm from the median antecubital veins	18- to 22-gauge, usually over-the-needle catheter	Area has many nerve endings and should be avoided Infiltration occurs easily.

TABLE 8–3. **SELECTING AN INSERTION SITE FOR THE SUPERFICIAL VEINS OF THE ARM** (*Continued*)

Vein	Location	Insertion Device	Considerations
Median basilic	Ulnar portion of the forearm	18- to 22-gauge, usually over-the-needle catheter	Good site for I.V. therapy
Median cubital	Radial side of forearm; crosses in front of the brachial artery at the antecubital space	18- to 22-gauge, usually over-the-needle catheter	Good site for I.V. therapy
Antecubital	In the bend of the elbow	All sizes especially 16- to 18-gauge; used for midline catheters and peripherally inserted central catheters	Should be reserved for blood draws for laboratory analysis only, unless in an emergency Uncomfortable placement site, owing to the arm extending in an unnatural position Area difficult to splint with armboard If used in an emergency situation, change site within 24 hours

SUMMARY WORKSHEET 1: Superficial Veins of the Upper Extremities

FILL IN THE SUPERFICIAL VEINS OF THE UPPER EXTREMITIES

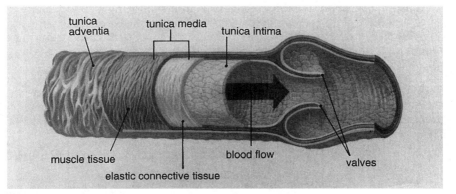

Figure 8–2. Anatomy of a vein. (Source: Medical Economics Publishing, Montvale, New Jersey, with permission.)

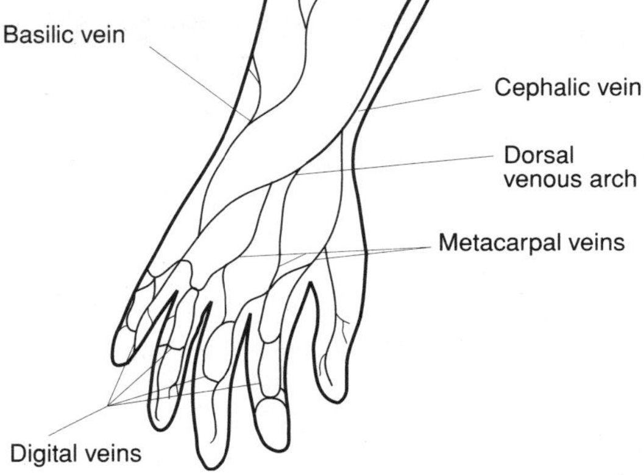

Figure 8–3. Superficial veins of the hand. (Courtesy of Becton-Dickinson Vascular Access, Sandy, Utah.)

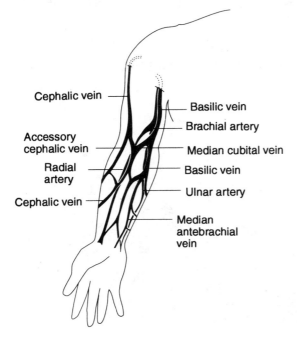

Figure 8–4. Superficial veins of the forearm. (Courtesy of Becton-Dickinson Vascular Access, Sandy, Utah.)

Labels in figure:
- Cephalic vein
- Basilic vein
- Brachial artery
- Accessory cephalic vein
- Median cubital vein
- Radial artery
- Basilic vein
- Ulnar artery
- Cephalic vein
- Median antebrachial vein

TABLE 8–4. **PHILLIPS 15-STEP VENIPUNCTURE METHOD**

Precannulation
1. Checking physician's order
2. Handwashing procedure
3. Equipment preparation
4. Patient assessment and psychological preparation
5. Site selection and vein dilation

Cannulation
6. Needle selection
7. Gloving
8. Site preparation
9. Vein entry, direct versus indirect
10. Catheter stabilization and dressing management

Postcannulation
11. Labeling
12. Equipment disposal
13. Patient education
14. Rate calculations
15. Documentation

APPROACHES TO VENIPUNCTURE

Performing a successful venipuncture requires mastery and knowledge of infusion therapy as well as psychomotor clinical skill. Many aseptic approaches to venipuncture techniques provide safe parenteral therapy. The Phillips 15-step venipuncture method, outlined in Table 8–4 and explained in detail in the following text, is an easy-to-remember step approach for the beginning practitioner.

Precannulation

Before initiating cannulation, you must follow steps 1 through 5: checking the physician's order, handwashing, preparing the equipment, assessing and preparing the patient, and selecting the vein and the site of insertion.

Step 1: Checking the Physician's Order

A physician's order is necessary to initiate I.V. therapy. The physician's order should be clear, concise, legible, and complete. All I.V. solutions should be checked against the physician's order. The physician's order should include:

Solution
Medication (if an additive is needed)
Dosage
Volume
Rate
Frequency
Route

Verbal orders must be written in the medical record within 24 hours.

Step 2: Handwashing Procedure

Handwashing has been shown to significantly decrease the potential risk of contamination and cross-contamination. Touch contamination is a common cause of transfer of pathogens. Soap and water are adequate for handwashing prior to insertion of cannula however, an antiseptic solution such as chlorhexidine may be used. Wash hands for 15 to 20 seconds before equipment preparation and before insertion of catheter. Do not apply hand lotion following handwashing (CDCP, 1995). The agent that you use for washing has an effect on efficiency. Bar, powdered, leaflet, or liquid soaps that do not contain an antibacterial agent are unacceptable for surgical scrubs (Larson, 1984). Agents recommended for handwashing are antiseptic soaps containing chemicals of iodine or chlorhexidine. Avoid wearing false fingernails, which can increase the number of hand-carried microorganisms (INS, 1985).

Step 3: Equipment Preparation

Inspect the infusate container at the nurses' station, in the clean utility, or in the medication room. In modern practice, two systems are available—glass system (open or closed) and plastic system (rigid or soft).

To check the glass system, hold the container up to the light to inspect for cracks as evidenced by flashes of light. Glass systems are crystal clear. Rotate the container and look for particulate contamination and cloudiness. Inspect the seal and check the expiration date.

239

To check a plastic system squeeze the soft plastic infusate container to check for breaks in the integrity of the plastic; squeeze the system to detect pinholes. Observe for any particulate contamination and check the expiration date. The plastic systems are not crystal clear. The outer wrap of the soft plastic systems should be dry.

Select either a vented or nonvented primary tubing set or a secondary set, depending on the rationale for infusion. It is wise to **spike** the solution container and **prime** the administration set at the nurses' station to detect defective equipment. Choose the correct tubing to match the solution container. For closed glass use vented only; for plastic use vented or nonvented. See Chapter 7 for more detailed information on I.V. equipment.

Step 4: Patient Assessment and Psychological Preparation

First, provide privacy for the patient. Explain the procedure to decrease anxiety, and instruct the patient regarding the purpose of the I.V. therapy, the procedure, what the physician has ordered in the infusate and why, and the limitations.

Evaluate the patient's psychological preparedness for the I.V. by talking with the patient before assessing the vein. The therapist should consider aspects such as autonomy and independence, along with invasion of personal space when I.V. placement is necessary. Often the patient has a fear of pain associated with venipuncture because of the lack of understanding related to necessity of the therapy (Delaney & Lauer, 1988).

Step 5: Site Selection and Vein Dilation

Site Selection

Several factors should be considered before a venipuncture is attempted (Table 8–5). These factors help the therapist to make a competent choice of location for the infusion.

1. **Type of solution:** Fluids that are hypertonic, more than 340 mOsm, such as antibiotics and potassium chloride, are irritating to vein walls. Select a large vein in the forearm to initiate this therapy. Start at the best, lowest vein.
2. **Condition of vein:** A soft, straight vein is the ideal choice for venipuncture. Palpate the vein by moving the tips of the fingers down the vein to observe how it refills. The dorsal metacarpal veins in elderly patients are a poor choice because blood extravasation (hematoma) occurs more readily in small thin veins. When a patient is hypovolemic, peripheral veins collapse more quickly than larger veins (Weinstein, 1993).

TABLE 8–5. **TIPS FOR SELECTING VEINS**

A suitable vein should feel relatively smooth, pliable with valves well spaced.
Veins will be difficult to stabilize in a patient who has recently lost weight.
Debilitated patients and those taking corticosteroids have fragile veins that bruise easily.
Sclerotic veins are common among narcotic addicts.
Sclerotic veins are common among the elderly population.
Dialysis patients usually know which veins are good for venipuncture.
Start with distal veins and work proximally.
Veins that feel bumpy like running your finger over a cat's tail are usually thrombosed or extremely valvular.

Avoid:
Bruised veins
Red swollen veins
Veins near previously infected areas
Sites near a previously discontinued site (Steele, 1988)

3. **Duration of therapy:** Choose a vein that supports I.V. therapy for at least 72 hours. Start at the best, lowest vein. Use the hand only if a nonirritating solution is being infused. Long courses of infusion therapy make preservation of veins essential. Perform venipuncture distally with each subsequent puncture proximal to previous puncture and alternate arms.
   Avoid:
   A joint flexion
   A vein too small for cannula size

4. **Cannula size:** Hemodilution is important. The gauge of the cannula should be as small as possible. When performing transfusion therapy, an 18-gauge catheter is preferred so the cellular portion of blood will not be damaged during infusion.

5. **Patient age:** Infants do not have the accessible sites that older children and adults have owing to increased fat. Veins in the hands, feet, and antecubital region may be the only accessible sites. Veins in the elderly are usually fragile. Approach venipuncture gently and evaluate the need for a tourniquet (Fabian, 1995).

✎ **NOTE:** Fragile veins can be penetrated with less extravasation of blood if a tourniquet is not used and an indirect (2-step) method is used.

6. **Patient preference:** Consider the patient's personal feelings when determining the catheter placement site. Evaluate the extremities taking into account the dominant hand.

7. **Patient activity:** Ambulatory patients using crutches or a walker will need cannula placement above the wrist so that the hand can still be used.

8. **Presence of disease or prior surgery:** Patients with vascular disease or dehydration may have limited venous access. Avoid phlebitis-infiltrated sites or a site of infection. If the patient has a condition with poor vascular venous return, the affected side *must be avoided.* Examples are cerebrovascular accident, mastectomy, amputation, orthopedic surgery of hand or arm, and plastic surgery of hand or arm (INS, 1996).

9. **Presence of shunt or graft:** *Do not* use a patient's arm or hand that has a patent graft or shunt for dialysis.

Vein dilation

There are many ways to increase the flow of blood in the upper extremities. Factors affecting the capacity for dilation are blood pressure, presence of valves, sclerotic veins, and multiple previous I.V. sites.

Ways in which veins can be dilated are:

1. **Gravity:** Position the extremity lower than the heart for several minutes.
2. **Fist clenching:** Instruct the patient to open and close the fist. Squeezing a rubber ball or rolled wash cloth works well.
3. **Tapping:** Using thumb and second digit, flick the vein; this releases histamines beneath the skin and causes dilation.
4. **Warm compresses:** Apply warm towels to the extremity for 10 minutes. Do not use a microwave to heat towels; the temperature can become too hot and cause a burn.

5. **Blood pressure cuff:** This is an excellent choice for vein dilation. Pump up the cuff between the systolic and diastolic pressure (e.g., if blood pressure is 120/80 mm Hg, cuff pressure would be 100 mm Hg). This method prevents constriction of the arterial system.

✎ **NOTE:** Care must be used when using a blood pressure cuff not to start the I.V. too close to the cuff owing to excessive back pressure.

6. **Tourniquet:** A Velcro strap or rubber tubing can be used. Apply the tourniquet 6 to 8 in above the venipuncture site if the blood pressure is within normal range. If the patient is hypertensive, the tourniquet should be placed high on the extremity; occasionally, the tourniquet is not needed with severely hypertensive patients. With hypotensive patients, move the tourniquet as close as possible to the venipuncture site without contamination of prepped area (see Chapter 10 for multiple tourniquet techniques).

✎ **NOTE:** Use the tourniquet only once; using the same tourniquet on more than one patient leads to cross-contamination.

Cannulation

Cannulation involves steps 6 through 10: selecting the needle, gloving, preparing the site, direct or indirect entry into the vein, and stabilizing the catheter and managing the dressing.

Step 6: Needle Selection

Infusions may be delivered with a plastic or steel cannula (see Chapter 7 for needle choice and sizes). The choice of catheter depends on the purpose of the infusion and the condition and availability of the veins. Steel needles are generally avoided except for bolus injections or infusions lasting only a few hours. Inflexible steel needles greatly increase the risk of vein injury and infiltration (Millam, 1992).

Catheters are made of polyethylene, Teflon, Vialon, and Aquavene. Radiopaque over-the-needle catheters are the best quality . Most hospitals, clinics, and home care agencies have policies and procedures for selection of catheters. Recommended are:

18 to 20 gauge for infusion of hypertonic or isotonic solutions with additives
18 to 20 gauge for blood administration
22 to 24 gauge for pediatric patients
22 gauge for fragile veins in the elderly, if unable to place a 20-gauge catheter

The tip of the catheter should be inspected for integrity prior to venipuncture to note the presence of burrs on the needle, peeling of catheter material, or other abnormalities.

✎ **NOTE:** Only two attempts at venipuncture are recommended because multiple unsuccessful attempts cause unnecessary trauma to the patient and limit vascular access. When aseptic technique is compromised (emergency situation), the cannula is also considered compromised and a new catheter should be placed within 24 hours.

Step 7: Gloving

The Centers for Disease Control and Prevention (CDCP, 1995) recommends following universal precautions whenever exposure to blood or body fluids is likely. Latex and vinyl gloves protect the wearer from contact with blood and body fluids. However, latex, a natural material, is more flexible then vinyl and molds to the wearer's hand, allowing freedom of movement. Its lattice-type structure allows tiny punctures to reseal automatically.

✎ **NOTE:** Latex and the powder used in the gloves are associated with potentially severe allergic reactions in susceptible persons. Avoid using this material if you have experienced any reactions to their use (for more information on latex allergy, see Chapter 2).

Gloves made of polyvinyl chloride, the synthetic rubber known as vinyl, do not reseal, are less flexible and less durable, and are of limited usefulness in high-risk, heavy-usage situations (Korniewicz, Kirwin, & Larson, 1991).

Step 8: Site Preparation

Cleansing the insertion site reduces the potential for infection. The following antimicrobial solutions may be used to prepare the cannula site:

Tincture of iodine 1% to 2%
Iodophor (povidone-iodine)
70% Isopropyl alcohol
Chlorhexidine

Aqueous benzalkonium-like compounds and hexachlorophene should not be used as preparatory solutions prior to venipuncture.

In preparing the site use a vigorous circular motion working from the center outward to a diameter of 2 to 3 in for *20 seconds*. The solutions should be allowed to air dry. Use 70% alcohol as a defatting agent before application of the povidone-iodine. If the patient is allergic to iodine, use 70% alcohol with friction for at least *30 seconds*. Shaving to remove hair is not recommended; instead hair should be clipped with scissors. Shaving is not recommended because of microabrasions, which increase the risk of infection.

Step 9: Vein Entry

Gloves should be in place before venipuncture and kept on until after the cannula is stabilized. Gloves should be removed only *after* the risk of exposure to body fluids has been eliminated. Venipuncture can be performed using with a *direct* (1-step) or *indirect* (2-step) method. The direct method is appropriate for small-gauge needles, fragile hand veins, or rolling veins and carries an increased risk of causing a hematoma. The indirect method can be used for all venipunctures.

PROCEDURE FOR VENIPUNCTURE
1. Pull skin below puncture site to stabilize the skin and prevent the rolling of the vein.
2. Grasp flashback chamber.
3. Insert the needle of choice bevel-up at a 30° to 45°-degree angle, depending on the vein location and catheter, while applying traction on the vein to keep skin taut.
4. Insert the catheter by direct or indirect method with a steady motion (Fig. 8–5 and Table 8–6). Jabbing, stabbing, or quick thrusting should be avoided because such actions may cause rupture of delicate veins (Enrich, 1991). For performing a venipuncture on difficult veins, see Table 8–7.
5. After the bevel enters the vein and blood flashback occurs, lower the angle of the catheter and stylet (needle) as one unit and advance into the vein. After the catheter tip and bevel are in the vein, advance the catheter forward off the stylet and into the vein $\frac{1}{4}$ to $\frac{1}{3}$ in. A *steady* backflow of blood indicates a successful entry. If the catheter is shorter than the needle, backflow may occur before the catheter tip is fully in the vein.

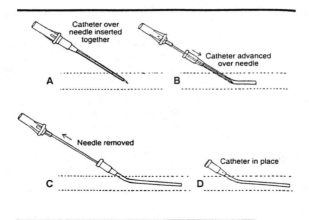

Figure 8–5. Direct entry. (Courtesy of American Heart Association, Dallas, Texas.)

6. Once the vein is entered, cautiously advance the cannula into the vein lumen. Hold the catheter hub with thumb and middle finger and use the index finger to advance the catheter, maintaining skin traction. A one-handed technique is recommended to advance the catheter off the stylet so that the opposite hand can maintain proper traction on the skin and maintain vein alignment (Weinstein, 1993). (A two-handed technique can be used, but increases the risk of vessel rupture during threading of a rigid cannula in a nonstabilized vein [Millam, 1992]).
7. While the stylet is still partially inside the catheter, release the tourniquet.
8. Remove the stylet.
9. Connect the adaptor on the administration set to the hub of the catheter.

✎ **NOTE:** Blood may ooze from the catheter, depending on the brand of needle used. If there is no blood, the catheter may not be placed correctly or may have penetrated the vein wall. If this is the case, remove the catheter and restart with a sterile cannula.

✎ **NOTE:** If the vein has sustained a through and through puncture and a hematoma develops, immediately remove the catheter and apply direct pressure to the site. Do not reapply a tourniquet to an extremity immediately after a venipuncture because a hematoma will form (Weinstein, 1993).

TABLE 8–6. **TWO METHODS OF PERFORMING A VENIPUNCTURE**

Direct Method: One Step	Indirect Method: Two Step
Insert the cannula directly over the vein at a 30- to 45-degree angle. Penetrate all layers of the vein with one motion.	Insert the cannula at a 30- to 45-degree angle to the skin alongside the vein; gently insert the cannula distal to the point at which the needle will enter the vein. Maintain parallel alignment and advance through the subcutaneous tissue. Relocate the vein and decrease the angle as the cannula enters the vein.

TABLE 8–7. TROUBLESHOOTING DIFFICULT VEINS

Problem	Intervention
Paper-thin transparent skin or delicate veins	Use smallest catheter possible (preferably 22 gauge); use direct entry; decrease angle of entry to 15 degrees; apply minimal tourniquet pressure
Obese patient, unable to palpate or see veins	Create a visual image of venous anatomy; select a longer catheter (preferably 2 in)
Vein rolls when venipuncture attempted	Apply traction to vein with thumb during venipuncture, keeping skin taut; leave tourniquet on to promote venous distention; use a blood pressure cuff for better filling of the vein; use 16- or 18-gauge catheter

Step 10: Cathether Stabilization and Dressing Management

Catheter Stabilization

The catheter should be stabilized in a manner that does not interfere with visualization and evaluation of the site. Stabilization reduces the risk of complications related to I.V. therapy such as phlebitis, infiltration, sepsis, and cannula migration. Junctions should be secured to aid in the reduction of complications (INS, 1996).

There are three methods appropriate for stabilization of the catheter hub: the U method, the H method, and the chevron method (Table 8–8).

TABLE 8–8 STABILIZING THE CATHETER*

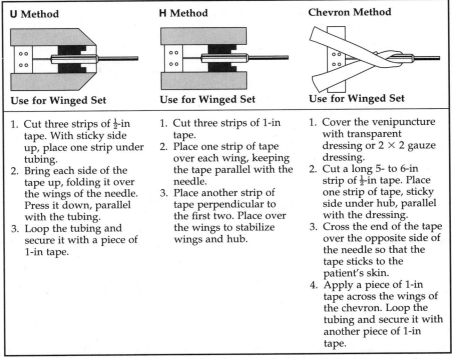

U Method	H Method	Chevron Method
Use for Winged Set	Use for Winged Set	Use for Winged Set
1. Cut three strips of ½-in tape. With sticky side up, place one strip under tubing. 2. Bring each side of the tape up, folding it over the wings of the needle. Press it down, parallel with the tubing. 3. Loop the tubing and secure it with a piece of 1-in tape.	1. Cut three strips of 1-in tape. 2. Place one strip of tape over each wing, keeping the tape parallel with the needle. 3. Place another strip of tape perpendicular to the first two. Place over the wings to stabilize wings and hub.	1. Cover the venipuncture with transparent dressing or 2 × 2 gauze dressing. 2. Cut a long 5- to 6-in strip of ½-in tape. Place one strip of tape, sticky side under hub, parallel with the dressing. 3. Cross the end of the tape over the opposite side of the needle so that the tape sticks to the patient's skin. 4. Apply a piece of 1-in tape across the wings of the chevron. Loop the tubing and secure it with another piece of 1-in tape.

*For all methods, include on the last piece of tape the date, time of insertion, size of gauge, length of needle or catheter, and your initials.

Using an armboard to stabilize the catheter site is not usually necessary with over-the-needle catheters. If it is necessary because of erratic flow rate from the patient's frequent change of position, use a disposable lightweight armboard. To absorb perspiration, cover the armboard with a washcloth or a paper cover (usually provided with armboards). Secure the armboard with two to three pieces of double-backed tape to protect the patient's skin. Do not tape over the site, and leave the patient's fingers free for movement (Millam, 1992).

Dressing Management

There are two methods for dressing management. One is the use of a gauze dressing secured with tape; the other is the use of a transparent semipermeable membrane dressing (TSM).

1. A sterile gauze dressing can be applied aseptically with edges secured with tape. Using a adhesive bandage strip in place of a gauze dressing is *not* recommended because it does not adequately cover and protect the site. Gauze dressings should be changed every 48 hours on peripheral sites or when integrity of the dressing is compromised. To apply the gauze dressing, (1) cleanse area of excess moisture after venipuncture before applying tape; (2) secure cannula hub; and (3) apply dressing.
2. TSM dressings should be applied aseptically and changed every 48 to 72 hours, depending on the standard of practice within the institution. The dressing and catheter should be replaced together, unless the integrity of the dressing is impaired; then removal of the dressing with replacement of a new sterile TSM is required. Do not use ointment of any kind under a TSM dressing. Adhesive-coated semipermeable film is available from many manufacturers. The TSM dressing should be applied only to the cannula hub and wings.

To apply a TSM, (1) cleanse area of excess moisture after venipuncture; (2) center transparent dressing over cannula site and partially over the hub; (3) press dressing down, sealing catheter site; and (4) apply tape to secure administration set. Do not put tape over the transparent film because it is difficult to remove the transparent film when the dressing needs to be changed.

ADVANTAGES OF TSM DRESSINGS
Continuous observation of site
Effective protection against infection
Cost-effectiveness (Byers, 1986; Katich & Band, 1985; Maki & Ringer, 1987)

✎ **NOTE** The use of a Band-Aid in place of gauze dressing is *not* recommended because it does not adequately cover and protect site.

Postcannulation

After you have successfully performed the cannulation, follow steps 11 through 14: labeling the I.V. setup, disposing of the equipment, educating the patient, calculating the rate of the infusion, and documenting the procedure.

Step 11: Labeling

The I.V. setup should be labeled in three spots. The insertion site, the tubing, and the solution container should be time-stripped.

1. The venipuncture site should be labeled on the side of the transparent dressing or across the hub. Do not place the label over the site, because this obstructs visualization of the site. Include on the label the (1) date and time, (2) the type and length of the catheter (e.g., 20-gauge; 1 in), and (3) the nurse's initials.
2. Label the tubing according to agency policy and procedure so that practitioners on subsequent shifts will be aware when the tubing must be changed.
3. Place a time strip on the solution container with the name of the solution, additives, initials of the nurse, and the time solution was started. Time strips are helpful for assessing whether the solution is on schedule.

Step 12: Equipment Disposal

Recapping needles increases the risk of needle-stick injuries to the practitioner. Needles and stylets should be disposed of in nonpermeable tamper-proof containers. Needles and stylets should not be recapped, broken, or bent, in accordance with the Occupational Safety and Health Administration (OSHA) and the Joint Commission on Accreditation of Healthcare Organizations (JCAHO, 1995) (CDC, 1995). After venipuncture is complete, dispose of all paper and plastic equipment in a container suitable for burning.

Step 13: Patient Education

After the catheter is stabilized, the dressing applied, and the labeling complete:

- Inform the patient of any limitations on movement or mobility.
- Explain all alarms if an electronic control device is used.
- Instruct the patient to call for assistance if the venipuncture site becomes tender or sore, or if redness or swelling develops.
- Advise the patient that the venipuncture site will be checked by the nurse.

Step 14: Rate Calculations

Although unit dose systems have largely replaced individual preparation of I.V. solutions, skilled rate calculation is still essential. Because many clinical environments require delivery of I.V. medications or unusual rates the I.V. therapist must be capable of accurate mathematic calculations. Calculating the proper I.V. rate for medication and solution delivery can be time-intensive. Two key components must be understood before using the following formula.

1. Drip rate of the I.V. administration set to be used.
2. Amount of solution to be infused over 1 hour.

Determining the Drip Rate

To correctly calculate the drip rate, note the drop factor of the tubing as listed on the side, front, or back of the administration package. Drip rates provided by administration sets are either macrodrip sets, which include primary and secondary sets, and microdrip sets, which include pediatric sets.

PRIMARY SETS
10 drops = 1 mL
15 drops = 1 mL
20 drops = 1 mL

SECONDARY SETS
10 drops = 1 mL
15 drops = 1 mL
20 drops = 1 mL

PEDIATRIC SETS
60 drops = 1 mL

BLOOD SETS
10 drops = 1 mL

Determining the Amount of Solution to Be Infused

The physician orders the amount of solution to be infused. Orders are written in one of two ways: (1) in total amount over a specified length of time, such as 1000 mL over 8 hour; or (2) in amount to be delivered per hour (e.g., 125 mL/hour). After both of these factors are obtained, determine the flow rate using the following formula:

FORMULA

$$\frac{\text{Drops per mL (drop factor)}}{60 \text{ (minutes in an hour)}} \times \text{mL per hour} = \text{drops per minute}$$

Calculations are particularly important when an electronic rate control device is not being used or when an electronic controller is used that does not have a mechanism to dial in mL per hour.

Example
Physician orders are for 125 mL/hour and a primary tubing selected has a drop factor of 15.

$$\text{Step 1} = \frac{15 \times 125}{60} = \text{drops per minute}$$

$$\text{Step 2} = \frac{1 \times 125 \text{ mL}}{4} = 31 \text{ drops per minute}$$

When using microdrip (pediatric tubing) that is 60 drops/1 mL, the = 1, so the drops per minute equal the mL per hour.

Example
The physician orders 35 mL of solution per hour on a 2-year-old girl. You would set up your rate calculation as follows:

$$\text{Step 1} = \frac{60 \times 35 \text{ mL}}{60} = \text{drops per minute}$$

$$\text{Step 2} = 1 \times 35 \text{ mL} = 35 \text{ drops per minute}$$

Try the practice problems in Worksheet No. 2 to test your comprehension of rate calculation. The conversion chart in Table 8–9 can assist in rate calculation.

Step 15: Documentation

Documentation of I.V. therapy generally includes the date of insertion, the location, the gauge and length of cannula, and the name of the person inserting the device.

TABLE 8–9. CONVERSION CHART: RATE CALCULATION

Order: mL/hour	Drop Factors			
	10 drops/mL	15 drops/mL	20 drops/mL	60 drops/mL
10	2	3	3	10
15	3	4	5	15
20	3	5	7	20
30	5	8	10	30
50	8	13	17	50
75	13	19	25	N/A
80	13	20	27	N/A
100	17	25	33	N/A
120	20	30	40	N/A
125	21	31	42	N/A
150	25	38	50	N/A
166	27	42	55	N/A
175	29	44	58	N/A
200	33	50	67	N/A
250	42	63	83	N/A
300	50	75	100	N/A

Microdrip tubing is not appropriate for rates over 50 mL/hour.

Patient education is lacking in most audits of charts; therefore, documentation of patient response to the procedure needs to be included in the charting format. This needs to be addressed in narrative charting or in a check-off format, which includes the status of the patient, the reason for restart, the procedure, and comments.

SUMMARY OF STEPS IN INITIATING I.V. THERAPY

Precannula Insertion

1. Check physician order; confirm all parts of the order for accuracy.
2. Wash hands for 15 to 20 seconds using bacteriocidal soap. Prepare equipment: Check for breaks in integrity, and expiration date; spike and prime the infusion system.
3. Provide privacy. Explain procedure to patient. Evaluate patient psychological preparation of I.V. therapy.
4. Make assessment of site and vein dilation.
5. Assess both arms keeping the factors for vein selection in mind. Make a choice whether to use blood pressure cuff or tourniquet for dilation. Use other methods for venous distension, such as warm packs, gravity, or tapping, if necessary.

Cannula Insertion

6. Choose the appropriate catheter for duration of infusion and type of infusate based on facility policy and procedure. Rewash hands.
7. Use gloves following universal precautions for exposure to blood or body fluids.

249

8. Prepare site by using 70% alcohol to cleanse the site, followed by a 20-second scrub with povidone-iodine, or chlorhexidine. Let the povidone-iodine or chlorhexidine air dry. Do not remove. If patient is allergic to iodine use alcohol for a 30-second vigorous scrub as a substitute. Do not retouch. Put on gloves before venipuncture.
9. Insert over the needle catheter via the direct or indirect method. Thread the catheter while removing the stylet needle. Connect the catheter hub to I.V. tubing or insert a locking device (PRN device).
10. Stabilize the catheter hub with the chevron taping method or use transparent dressing directly over hub and site. There are two methods of dressing management: *Gauze*—2-in × 2-in gauze with all edges taped; change every 48 hours or, *TSM*—Transparent film applied with aseptic technique and changed every 48 to 72 hours, or if integrity of dressing compromised.

Postcannula Insertion

11. Label the insertion site with cannula size, date, time and initials, the tubing with date, and time strip the solution.
12. To facilitate equipment disposal use OSHA and JCAHO standards for disposal of the needle.
13. Explain to the patient their limitations, the equipment in use, and give instructions for observation of the site.
14. Remember when doing rate calculations, if a roller clamp or electronic controller is used the drops per minute will need to be calculated based on the drop factor.
15. Document on the patient's chart the procedure performed, how patient tolerated the venipuncture, and what instructions were given to the patient.

SUMMARY WORKSHEET 2: Rate Calculations

1. The physician orders 1000 mL of 5% dextrose in water at 100 mL/hour. You have available 20 drop-factor tubing: Calculate the drops per minute.

$$\frac{1000 \cancel{20}}{5\cancel{100}} = 200$$

2. The physician orders 1000 mL of 5% dextrose and 0.45% sodium chloride at 150 mL/hour. You have available 15-drop factor tubing. Calculate the drops per minute.

3. The physician orders 250 mL (1 U) of packed cells over 4 hours. Remember, blood tubing is always 10 drop factor. Calculate the drops per minute.

4. The physician orders 45 mL/hour of 0.50% sodium chloride solution on an 8-month-old baby. Calculate the drops per minute if you have to use a controller that is drops per minute. (Remember, use microdrip tubing.)

5. The physician orders 3000 mL of a multiple electrolyte fluid over 24 hours. Calculate the drops per minute using 20 drop-factor tubing.

6. The physician orders 250 mL of packed cells to be administered over 2 hours. Calculate the drops per minute.

7. The physician orders 500 mL of 5% dextrose/0.25% sodium chloride to be administered at 75 mL/hour. You have available 15 drop-factor tubing.

8. Calculate problem #7 using 20 drop-factor tubing.

9. A physician orders 50 mL/hour of 5% dextrose in water to rehydrate an 85-year-old woman. You assess the patient and find her cardiovascular status compromised. What tubing do you choose? Microdrip or macrodrip, and why? Calculate the drops per minute using 20 drop-factor tubing and 60 drop-factor tubing.

10. The physician orders a fluid challenge of 250 mL of sodium chloride over 45 minutes. You have 20 drop-factor tubing available. Calculate the drops per minute in order to accurately deliver the 250 mL over 45 minutes.

RECOMMENDATIONS FOR USE OF PERIPHERAL VENOUS CATHETERS

Both the Intravenous Nurses Society and the CDCP have developed recommendations for safe use of peripheral venous catheters for I.V. therapy. In addition, it is important to follow the institutional policy.

Centers for Disease Control and Prevention (1995)

Peripheral Venous Catheters

In adults, change catheter and rotate site every 48 to 72 hours.
Replace catheters inserted under emergency conditions within 24 hours.
Leave dressing in place until the catheter is removed or changed, or the dressing becomes damp, loosened, or soiled.
Change administration sets including "piggyback" tubing no more frequently than every 72 hours.
No recommendation is made for the "hang time" of I.V. fluids other than parenteral nutritional fluids.
No recommendation is made for the routine application of antimicrobial ointments to the catheter site.

Midline Catheters

No recommendation is made regarding how frequently to change catheter.
Leave dressing in place until catheter in place is removed or changed, or the dressing becomes damp, loosened, or soiled.
Change administration sets including "piggyback" tubing no more frequently than every 72 hours.
No recommendation is made on "hang time" of I.V. fluids other than parenteral nutritional fluids.

DISCONTINUATION OF I.V. CANNULA

I.V. therapy should be discontinued if the integrity of the cannula is compromised or the physician orders the discontinuation of therapy.

Procedure

1. Put on gloves.
2. Obtain a dry 2-in × 2-in gauze pad. Avoid one with alcohol because it causes stinging and promotes bleeding.
3. Loosen the tape and apply the 2-in × 2-in gauze pad loosely over the site.
4. Remove the cannula and transparent dressing as one unit, without pressure over the site.
5. After the catheter is removed, apply direct pressure with the sterile 2-in × 2-in gauze pad over the site.
6. An adhesive bandage may be applied to the venipuncture site after bleeding is controlled.
7. Document the site appearance, how the patient tolerated the procedure, and the intactness of the cannula.

LATEX RESEALABLE LOCKS (PRN DEVICES)

Latex resealable locks, also called PRN devices, intermittent I.V. lock devices, and heparin locks have been a standard of practice in most hospitals for over a decade. Maintaining these devices is typically accomplished by flushing with dilute heparinized saline at the end of an infusion and between injections. Controversies have arisen regarding standardization of heparin flushing protocols and the use of saline flushes for maintaining patency of peripheral lines (Fry, 1992).

Resealable locks consist of a cap that fits over the proximal end of the I.V. catheter with a resealable latex diaphragm. A number of sets are available commercially. Originally, heparin locks were used for pediatric and geriatric patients.

ADVANTAGES

Provide access to the vascular system, allowing for more flexibility than hanging I.V. fluids

Allow for reduced volume of fluid administered, which can be important for a cardiac patient

Can be used to collect blood samples for glucose tolerance tests, eliminating multiple puncture sites

Provide access for delivery of emergency medications

DISADVANTAGES

Occlusion or blood clotting within the lock

Possibility of speed shock and damage from drug being rapidly introduced into the circulation

HEPARIN FLUSH VERSUS SALINE FLUSH

How a device is kept patent is determined by institution policy. Flushing either with a heparin solution or with saline can be done. See Table 8–10 for flush procedure.

Heparin Lock Flush

Heparin inhibits reactions that lead to blood coagulation and the formation of fibrin clots in vitro and in vivo. The anticoagulant effect of heparin is almost immediate.

TABLE 8–10. **COMPARISON OF PROCEDURE FOR HEPARIN LOCK FLUSH AND SALINE LOCK FLUSH**

Heparin Lock Flush*	Saline Lock Flush
1. Check patency of lock.	1. Check patency of the lock.
2. Flush lock with 1 mL saline to clear lock of any bioincompatibility.	2. Flush with 1 mL of 0.9% sodium chloride.
3. Administer medication.	3. Administer medication.
4. Flush with saline again to clear lock of any bioincompatibility.	4. Flush with 1 mL of 0.9% sodium chloride.
5. Heparinize with 10 to 100 units of heparin in 1 mL saline to reseal the lock.	

*This is the SASH method: saline = administration = saline = heparin..

Heparin acts indirectly by means of a plasma cofactor, thereby neutralizing several activated clotting factors. Because of these properties, it can be used therapeutically as a flushing agent.

The INS currently recommends the use of 1 mL of heparin lock flush solution containing heparin sodium, 10 or 100 U, to maintain patency of indwelling venipuncture devices. This solution is injected into the diaphragm (hub) of the device after each use or every 8 hours if not in use (Fry, 1992); (Goode, Titler, & Rakel, 1991). A study by Andersen and Holland (1992) found that 10 U/mL heparin was as effective as 100 U/mL heparin in maintaining patency of peripherally inserted central catheters.

The use of heparinized saline has been successful for many years and is a recognized standard of practice in the medical community. It is recommended that the lowest possible concentration of heparin be used.

ADVANTAGES
Reduced risk of phlebitis
Low incidence of side effects when properly used
Low risk of tort liability with heparin flushing practices

The literature contains well-documented studies supporting the use of heparin in small amounts as an effective way to maintain the lock device.

One dose of heparin solution will maintain anticoagulation within the lumen of the device for up to 4 hours. Omission of heparin is thought to allow the formation and accumulation of fibrin material within the lumen of the needle or catheter or both, thus causing loss of patency and leading to the development of phlebitis.

Despite pressures to reduce costs by eliminating the flush, hospitals legally and ethically can support only policies that benefit or at least have no adverse effect on the patient.

DISADVANTAGES
Must be used with caution in patients with known hypersensitivity to pork and beef
Local and systemic allergic-type reactions with the use of multidose vial preparations thought to be associated with a preservative hypersensitivity
Has one extra step
Entails increased cost to patient
Complications, including hypersensitivity reactions, transient increases in activated partial thromboplastin time, and delayed fibrinolysis with platelet aggregation and thrombocytopenia (Baldwin, 1989; Chang, 1987)
Has bioincompatibilities (Nelson, Young, & Lammin, 1987)

✎ NOTE: When flushing the device, positive pressure within the lumen of the catheter must be maintained during and after administration of the flush solution to prevent reflux of blood into the cannula lumen.

Saline Lock Flush

Cost-effectiveness is a driving factor influencing the choices of practice in today's health care field. Use of saline rather than heparin to maintain heparin locks has been investigated as a way of reducing cost. At the present time, data supporting the proposition that 0.9% sodium chloride may be as effective as heparinized saline in maintaining patency of intermittent I.V. devices is inconclusive (Goode, Titler, & Rakel, 1991).

ADVANTAGES

Fewer steps

Lower cost

Takes 2 minutes for a nurse to administer and document a flush (eliminating two thirds of the flushes per year saves nursing time)

According to a study by Epperson (1984), no statistically significant difference in the rate of site loss among the patients who received normal saline flushes and those who received heparin flushes

DISADVANTAGES

Further controlled studies in larger numbers of patient needed to confirm results that heparin and saline are equally effective

Possible complications associated with use of saline flush alone include loss of patency, phlebitis, and increased patient stress caused by catheter starts (Cyganski, Donohue, & Heaton, 1987)

Flushing with saline solution may loosen, and embolize, clots formed at the tip of nonheparinized catheters (Morris, 1989)

CONTROVERSIAL PRACTICES

Controversy exists in the administration of anesthetics either on or in the skin prior to venipuncture. These include the use of xylocaine hydrochloride intradermal injection as well as transdermal application of xylocaine (EMLA cream) and topical nitroglycerin.

Lidocaine

Lidocaine (xylocaine hydrochloride) has been used in clinical practice since 1948 and is one of the safest anesthetics. Lidocaine is an amide that works by stopping impulses at the neural membrane. The anesthetized site is numb to pain, but the patient perceives touch and pressure and control of muscles. The anesthetic becomes effective within 15 to 30 seconds and lasts 30 to 45 minutes (Millam, 1992). The use of lidocaine is a simple process:

1. Check for patient allergy—lidocaine sensitivity.
2. Select appropriate arm, apply tourniquet, and select suitable vein.
3. Draw up 0.1 cc of 1% lidocaine (plain) in a TB syringe. Greater than 0.1 cc increases the risk for vasospasm.
4. Don gloves.
5. Prep site with alcohol for 30 seconds and allow to dry.
6. Reapply tourniquet. The vein should be fully dilated, pulled taut by stretching, and stabilized while the local anesthetic is administered.
7. Insert the needle at a 15- to 25-degree angle, inject the lidocaine intradermally into the side of the vein next to the desired insertion site. Do not nick vein.
8. Withdraw needle—allow 5 to 10 seconds for anesthetic to take effect.
9. Continue with steps in starting I.V. (e.g. prep skin with Betadine).

✎ NOTE: Local anesthetics should not be injected into the vein because of the possibility of an undesirable systemic effect. The local anesthetic will not "freeze" the venipuncture site if it is injected into the vein (Fig. 8–6).

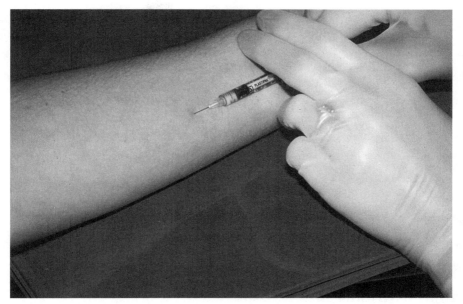

Figure 8–6. Intradermal lidocaine administered before ventipuncture using 0.1 to 0.2 mL of 1% lidocaine and a tuberculin syringe entering the skin at a 15- to 25-degree angle.

✎ **NOTE:** Some clinicians believe administration of lidocaine prior to catheter insertion increases patient comfort and decreases anxiety. However, lidocaine may expose the patient to complications that include but are not limited to allergic reaction, anaphylaxis, inadvertent injection of the drug into the vascular system, and obliteration of the vein.

The nurse must have knowledge of the actions and side effects associated with lidocaine. A history of previous allergies precludes the administration of lidocaine.

Transdermal Analgesia

EMLA cream is a mixture of two local anesthetics (lidocaine 2.5% and prilocaine 2.5%). When EMLA is applied to the skin under an occlusive dressing, analgesia is provided by a release of lidocaine and prilocaine from the cream into the epidermal and dermal layers of the skin. The two agents stabilize neuronal membranes by inhibiting the conduction of impulses, therefore effecting local anesthetic action (Astra, 1992) (Fig. 8–7).

Follow these steps in the application of EMLA cream:

1. Apply 2.5 g in a thick layer at the intended site of the venipuncture.
2. Place an occlusive dressing over the EMLA cream and smooth down the edges. Be sure to write the time of application on the dressing.
3. Remove the occlusive dressing and cleanse the skin with an antiseptic and prepare the patient for the venipuncture.

In a study by Cooper, Gerrish, Harwick and Kay (1987), it was found that EMLA cream reduced the pain associated with venipuncture in children when a 25-gauge needle was used. Sixty minutes are required to achieve effective analgesia.

257

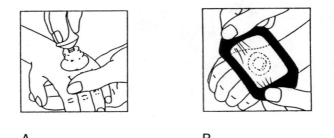

A	B

Figure 8–7. (A) Application of EMLA cream to the intended venipuncture site. (B) Placement of an occlusive dressing over the cream. (Courtesy of Astra Pharmaceutical Products, Inc., Westborough, Massachusetts.)

✎ **NOTE:** Apply EMLA cream under occlusive dressing for 1 hour prior to venipuncture.

✎ **NOTE:** EMLA cream is contraindicated in patients with known history of sensitivity to local anesthetics of the amide type.

Topical Nitroglycerin

The use of 1 to 2 mg of nitroglycerin rubbed topically into the skin area has been studied as a method of dilating veins prior to venipuncture. This technique has been studied in Australia by Hecker, Lewis, and Stanley (1983). The study, which needs replication, found that the use of topical Nitrobid distended the veins without the need for other adjuncts such as tapping, swabbing, or clenching the fist.

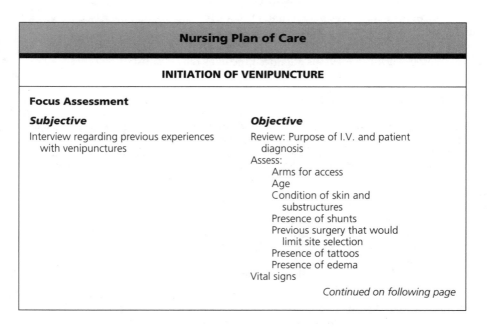

Nursing Plan of Care

INITIATION OF VENIPUNCTURE

Focus Assessment

Subjective	*Objective*
Interview regarding previous experiences with venipunctures	Review: Purpose of I.V. and patient diagnosis Assess: 　　Arms for access 　　Age 　　Condition of skin and 　　　substructures 　　Presence of shunts 　　Previous surgery that would 　　　limit site selection 　　Presence of tattoos 　　Presence of edema Vital signs

Continued on following page

Patient Outcome Criteria
The patient will:
Demonstrate improved fluid balance.
Verbalize understanding of need for I.V. access and consent to procedure.
Be free of complications associated with intravenous therapy.

Nursing Diagnoses
Anxiety (mild, moderate, or severe) related to threat to or change in health status; misconceptions regarding therapy
Fear related to insertion of cannula
Knowledge deficit related to new procedure and maintaining I.V. therapy
Impaired physical mobility related to pain or discomfort resulting from placement and maintenance of I.V. cannula
Impaired skin integrity related to I.V. cannula; I.V. solution
Pain related to physical trauma (e.g., cannula insertion)
Risk of infection related to broken skin or traumatized tissue

Nursing Management: Critical Activities
Verify physician's order for I.V. therapy.
Instruct patient about procedure.
Maintain universal precautions.
Use strict aseptic technique during insertion of cannula.
Examine solution for type, amount, expiration date, character of solution, and integrity of container.
Select and prepare an I.V. infusion pump as indicated.
Administer I.V. fluids at room temperature.
Monitor I.V. flow rate and I.V. site during infusion, following protocol.
Monitor for I.V. therapy complications (e.g., phlebitis, infiltration, site infection).
Replace I.V. cannula, and administration every 48 to 72 hours.
Maintain integrity of occlusive dressing.

PATIENT EDUCATION

Instruct on purpose of I.V. therapy.
Educate regarding limitations of movement.
Instruct to notify the nurse if pump alarms.
Instruct to report discomfort at the infusion site.

HOME CARE ISSUES

Home care issues for initiation and maintenance of I.V. therapy revolve around technical procedures, as well as the monitoring of therapy. The technical procedures that the patient is expected to learn and perform depend on cognitive ability, willingness to learn, and the specific technique being taught. Another home care issue is the number of visits that will be required to maintain the line and the proximity of the patient's home to a health care facility.

PATIENT OR THEIR CAREGIVERS ARE OFTEN EXPECTED TO:
Administer solutions or medications.
Change dressings.

259

Change administration sets.
Set up or monitor pump equipment.

Patient and/or family must be taught universal precautions and aseptic technique in the home care setting.

✎ **NOTE:** The nursing staff would be responsible for the routine restarts of peripheral I.V. or blood draws.

COMPETENCY CRITERIA: Peripheral I.V. Therapy

Competency Statement: The competent I.V. therapy nurse will be able to perform I.V. therapy using aseptic technique.

PERFORMANCE CRITERIA

	Skilled	Needs Education
1. Describes the anatomy and physiology of the vascular system:		
Skin		
Tissue layers of vein		
Venous and arterial system		
2. Determines appropriate placement of venous device:		
Length and type of therapy		
Age and size of patient		
Factors influencing site selection		
3. Verifies appropriate fluid type, rate, and volume of delivery:		
Isotonic, hypotonic, hypertonic		
Appropriate rate and volume for patient		
4. Inspects equipment for integrity:		
Fluid containers		
Administration set		
Cannula		
5. Performs successful venipuncture (85% to 95%) on initial attempt:		
One attempt per device		
6. Initiates I.V. standards of practice maintenance:		
Gauze dressings		
Transparent semipermeable dressing		
Site rotation		
Administration set		

7. **Documents changes appropriate to institutional policy:**
   Assessment of site
   Size and length of cannula
   Placement of cannula
   Number attempts
   Solution

8. **Educates patient/family concerning I.V. therapy:**
   Psychosocial support
   Signs and symptoms of complications
   Precautions and limitations
   Nursing care

SUGGESTED EVALUATION CRITERIA

Performance demonstration on model
Performance demonstration on patient
Review of documentation

KEY POINTS

The first step is an understanding of the anatomy and physiology of the venous system. The five layers in the approach to successful venipuncture are:
   Epidermis
   Dermis
   Tunica adventitia
   Tunica media
   Tunica intima

A working knowledge of the veins in the hand and forearm is vital so the practitioner can successfully locate an acceptable vein for venipuncture and cannula placement. The factors affecting vein selection in summary are:
   Type of solution
   Condition of vein
   Duration of therapy
   Patient age
   Patient preference
   Patient activity
   Presence of disease/prior surgery
   Presence of shunts or grafts

The steps in performing the placement of a catheter which can support I.V. therapy for 48 to 72 hours are as follows:

Precannulation
    Step 1: Check physician's order
    Step 2: Wash hands
    Step 3: Prepare equipment
    Step 4: Patient assessment and psychological preparedness
    Step 5: Site selection and vein dilation
Cannula Placement
    Step 6: Needle selection
    Step 7: Gloving
    Step 8: Site preparation
    Step 9: Vein entry
    Step 10: Catheter stabilization and dressing management
Postcannulation
    Step 11: Labeling
    Step 12: Equipment disposal
    Step 13: Patient instructions
    Step 14: Rate calculation
    Step 15: Documentation

The choice of using heparin or saline to maintain latex injection ports (locks) is determined by the agency's policies and procedures and the physician's order. Check these before using the steps in heparin/saline lock flush.

Heparin Lock Flush
    1. Check for patency
    2. Flush lock with sodium chloride 1 mL
    3. Administer medication
    4. Flush lock with sodium chloride 1 mL
    5. Inject 1 mL of 10 to 100 unit of heparin with positive pressure to fill the lock.

Saline Lock Flush
    1. Check patency of catheter
    2. Flush with 1 mL of 0.9% sodium chloride
    3. Administer medication
    4. Flush with 1 mL of sodium chloride

NOTE: Locks must be flushed every 8 hours if not being utilized for medication administration.

Controversial issues
    Use of xylocaine hydrochloride prior to venipuncture
    Use of nitroglycerine topical agent prior to venipuncture
    Use of EMLA cream

CRITICAL THINKING ACTIVITY

1. Check the policy and procedure manual at your facility to check the procedure for:

   Flushing an intermittent infusion device
   Recommendations for tubing changes
   Recommendations for catheter replacement

2. Do you feel checking for patency is necessary prior to flush procedure? Why?

3. Check the I.V. setups in your agency and check for labeling practices. What did you find?

4. Identify techniques, which you have observed, that might contribute to contamination of an I.V. site.

POST-TEST, CHAPTER 8

1. List the five layers that must be penetrated during a venipuncture.

   A. _____

   B. _____

   C. _____

   D. _____

   E. _____

2. List three of the nine factors that affect site selection.

   A. _____

   B. _____

   C. _____

Match the definition in column II to the term in column I.

Column I

3. _____ antimicrobial

4. _____ cannula

5. _____ bevel

6. _____ prime

7. _____ spike

Column II

A. Hollow plastic tube made of Teflon, Aquavene, or Vialon used for accessing the vascular system

B. Slanted portion of cannula device or needle

C. To fill the administration set with infusate for the first time

D. To insert the administration set into the infusate container

E. An agent that destroys or prevents development of microorganisms

8. List the five steps in a heparin flush of an intermittent infusion device.

   A. _____

   B. _____

   C. _____

   D. _____

   E. _____

9. List the 15-step approach in initiating I.V. therapy.

Precannulation

Step 1: _____

Step 2: _____

(How?) _____

Step 3: _____

(List what to check.)

Step 4: _____

Step 5: _____

265

Cannulation

Step 6: _____

Step 7: _____

(How?) _____

Step 8: _____

Step 9: _____

Step 10: _____

Postcannulation

Step 11: _____

(What three sites?) _____

Step 12: _____

Step 13: _____

Step 14: _____

Step 15: _____

10. State one controversial practice:

   _____

11. Before equipment setup and venipuncture, how many seconds of handwashing with an antimicrobial soap are recommended?
   A. 10 to 30
   B. 15 to 20
   C. 30 to 60
   D. 45 to 60

12. Labels should be on what areas?
   A. Catheter site, tubing, and solution container
   B. Tubing, solution container, and chart
   C. Solution container, catheter site, and patient's armband

ANSWERS TO CHAPTER 8

PRE-TEST

1. B	5. D	9. C	13. E
2. E	6. A	10. A	14. B
3. C	7. B	11. C	
4. B	8. B	12. D	

POST-TEST

1. A. Epidermis
   B. Dermis
   C. Tunica adventitia
   D. Tunica media
   E. Tunica intima
2. A. Type of solution
   B. Condition of vein
   C. Duration of therapy
   D. Cannula size
   E. Patient size
   F. Patient preference
   G. Patient activity
   H. Presence of disease or prior surgery
   I. Presence of shunts or grafts
3. E
4. A
5. B
6. C
7. D
8. A. Check for patency
   B. Flush with saline
   C. Administer medication
   D. Flush with saline
   E. Heparin 10 to 100 U to fill the lock
9. **Precannulation**
   Step 1: Checking physician's order
   Step 2: Washing hands for 15 to 20 seconds with antimicrobial soap

Step 3: Preparing equipment check for clarity, expiration date, and integrity of glass or plastic
Step 4: Assessing and psychologically preparing the patient
Step 5: Selecting site and dilating vein
Cannulation
Step 6: Selecting catheter
Step 7: Gloving
Step 8: Preparing site for 20 seconds with povidone-iodine circular motion from inside out
Step 9: Vein entry (direct or indirect)
Step 10: Catheter stabilization and dressing management
Postcannulation
Step 11: Site, tubing, and solution container labeling
Step 12: Disposing of equipment in appropriate receptacle
Step 13: Instructing patient
Step 14: Calculating drop rate
Step 15: Documentation
10. Use of lidocaine or use of nitroglycerin ointment before venipuncture
11. B
12. A

REFERENCES

American Heart Association (1994). Guidelines for cardiopulmonary resuscitation and emergency cardiac care, III: Adult advanced cardiac life support. Dallas: American Heart Association, 6-1–6-12.

Anderson, M., & Holland, J. (1992). Maintaining the patency of peripherally inserted central catheters with 10 units/cc heparin. *Journal of Intravenous Nursing, 15* (2), 84–88.

Astra Pharmaceutical Products. (1992). *EMLA cream package insert.* Wesborough, MA: ASTRA.

Baldwin, D.R. (1989). Heparin-induced thrombocytopenia. *Journal of Intravenous Nursing, 12* (6), 378–382.

Byers, P.H. (1986). Comparison of application factors among three brands of transparent semipermeable films for peripheral I.V.'s *National Intravenous Therapy Association, 8* (4), 315–318.

Centers for Disease Control and Prevention. (1995). *Centers for Disease Control and Prevention intravascular device-related infections prevention; Guideline availability; notice.* Atlanta: US Department of Health and Human Services.

Chang, J.C. (1987). White clot syndrome associated with heparin-induced thrombocytopenia: A review of 23 cases. *Heart Lung, 16,* 403–407.

Cooper, C.M., Gerrish, S.P., Hardwick, M., & Kay, R. (1987). EMLA cream reduces the pain of venipuncture in children. *European Journal of Anaesthesiology, 4,* 441–448.

Cyganski, J.M., Donahue, J.M., & Heaton, J.S. (1987). The case for the heparin flush. *American Journal of Nursing, 87,* 796–797.

Delaney, C.W., & Lauer, M.L. (1988). *Intravenous therapy: A guide to quality care.* Philadelphia: J.B. Lippincott.

Enrich, M. (1991). Performing venipuncture in elderly patients. *Nursing 91,* 21.

Epperson, E.L. (1984). Efficacy of 0.9% sodium chloride injection with and without heparin for maintaining indwelling intermittent injection sites. *Clinical Pharmacy, 3,* 626–629.

Fabian, B. (1995). Intravenous therapy in the older adult. In Terry, J., Baranowski, L., Lonsway, R., & Hedrick, C. (Eds.). *Intravenous therapy: Clinical principles and practice. Intravenous Nurses Society* (pp. 495–504). Philadelphia: W.B. Saunders.

Fry, B. (1992). Intermittent flushing protocols: A standardization issue. *Journal of Intravenous Nursing, 15* (3), 160–163.

Goode, C.J., Titler, M., & Rakel, B. (1991). A meta-analysis of effects of heparin flush and saline flush: Quality and cost implications. *Nursing Research, 40* (6), 324–330.

Guyton, A.C. (1991). *Textbook of medical physiology (8th ed.).* Philadelphia: W.B. Saunders.

Hecker, J.F., Lewis, G.B., & Stanley, H. (1983). Nitroglycerine ointment as an aide to venipuncture, *Lancet, 2,* 332–333.

Katich, M., & Band, J. (1985). Local infection of the intravenous-cannula wound associated with transparent dressings. *Journal of Infectious Diseases, 151* (5), 971–972.

Korniewicz, D.M., Kirwin, M., & Larson, E. (1991). Do your gloves fit the task? *American Journal of Nursing, 91* (6), 38–39.

Maki, D.G., Botticelli, J.T., LeRoy, L.L., & Thielke, T.S. (1987). Prospective study of replacing administration sets for intravenous therapy at 48 vs 72 hour intervals. 72 Hours is safe and cost effective. *JAMA, 258* (13), 1777–1781.

Maki, D.G., & Ringer, M. (1987). Evaluation of dressing regimens for prevention of infection with peripheral intravenous catheters. *JAMA, 58,* 2396.

Mathewson-Kuhn, M. (1994). *Pharmacotherapeutics: A nursing process approach* (3rd ed.). Philadelphia: F.A. Davis, 180–182.

Millam, D.A. (1992). Starting I.V.s: How to develop your venipuncture expertise. *Nursing 92, 9,* 33–45.

Millam, D.A., & Warren, J. (1985). Using local anesthetic for I.V. insertion: Pro & con. *Nursing Life.*

National Intravenous Therapy Association Editorial. (1985). Infection traced to false fingernails, *Journal of Intravenous Nursing, 6* (6), 5.

Nelson, R.W., Young, R., & Lamnin, M. (1987). Visual incompatibility of dacarbazine and heparin. *American Journal of Hospital Pharmacy, 44,* 71–73.

Pauley, S. (1985). Nitro vein dilation. *National Intravenous Therapy Association, 6* (2), 5.

Perucca, R. (1995). Obtaining vascular access. In Terry, J., Baranowski, L., Lonsway, R., & Hedrick, C. (Eds.). *Intravenous therapy: Clinical principles and practice. Intravenous Nurses Society* (pp. 370–399). Philadelphia: W.B. Saunders.

Peterson, F.Y., & Kirchhoff, K.T. (1991). Heparinized versus nonheparinized intravenous lines. *Heart & Lung 20* (6), 631–637.

Smeltzer, S.C., & Bare, B.G. (1992). *Brunner and Suddarth's textbook of medical-surgical nursing* (7th ed.). Philadelphia: J.B. Lippincott.

Steele, J. (1988). *Practical I.V. therapy.* Springhouse, PA: Springhouse Corporation.

Weinstein, S. (1993). *Plumers' principles and practice of intravenous therapy (5th ed.).* Philadelphia: J.B. Lippincott.

Complications of Intravenous Therapy

CHAPTER CONTENTS

GLOSSARY
LEARNING OBJECTIVES
PRE-TEST, CHAPTER 9
LOCAL COMPLICATIONS
Hematoma
Thrombosis
Phlebitis
Thrombophlebitis
Infiltration
Extravasation
Local Infection
Venous Spasm
SUMMARY WORKSHEET #1: LOCAL
    COMPLICATIONS
SYSTEMIC COMPLICATIONS
Septicemia
Circulatory Overload
Pulmonary Edema
Air Embolism

Speed Shock
Catheter Embolism
SUMMARY WORKSHEET #2: SYSTEMIC
    COMPLICATIONS
ERRATIC FLOW RATES
NURSING PLAN OF CARE: PREVENTION OF
    COMPLICATIONS
PATIENT EDUCATION
HOME CARE ISSUES
COMPETENCY CRITERIA; PREVENTION OF
    COMPLICATIONS OF I.V. THERAPY
KEY POINTS
CRITICAL THINKING ACTIVITY
POST-TEST, CHAPTER 9
ANSWERS TO CHAPTER 9
Pre-Test
Post-Test
REFERENCES

GLOSSARY

Ecchymosis A bruise; a "black and blue spot" on the skin caused by escape of blood from injured vessels

Embolism A sudden obstruction of a blood vessel by a clot or foreign material formed or introduced elsewhere in the circulatory system and carried to the point of obstruction by the bloodstream

Extravasation Escape of fluid from a vessel into the surrounding tissue

Hematoma A localized mass of blood outside of the blood vessel, usually found in a partially clotted state

Hemodilution Increase in the plasma content of the blood with resulting decrease in the concentration of red blood cells

Infiltration Process of seepage or diffusion into tissue of I.V. infusate

Phlebitis Inflammation of the intima of a vein associated with chemical irritation (chemical phlebitis), mechanical irritation (mechanical phlebitis), or bacterial infection (bacterial phlebitis); postinfusion, inflammation of the intima of a vein within 48 to 96 hours of cannula removal

Septicemia Systemic disease caused by the presence of pathogenic microorganisms in the body

Speed shock Systemic reaction that occurs when a substance foreign to the body is rapidly introduced into the circulation

Thrombosis Formation or presence of a blood clot; venous, arrest of circulation in the vein by a blood clot; also called *phlebemphraxis*

Vasospasm Contraction of the muscular coats of the blood vessels; also called *angiospasm*

Vesicant Any agent that produces blisters

LEARNING OBJECTIVES

Upon completion of this chapter, the reader will be able to:

- Define terms related to the hazards associated with I.V. therapy.
- Differentiate between local and systemic complications.
- Identify prompt treatment for each local and systemic complication.
- Document assessment of each local and systemic complication.
- Identify the most hazardous local complication.
- Describe the signs and symptoms of eight local complications.
- List three risk factors for phlebitis.
- Use phlebitis criteria chart for identifying and rating postinfusion phlebitis.
- Apply the dilution guideline rate for minibag admixtures as an intervention to decrease phlebitis.
- Compare erratic flow rates as they relate to the hazards associated with I.V. therapy.
- Identify organisms responsible for most cases of septicemia related to infusion therapy.
- Identify prevention techniques for the six systemic complications.
- Identify Centers for Disease Control.
- Give recommendations for prevention of complications involving intravascular devices.
- Use the nursing process in assessment, prevention, and treatment of complications associated with I.V. therapy.

PRE-TEST, CHAPTER 9

Match the definition in column II to the term in column I.

Column I

1. _____ colonization
2. _____ extravasation
3. _____ bacterial phlebitis
4. _____ septicemia
5. _____ hematoma
6. _____ chemical phlebitis
7. _____ postinfusion phlebitis

Column II

A. A localized mass of blood outside of the blood vessel

B. Forming a compact group, or colony, of the same organization

C. Systemic disease caused by the presence of pathogenic microorganisms

D. Inflammation of the intima of a vein associated with infection

E. Escape of fluid from a vessel into the surrounding tissue

F. Inflammatory response of the intima of a vein to certain chemicals

G. Inflammation of a vein occurring 48 to 96 hours after removal of cannula

8. The risk of phlebitis is increased in which of the following patients?
   A. Patients receiving total parenteral nutrition
   B. Immunosuppressed patients
   C. Patients with burns
   D. Patients who have multiple I.V. manipulations
   E. All of the above

Match the type of complication (local or systemic) in column II to the complication in column I.

Column I

9. _____ thrombosis

10. _____ septicemia

11. _____ speed shock

12. _____ catheter embolus

13. _____ phlebitis

14. _____ vasospasm

15. _____ thrombophlebitis

16. _____ hematoma

Column II

A. Local

B. Systemic

17. The recommended treatment of phlebitis stage 2+ is to:
   A. Discontinue the cannula and apply heat to site
   B. Watch the site and document observations
   C. Leave the cannula in place and apply heat to site
   D. Flush cannula with 0.9% sodium chloride

18. The first symptoms of venous vasospasm is:
   A. Sharp pain extending from the site of infusion
   B. Redness along the vein
   C. Increased temperature
   D. Cold feeling in the extremity

19. The organism responsible for most cases of septicemia related to infusion is
   A. *Proteus*
   B. *Escherichia coli*
   C. Coagulase-negative staphylococci
   D. *Pseudomonas*

True-False

20. **T F** I.V. push drugs should be administered over at least 1 minute to prevent speed shock.

21. **T F** Use of hypertonic fluids increases the risk of phlebitis.

22. **T F** The phlebitis criteria, according to the Intravenous Nursing Society, have three stages.

23. **T F** To prevent local complications, it is necessary to use a good aseptic technique when starting or maintaining an infusion.

The most important practical lesson that can be given to nurses is to teach them what to observe—how to observe—what symptoms indicate improvement—what the reverse—which are of importance—which are of none—which are the evidence of neglect—and of what kind of neglect.

FLORENCE NIGHTINGALE, 1859

Since the nursing profession assumed the role of I.V. care in the 1940s, a large body of knowledge has been gathered about I.V. therapy. Complications such as embolism, catheter dislodgment or perforation, metabolic imbalance, hypervolemia, and nosocomial infections have been documented. The fact that 90% of hospitalized patients receive I.V. fluids and medications puts patients at risk for developing complications associated with this form of therapy.

LOCAL COMPLICATIONS

Local complications of I.V. therapy occur as adverse reactions or trauma to the surrounding venipuncture site (Table 9–1). Local complications are rarely of a serious nature. These complications can be recognized early by objective assessment. Assessing and monitoring are the key components in early intervention. Good venipuncture technique is the main factor related to the prevention of most local complications associated with I.V. therapy.

Hematoma

The formation of a *hematoma* at the venipuncture site is usually related to nursing venipuncture technique. Patients who bruise easily can develop a hematoma when large cannulas are used to initiate I.V. therapy, owing to trauma to the vein during insertion (Fig. 9–1). Hematomas are most often related to:

Nicking the vein during an unsuccessful venipuncture attempt

Discontinuing of I.V. cannula or needle without pressure held over site after removal of needle

Applying a tourniquet too tightly above a previously attempted venipuncture site

TABLE 9–1. **LOCAL COMPLICATIONS**

1. Hematoma
2. Thrombosis
3. Phlebitis
    Mechanical
    Chemical
    Bacterial
    Postinfustion
4. Thrombophlebitis
5. Infiltration
6. Extravasation
7. Local infection
8. Venous system

272

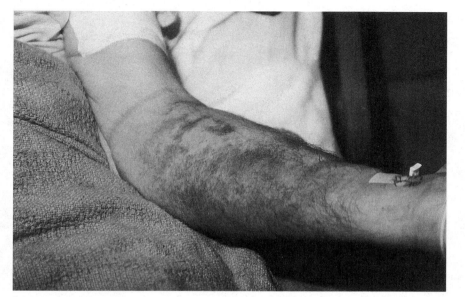

Figure 9–1. Hematoma. (Courtesy of Beth Fabian, CRNI Veterans Administration Medical Center, Ann Arbor, Michigan.)

Signs and symptoms of hematoma are:

- Discoloration of the skin surrounding the venipuncture (immediate or slow)
- Site swelling and discomfort

Prevention

Techniques for prevention of hematoma formation include:

1. Use an indirect method for starting an I.V. until technique is perfected for direct sticks. This will decrease the chance of piercing through the vein causing seepage of blood into the subcutaneous tissue (see Chap. 7 for techniques for venipuncture).
2. Apply the tourniquet just before venipuncture.

For elderly patients, patients on corticosteroids, or patients with paper-thin skin, use a small needle or catheter, preferably 20 or 22 gauge. Use a blood pressure cuff rather than a rubber tourniquet to fill the vein so that you have better control of the pressure exerted on the vein. Be very gentle in your venipuncture technique.

✎ **NOTE:** The presence of both ecchymosis and hematomas limits veins from future use (Perdue, 1995).

Treatment

1. Apply direct pressure with sterile 2 × 2 gauze over site, after catheter or needle is removed.
2. Have patient elevate the extremity over head or on pillow to maximize venous return.

273

Documentation

Document observable ecchymotic areas. Be sure to document the nursing interventions you used for care of the site.

Thrombosis

Trauma to the endothelial cells of the venous wall cause platelets to adhere to the vein wall, which may lead to formation of a clot. The *thrombosis* usually occludes the circulation of blood. Thrombus formation is manifested by the flow of the I.V. solution: the drip rate slows, or the line does not flush easily and resistance is felt, especially in a lock device. The I.V. site may appear healthy. There are two areas of great concern in assessing for a thrombosis. First, do not propel the clot into the bloodstream with pressure from a syringe, and, second, keep in mind that a thrombus within the vein can trap bacteria.

The causes of thrombosis formation are:

1. Blood backing up in the system of a hypertensive patient
2. Low flow rate, which limits fluid movement to maintain patency
3. Location of the I.V. cannula (catheter placed in a flexor area may occlude when position is changed)
4. Obstruction of flow rate due to patient compressing
5. I.V. line dry for an extended period of time
6. Trauma to the wall of the vein by the cannula

Thrombosis, along with thrombophlebitis, can lead to a systemic embolism.

✎ **NOTE:** The therapist must avoid injuring the vein wall, performing multiple punctures, and performing through-and-through punctures.

Prevention

Techniques for the prevention of a thrombosis include:

1. Use pumps and controllers for managing rate control. Rate control devices prevent blood from backing up in the tubing and produce an alarm when the I.V. line is dry.
2. Choose microdrip tubing, 60 drops/mL, when gravity flow I.V. rates are below 50 mL/hour. Remember, more drops mean more movement.
3. Avoid flexion areas for placement of I.V. cannulas.
4. Use of filters.
5. Avoid cannulation of lower extremities.

Treatment

1. Discontinue the cannula and restart with new catheter in a different site.
2. Apply cold compresses to the site to decrease the flow of blood and increase platelet adherence to the clot that has already formed (Perdue, 1995).
3. Notify physician and assess site for circulatory impairment.

✎ **NOTE:** If an occlusion occurs, *do not irrigate.* Irrigation of an occluded line with saline can propel the clot into the circulatory system causing an embolism. Follow the steps in Table 9–2.

TABLE 9–2. STEPS FOR CHECKING SLOWED INFUSION

Check tubing for kinks → Yes → Unkink and check flow rate → Ok → Stop
   ↓
  No
   ↓
Check catheter: Is it taped too tightly? → Yes → Retape and milk tubing to restart flow rate
→ Ok → Stop
   ↓
  No
   ↓
Suspect Clot
Milk the tubing using the side of pen or pencil OR
Strip tubing (*above lowest medicinal entry*) toward the patient with fingers.
NOTE: Stripping the tubing moves the catheter from the vein wall with minimal pressure.
   ↓   ↓
  No   Yes
Use 3-mL syringe filled with 2 mL of saline to attempt to   Blood return
aspirate clot (never use a 1 mL syringe because it generates   Flush with Saline → Ok
too much pressure)
   ↓
  No
Discontinue the I.V. and restart

Urokinase, a fibrinolytic drug, is being studied to remove occlusions from catheters and maintain patency. Urokinase works by lysing blood clots, but it does not work instantly. Often it must be left in the catheter 15 minutes or longer before aspirating. A study using urokinase in 1600 occluded central venous cathethers resulted in a success rate of 98.6% with no adverse reaction reported. Check your hospital protocol for specific policy and procedure (Barrus & Danek, 1987).

Documentation

Document the change of infusion rate, the steps taken to solve the problem, and the end result. Be sure to chart the new I.V. site, its patency, and the size catheter used for restart. Document how the occluded site appears.

Phlebitis

Phlebitis is a commonly reported complication of I.V. therapy. The fact that 27% to 70% of patients receiving I.V. therapy develop some stage of phlebitis makes this local complication one of the most common hazards associated with over-the-needle catheters in today's practice (Maki & Ringer, 1991). Phlebitis is an inflammation of the vein in which the endothelial cells of the venous wall become irritated and cells roughen, allowing platelets to adhere and predispose the vein to inflammation-induced phlebitis (Harrigan, 1984). The site is tender to touch and can be very painful. At the first sign of redness or complaint of tenderness, the I.V. site should be checked. Phlebitis can prolong hospitalization unless treated early.

Signs and symptoms associated with phlebitis are:

- Redness at site
- Site warm to touch
- Local swelling
- Palpable cord along the vein
- Sluggish infusion rate
- Increase in basal temperature

The process of phlebitis formation involves an increase in capillary permeability, which allows proteins and fluids to leak into the interstitial space. The traumatized tissue continues to be irritated mechanically or chemically. The immune system causes leukocytes to gather at the inflamed site. When leukocytes are released, pyrogens stimulate the hypothalamus to raise body temperature. Pyrogens also stimulate bone marrow to release more leukocytes. Redness and tenderness increase with each step of the phlebitis (Maki & Ringer, 1991). According to Hecker (1988), when local inflammation was viewed under a microscope histologic changes were marked, with loss of endothelial cells, edema, and presence of neutrophils in the vein wall. Inspection of the affected site reveals a similar appearance, regardless of the underlying cause (see Fig. 9–2).

Factors Affecting Phlebitis Formation

Factors that influence the development of phlebitis include but are not limited to insertion techniques; condition of patient; vein condition; compatibility; type and pH of medication or solution; ineffective filtration, and gauge, size, length, and material of cannula (Table 9–3). The phlebitis scale is recommended to establish a uniform standard for measuring degrees of phlebitis (Table 9–4). Phlebitis is classified according to the causative factors, which can be chemical, mechanical or bacterial (Perdue, 1995).

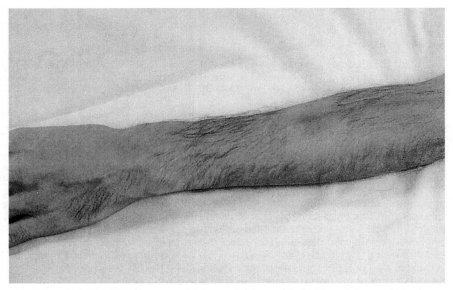

Figure 9–2. Phlebitis. (Courtesy of Johnson & Johnson Medical Inc., Arlington, Texas.)

TABLE 9–3. FACTORS AFFECTING PHLEBITIS FORMATION

1. Catheter material
   Polypropylene > Teflon
   Silicone elastomer > polyurethane
   Teflon > polyurethane
   Teflon > steel needles
2. Catheter size
   Large bore > small bore
3. **Insertion in emergency room > inpatient unit**
4. **Increasing duration of catheter placement**
5. Infusate
   Low pH
   Potassium chloride
   Hypertonic glucose, amino acids, lipids
   Antibiotics (especially β-lactams, vancomycin, metronidazole)
   High flow rate of I.V. fluid (> 90 mL/h)
6. Daily I.V. dressing changes > dressing changes every 48 hours
7. Host factors
   Poor-quality peripheral veins
   Insertion in the upper arm or wrist > hand
8. Age
   Children: older > younger
   Adults: younger > older
   Women > men
   White > Black
9. **Individual biologic vulnerability**

> denotes a significantly greater risk for phlebitis.
Terms in bold print are significant predictors of risk in this study.
Source: Adapted from Maki, D.G., & Ringer, M. (1991). Risk factors for infusion-related phlebitis with small peripheral venous catheters: A randomized controlled trial. *Annals of Internal Medicine,* 114, 845–854. By permission.

Mechanical Phlebitis

Mechanical irritation, causing a phlebitis or inflammation of the vein can be attributed to use of too large a cannula in a small vein. A large cannula placed in a vein with a smaller lumen than the cannula irritates the intima of the vein, causing inflammation and phlebitis. Large veins with thick walls hold up better during an infusion. Also, veins higher on the forearm are less likely to develop phlebitis. The other cause of mechanical phlebitis is improper taping, in which the catheter tip rubs the vein wall damaging the endothelial cell. Manipulation of the catheter during infusion causes irritation of vein wall. Securely affix catheter hub and tubing using the chevron method to prevent wiggling of the catheter.

TABLE 9–4. INFUSION PHLEBITIS SCALE

Rating	Signs and Symptoms
1+	Pain at site, erythema, or edema; no streak; no palpable cord
2+	Pain at site, erythema, or edema; streak formation; no palpable cord
3+	Pain at site, erythema, or edema; streak formation; palpable cord

Source: From Standards of Practice by the Intravenous Nurses Society, 1990, Philadelphia: JB Lippincott Company. Copyright 1990 by J.B. Lippincott Company. Reprinted by permission.

277

Chemical Phlebitis

Several factors contribute to chemical phlebitis. Generally, these include administration of:

Irritating medications or solutions
Improperly mixed or diluted medications
Too-rapid infusion
Presence of particulate matter in solution

The more acidic the I.V. solution, the greater is the risk of chemical phlebitis. I.V. solutions have a pH of 3 to 6, which helps to prevent them from caramelizing during sterilization and to maintain stability. Dextrose solutions have a pH of 3.5 to 6.5 or lower, whereas saline solutions have a pH of 5.5 (United States Pharmacopeia, 1995). The pH falls further with storage; pH values of 3.4 have been found in date-expired 5% dextrose solutions (Hecker, 1988). Additives can further decrease the pH such as vitamin C, doxorubicin (Adriamycin), and cimetidine. Some drugs, such as heparin, which has a pH of 5 to 7.5, can raise the pH. Hypertonic fluids such as 10% dextrose, which have a tonicity of greater than 375, increase the hazards of phlebitis. An increase in electrolytes also add to the increased tonicity of the solution.

✎ **NOTE:** Heparin infusions rarely cause phlebitis (Millam, 1988).

Potassium chloride (KCL) is the most common medication added to I.V. fluids according to Gong and King (1983). An association with infusion phlebitis has been reported with KCL. For example, Jones (1982) found that phlebitis developed in 27.2% of patients who received continuous infusion of KCL in addition to intermittent medications. It was reported that patients who received greater than 30 mEq of KCL/L of solution have a greater risk of phlebitis.

Another factor contributing to chemical phlebitis is particulate matter in a solution, such as drug particles that do not fully dissolve during mixing and are not visible to the eye. It has been found in many studies that the use of a 0.22-micron in-line or final filter will remove not only air and bacteria but also harmful particles (DeLuca, Rapp, Bivins, McKean, & Griffen, 1975; Jemison-Smith & Thrupp, 1982). In addition, increasing exposure of the vein lumen to irritating particles may increase the incidence of infusion phlebitis by as much as 50% to 60% (Ervin, 1987).

Intermittent infusions with heparin locks cause less irritation to the vein wall over time than continuous infusions. The slower the rate of infusion, the less irritating the solution will be to the vein wall, because cells of the vein are exposed for a shorter period of time to solutions with less than normal pH. The fact that heparin is used to maintain the lock might have further significance in the reduction of phlebitis rates.

How to prevent chemically induced phlebitis presents a problem in I.V. therapy. The use of 0.9% sodium chloride or 5% dextrose in water are usually recommended for admixtures. A study on admixtures and dilution rates by Harrigan (1984) concluded that increasing dilution rates decreased the amount of chemically induced phlebitis. Also noted in this study was that the amount of diluent must be increased when multiple medication therapy is administered. Harrigan suggested diluting irritating drugs in the following manner; drugs with a pH of 5 to 10 should be diluted in 100 mL of solution; drugs with a pH range of 3.5 to 6 should be diluted in 150 mL

278

TABLE 9–5. FREQUENTLY ADMINISTERED I.V. DRUGS: pH AND RECOMMENDED DILUTION

Drug	pH Range	Minimal Dilution Rate (mL)
Amikacin (Amikin)	4.5	150
Amphotericin B (Fungizone)	5–7	100
Cimetidine (Tagamet)	3.8–6	150
Doxycycline (Vibramycin)	2.6	200
Dopamine (Dopastat)	3.0–4.5	200
Cefazolin (Ancef)	4.5–5.5	150
Gentamicin (Garamycin)	3.0–5.5	150
Morphine	3.0–6.0	150
Nafcillin (Unipen)	6.0–6.5	100
Norepinephrine (Levophed)	3.0–4.5	200

Source: Adapted from Harrigan, C. A. (1984). A cost-effective guide for the prevention of chemical phlebitis caused by the pH of pharmaceutical agents. *Journal of Intravenous Nursing, 7*, 478–482. With permission.

of solution; and drugs with a pH range of 2.6 to 5.5 should be diluted in 200 to 250 mL of solution. See Table 9–5 for frequently administered I.V. drugs, their pH values, and recommended dilution rates.

Bacterial Phlebitis

Bacterial phlebitis, also referred to as septic phlebitis, is the least common type of phlebitis. It is an inflammation of the intima of a vein that is associated with a bacterial infection. Factors contributing to the development of bacterial phlebitis include poor aseptic technique, failure to detect breaks in the integrity of the equipment, poor cannula insertion technique, inadequately taped cannula, and failure to perform site assessments.

Bacterial phlebitis can be prevented by preparing solutions aseptically under a laminar flow hood. All solution containers should be inspected carefully before hanging; in addition, washing hands and preparing skin carefully are necessary to prevent bacterial phlebitis.

Handwashing is the most important procedure for preventing nosocomial infection and thus bacterial phlebitis (Wenzel, 1993). All equipment should be inspected for integrity, particulate matter, cloudiness, and any signs indicating a break in sterility.

✎ **NOTE:** Shaving is not recommended because of the potential for microabrasion, which allows microorganisms to enter the vascular system.

Postinfusion Phlebitis

Postinfusion phlebitis is associated with inflammation of the vein that usually becomes evident within 48 to 96 hours after the cannula has been removed. Factors that contribute to its development are cannula insertion technique, condition of vein used, type, compatibility, and pH of solution or medication being infused, gauge, size, length, and material of cannula, and cannula indwelling time.

Postinfusion phlebitis can occur without the usual signs or symptoms. There is no way to anticipate this type of phlebitis; however, once it appears, the treatment is the same as for any other phlebitis (Bohony, 1993).

279

Prevention

Techniques for prevention of phlebitis include:

1. Use larger veins for hypertonic solutions.
2. Use central lines or long-arm catheters for long-term hypertonic solutions.
3. Choose the smallest I.V. cannula appropriate for the infusate.
4. Rotate I.V. site every 72 hours, a practice that has been shown to significantly decrease the risk of phlebitis.
5. Stabilize the catheter to prevent mechanical irritation.
6. Use a 0.22-micron in-line final filter, which will remove air and bacteria, as well as harmful particulate matter (Millam, 1988).
7. Venipuncture should be performed by a skilled professional.
8. Observe good handwashing practices.
9. Add a buffer to known irritating medication and to hypertonic solutions.
10. Change solution containers every 24 hours.

Be aware that:

- Phlebitis risk factors in I.V. therapy increase after 24 hours.
- All peripheral I.V.s should be changed every 48 to 72 hours.
- A 3+ phlebitis takes from 10 days to 3 weeks to heal.
- Dextrose solutions, KCL, antibiotics, and vitamin C have lower pH and are associated with a higher risk of phlebitis.

✎ **NOTE:** According to *Nurse's Drug Alert*, use of in-line final filters decreases phlebitis by 66%.

Treatment

Apply hot or cold compresses to the affected site. Cold significantly decreases intradermal skin toxicity for 45 minutes (Rudolph & Larson, 1987).
   A physician must be notified for 3+ phlebitis.

Documentation

Documentation is critical when phlebitis has been detected. Document the site assessment, the phlebitis rating (1+, 2+, or 3+), whether the physician was notified, and the treatment used.

Thrombophlebitis

Thrombophlebitis denotes a twofold injury: thrombosis and inflammation. A painful inflamed vein promptly develops from the point of thrombosis. Signs and symptoms of thrombophlebitis are sluggish flow rate, edema in the limb, tender and cordlike vein, site warm to touch, and a visible red line above venipuncture site.
   Thrombophlebitis causes the patient unnecessary discomfort (Weinstein, 1993). Chemical or mechanical phlebitis can also precipitate a thrombophlebitis.

✎ **NOTE:** If the inflammation is the result of bacterial phlebitis, a much more serious condition leading to septicemia may develop if not treated.

Prevention

Techniques to prevent thrombophlebitis include:

1. Use veins in forearm rather than in hands when infusing any medication.
2. Do not use veins in joint flexion areas.

280

3. Check the infusion site at least every 4 hours in an adult and every 2 hours in a pediatric patient for signs and symptoms of redness, swelling, or pain at the site.
4. Anchor the cannula securely to prevent mobility of catheter tip.
5. Infuse solutions at prescribed rate. Do not attempt to catch up on delayed infusion time.
6. Use the smallest size catheter that meets needs of the patient.
7. Dilute irritating medications.

Septic thrombophlebitis can be prevented with:

1. Appropriate skin preparation
2. Aseptic technique in maintenance of infusion
3. *Good handwashing*

✎ **NOTE:** Thrombophlebitis can lead to a potential embolism owing to the thrombus formation in the vein wall.

Treatment

Remove entire I.V. catheter and restart with fresh equipment in opposite extremity.
Notify the physician.
Apply warm, moist compresses for 20 minutes to provide comfort.

✎ **NOTE:** You must discontinue the infusion and restart the infusion to prevent progression of thrombophlebitis.

Documentation

Document all observable symptoms and patient's subjective complaints such as "feels tender to touch, hurts." State your actions to resolve the problem and the time at which you notified the physician. State the site in which you restarted I.V. therapy.

Infiltration

Infiltration is the seepage of a nonvesicant solution or medication into surrounding tissue. Infiltration occurs from the dislodgment of the cannula from the intima of a vein. It can also occur from phlebitis, causing the vein to become threadlike when the lumen along the cannula shaft narrows, so that fluid leaks from the site where the cannula enters the vein wall (Hecker, 1988). Infiltration is second to phlebitis as a cause of I.V. therapy morbidity (Lewis & Hecker, 1991).

Signs and symptoms of infiltration are:

- Coolness of skin around site
- Taut skin
- Dependent edema
- Backflow of blood absent
- A "pinkish" blood return
- Infusion rate slowing but continuing to infuse

Assessment of Site

Checking for a blood return, or backflow of blood, is not a reliable method of determining patency of a cannula. A blood return may be present when small veins are used, because they may not permit blood flow around the cannula. Use of veins that

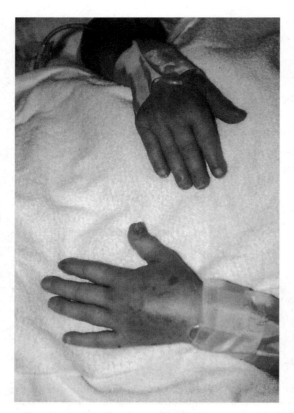

Figure 9–3. Infiltration and swelling below the I.V. site because of hands underneath patient during turning. Occlusion or restriction of blood flow caused fluid to back up in the vessels, resulting in infiltration and dependent edema below the I.V. site rather than above. (Courtesy of Beth Fabian, CRNI Veterans Administration Medical Center, Ann Arbor, Michigan.)

have had previous punctures or veins that are very fragile may seep fluid at the site above or below the vein cannula entry point; a blood return may be present, yet an infiltration is occurring (Fig. 9–3). The most accurate method of checking for infiltration is assessment of the site: With infusion running, apply pressure 3 inches above the catheter site in front of the catheter tip. If infusion continues to run, suspect infiltration. When the vein is compressed and the catheter is in proper alignment in the vein, the I.V. solution will stop owing to occlusion. Also, compare both arms when assessing for infiltration (Fig. 9–4).

✎ **NOTE:** The immobilized patient or the patient with muscular weakness or paralysis of an extremity may have edema of an extremity that is not related to infiltration of an I.V. site. Accurate assessment of the cannula and infusion site is the key to differentiation (Millam, 1988).

Extravasation

Extravasation refers to infiltration of a vesicant medication. A vesicant solution is a fluid or medication that causes the formation of blisters, with subsequent sloughing of tissues occurring from the tissue necrosis (Tabor, 1993) (Figs. 9–5 and 9–6). Some patients have a high risk for extravasation injury (Table 9–6).

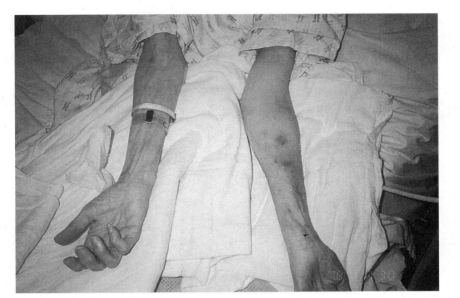

Figure 9–4. Infiltration. Compare both arms when assessing for infiltration (note left arm is swollen compared with right).

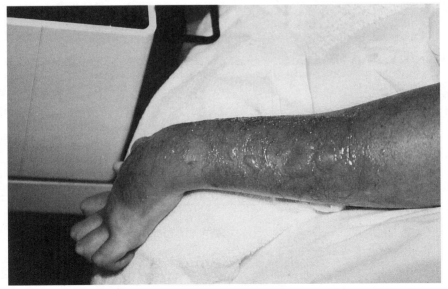

Figure 9–5. Infiltration of vancomycin into subcutaneous tissue, causing blistering of skin. (Courtesy of Beth Fabian, CRNI Veterans Administration Medical Center, Ann Arbor, Michigan.)

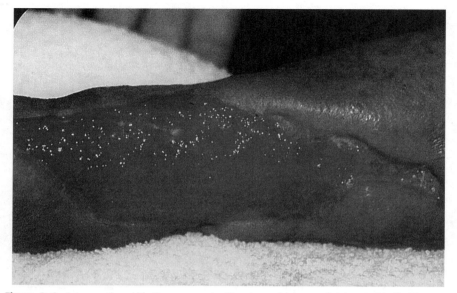

Figure 9–6. Extravasation with tissue necrosis. (Courtesy of Johnson & Johnson Medical Inc., Arlington, Texas.)

Sign and symptoms of extravasation include:

- Complaints of pain or burning
- Skin tightness at venipuncture site
- Blanching and coolness of skin
- Slow or stopped infusion
- Dependent edema of affected extremity

✎ **NOTE:** Never increase the flow rate to determine the infiltration of a vesicant. Checking for blood return is not a reliable method of determining an infiltration (Perdue, 1995).

TABLE 9–6. **FACTORS AFFECTING RISK FOR EXTRAVASATION INJURY**

Age
    Neonate
    Geriatric patient

Condition
    Oncology patient
    Comatose patient
    Anesthetized patient
    Patients with peripheral or cardiovascular disease
    Diabetic patient

Equipment
    High-pressure infusion pumps

The severity of damage is directly related to the type, concentration, and volume of fluid infiltrated into the interstitial tissues. The endothelium is particularly sensitive to pH and osmolarity differences found in physiologic and nonphysiologic solutions. These fluids may induce cellular injury through irritation, stimulating the inflammatory process. The damaged tissues release precipitating proteins with an increase in capillary permeability, which allows fluid and protein shifts to interstitial space. Edema, ischemia, vasoconstriction, pain, and erythema are responses to these cellular changes and may lead to tissue necrosis (Hastings-Tolsma, Yucha, Tompkins, Robson, & Szeverenyi, 1993).

The most harmful vesicant medications are antineoplastic agents (doxorubicin [Adriamycin] causing the most severe tissue necrosis), dopamine hydrochloride (Dopastat, Intropin), norephinephrine (levarterenol bitartrate, Levophed), potassium chloride in high doses, amphotericin B (Fungizone), calcium, and sodium bicarbonate in high concentrations.

Prevention

To prevent infiltration or extravasation, follow these 11 rules of proper technique:

1. Choose veins that avoid the dorsum of the hand, wrist, and digits. Avoid the median basilic vein above the elbow, which is too close to artery and nerves.
2. Avoid the antecubital area.
3. Avoid areas of multiple venipunctures.
4. Apply armboard or restraints to prevent excessive movement.
5. Dilute all medications as indicated in the literature.
6. Secure the cannula so that the site is visible.
7. Avoid the use of high-pressure infusion pumps when administering highly vesicant drugs. Pumps continue infusing solutions when infiltration is present until occlusion pressure is reached and an alarm goes off. (Older pumps have a higher pressure, usually greater than 20 pounds [Millam, 1988].)
8. Only qualified registered nurses who have been trained in venipuncture and drug administration skills and who have knowledge of medications with vesicant potential should be allowed to administer a vesicant fluid or medication.
9. Check for patency before flushing with sodium chloride solutions.
10. Monitor the I.V. site routinely for edema.
11. Educate the patient to report any feelings of burning (Ford, 1990).

✎ **NOTE:** Restraints must be applied with extreme caution and within the guidelines established by Joint Commission on Accreditation of Healthcare Organizations (JCAHO) and by the Food and Drug Administration (FDA). Immobilization devices should be well padded and applied so that they do not cause nerve damage, constrict circulation, or cause pressure areas; they should be removed at frequent intervals, and nurse-assisted range-of-motion exercises should be performed. Inadequate or improper use of immobilization devices can cause very serious complications; policies and procedures should be established to guide their use (JCAHO, 1995; FDA, 1992).

Treatment

To treat infiltration, discontinue the infusion, elevate the extremity, and apply warm compresses to aid in the resolution of infiltrated fluid (Hastings-Tolsma, Yucha,

285

Tompkins, Robson, & Szevernyi, 1993). The most effective treatment for extravasation is prevention. However, if extravasation is suspected:

1. Stop I.V. flow and leave cannula in place until after any residual medication and blood are aspirated and an antidote particular to the vesicant is instilled into the tissues.
2. Administer prescribed antidote (this cannot be delayed).
3. Remove the cannula.
4. Photograph the suspected area of extravasation according to institutional policy.
5. Apply warm or cold compresses as indicated for the specific agent extravasated.
6. Elevate the arm.
7. Notify the physician (request a plastic surgery consultation if a vesicant drug has infiltrated (Tipton & Skeel, 1995).

Documentation

It is important to document the following when extravasation occurs:

- Date, time, cannula type, and size
- Insertion site: location and description
- Number and location of previous venipuncture attempts
- Any difficulty in previous venipuncture
- Drugs (in order of administration)
- Any difficulty in drug administration
- Symptoms reported by patient
- Nursing interventions and patient's response
- Time physician was notified and name of physician
- Follow-up instructions given to patient (orally and in written form)
- Date of scheduled return visit for follow-up evaluation
- Photos of the insertion site and entire extremity (Wood & Gullo, 1993)

✎ NOTE: Soft tissue damage from extravasation can lead to prolonged healing, potential infections, necrosis, multiple debridment surgeries, cosmetic disfiguration, loss of limb function, and amputation.

Antidotes

Antidotes (Table 9–7) for extravasation injury fall into four categories: (1) those that alter local pH, (2) those that alter DNA binding, (3) those that chemically neutralize, and (4) those that dilute extravasated drug (Ford, 1990).

If you are going to instill an antidote, do so through the existing I.V. catheter. Or, use a 1-mL tuberculin syringe, injecting small amounts subcutaneously in a circle around the infiltrated area.

✎ NOTE: If you work with high-risk patients a copy of Table 9–7 could be posted in the medication area for quick reference.

Local Infection

The 1962 edition of American Hospital Association's *Control of Infections in Hospitals*, provides no mention that infections due to I.V. therapy may be hazardous (Lenox,

TABLE 9–7. ANTIDOTES FOR EXTRAVASATED DRUGS

Extravasated Drug	Antidote (Dose)	Nursing Tips	Side Effect of Antidote
Protein Enzyme			

Calcium solutions
Contrast media
20%, 50% dextrose
Nafcillin
Hyperalimentation
  solutions
Potassium solutions
Vinblastine (Velban)
Vincristine (Oncovin)
Vindestine (Eldisine)
	Hyaluronidase (Wydase), 15
	  U/mL 0.2 mL × 5
	  subcutaneously
		Use 27- to 25-gauge needle.
		Use moist *warm* compresses
		  and elevate the extremity.
			Rash, urticaria (10%)

Adrenergic Blocker			

Dobutamine
  (Dobutrex)
Dopamine (Dopastat)
Epinephrine
Metaraminol biturate
  (Aramine)
Norepinephrine
	Phentolamine hydrochloride
	  (Regitine), 5–10 mg
	  subcutaneously diluted in
	  10–15 mL of sodium
	  chloride.
		Treatment must start
		  immediately with this
		  group of vesicants. Use
		  warm compresses.
			Cardiovascular:
			  hypotension,
			  tachycardia, flushing
			Gastrointestinal:
			  nausea and
			  vomiting

Alkalization Agent			

Mechlorethamine
(Nitrogen Mustard)
Sodium
  nitroprusside
  (Nipride)
	Sodium thiosulfate
	Dilute 4 mL with 6 mL *sterile*
	  water for injection.
	Administer 10 mL I.V. push
	  over 10 min.
		Use *ice* compresses.	Rash, hypersensitivity

Glucocorticoid Steroid			

Doxorubicin
  (Adriamycin)
Vincristine (Oncovin)
Daunorubicin
  (Cerubidine)
Dacarbazine (DTIC)
Dactinomycin
  (Actinomycin)
Plicamycin
  (Mithracin)
	Hydrocortisone sodium
	  succinate, 100 mg/mL.
	Give 25–50 mg/mL of
	  extravasate.
	Dexamethasone, long-
	  acting is also used.
		After long-acting steroid
		  given, apply 1% topical
		  hydrocortisone cream. Use
		  cool moist compresses.
			Delayed wound
			  healing, various skin
			  eruptions

1990). I.V.-related infections consist of those related to microbial contamination of the cannula or infusate. Cannula contamination is the most common source of local infections. Local infections are preventable by maintaining aseptic technique and following guidelines established by the INS or CDC for duration of infusion, length of time of catheter placement, and tubing change criteria. Local infections are difficult to control in the immunosuppressive patient.

Signs and symptoms of local infection include:

- Redness and swelling at the site
- Possible exudate of purulent material
- Increased white blood cells
- Elevated temperature (chills are not associated with local infection)

The ways in which a catheter tip may acquire bacteria are:

During introduction of venipuncture
During removal of stylet
From colonization from skin
From contaminated I.V. solutions
From air inlet filter malfunction
From microorganisms entering system at catheter or administration set junction.

Prevention

Techniques to prevent local infections include:

1. Inspect all solution containers for cracks and leaks before hanging.
2. Change solution containers every 24 hours.
3. Maintain aseptic technique during cannula insertion, I.V. therapy, and catheter removal (Perdue, 1995).

Risk of local infection is affected by choice and preparation of site. The venipuncture site should be scrubbed with 70% alcohol to remove blood or dirt, which can interfere with disinfectant prepping solution. Then, a 20-second circular preparation with 1–2% tincture of iodine, iodophor; 70% isopropyl alcohol or chlorhexidine, allowing the site to dry has excellent bactericidal activity. If the patient is allergic to iodine, use 70% alcohol for a 1-minute *vigorous* scrub. I.V. cannulas contaminated during time of insertion by microorganism on the hands of hospital personnel contribute significantly to local infections. Washing hands with soap and water with mechanical friction for at least 15 seconds removes most transient acquired bacteria (Wenzel, 1993).

✎ **NOTE:** Thrombus formation appears to be related to the presence of microorganisms on a catheter tip (Stratton, 1982). Presence of phlebitis connotes an 18-fold increased risk of sepsis compared with absence of phlebitis (Jemison-Smith & Thrupp, 1982).

See Chapter 6 for further information on infections at cannula site.

Documentation

Document assessment of site, culture technique, and sources of culture, notification of physician, and any treatment initiated. Culture techniques are discussed in Chapter 6.

Venous Spasm

Venous spasm can occur suddenly and for a variety of reasons. The spasm usually results from the administration of a cold infusate, an irritating solution, or a too-rapid administration of I.V. solution or viscous solution such as a blood product.

Signs and symptoms of venous spasms include (1) sharp pain at I.V. site traveling up the arm, caused by a piercing stream of fluid that irritates or shocks the vein wall and (2) slowing of infusion.

Prevention

Techniques to prevent vasospasm include:

1. Dilute medication additive adequately.
2. Keep I.V. solution at room temperature.
3. Wrap extremity with warm compresses during infusion.
4. Administrative solution at prescribed rate.

✎ **NOTE:** If a rapid infusion rate is desired, use a larger cannula.

Treatment

1. Apply warm compresses to warm the extremity and decrease flow rate until spasm subsides.
2. Restart the I.V. if venospasm continues.

Documentation

Document patient complaints, duration of complaints, treatment, and length of time to resolve the problem. Document whether the I.V. site needed to be rotated to resolve the problem.

KEY TIPS—PREVENT LOCAL COMPLICATIONS

1. Maintain INS guidelines on tubing change, cannula change, and length of time IV solutions remain hanging.
2. Follow aseptic technique in skin preparation and venipuncture techniques.
3. *Wash hands*.
4. Choose appropriate dressing.
5. Secure tubing and cannula with good taping technique.
6. Use 0.22-micron in-line filter as extra safeguard.
7. Keep solutions at prescribed rate.
8. Document observed I.V. site every 4 hours for adults and every 2 hours for infants and children.

289

SUMMARY WORKSHEET 1: Local Complications

Complication	Signs and Symptoms	Treatment
Hematoma		
Thrombosis		
Phlebitis		
Thrombophlebitis		
Infiltration		
Extravasation		
Local infection		
Venous spasm		

SYSTEMIC COMPLICATIONS

Systemic complications can be life-threatening. Such complications include septicemia, circulatory overload, pulmonary edema, air embolus, speed shock, and catheter embolus.

Septicemia

In 1986, approximately 70% of the 40 million patients hospitalized in the United States received some form of infusion therapy. This therapy was assumed to be responsible for 50,000 to 100,000 cases of septicemia nationwide each year (Maki, 1990). Neither the intravascular device nor the infusate are cultured in most of these infections; consequently, the source remains unknown. Septicemia can occur when microorganisms migrate into the bloodstream. The nurse must be aware of risk factors, prevention techniques, and the presence of an infected catheter tip because bacteremia, fungemia, or septicemia could occur.

Septicemia is related to poor aseptic techniques and contaminated equipment during manufacturing and storage or use. In addition, peripheral I.V. infusions are contaminated less frequently than infusions used for central venous access or total parenteral nutrition. Infusions to intensive care unit (ICU) patients with both peripheral and central venous lines are more frequently contaminated than infusions to patients on medical-surgical units (Maki & Ringer, 1991). Factors that increase the risk of septicemia are presented in Table 9–8. Irrigation of clogged I.V. catheters can propel a clot, which is a high source of bacterial contamination, into the systemic circulation. Organism growth can lead to overwhelming infection, which in turn leads to hypotension, vascular collapse, shock, and death.

TABLE 9–8. **RISK FACTORS ASSOCIATED WITH SEPTICEMIA**

Patient Susceptibility
    Age
    Alteration in host defense
    Underlying illness
    Presence of other infectious processes

Infusion-Related Sources
    Solution container
    Stopcocks
    Catheter material and structure
    Insertion site
    Hematogenous seeding
    Manipulation of infusion system
    Certain transparent dressings
    Duration of cannulation

Source: From Maki, D.G., & Ringer, M. (1991). Risk factors for infusion-related phlebitis with small peripheral venous catheters. *Annals of Internal Medicine, 114,* 845–854.

Signs and symptoms of septicemia include:

- Fluctuating fever—tremors, chattering teeth
- Profuse cold sweat
- Nausea and vomiting
- Diarrhea—sudden and explosive
- Abdominal pain
- Tachycardia

See Chapter 6, Table 6-5 for a list of microbial pathogens associated with intra-vascular line-related infections.

Prevention

Techniques to prevent septicemia include:

1. Good handwashing! Handwashing and sterile technique are imperative to minimize the risk of technique-induced septicemia.
2. Carefully inspect solutions for abnormal cloudiness, cracks, and pinholes.
3. Use only freshly opened solutions.
4. Protein solutions, such as albumin and protein hydrolysates, should be used as soon as the seal is broken.
5. Use iodine-containing antiseptics (rather than alcohol-containing antiseptics), which have a superior spectrum of antimicrobial activity. It is inexpensive, well tolerated, and highly reliable.
6. Use the smallest needle possible for accessing an injection port, such as a 25- to 20-gauge needle that does not exceed 1 in. in length.
7. Use Luer-lock connections when possible.
8. Cover infusion sites with a sterile dressing.
9. Tape cannulas to prevent an in-and-out movement.
10. Limit use of add-on devices.
11. Inspect the site and assess the patient routinely to ensure early recognition of symptoms.
12. Change peripheral cannulas according to Intravenous Nursing Standards of Practice.

✎ **NOTE:** The key to prevention of septicemia is staff education.

Treatment

It is sometimes difficult to identify infusion-associated sepsis from septicemia of other causes, unless associated with phlebitis (Maki, 1992). Steps in treating suspected septicemia based on patient signs and symptoms are:

1. Notify physician.
2. Restart new I.V. system in opposite extremity.
3. Obtain cultures from:
   Administration set
   Container
   Catheter tip
   Site
   Blood
4. Initiate antimicrobial therapy as ordered.
5. Monitor the patient closely.
6. Determine whether the patient's condition requires transfer to ICU.

Documentation

Document the signs and symptoms assessed, the time you notified the physician, and all treatments instituted. Document the time of transfer to ICU, the time the new I.V. system was inserted, and how the patient is tolerating interventions.

✎ **NOTE:** Fluids temporarily discontinued to administer blood components should be discarded and fresh solutions restarted after transfusion is terminated.

Circulatory Overload

Circulatory overload is caused by infusing excessive amounts of sodium chloride solution too rapidly, failure to monitor the I.V. infusion, or too rapid of an infusion of any fluid in a patient compromised by cardiopulmonary or renal disease.

Signs and symptoms of circulatory overload include:

- Weight gain
- Edema
- Puffy eyelids
- Hypertension
- Wide variance between intake and output
- Rise in central venous pressure (CVP)
- Shortness of breath and rales (crackles)
- Distended neck veins

Prevention

Techniques to prevent circulatory overload include:

1. Monitor the infusion, especially sodium chloride, and know the solution's physiologic effects on the circulatory system.
2. Maintain flow at prescribed rate.
3. Do not "catch up" on I.V. solutions that are behind schedule.
4. Monitor intake and output on all patients receiving I.V. fluids.
5. Know the patient's cardiovascular history.

Treatment

Notify the physician if you suspect circulatory overload.

1. Decrease I.V. flow rate.
2. Raise the head of the bed.
3. Keep the patient warm to promote peripheral circulation.
4. Monitor vital signs.
5. Administer oxygen as ordered.

Documentation

Document patient assessment, notification of physician, and treatments instituted by physician order. Monitor the patient and record vital signs on an interval flow sheet.

Pulmonary Edema

Circulatory overload can lead to pulmonary edema. Fluids too rapidly infused increase venous pressure and lead to pulmonary edema. Pulmonary edema is an ab-

293

normal accumulation of fluid in the lungs. In pulmonary edema, fluid leaks through the capillary wall and fills the interstitium and alveoli. "The pulmonary vascular bed has received more blood from the right ventricle than the left can accommodate and remove. The slightest imbalance between inflow on the right side and outflow on the left side may have drastic consequences" (Smeltzer & Bare, 1992). Patients at risk for pulmonary edema are patients with cardiovascular disease, patients with renal disease and the elderly. It is important to identify patients at risk for pulmonary edema and provide nursing care that decreases the heart's workload. Sodium chloride given to correct profound sodium deficits can lead to pulmonary overload and must be monitored closely (Metheny, 1996).

Initial signs and symptoms of pulmonary edema include:

- Restlessness
- Slow increase in pulse rate
- Headache
- Shortness of breath
- Cough
- Flushing

As fluid builds in the pulmonary bed, later signs and symptoms include hypertension, severe dyspnea, gurgling respirations, coughing up frothy fluid, and moist crackles.

Prevention

Techniques to prevent pulmonary edema include:

1. Obtain a baseline assessment before starting I.V. therapy.
2. Review history of cardiac or respiratory problems before starting I.V. therapy.
3. Maintain consistent infusion rate.
4. Monitor lung sounds for crackles.

Treatment

Notify the physician if you suspect pulmonary edema. Treatment is the same as for circulatory overload.

Documentation

Document patient assessment, notification of physician and treatments that are instituted by physician order. Monitor the patient and record vital signs on an interval flow sheet.

Air Embolism

Air embolism is a rare but lethal complication, especially involving vascular access devices (VAD). The problem is treatable with prompt recognition, but prevention is the key. The pathophysiologic consequences of air emboli are a result of air entering the central veins, which is quickly trapped in the blood as it flows forward. Trapped air is carried to the right ventricle, where it lodges against the pulmonary valve and blocks the flow of blood from the ventricle into the pulmonary arteries (Richardson & Bruso, 1993). Less blood is ejected from the right ventricle, and the right heart overfills. The force of right ventricular contractions increases in an attempt to eject blood past the occluding air pocket. These forceful contractions break small air bubbles loose from the air pocket. Minute air bubbles are subsequently pumped into the pulmonary circulation, causing even greater obstruction to the forward flow of blood as well as local pulmonary tissue hypoxia. Pulmonary hypoxia results in vasocon-striction in the lung tissue, which further increases the workload of the right ventricle and reduces blood flow out of the right heart. This leads to diminished cardiac output, shock, and death (Lambert, 1982).

The same intrathoracic pressure changes that allow for pulmonary ventilation are responsible for air emboli associated with subclavian line removal. Pressure in the central veins decreases during inspiration and increases during expiration. If an opening into a central vein exposes the vessel to the atmosphere during the negative inspiratory cycle, air can be sucked into the central venous system in much the same manner that air is pulled into the lungs (Thielen & Nyquist, 1991). The causes of air embolism include:

Allowing the solution container to run dry
Infusing air in tubing, which gets infused into the patient
Loose connections allowing air to enter the system
Poor technique in dressing and tubing changes for central lines

Initial signs and symptoms of air embolism include:

- Patient complaints of palpitations, light-headedness, and weakness
- Pulmonary findings: dyspnea, cyanosis, tachypnea, expiratory wheezes, cough, and pulmonary edema
- Cardiovascular findings: "mill wheel" murmur, weak thready pulse, tachy-cardia, substernal chest pain, hypotension, and jugular venous distention
- Neurologic findings: Change in mental status, confusion, coma, anxiousness, and seizures

If untreated, these signs and symptoms lead to hemiplegia, aphasia, generalized sei-zures, coma, and cardiac arrest.

Prevention

Techniques to prevent air embolism include:

1. Wrap tubing around a pencil to force air bubbles upward into drip chamber infusing.
2. Use a clamp on the patient side of an injection port if removal of air by a needle is used at the injection port (Table 9–9 and Fig. 9–7).
3. Use a 0.22-micron air eliminating filter.
4. Tape all connectors, especially on central lines.
5. Follow protocol for dressing and tubing changes of central lines.
6. Superimpose I.V. solutions before the previous solution runs completely dry.
7. Attach piggyback medications to high injection port, so that check valve will prevent air from being drawn into the line after the infusion of medication.
8. Use Luer-lock connectors whenever possible.
9. *Do not* bypass "pump housing" of electric volumetric pump.

TABLE 9–9. REMOVAL OF AIR FROM PRIMARY SET

Steps
1. Clamp tubing to patient, distally to the lowest medicinal entry port. (prevents air from entering patient).
2. Swab medicinal port with alcohol.
3. Insert 20-gauge 1-in needle without syringe into medicinal entry. This will vent all air out of primary line.
4. When all air has been removed, remove needle; then unclamp.

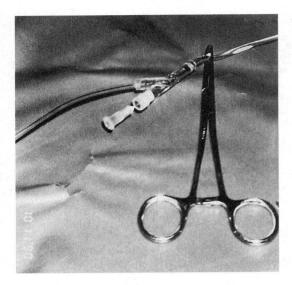

Figure 9–7. Removal of air from primary set.

Treatment

If you suspect an air embolus, do the following:

1. Call for help.
2. Place patient in Trendelenburg's position on left side (left lateral decubitus position), head down. This causes the air to rise in the right atrium, preventing it from entering the pulmonary artery.
3. Administer oxygen.
4. Monitor vital signs.
5. Have emergency equipment available.
6. Notify physician immediately.

✎ **NOTE:** A pathognomonic indicator of an air embolism is a loud, churning, drum-like sound audible over the precordium, called a *mill wheel murmur*. This symptom may be absent or transient (O'Quin & Lakshminaayan, 1982).

Documentation

Document patient assessment, nursing interventions to correct the cause of embolism if apparent, notification of physician, and treatment. If emergency treatment was necessary use an interval flow sheet to document management of the air embolism, record interval vital signs, and indicate patient response.

Speed Shock

Speed shock occurs when a foreign substance, usually a medication, is rapidly introduced into the circulation. Rapid injection permits the concentration of medication in the plasma to reach toxic proportions, flooding the organs rich in blood—the heart and the brain. Syncope, shock, and cardiac arrest may result.

Signs and symptoms of speed shock include dizziness, facial flushing, headache, tightness in the chest, and hypotension, irregular pulse, and progression of shock.

Prevention

Techniques to prevent speed shock include:

1. Reduce the size of drops by using microdrop sets for medication delivery.
2. Use an electronic flow control with high-risk drugs.
3. Monitor the infusion rate for accuracy before piggybacking in the medication.
4. Be careful not to manipulate the catheter; cannula movement may speed up flow rate.

✎ **NOTE:** Prevention of speed shock is the key. When giving I.V. push drugs, give *slowly* and according to manufacturer's recommendations.

Treatment

If you suspect speed shock, do the following:

1. Get help.
2. Give antidote or resuscitation medications as needed.
3. If giving I.V. narcotics have naloxone (Narcan) available on the unit.

✎ **NOTE:** See Chapter 11 for steps in delivery of I.V. push medications.

Documentation

Document the medication or fluid administered and the signs and symptoms that the patient reported and those assessed. Document that the physician was notified and the treatment initiated, and the patient response.

Catheter Embolism

Catheter embolism is an infrequent systemic complication of over-the-needle catheters. In this situation, a piece of the catheter breaks off and travels through the vascular system. It may migrate to the chest and lodge in the pulmonary artery or the right ventricle.

Signs and symptoms include sharp sudden pain at I.V. site, minimal blood return, short, rough, and uneven catheter noted on removal, cyanosis, chest pain, tachycardia, and hypotension.

Pulmonary embolism, cardiac dysrythmia, sepsis, endocarditis, thrombosis, and death may result if the catheter embolism migrates to the chest and lodges in the pulmonary artery or the right ventricle (Feldstein, 1986).

Prevention

Techniques to prevent catheter embolism include:

1. Never reinsert a needle in a catheter (over-the-needle) after removal.
2. Avoid inserting the catheter over joint flexion where movement causes catheter to bend back and forth.
3. Splint arm if the patient is restless.
4. Do not apply pressure over site while removing a catheter.

✎ **NOTE:** Always use radiopaque catheters, so that the catheter will be detectable on x-ray.

Treatment

Have the patient apply digital pressure on the vein above the insertion site if the patient is cooperative. This may prevent the catheter from migrating. Other techniques include:

1. Apply tourniquet above the elbow.
2. Contact physician and radiologist.
3. Start a new I.V. line.
4. Prepare patient for x-ray examination.
5. Measure remainder of the catheter tip to determine the length of the embolized tip.

✎ **NOTE:** Be sure to assess circulation of extremity while tourniquet is on the arm.

Documentation

Document the patient's subjective complaints in quotes. Document discontinuation of catheter, technique, and length of catheter removed. State the nursing interventions and the time the physician was notified.

SUMMARY WORKSHEET 2: Systemic Complications

Complication	Signs and Symptoms	Treatment
Septicemia		
Circulatory Overload		
Pulmonary Edema		
Air Embolism		
Speed Shock		
Catheter Embolism		

ERRATIC FLOW RATES

Free-flow incidents are common occurrences in delivery of infusion therapy according to a survey. In this survey of more than 400 nurses, 42% knew of free-flow incidents at their institutions (Cohen, 1993).

There are many factors to consider in determining flow rate (Table 9–10). These include body size, fluid type, patient's age and condition, physiologic responses as reflected by urinary output, pulmonary status, and specific drugs being infused. The very young and the very old often need a slower rate of infusion and small volumes of solution (ECRI, 1992). Patients with cardiac or renal disease may also have problems tolerating large fluid volumes or fast rates. Situations in which flow rates have been poorly regulated can have serious consequences, especially with I.V. solutions containing medications such as: epinephrine, theophylline, meperidine, lidocaine, sodium bicarbonate, amphotericin B, potassium chloride magnesium, and heparin (Cohen 1993). Accurate flow rate is imperative when a drug level must be kept constant. If the rate is too *slow:*

- The patient is not receiving the desired amount of drug or solution.
- A too-slow rate can lead to clogged I.V. needle or catheter and perhaps the loss of a premium vein.

If the rate is too *fast:*

- Hypotonic solutions can lead to pulmonary edema or congestive heart failure.
- Rapid infusion of hypertonic glucose can result in osmotic diuresis, leading to dehydration.
- Hypertonic solutions are also irritating and phlebitis can result.
- Free-flow administration of drugs cause serious cardiovascular and respiratory complications

✎ **NOTE:** A fast rate is considered more dangerous than a rate that is too slow.

Prevention

Prevention of erratic flow rates and the complications they cause include:

1. Only experienced nurses should set up, adjust, or remove I.V. administration sets.
2. Use pumps that provide free-flow protection; check with each manufacturer.
3. Properly close clamps if removing administration set from pump.

TABLE 9–10. **FACTORS IN FLOW-RATE CONTROL**

Patient-Related	*Vein-Related*
Patient or family intervention	Infiltration
Patient blood pressure	Phlebitis
	Venous spasm
Tubing-Related	
"Cold flow" of plastic tubing	*Clot formation*
Drop formation rate	*needle or catheter position*
Final in-filters kinked or pinched tubing	
Rate of fluid flow	*Other*
Slipping of roller clamp	Height of I.V. standard
Electronic infusion device malfunction	Bed position

Source: Adapted from Steele, J. (1983). Too fast or too slow: The erratic I.V. *American Journal of Nursing, 6,* 898–900, with permission.

4. Check or recalculate infusion rates.
5. Provide or attend staff development education on electronic infusion devices.
6. Report all free-flow incidents.

Treatment

Treatment techniques for erratic flow rates include the following: (1) stop flow and recalculate; (2) treat the patient symptomatically; and (3) notify the physician. In addition, notify product evaluation committee or central services if cause of erratic flow is an electronic infusion device.

Nursing Plan of Care

PREVENTION OF COMPLICATIONS

Focus Criteria for Assessment

Subjective	*Objective*
Patient reports signs and symptoms of discomfort the I.V. site.	Assess cardiac and renal function.
Evaluate for anxiety or fear.	Assess for age-related risks.
Assess intake and output ratios	Determine baseline weight.
	Assess vital signs.
	Inspect skin for integrity.

Nursing Diagnosis
1. Anxiety (mild, moderate, severe) related to threat to or change in health status; misconceptions regarding therapy
2. Altered tissue perfusion (peripheral) related to infiltration of fluid or medication
3. Decreased cardiac output related to sepsis contamination; infusion of isotonic or hypertonic fluids
4. Fear related to insertion of catheter; fear of "needles."
5. Hyperthermia related to increased metabolic rate; illness; dehydration
6. Impaired gas exchange related to ventilation-perfusion imbalance; embolism
7. Impaired skin integrity related to I.V. catheter; irritating I.V. fluids, inflammation; infection; infiltration
8. Impaired tissue integrity related to altered circulation; fluid deficit or excess; irritating I.V. fluids; inflammation; infection; infiltration
9. Impaired physical mobility related to pain or discomfort resulting from placement and maintenance of I.V. infusion
10. Alteration in comfort, pain, related to physical trauma (e.g., catheter insertion)
11. Risk of infection related to broken skin or traumatized tissue

Patient Outcome Criteria
The patient will:
Express fears related to infusion therapy.
Remain free of complications related to the administration of I.V. therapy.
Report any changes in comfort of I.V. site.
Demonstrate care in maintaining the I.V. system.

Nursing Management: Critical Activities
Maintain strict aseptic technique.
Examine the solution for type, amount, expiration date, character of the fluid, and lack of damage to container.

Continued on following page

> **Nursing Management: Critical Activities**
> Select and prepare an electronic infusion device as indicated.
> Administer fluids at room temperature.
> Administer I.V. medications at prescribed rate and monitor for results.
> Monitor intravenous flow rate and site during infusion.
> Replace I.V. cannula, administration set, and dressing every 48–72 hours.
> Maintain occlusive dressing.
> Perform I.V. site checks and document at regular intervals.
> Limit intravenous potassium to 20 mEq per hour or 200 mEq per 24 hours as appropriate.
> Record intake and output.
> Use serial weight to assess for fluid overload.
> Tape cannula sites securely to prevent movement (McCloskey & Bulechek, 1992).

PATIENT EDUCATION

Instruct to perform routine activities—bathing, movement in bed, and ambulation to maintain I.V. system.

Instruct to report any signs or symptoms of common local complications, (e.g., redness, swelling, pain at site).

Instruct to report any interruption in flow rate.

Instruct on purpose of electronic infusion device.

HOME CARE ISSUES

Same as for Patient Education.

The new JCAHO standards address the broad range of home health care services: P.L. 100-203 establishes mandates affecting the home health industry.

Establish home health hotlines in each state.

Place more emphasis on client outcomes.

Document questions about complaints.

Develop, maintain, and update a database containing the results of each agency's certification and survey.

The home care practitioner must be aware of the potential danger that exists in I.V. drug administration and must be able to handle emergency situations. Adverse reactions, such as drowsiness, dizziness, nausea, and diarrhea, as well as local and systemic complications, can occur with delivery of medications in the home setting.

Allergic reactions from hypersensitivity to a specific antigen can also occur. An emergency kit, including epinephrine, dipenhydramine (Benadryl), and dexamethasone (Decadron) or hydrocortisone (Solu-Cortef) should be available to the clinician delivering medication in the home setting. The emergency kit should also include an airway, unused tubing, and additional catheters in the event that a new I.V. access must be established (Moser, 1991).

Potential problems and complications encountered in home infusion therapy include:

Mechanical problems
  Nonrunning I.V. line
  Inability to flush line
  Electronic infusion device alarms
Local complications
  Redness or swelling at site
  Pain along cannulated vein
  Difficulty flushing line

Systemic complications
    Signs and symptoms associated with fluid overload, sepsis
    Allergic reactions
Provide the patient or caregiver education on aseptic technique and the importance of handwashing prior to working with I.V. equipment.
Documentation
    Nursing assessments at each visit specific to signs and symptoms of local or systemic complications
    Assessment of presence of adverse drug reactions
    Self-care education relating to reporting signs and symptoms of complications
    Care provided directly by nurse

COMPETENCY CRITERIA: Prevention of Complications of I.V. Therapy

Competency Statement: The competent I.V. therapy nurse will be able to: Assess for complications associated with I.V. therapy.

PERFORMANCE CRITERIA

	Skilled	Needs Education
1. Demonstrates aseptic technique when performing venipuncture, maintaining infusion, or performing flush procedure:		
Scrubs 15–20 seconds		
Uses no-touch technique		
Maintains sterility of equipment		
2. Documents appropriate assessments of site.		
3. Describes insertion site assessments:		
Erythema		
Palpable cord		
Purulent drainage		
Emergency cannulations replaced within 24 hours		
4. Recognizes signs and symptoms of complications of peripheral line placement:		
Phlebitis		
Postinfusion phlebitis		
Infiltration		
Extravasation		
Infection/septicemia		
5. Checks route, indications, side effects, adverse reactions of medication delivery:		
Vesicant/nonvesicant		
6. Inspects fluids and equipment for abnormalities, radiopaque catheter compatibility, extrinsic/intrinsic contamination.		

SUGGESTED EVALUATION CRITERIA

Documentation by nurse of site assessments, care of infusion

Observation of maintenance of good aseptic technique

Written test on complications associated with infusion therapy

KEY POINTS

After reading this chapter you have increased your awareness about the risks to the patient who is receiving I.V. therapy. Remember you have observation skills to assess for local complications, as well as cognitive skills to assess for systemic complications.

Local complications

Hematoma

Observe the skin for swelling and discoloration. Prevent a hematoma by use of indirect method of venipuncture, apply a tourniquet just prior to venipuncture, and use microdrip tubing with rates below 50 mL. Observe for slowed drip rate or resistance when attempting to flush the catheter with sodium chloride. Prevent by use of pump or controller.

Phlebitis

Observe the I.V. site for warmth, increased temperature, redness, and sluggish flow rate or a palpable cord. Prevent phlebitis by use of large veins, change I.V. site every 72 hours, and document observations every shift.

Thrombophlebitis

Observations are the same as for phlebitis with the addition of observing for a red line above venipuncture site, edema of the limb, and increase in basal temperature. Prevention includes the use of 0.22-micron filter, site checks, dilution of irritating medication, and good handwashing technique.

Infiltration

Observe the venipuncture site for coolness of the skin, taut skin, dependent edema, and backflow of blood. Prevent by early recognition, use of appropriate veins, and checking for patency before administration of drug. Extravasation may occur with vesicant drugs. Care must be taken to observe for a patent I.V. with vesicant materials and to know the antidote if extravasation should occur.

Local infection

Observe the site for redness and exudate at site. Monitor the WBC level and vital signs. Prevent local infection with good aseptic technique, handwashing, and safe standards of practice. Inspect all solutions for cracks, leaks, or discoloration.

Venous spasm

Observe for slowed I.V. rate. The patient may complain of a sharp pain at site traveling up the arm. Prevent venous spasm by infusing solutions at room temperature and administration of solution at prescribed rate.

Systemic complications

Septicemia

Observe for signs and symptoms of septicemia, including

- Fluctuating fever
- Profuse sweating

305

- Nausea and vomiting
- Diarrhea
- Decreasing BP

Prevent septicemia by inspection of all solutions, use of aseptic techniques, and following proper standards of practice for site care.

Circulatory overload

Signs and symptoms of circulatory overload include: weight gain, edema, puffy eyes and increased BP, a variance in intake and output records. Know the cardiovascular history of your patients. Prevent circulatory overload by taking time to know your patient and keeping the I.V. rate at the prescribed rate.

Pulmonary edema

In addition assessing for signs and symptoms of circulatory overload, assess for pulmonary edema by listening to your patient's lungs for crackles. Prevent pulmonary edema by using extreme caution when giving hypertonic solutions such as 5%D/0.9NACL and isotonic saline. Use less fluid volume with CHF patients.

Air embolism

Observe for signs of hypoxia, hypotension, and respiratory distress. Prevent this complication with a 0.22-micron air venting filter, use of leur-lock connectors, and maintenance of drip rate.

Speed shock

Observe for signs and symptoms of syncope, shock, and cardiac arrest. Prevention is the *key*! Give all I.V. drugs according to manufacturer's recommendation for administration.

Catheter embolism

Observe for patient reporting of sudden pain. Check catheter for signs of a blood return. Upon removal of a catheter, if the end is rough and uneven report findings to the physician. Prevent catheter embolism by *never* reinserting the needle of an over-the-needle catheter after it has been removed. Do *not* apply pressure over the site during removal of a catheter.

Erratic flow rates

Too slow rate is caused by clogged I.V. needle or loss of integrity of the vein. Too fast rates are caused by poorly regulated flow, cold flow of administration set, miscalculation of dose, and equipment which is not functioning accurately. To prevent erratic flow rates, use pumps with free flow protection, close clamps properly when removing administration sets, check or recalculate rates, and instruct or seek instruction on electronic infusion devices.

CRITICAL THINKING ACTIVITY

1. Check the policy and procedure manual in the facility in which you are working. Is there a policy which addresses:
   a. Length of time the I.V. catheter is to be left in the patient
   b. Frequency of tubing changes
   c. Type of solution used for preparing site before venipuncture

2. Do you feel that more attention should be paid to the quality management of the I.V.s in your hospital, extended care facility, or home care setting?   Why?

   If yes, how can you contribute to safer I.V. therapy?

3. Have you ever detected a case of phlebitis? Describe the changes that you found.

POST-TEST, CHAPTER 9

Match the definition in column II with the term in column I.

Column I

1. _____ vasospasm
2. _____ ecchymosis
3. _____ thrombosis
4. _____ extravasation
5. _____ speed shock

Column II

A. Foreign substance injected into body too rapidly

B. Escape of fluid from vessel

C. Contraction of muscular coat of the blood vessels

D. Formation or presence of blood clot

E. Bruise

6. Which of the following are local complications associated with I.V. therapy?
   A. Speed shock, septicemia, and venous spasm
   B. Phlebitis, venous spasm, and hematoma
   C. Septicemia, thrombophlebitis, and hematoma
   D. Phlebitis, pulmonary edema, and speed shock

7. The nurse can avoid a thrombosis formation by:
   A. Avoiding injury to the vein wall
   B. Avoiding multiple punctures
   C. Avoiding through-and-through punctures
   D. All of the above

8. Mr. Jenkins states that his I.V. site is sore. You assess the site and note redness and swelling, but no signs of palpable cord or streak. Using the criteria for infusion phlebitis, what is the severity of this phlebitis?
   A. 3+
   B. 1+
   C. 2+
   D. 0

9. The highest risk factor for phlebitis is among patients who are:
   A. Immunosuppressed
   B. Neonates
   C. Receiving total parenteral nutrition
   D. Receiving medications through multiple lines
   E. All of the above

10. A patient has a fluctuating fever, profuse sweating, nausea, and a lower-than—normal blood pressure. You would suspect:
    A. Local infection
    B. Septicemia
    C. Venous spasm
    D. Circulatory overload

11. The I.V. container runs dry and you superimpose a new solution. There is air in the tubing. How would you safely remove the air from the tubing? Give four steps.

    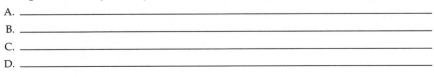

    A. _____

    B. _____

    C. _____

    D. _____

12. List two of the four ways a catheter tip may acquire bacteria.

    A. _____

    B. _____

13. List two of the three prevention techniques for avoiding phlebitis.

    A. _____

    B. _____

14. The infusion slows on your patient. What is the first step in checking on or managing this situation?

    _____

15. Name the three types of phlebitis.

    A. _____

    B. _____

    C. _____

16. A patient needs an I.V. for rehydration. You attempt an I.V. with a 20-gauge catheter but are unsuccessful. A large hematoma forms over the venipuncture site. Give two treatments for this tissue injury.

    A. _____

    B. _____

17. In the foregoing situation, what nursing tip could be used to decrease the risk of hematoma formation?

    _____

18. Of the six causes of thrombosis formation, list two.

    A. _____

    B. _____

19. While a solution is infusing, what treatment can be given for venous spasm?

20. What is the initial treatment for a suspected air embolism?

ANSWERS TO CHAPTER 9

PRE-TEST

1. B	7. G	13. A	19. C
2. E	8. E	14. A	20. T
3. D	9. A	15. A	21. T
4. C	10. B	16. A	22. T
5. A	11. B	17. A	23. T
6. F	12. B	18. A	

POST-TEST

1. C
2. E
3. D
4. B
5. A
6. B
7. D
8. B
9. E
10. B
11. A. Clamp tubing.
    B. Swab lowest Y port with alcohol
    C. Insert a 20-gauge 1-in needle and turn on roller clamp.
    D. When all air is vented, remove needle and then unclamp.
12. A. During venipuncture
    B. Colonization from skin
    C. Contaminated I.V. solution
    D. During removal of catheter
13. A. Use larger veins for hypertonic solutions
    B. Rotate sites every 72 hours
    C. Use 0.22-micron filter
14. Check tubing for kinks.

15. A. Chemical
    B. Mechanical
    C. Bacterial
16. A. Apply pressure with 2 × 2 gauze.
    B. Elevate extremity.
17. A. Use small-gauge needle for elderly patients or patients with thin skin.
    B. Use blood pressure cuff instead of tourniquet.
18. A. Blood backing up system in hypertensive patient
    B. Not enough fluid movement to maintain patency
    C. I.V. site in flexor area
    D. I.V. solution running dry
    E. Traumatization of wall of vein by cannula
    F. Flow rate due to patient compression
19. Wrap extremity with warm compress.
20. A. Place patient in Trendelenburg's position.
    B. Position on left side.
    C. Administer 100% oxygen.
    D. Monitor vital signs.
    E. *Get help.*

REFERENCES

Barrus, D.H., & Danek G. (1987). Should you irrigate an occluded I.V. line? *Nursing 87, 3,* 63–64.

Bohony, J. (1993). 9 Common I.V. complications and what to do about them. *American Journal of Nursing, 93* (10), 45–49.

Brunner, L.S., & Suddarth, D.S. (1992). *Textbook of medical-surgical nursing* (7th ed). Philadelphia: J.B. Lippincott.

Centers for Disease Control and Prevention. (1995). Guideline for prevention of intravascular infections. Atlanta: US Department of Health and Human Services.

Cohen, M.R. (1993). Recognizing the dangers of free flow. *Nursing 93, 6,* 56–59.

DeLuca, P.P., Rapp R.P., Blevins B., McKean H.E., & Griffen, W.O. (1975). Filtration and infusion phlebitis: A double blind prospective clinical study. *American Journal Hospital Pharmacy, 32,* 1001–1007.

ECRI. (1992). Emergency Care Research Institute. IV free flow still a cause for alarm 21(9) 323–328.

Ervin, S.M. (1987). The association of potassium chloride and particulate matter with the development of phlebitis. *National Intravenous Therapy Association, 10* (2), 145–149.

Feldstein, A. (1986). Detect phlebitis and infiltration before they harm your patient. *Nursing 86* (1), 44–46.

Food and Drug Administration. (1992). FDA safety alert: Potential hazards with restraint devices. *Food and Drug Administration, 7.*

Ford, C.D. (1990). *Extravasation.* Paper presented at the annual meeting of the Intravenous Nursing Society. Reno, Nevada.

Gong, H., & King, C. (1983). Inadequate drug mixing: A potential hazard in continuous intravenous administration. *Heart Lung, 12,* 528–532.

Harrigan, C.A. (1984). A cost-effective guide for the prevention of chemical phlebitis caused by the pH of the pharmaceutical agent. *Journal of Intravenous Therapy, 7,* 478–482.

Hastings-Tolsma, M.T., Yucha, C.B., Tompkins, J., Robson, L. & Szevernyi, N. (1993). Effect of warm and cold applications on the resolution of I.V. infiltrations. *Research in Nursing & Health, 16,* 171–178.

Hecker, J. (1988). Improved technique in I.V. therapy. *Nursing Times, 84* (34), 28–33.

Intravenous Nursing Society (1996). *Standards of Practice*. Philadelphia: J.B. Lippincott.

Jemison-Smith, P., & Thrupp, L.D. (1982). Phlebitis, infections and filtration. *Journal of Intravenous therapy, 6* (5), 328–335.

Joint Commission on Accreditation of Health Care Perspective. (1995). Joint commission perspectives: Interpretations: Limitations on hospital patient movement that constitute restraint. *Joint Commission on Accreditation of Health Care Organizations, 11–12, 15–16.*

Jones, E. (1982). Relationship between pH of intravenous medications and phlebitis: An experimental study. *National Intravenous Therapy Association, 5* (4), 273.

Lambert, M.J. (1982). Air embolism in central venous catheterization: Diagnosis, treatment and prevention. *Southern Medical Journal, 75* (10). 1189–1191.

Lenox, A.C. (1990). I.V. therapy reducing the risk of infection. *Nursing 90, 3,* 60–61.

Lewis, G.B.H., & Hecker, J.F. (1991). Radiological examination of failure of intravenous infusion. *British Journal of Surgery, 78,* 500–501.

Lonsway, R.A. (1987). Research, standards and infection control: The impact on I.V. nursing. *National Intravenous Therapy Association, 10* (2), 106–109.

Maki, D.G. (1990). The epidemiology and prevention of nosocomial bloodstream infections. In *Program and abstracts of the third international conference on nosocomial infection.* Atlanta: Centers for Disease Control.

Maki D.G. (1992). Infections due to infusion therapy. In Bennett, J.V., & Brachman, P.S. (eds.). *Hospital Infections (3rd ed.).* Boston: Little, Brown.

Maki, D.G., & Ringer, M. (1991). Risk factors for infusion-related phlebitis with small peripheral venous catheters. *Annals of Internal Medicine, 114,* 845–854.

McCloskey, J.C., & Bulechek, G.M. (1992). *Iowa intervention project: Nursing intervention classification (NIC).* St Louis: Mosby-Year Book, p. 320.

Messner, R.L., & Pinkerman, M.L. (1993). Preventing a peripheral I.V. infection. *Nursing 93, 6,* 34–41.

Metheny, N.M. (1996). *Fluid and electrolyte balance: Nursing considerations (3rd ed.).* Philadelphia: J.B. Lippincott.

Millam, D.A. (1988). Managing complications of I.V. therapy. *Nursing 88, 18* (3), 34–42.

Moser, L.C. (1991). Anaphylaxis: A preventable complication of home infusion therapy. *Journal of Intravenous Nursing, 14* (2), 108–112.

Nightingale, F. (1859). *Notes on nursing: What it is, and what it is not.* London: Harrison, 59, Pall Mall, 59.

Nursing Drug Alert. (1985). In-line filters can prevent much infusion-related phlebitis. 4, 27–28.

O'Quin, R.J., & Lakshminaayan, S. (1982). Venous air embolism. *Archives of Internal Medicine, 142* (12), 2173–2176.

Perdue, M. (1995). Intravenous complications. In Terry, J., Baranowski, L., Hedrick, C., & Recker, D. (1992). Catheter-related sepsis: An analysis of the research. *Research Analysis, 11* (5), 249–261.

Richardson, D., & Bruso, P. (1993). Vascular access devices: Management of common complications. *Journal of Intravenous Nursing, 16* (1), 44–48.

Rudolph, R., & Larson, D.L. (1987). Etiology and treatment of chemotherapeutic agent extravasation injuries: A review. *Journal of Clinical Oncology, 5,* 1116–1126.

Steel, J. (1983). Too fast or too slow: The erratic I.V. *American Journal of Nursing, 6,* 898–900.

Stratton, C.W. (1982). Infection related to intravenous infusion. *Heart & Lung, 11* (2), 123–137.

Tabor, C.L. (1993). Tabor's cyclopedic medical dictionary (17th ed.). Philadelphia: F.A. Davis, p. 531, 1277.

Teplitz, L. (1992). Responding to an air embolism. *Nursing 92, 7,* 33.

Thielen, J.B., & Nyquist, J. (1991). Subclavian catheter removal nursing implications to prevent air emboli. *Journal of Intravenous Nursing, 14* (2), 114–118.

Tipton, J.M., & Skeel, R.T. (1995). Management of acute side effects of cancer chemotherapy. In Tipton, J.M., & Skeel, R.T. (1995). In Skeel, R.T., & Lachant, N.A. (eds.). *Handbook of cancer chemotherapy (4th ed.).* Boston: Little, Brown, 573–574.

Weinstein, S. (1993). *Plumer's principles and practices of intravenous therapy.* Philadelphia: J.B. Lippincott.

Wenzel, R.P. (1993). Prevention and control of nosocomial infection (2nd ed.). Baltimore: Williams & Wilkins, 450–451.

Wood, L.S. & Gullo, M. (1993). IV vesicants: How to avoid extravasation. *American Journal of Nursing, 93* (4), 42–45.

Intravenous Therapy: Special Problems

CHAPTER CONTENTS

GLOSSARY
LEARNING OBJECTIVES
PRE-TEST, CHAPTER 10
PEDIATRIC I.V. THERAPY
Physiologic Characteristics
Physical Assessment
Site Selection
Selecting the Equipment
Venipuncture Techniques
Medication Administration
Alternative Administration Routes
GERIATRIC I.V. THERAPY
Physiologic Changes
Venipuncture Techniques
SPECIAL PROBLEMS
Alterations in Skin Surfaces

Hard Sclerosed Vessels
Obesity
Edema
NURSING PLAN OF CARE: THE PEDIATRIC
   CLIENT
PATIENT EDUCATION
HOME CARE ISSUES
COMPETENCY CRITERIA
KEY POINTS
CRITICAL THINKING ACTIVITY
POST-TEST, CHAPTER 10
ANSWERS TO CHAPTER 10
Pre-Test
Post-Test
REFERENCES

GLOSSARY

Body surface area   Surface area of the body determined through use of a nomogram
Caloric method   Calculation of metabolic expenditure of energy
Catabolism   Breakdown of chemical compounds into more elementary principles by the body; an energy-producing metabolic process
Ecchymoses   Bruising caused by escape of blood from injured vessels
Infant   Child under the age of 2 years
Intraosseous infusion   Infusion within the bone marrow cavity
Meter square method   Use of a nomogram to determine surface areas of a patient
Neonate   Infant in the period of extrauterine life up to the first 28 days after birth
Oncotic   Within the tissue, tissue pressure
Purpura   Condition in which spontaneous bleeding occurs in the subcutaneous tissue, causing purple patches to appear on the skin
Tangential lighting   Light touching a curve, indirect lighting
Weight method   Formula based on weight in kilograms to estimate the fluid needs

LEARNING OBJECTIVES

Upon completion of this chapter, the reader will be able to:

- Describe terms related to delivery of I.V. therapy to pediatric and geriatric patients.
- Identify physiologic characteristics of a neonate, infant, children, and geriatric patients related to venous structure.
- Locate common sites for venipuncture in the pediatric and geriatric patient.
- Identify common reasons for neonate and infant infusions.
- List the formulas available for calculating fluid needs of an infant.
- Contrast the stages of development and fears through the life span as related to performance of invasive procedures.
- Identify types of needles and catheters available for the pediatric patient.
- Describe special considerations for successful venipuncture of neonates, infants, and the geriatric patient.
- Describe the use of intraosseous infusions in the pediatric patient.
- Identify the complications related to intraosseous infusions.
- List the risk factors associated with pediatric and geriatric infusions.
- Describe techniques for venipuncture in patients with sclerotic veins, alterations in skin integrity, obesity, and edema.
- Use the nursing plan of care for the pediatric patient.

PRE-TEST, CHAPTER 10

Match the definition in column II to the term in column I.

Column I

1. _____ ecchymosis
2. _____ intraosseous
3. _____ weight method
4. _____ caloric method
5. _____ neonate
6. _____ body surface area

Column II

A. Infant in the first 28 days of life
B. Calculation of metabolic expenditure of energy
C. Bruise
D. Within the bone marrow cavity
E. Formula based on kilograms of weight
F. Surface area determined through use of nomogram

7. Risk factors affecting the need for infusion therapy in the neonate include:
   A. Prematurity
   B. Catabolic disease
   C. Hypothermia
   D. Acid-base imbalance
   E. All of the above

8. Identify the three methods for assessment of 24-hour fluid needs in the infant:
   A. Meter square, diaper weight, and urinary output
   B. Meter square, weight, and caloric methods
   C. Meter square, specific gravity, and head circumference

9. Common sites for venipuncture in infants less than 9 months of age include:
   A. Antecubital space, dorsum of the foot, and scalp veins
   B. Dorsum of the foot, external jugular vein, and saphenous vein
   C. Dorsum of the hand, dorsum of the foot, and external jugular vein
   D. Scalp veins, antecubital space, and external jugular vein

10. Intraosseous infusions are useful for:
    A. Emergency delivery of medication and fluids
    B. Long-term nutritional support
    C. Home antibiotic therapy

11. Disadvantages of intraosseous infusions include:
    A. Potential osteomyelitis
    B. Potential cellulitis
    C. Potential damage to epiphyseal plate
    D. All of the above

12. The physiologic changes in the geriatric patient that affect I.V. placement include:
    A. Arteriosclerosis
    B. Increased density and amount of collagen in the vessel walls
    C. Loss of subcutaneous fat
    D. Thinning of the skin
    E. All of the above

13. How many superficial veins in the infant's head are accessible for venipuncture?
    A. 1
    B. 2
    C. 4
    D. 6

14. to perform an I.V. infusion on a preschool child, the nurse should:
    A. Explain the procedure in simple terms
    B. Explain the procedure completely
    C. Restrain the child to perform the venipuncture
    D. Provide reading materials before performing venipuncture

15. To perform a venipuncture on a toddler, it is helpful if the nurse:
    A. Provides pictures to color during the procedure
    B. Provides a doll or stuffed animal in which to start the I.V. infusion prior to venipuncture
    C. Has assistance for the venipuncture
    D. Has parents assist with the procedure

16. Tangential lighting should be used with patients who have:
    A. Alterations in skin surfaces
    B. Burned skin surfaces
    C. Edematous tissue
    D. Easily palpable and visible veins

17. The use of multiple tourniquets can be helpful with:
    A. Pediatric patients
    B. Frail geriatric patients, to distend veins
    C. Patients with sclerosed veins
    D. Patients with dark skin

True-False

18. **T F** Digital pressure to displace edematous fluid allows for visualization of the vein.

19. **T F** Minor trauma can easily cause bruising in the frail geriatric patient.

20. **T F** Hard sclerosed veins are found in patients in renal failure, who have sickle cell anemia, and who are intravenous drug abusers.

Children are not little adults.

VIRGINIA TURNER, 1995

Children, older adults, and persons with certain disorders can create a challenge to safe administration of I.V. therapy. Understanding those problems and ways to overcome them can help you ensure safe delivery with minimal risk to the client.

PEDIATRIC I.V. THERAPY

I.V. therapy for the pediatric patient requires special considerations to safeguard the child. When assessing the child before administration, the practitioner must be aware of the body composition of an infant and the homeostatic differences between children and adults. Also, the calculation of small doses, low infusion rates, and choice of appropriate venipuncture site and equipment, need to be taken into consideration.

Physiologic Characteristics

A neonate is defined as a child in the period of extrauterine life up to the first 28 days after birth. Low-birth-weight and premature infants have decreased energy stores and increased metabolic needs, compared with those of a full-term, average-weight newborn.

The premature infant's body is made up of approximately 90% water; the newborn infant's 70% to 80%, and the adult's about 60%. Infants have proportionately more water in the extracellular compartment than do adults. Therefore, any depletion in these water stores may lead to dehydration. As the infant becomes older, the ratio of extracellular to intracellular fluid volume decreases.

Although infants have a relatively greater total body water content, this does not protect them from excessive fluid loss. Infants are more vulnerable to fluid volume deficit because they ingest and excrete a relatively greater daily volume of water than adults (Metheny, 1996). Any condition that interferes with normal water and electrolyte intake or that produces excessive water and electrolyte losses will produce a more rapid depletion of water and electrolyte stores in the infant than it will in the adult.

Illness, increased muscular activity, thermal stress, congenital abnormalities, and respiratory distress syndrome influence metabolic demands as well. The metabolic demand of an infant is two times higher per unit of weight than that of adults (Whaley & Wong, 1991).

In most cases, 100 to 120 calories/kg per day will maintain the normal infant and provide sufficient calories for growth. For high-risk infants who require increased handling for procedures, the calorie requirement is up to 100% higher than that of the normal newborn. Heat production increases calorie expenditure by 7% per degree of temperature elevation. The infant and young child cannot store protein as well as adults; therefore, preventive nutritional support is needed.

Young children have immature homeostatic regulating mechanisms that need to be considered when water and electrolyte replacement is needed. Renal functioning, acid-base balance, body surface area differences, and electrolyte concentrations all must be taken into consideration when planning fluid needs.

The newborn's renal function is not yet completely developed. The infant's kidneys appear to become mature by the end of the neonatal period. An infant's kidneys have a limited concentrating ability and require more water to excrete a given amount of solutes. The infant is less likely to be able to regulate fluid intake and output.

The buffering capacity to regulate acid-base balance is less in the newborn than in older children. Neonates, with an average pH of 7.0 to 7.38, are slightly more acidotic than adults. This base bicarbonate deficit is thought to be related to high metabolic acid production and to renal immaturity.

The integumentary system in the neonate is an important route of fluid loss, especially in illness. This must be considered when determining fluid balance in infants and young children, since their body surface area is greater than that of older children and adults. Any condition that produces a decrease in intake or output of water and electrolytes affects the body fluid stores of the infant. Because the gastrointestinal membranes are an extension of the body surface area, relatively greater losses occur from the gastrointestinal tract in the sick infant (Wong, 1995).

Plasma electrolyte concentrations do not vary strikingly among infants, small children, or adults. The plasma sodium concentration changes little from birth to adulthood. The potassium and chloride concentrations are higher in the first few months of life than at any other time.

Magnesium and calcium are both low in the first 24 hours after birth. The serum phosphate level is elevated in the early months of infancy, which contributes to a low calcium level. The newborn infant is vulnerable to disrupted calcium homeostasis when stressed by illness or by an excess phosphate load and is at risk for hypocalcemia (Metheny, 1996) Table 10–1 provides normal laboratory values in the newborn.

TABLE 10–1. NORMAL LABORATORY VALUES FOR CHILDREN

Laboratory Value	Neonate	Infant	2–5 years	6–12 years	Adolescent
Blood Count					
Red blood cells (million/μL)		2.7–5.4	4.27	4.31	4.60
Whole blood cells (per μL)		6000–17,000	5000–15,500	4500–13,500	4500–11,000
Platelet count (per μL)	84,000–479,000	150,000–400,000/mm all remaining ages			
Partial thromboplastin time and prothrombin time		<17 s		18–22 s	
Hemoglobin (g/dL)	14.5	9.0–14.0		11.5–15.5	Male 13–16 Female 12–16
Serum Electrolytes					
Sodium (mEq/L)		139–146	138–145		136–146
Potassium (mEq/L)		4.1–5.3		3.4–4.7	3.5–5.1
Magnesium (mEq/L)		1.4–1.9 . . . same for all ages			
Calcium (mg/dL)	7.5–11	8.8–10.8			8.4–10.8
Chloride (mEq/L)		98–106 . . . same for all ages			
Phorphorus (mg/dL)	4.0–10.5			5.0–7.8	

Physical Assessment

A physical assessment should be performed on the pediatric patient prior to I.V. therapy. (Table 10–2 lists the components of a pediatric assessment.) Risk factors that must be considered during the assessment phase include prematurity, *catabolic* disease state, hypothermia, hyperthermia, metabolic or respiratory alkalosis or acidosis, and other metabolic derangements.

Candidates for neonatal I.V. therapy include those with:

Congenital cardiac disorder
Gastrointestinal defects
Neurologic defects

Candidates for infant I.V. therapy include those with:

Fluid volume deficit (dehydration)
Electrolyte imbalance (diarrhea)
Antibiotic therapy for treatment of serious infections
Need for nutritional support for maintenance of growth and development
Antineoplastic therapy for treatment of cancer

Assessment of Fluid Needs

There are three methods for assessment of 24-hour maintenance of fluids: meter square, caloric, and weight methods.

Meter Square Method

The nomogram (Appendix A) is used to determine the surface area of the patient in the meter square method. To use a nomogram in this method, draw a straight line between the point representing the patient's height on the left vertical scale to the point representing the patient's weight on the right vertical scale. The point at which the line intersects indicates the body surface area in square meters (Weinstein, 1990).

ADVANTAGES
Provides calculation of body surface area to help determine the amount of fluid and electrolytes to be infused and assists with computing rate of infusion
Helps to calculate adult and pediatric dosages of I.V. medications
Is simple to calculate

DISADVANTAGE
Difficulty in accessibility to visual nomogram

TABLE 10–2. **COMPONENTS OF THE PEDIATRIC PHYSICAL ASSESSMENT**

Measurement of head circumference (up to 1 year)
Height or length
Weight
Vital signs
Skin turgor
Presence of tears
Moistness and color of mucous membranes
Urinary output
Characteristics of fontanelles
Level of child's activity related to growth and development

To calculate the maintenance of fluid requirements, use the following:

FORMULA

$$1500 \text{ mL/m}^2 \text{ per 24 hours}$$

Example
If child's surface area is 0.5^2, then 1500 mL $\times$ 0.5 m^2 = 750 mL/24 hours.

Weight Method

The weight method uses the child's weight in kilograms to estimate fluid needs. This method uses 100 to 150 mL/kg for estimating maintenance fluid requirements and is most useful in children weighing less than 10 kg. (Use of the square meter method is recommended in children weighing more than 10 kg.)

ADVANTAGE
Simple to use

DISADVANTAGE
Inaccurate in a child who weighs more than 10 kg

Example
In a child weighing 10 kg, 100 $\times$ 10 kg = 1000 mL in 24 hours.

Caloric Method

The caloric method calculates the usual metabolic expenditure of fluid. It is based on the following metabolic expenditure:

Child weighing 0 to 10 kg expends approximately 100 calories/kg per day.
Child weighting 10 to 20 kg expends approximately 1000 calories, plus 50 calories/kg for each kg over 10 kg.
Child weighing 20 kg or more expends approximately 1500 calories, plus 20 calories/kg for each kg over 20 kg.

ADVANTAGE
Simple to calculate

DISADVANTAGE
Not totally accurate unless actual calorie requirements and energy intake are continuously assessed

The formula for calculating fluid requirement is 100 to 150 mL/100 calories metabolized.

Example
If the weight of the child is 30 kg and the child expends 1700 calories/day, fluid requirement is 1700 to 2550 mL/24 hours.

Factors Affecting Fluid Needs in the Pediatric Patient

The most common cause of increased fluid and calorie needs in children is temperature elevation. An increase in temperature of 1°C increases a child's calorie needs by 12%. Fluid requirements of a child who is hypothermic decrease by 12% (Weinstein, 1993). In children, loss of gastrointestinal fluids, ongoing diarrhea, and small intestinal drainage can seriously affect fluid balance.

319

✎ **NOTE:** To ensure accuracy of fluid needs, most pediatric patients should be on strict intake and output monitoring, including diaper weighing

Diaper Weighing

When weighing the infant's diaper, consider the weight of the diaper before it was wet. The weight difference in a dry and a wet piece of linen represents the amount of liquid that it has absorbed. The weight of the fluid measured in grams is the same as the volume measured in milliliters (Marlow & Redding, 1988).

Site Selection

When selecting the venipuncture site, keep in mind that the main goal of I.V. therapy is to provide the treatment with safety and efficiency, while meeting the child's emotional and developmental needs (Wheeler & Frey, 1995). Consider the following factors before selecting a site for venipuncture:

Age of child
Size of child
Condition of veins
Reason for therapy
General patient condition
Mobility and level of activity of child
Gross and fine motor skills (e.g., sucks fingers, plays with hands, holds bottle, draws)
Sense of body image
Fear of mutilation
Cognitive ability of the child (i.e., understands and follows directions) (Wheeler & Frey, 1995).

Peripheral Routes

Peripheral routes for pediatric I.V. therapy include scalp veins and the veins in the dorsum of the hand, forearm, and foot (Fig. 10–1).

Scalp Veins

The major superficial veins of the scalp can be used. Scalp veins can be used in children up to age 18 months; after that age the hair follicles mature and the epidermis toughens. There are four scalp veins used most commonly for I.V. access: frontal (best access), preauricular, supraorbital, and occipital.

✎ **NOTE:** The choice of scalp vein for placement of I.V. therapy is often traumatic for the parents because removal of hair may have cultural as well as religious significance. In addition, maintaining patency of this site can at times be difficult.

ADVANTAGES
Easily visualized
Readily dilates—no valves
Hands kept free
Head easily stabilizes

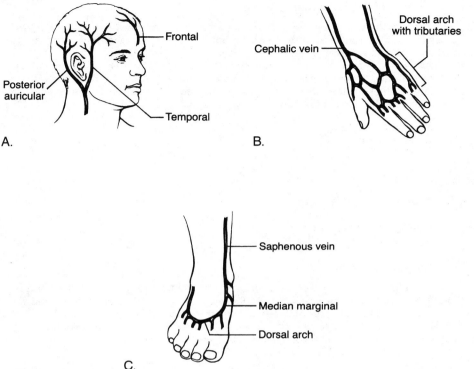

Figure 10–1. Superficial veins of the scalp (*A*) and dorsum of hand (*B*) and foot (*C*). (Mathewson-Kuhn, M. [1994]. *Pharmacotherapeutics: A nursing process approach* [3rd ed.] Philadelphia: FA Davis, with permission.)

DISADVANTAGES
Shaving of hair
Infiltrates easily
Disfigurement with infiltration
Difficult to secure device
Increased family anxiety

The I.V. needle must be placed in the direction of blood flow to ensure that the I.V. fluid will flow in the same direction as that of the blood returning to the heart. In the scalp, venous blood generally flows from the top of the head down.

✎ **NOTE:** A rubberband with a piece of tape attached can be used as a tourniquet (or pressure can be applied with the finger to distend the vein). Place the rubberband low on the forehead like a headband. It is also recommended that the rubberband be cut to decrease the chances of dislodging the I.V. after cannulation (Wheeler & Frey, 1995).

✎ **NOTE:** Shaving is not recommended; if necessary, clip the hair on the infant (Fabian, 1991).

321

Dorsum of the Hand and Forearm

Because the veins over the metacarpal area are mobile and not well supported by surrounding tissue, the limb must be immobilized with a splint and tape prior to cannulation. This site can be used in all ages.

The antecubital fossa should not be routinely used, because of the use of the antecubital area for blood drawing and the mobility problems resulting from use of this site. However, the antecubital area can be used for placement of peripherally inserted central catheters (PICC).

ADVANTAGES
Easily accessible
Readily visible
Large enough for a larger-gauge cannula
Bones act as natural splints

DISADVANTAGES
Increased nerve endings
Difficult to anchor cannula on infant
Interferes with child's activity

Dorsum of the Foot

The foot is used as a venipuncture site for infants and toddlers but should be avoided in children who are walking. The curve of the foot, especially around the ankle, makes entry and cannula advancement difficult. The veins used are the saphenous, median, and marginal dorsal arch. Because the neonate has very little subcutaneous adipose tissue, the veins are easily identified and cannulated just beneath the skin.

✎ **NOTE:** The foot should be secured on a padded board with normal joint position.

ADVANTAGES
Readily dilates
Hands kept free
Less rolling of vein
Increased visibility in chubby infants
Easy to splint

DISADVANTAGES
Decreased mobility in walking
Limited to smaller-gauge cannulas
Located near arteries
Difficult to advance cannula

Selecting the Equipment

The nurse must be aware of the special needs of the pediatric patient in selection of appropriate equipment for administration of fluids and medication. When choosing administration equipment, the safety of the child requires that the activity level, age, and size of the patient be considered. For safe delivery of I.V. therapy in the pediatric patient, the following equipment is recommended:

- An electronic infusion device for administration of therapy
- The volume of solution container used should be based on the age, height, and weight of the patient and should contain no greater than *500 mL* of fluid (preferably 250 mL

- Special pediatric equipment, such as volume control chamber for the delivery of therapy
- Plastic fluid containers (preferable to glass because of possible breakage)
- Microdrip tubing (60 drops/min)
- Monitoring at least every 2 hours and more frequently, depending on patient's age and size or type of therapy
- Visible cannula site

Needle Selection

The choice of needle depends on the site selected. Peripheral cannulas, gauges 26 to 21, can be used in children. A 27- to 19-gauge scalp vein (butterfly) needle is easy to insert but has the risk of infiltrating easily. The scalp vein needle has been replaced by more contemporary types of peripheral venous access devices.

Over-the-needle catheters 26- to 14-gauge, can also be used for pediatric patients. For neonates 26- to 24-gauge needles are used; for children 24- to 22-gauge are most common. Over-the-needle cannulas usually last longer than scalp vein needles but are more difficult to insert. These catheters are also easier to stabilize.

Venipuncture Techniques

The methods for venipuncture are the same for children as for adults (see Chapter 8); a direct or indirect method can be used. The following are tips on technique are unique to the pediatric patient:

- Venipuncture should be performed in a room separate from the child's room. The child's room is his or her "safe space."
- Use a pacifier for neonates and infants.
- Use mummy and clove-hitch immobilizers as needed. The infant should be covered with a blanket to minimize cold stress. If the dorsum of the hand is used, place the extremity on an armbard before venipuncture.
- A flashlight or transilluminator device placed beneath the extremity helps to illuminate tissue surrounding the vein; the veins are then outlined for better visualization (Wheeler & Frey, 1995).
- Warm hands by washing in hot water before gloving.
- Omit tourniquet use if possible. Use rubberband to dilate scalp veins.
- Use a saline-filled syringe with a scalp vein infusion device.
- Flush the needle immediately with saline upon backflow of blood.
- Use surgical lubricating jelly to help secure tape around a scalp I.V. by applying a small amount under the tape. Use only hypoallergenic or paper tape. When you are ready to remove the tape, apply warm water and the tape will lift off easily (Wheeler & Frey, 1995).
- Stabilize the cannula with a padded tongue blade.
- Collect laboratory specimens at the time of I.V. insertion.
- Use stickers or drawings on the I.V. site as a reward.
- *Always have extra help.*

✎ **NOTE:** When securing the child's extremity to an armboard, use clear tape for visualization of the I.V. site and digits or skin immediately adjacent to the site (Blatz & Paez, 1990; Delaney & Lauer, 1988; Tietjen, 1990).

✎ **NOTE:** Use of a paper cup if not recommended to cover the infusion site on the scalp (Jarmen, 1985). A clear medicine cup can offer the needed protection.

Stabilizing and maintaining patency of I.V. cannula sites can be a challenge. Poorly secured I.V. access sites may result in dislodgements or infiltrations requiring I.V.

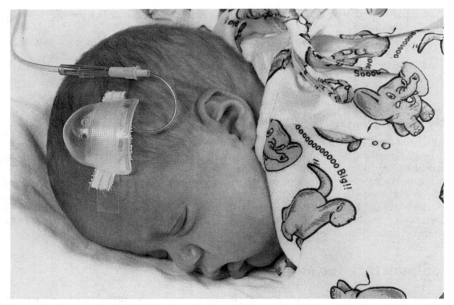

Figure 10–2. Protection of the I.V. site. Courtesy of Progressive IVs, Inc., Hazelwood, Missouri.)

restarts. Some commercial products are available to help protect I.V. sites. For example, the Bubbles and Boards System by Acme United Corporation is a three-piece system designed to meet the needs for I.V. cannula protection, site visibility, limb stabilization, and maintenance of skin integrity (Stifter & Shanahan, 1994). The I.V. House by Progressive IVs, Inc, is a one-piece unit that protects any I.V. site (Fig. 10–2).

For children, illness and hospitalization constitute a major life crisis. Children are vulnerable to the crises of illness and hospitalization because stress represents a change from the usual state of health and environmental routine and children have a limited number of coping mechanisms to resolve the stressful events.

Children's understanding of, reaction to, and method of coping with illness or hospitalization are influenced by the significance of individual stressors during each developmental phase. The major stressors are separation, loss of control, and bodily injury. See Table 10-3, which summarizes the principal behavioral responses to each stressor as related to the function of I.V. therapy.

Medication Administration

To deliver medication to children requires that the nurse have expert knowledge of the techniques for delivery of medication and for calculation of formulas. The most common methods of calculation are covered in the beginning of this chapter: body weight and body surface area are most frequently used. Dosages of pediatric medications are usually recommended in terms of body weight. The dose and volume can be different in children, and frequently drugs are calculated to the tenth of a milligram or milliliter (Wheeler & Frey, 1995).

324

TABLE 10–3. **NURSING INTERVENTIONS FOR THE CHILD REQUIRING I.V. THERAPY AS RELATED TO PHYSICAL AND PSYCHOLOGICAL DEVELOPMENT**

Age	Development/Stressor	Behavior	Intervention
Infant	Trust versus mistrust *Stressor:* Pain	Cries, screams, clings in protest Neonate: easily distracted—total body reaction Infant: localized reaction; often uncooperative	Consistency in assigning caregivers Encourage parents to assist with care Explain I.V. to parents Have assistance starting I.V.
Toddler	Autonomy versus shame and doubt *Stressor:* Loss of control Physical restriction Loss of routine and rituals Bodily injury and pain	Protests verbally Cries for parents Kicks, bites, tries to escape to find parents Resists Verbally uncooperative	Allow to express feelings Encourage parental help Allow as much mobility as possible in securing I.V. Encourage presence of favorite toy or blanket during procedure Use comfort after procedure
Preschool	Initiative versus guilt *Stressor:* Loss of control Sense of own power Bodily injury–intrusive procedure, mutilations	Protests less directly Anxiety, guilt, shame, physiologic responses Immature behavior	Allow child to express protest Provide play and diversional activity Encourage to play out feelings and fears Allow as much mobility as possible; limit invasive procedures Explain procedure in simple terms; start pretend I.V. on doll
School-age	Industry versus inferiority *Stressor:* Loss of control Enforced dependency Altered family roles Bodily injury and pain Illness and death—intrusive procedures in genital area	Loneliness, boredom, isolation, hostility, and frustration Depression and displaced anger Seeks information Passively accepts Communicates about pain	Allow to express feelings both verbally and nonverbally Involve in starting I.V. by tearing tape or holding tubing Encourage peer contacts Use diversional activities
Adolescent	Identity versus role diffusion *Stressor:* Loss of control Loss of identity Enforced dependency Bodily injury and mutilation	Rejection Uncooperativeness Self-assertion Overconfidence Boredom	Explore feelings regarding hospitalization Help to adjust to authority Explain all procedures Allow choices in sites Provide privacy

Source: From Wong, D.L. (1993). *Essentials of pediatric nursing*, 3rd ed. St. Louis: CV Mosley Company. Copyright 1993 by CV Mosley. Reprinted by permission.

Intermittent Infusions

The in-line calibrated chamber is commonly used in the general pediatric setting. The medication is injected into the in-line chamber and infused at a prescribed rate.

ADVANTAGE
Simplicity

DISADVANTAGES
Not practical for small infants
Necessity of drug compatibility with primary solution, or a second tubing setup is required
Flushing of the chamber with a certain volume is insufficient to clear chamber of medication

Retrograde Infusion

Retrograde infusion is used in the general pediatric area and neonatal intensive care units and often in infants or children who cannot tolerate a rapid infusion rate or additional fluid volume. A specific retrograde administration set is required for this purpose. The tubing volume varies but generally holds less than 1 mL. A three-way stopcock or access port is at each end of the tubing. To use retrograde infusion, follow these steps:

1. Attach the retrograde tubing and prime along with the primary administration set. The tubing functions as an extension set when it is not used to administer medication.
2. To administer the medication, attach a medication-filled syringe to the port proximal to the patient, and connect an empty syringe to the port most distal from the patient.
3. Make sure the clamp between the port and the child is closed, and inject the medication distally up the tubing. The fluid in the retrograde tubing is displaced upward into the tubing and the empty syringe.
4. Remove both syringes and open the lower clamp. The medication is then infused into the patient at the prescribed rate.

Syringe Pump

The syringe pump is an increasingly popular and accurate method of delivery of I.V. medications in children. It can be connected by an extension set into a primary line. See Chapter 7 for information on syringe pumps.

✎ **NOTE:** Parenteral nutrition and transfusion therapy are also frequently administered to the pediatric client; special considerations for delivery of blood products or parenteral nutrition are discussed in Chapters 13 and 15.

Formulas for Delivery of Pediatric Therapies

The following are formulas used in calculation of delivery of pediatric therapies.

Body weight. Dosages of drugs based on kilograms of body weight require that the nurse use the weight (in kg) of the child in dosage administration (1 kilogram (kg) = 2.2 lb). Many drugs are ordered as milligram per kilogram of body weight. Multiply the mg of the drug times the kg of body weight.

$$\text{mg of drug} \times \text{kg of child's body weight} = \text{Child's dose}$$

Body surface area (BSA). Dosages of drugs based on BSA are determined by multiplying the child's BSA (m²) times the recommended adult dose, divided by the adult's BSA (1.73 m²).

$$\frac{\text{BSA of child (m}^2) \times \text{recommended adult dosage}}{\text{BSA of adult (1.73 m}^2)} = \text{Child's dose}$$

Bastedo's rule. This rule determines the child's dose based on the child's age + 3, times the average adult dose, divided by 30.

$$\frac{\text{Age (years)} + 3 \times \text{Average adult dose}}{30} = \text{Child's dose}$$

Clark's rule. This rule determines the child's dose based on the child's weight in relation to the average adult body weight and dose.

$$\frac{\text{Weight (lb)} \times \text{Average adult dose}}{\text{(Average adult weight} = 150 \text{ lb)}} = \text{Child's dose}$$

Cowling's rule. This rule determines the child's dose based on the child's age and the average adult dose, divided by 24.

$$\frac{\text{Age (years on next birthday)} \times \text{Average adult dose}}{24} = \text{Child's dose}$$

Fried's rule. This rule determines the infant's dose based on the infant's age in relation to the average adult body weight and dose.

✎ NOTE: This rule is effective only for infants younger than 1 year.

Young's rule. This rule determines the child's dose based on the child's age and average adult dose, divided by the child's age + 12.

$$\frac{\text{Age in years} \times \text{Average adult dose}}{\text{Age (in years)} +12} = \text{Child's dose}$$

Alternative Administration Routes

Alternative routes for administration of I.V. therapy in the pediatric patient are intraosseous and umbilical veins and arteries.

Intraosseous Route

The intraosseous route is a safe alternative for fluid and drug administration in the infant or child. From 1940 to 1950, the intraosseous infusion for both adults and children was widely used. By the late 1950s, it was replaced by plastic catheters and newer infusion techniques (Peck & Altieri, 1988).

The revised standards and guidelines outlined in the *Textbook of Pediatric Advanced Life Support* by the American Heart Association (1992) recognize intraosseous infusion as an effective route for the administration of emergency medications or fluids to children under 6 years. These guidelines further emphasize the importance

327

of establishing and maintaining an infusion route during the resuscitation of critically ill children (Chameides, 1992).

Intraosseous infusion uses the rich vascular network of the long bones to transport fluids and medications from the medullary cavity to the circulation. The medullary cavity is composed of a spongy network of venous sinusoids that drain into a central venous canal. Blood exits the venous canal by the nutrient and emissary veins into the circulation. Fluids infused into the medullary space diffuse a short space, then are absorbed into the venous circulation; the distribution is similar to intravenous injection (Spivey, 1987) Fig. 10–3A).

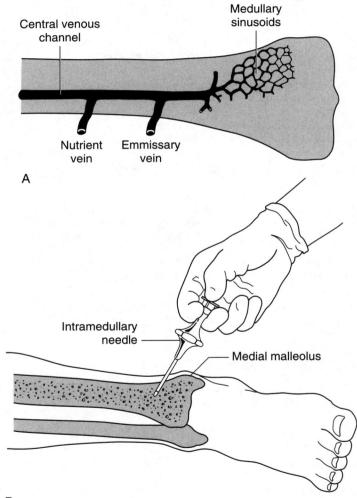

Figure 10–3. Intramedullary venous system (A) and placement of intraosseous needle (B). (From Spivey, W.H. [1987]. Intraosseous infusion. *Journal of Pediatrics, 111,* 639–644. Copyright 1987 by Mosby–Year Book. Reprinted by permission.)

ADVANTAGES

Provides a quick access in emergency cases when life-sustaining medication must be administered. In difficult-to-access patients, provides an accessible access for delivery of volume resuscitation. Useful in cardiac arrest, shock, trauma, or any situation in which the potential benefit of rapid venous access outweighs the low incidence of complications.

DISADVANTAGES

Potential for osteomyelitis (low incidence reported)

Potential for cellulitis; however, studies have reported only a 0.6% incidence of cellulitis (Rossetti & Thompson, 1985)

Potential damage to the epiphyseal plate is a concern

Potential embolus caused by fat dislodged from the marrow cavity is a risk

Intraosseous Insertion Technique

The appropriate sites for intraosseous infusion are the distal tibia, the proximal tibia, and the distal femur. The distal tibia is used most frequently because of the flat area proximal to the malleolus and the thin covering of bony cortex (Wheeler & Frey, 1995).

ASSEMBLE EQUIPMENT

Providone-iodine solution (Betadine)

Jamshidi Bone Marrow Biopsy Needle or 16- or 19-gauge straight-gauge needle with stylet, short shaft, and sturdy handle

Commercially prepared disposable intraosseous infusion needle by Cook Critical Care (Bloomington, IN)

One 10-mL syringe filled with saline

Fluid and medications to be administered with administration set

Tape or Elastoplast

Prepare the child's skin using povidone-iodine solution.

Wear gloves, mask, gown, and goggles.

Select site. Most common sites are the proximal tibia and the distal tibia. Use of the sternum in children is discouraged because it is too thin and poorly developed to guarantee safe placement.

Use local anesthesia, 1% lidocaine hydrochloride, if patient is awake and alert.

Insert the needle at a 30-degree angle with the point directed away from the epiphyseal plate (see Fig. 10–3B). A twisting or boring motion is used until penetration through the cortex is achieved.

Remove stylet.

Infuse saline by syringe to clear the needle of marrow, as well as to check for placement.

Start infusion of fluid or medications under gravity pressure.

Apply a sterile dressing.

Regulate infusion.

Chart the site, needle type and size, type of fluid and medication, as well as patient response to the treatment (Peck & Altieri, 1988).

✎ **NOTE:** This method of infusion should only be used in children under 6.

Contraindications

Patients who have areas of cellulitis or infected burns, or those with recently fractured bones should not undergo intraosseous infusion. Patients with osteogenesis imperfecta or osteoporosis are not good candidates for this route (Hodge, 1985).

Nursing Management

The nursing staff is responsible for managing the site and assessment, administration of the fluid or medication, proper use of I.V. equipment, and documentation.

✎ NOTE: After the needle is removed, a sterile gauze pad should be placed over the puncture site and direct pressure applied. The site should be inspected daily and redressed. After 48 hours, if no drainage is seen, the dressing may be removed (Wheeler, 1989).

Umbilical Vein and Arteries

There are three vessels in the umbilical cord: one vein and two arteries. These vessels provide alternative routes for vascular access in the neonate. These routes are reserved for emergency access in the delivery room and for hemodynamic monitoring in the neonatal intensive care unit.

The goals of arterial catheterization are different from those of venous catheterization. The main goals of arterial umbilical catheterization are:

- Monitoring arterial pressure
- Obtaining blood samples for arterial pH and blood gases
- Performing aortography
- Performing exchange transfusions

The vein of the umbilicus can be catheterized up to 4 days of life. However, it is usually inserted in the delivery room in a compromised infant. The goals of venous catheterization include:

- Emergency administration of medication and fluid
- Venous blood sampling
- Exchange transfusion (Wheeler, 1995)

There is a risk of vascular compromise, hemorrhage, air embolism, infection, thrombosis, and vascular perforation with umbilical catheterization. The risk of infection is greater with the venous catheter and becomes a significant risk after 24 hours. The umbilical venous catheter is removed as soon as an alternative access route has been established—usually within 48 to 72 hours.

GERIATRIC I.V. THERAPY

The United States Census Bureau (1990) projects that by the year 2030 there will be a higher proportion of persons over 65 years (23%) than persons under 18 years (18%) in the population. Those 85 and older constitute one of the largest-growing segments of the population. By the turn of the century, 50% of the older population will be age 75 years or older. This will place greater demands on the health care system (Smeltzer & Bare, 1992). Life expectancy in the United States is 75 years (Taylor, 1992). Health care practitioners need a heightened awareness and understanding of the special needs of the elderly.

Physiologic Changes

Aging occurs on all levels of bodily function: cellular, organic, and systemic. "Loss of cells and loss of physiologic reserve make up the dominant processes of aging" (Smeltzer & Bare, 1992). The major systems changes the nurse must be aware of related to infusion therapy are homeostatic changes, immune system and cardiovascular changes, and skin and connective tissue changes.

Homeostatis is the body's ability to maintain a stable internal environment. The homeostatic mechanism in the aging become less efficient, and reserve power is lost. For example, when external stressors such as trauma or infection occur, there is minimal reserve capacity. This creates a situation in which the person is more vulnerable to disease.

Two immune processes change with aging. (1) The immune system becomes hyporesponsive to foreign antigens (e.g., decreased numbers of circulating lymphocytes, cells have fewer receptors to decrease ability to generate energy). (2) The immune system becomes hyperresponsive to itself (Whitehouse, 1992).

Cardiovascular changes related to arteriosclerosis become clinically recognizable. With aging, the three functions of the heart affected are: the ability to oxygenate the cardiac muscle decreases, diastolic filling decreases, and left ventricular wall thickness increases. Arteries show progressive chemical and anatomic changes, with an increase in cholesterol, other lipids, and calcium. The intima increases, which increases resistance and decreases compliance of the vein or artery. The elastic fibers progressively straighten, fray, split, and fragment. There is an increase in density and amount of collagen fibers in the vessel walls, along with decreasing elasticity of the wall.

The skin is one of the first systems to show signs of the aging process. The epidermis and dermis are visible markers of aging and greatly affect placement of peripheral catheters. As a person ages, there is loss of subcutaneous supporting tissue and resultant thinning of the skin. The turnover rate for the production of new cells slows: at the age of 20, turnover of new cells take 3 weeks, at 30, 6 weeks, and after 30, 2 months (Whitehouse, 1992). Folds, lines, wrinkles, and slackness appear as the skin ages. *Purpura* and *ecchymoses* may appear owing to the greater fragility of the dermal and subcutaneous vessels and the loss of support for the skin capillaries. Minor trauma can easily cause bruising.

A common symptom in older people is pruritus or "itchiness." This is usually caused by dry skin and by medications and should be considered when preparing for parenteral therapy.

The dermis becomes relatively dehydrated and loses strength and elasticity. This layer has underlying papillae that hold the epidermis and dermis together; this means that as one ages, the older skin loosens. Older skin has decreased flexibility in the collagen fibers, increased fragility of the capillaries, and fewer capillaries. Older skin feels "dryer" because of loss of subcutaneous fat and decreased production of sebum and sweat (Whitehouse, 1992).

Fluid Balance in the Elderly

Fluid balance in the elderly is affected by the physiologic changes associated with aging. The older person does not possess the fluid reserves or the ability to adapt readily to rapid changes. Alterations in fluid and electrolyte balance frequently accompany illness.

Renal structural changes associated with the aging process result in decreased glomerular filtration rate. When fluid is restricted for any reason, the nurse must be aware that there will be a slower conservation of fluids in response to the fluid restriction.

The total body water is reduced by 6%, which creates a potential for fluid volume deficit. Gastrointestinal changes such as decreased volume of saliva, gastric juice and calcium absorption cause the mouth to be drier in the aged, in addition to the potential for sodium and potassium deficit during episodes of vomiting and gastric suction, and calcium deficit.

Cardiovascular and respiratory changes combine to contribute to a slower response to the stress of blood loss, fluid depletion, shock, and acid-base imbalances (Metheny, 1996). The elderly patient should be assessed for potential fluid volume disturbances (Table 10–4).

331

TABLE 10–4. ASSESSMENT GUIDELINES FOR FLUID VOLUME DISTURBANCES IN THE ELDERLY

Skin turgor of forehead or sternum
Temperature (normal body temperature often below 98.6° F)
Rate and filling of veins in hand or foot
Daily weight possibly a more accurate measure of patient's fluid balance (Pflaum, 1979)
Intake and output
Tongue—center should be moist, with observable pool of saliva beneath the tongue (even though the aged have decreased saliva, this method is useful in evaluating hydration) (Robinson & Demuth, 1985)
Orthostatic (postural) blood pressure changes
Swallowing ability
Functional assessment of patient's ability to obtain fluids

Venipuncture Techniques

The elderly patient requires special venipuncture techniques to successfully place and maintain I.V. therapy. The potential complications associated with trauma, surgery, or illness in the elderly, along with the physiologic changes, require that the nurse be knowledgeable in the special skills associated with delivery of care.

Vascular Access Device Selection

Consider the skin and vein changes of the older adult before initiating I.V. therapies. Also, consider catheter design and gauge size. Softer, more flexible materials and those that soften after insertion into the vein may allow increased indwelling time and prevent or reduce complications (Gaukroger, Roberts, & Manners, 1988).

The bevel-tip design of the peripheral catheter's needle may help to decrease trauma to vein.

✎ **NOTE:** Use of a 22- to 24-gauge catheter is appropriate for delivery of I.V. therapy in the elderly. These sizes help reduce insertion-related trauma (Fabian, 1995).

Selecting Administration Equipment

Because of the risk of overadministration or underadministration of I.V. therapy, the type of infusion equipment selected should provide safe, consistent delivery of medication and fluids.

Advanced technology provides uses of stationary and ambulatory electronic monitoring devices. Monitoring devices must have safety features to protect the high-risk patient from fluid volume overload.

✎ **NOTE:** To prevent fluid overload, use a microdrip administration set when appropriate.

✎ **NOTE:** Because of the fragile nature of the veins of the elderly, be aware of the potential complications associated with pressures generated from mechanical infusion devices (see Chapter 7 for a discussion of safety features associated with programmable pumps).

Selecting a Vein

Selecting a vein that can support I.V. therapy for at least 72 hours can be a challenge for the nurse. Initial venipuncture should be in the most distal portion of the extremity, allowing for subsequent venipunctures to move progressively upward. However, in the older adult, the veins of the hands may not be the best choice for initial site because of loss of subcutaneous fat and thinning of the skin. Physiologic changes in the skin and veins must be considered when a site is selected. Areas for I.V. access should have adequate tissue and skeletal support. Avoid flexion areas and areas with bruising, because the oncotic pressure is increased in these areas and cause vessels to collapse.

✎ **NOTE:** To enhance vein location, use adequate lighting. Bright, direct overhead examination lights may have a "washout" effect on the vein. Instead, use side lighting, which can add contour and "shadowing," which highlights the skin color and texture, and allows visualization of the vein shadow below the skin (Enrich, 1991).

Use a tourniquet to help distend and locate appropriate veins, but avoid applying it too tightly because it can cause vein damage when the vein is punctured. During venous distention, palpate the vein to determine its condition. Veins that feel ribbed or rippled may distend readily when a tourniquet is applied, but these sites are often impossible to access, causing pain for the patient (Fabian, 1995).

Valves become stiff and less effective with age. Bumps along the vein path—valves—may cause problems during attempts at vein access. Venous circulation may be sluggish, resulting in slow venous return, distention, venous stasis, and dependent edema. The catheter may not thread into a vein with stiff valves.

✎ **NOTE:** To thread a catheter through an inflexible valve, reduce the catheter size by several gauges.

Small surface veins appear as thin tortuous veins with many bifurcations (Fig. 10–4). Appropriate catheter gauge and length selection are critical to a successful I.V. access placement in these veins.

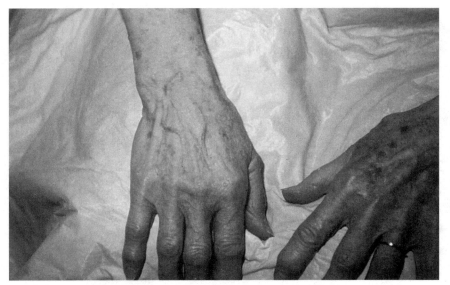

Figure 10–4. Fragile veins of the elderly patient.

Cannulation Techniques

In the elderly, stabilization of the vein is critical. The vessels may lack stability as a result of loss of tissue mass and may tend to roll (Coulter, 1992). Techniques to perform a venipuncture on the elderly include:

> Use of traction by placing the thumb directly along the vein axis about 2 to 3 inches below the intended venipuncture site. The palm and fingers of the traction hand serve to hold and stabilize the extremity. Using the index finger of the hand, provide traction to further stretch the skin above the intended venipuncture site. Maintain traction throughout venipuncture.
>
> Insert the catheter, using either direct or indirect technique. When direct technique is used, insert the catheter at a 20- to 30-degree angle in a single motion, penetrating the skin and vein simultaneously. Do not stab or thrust the catheter into the skin; this could cause the catheter to advance too deeply and accidentally damage the vein. Use the indirect method (two-step) for patients with small, delicate veins (Hadaway, 1991). An alternative method is to have another nurse apply digital pressure with the hand above the site of venipuncture and release it after the vein has been entered.
>
> For patients with very small spidery veins, preflush the catheter before access is attempted. Preflushing enhances the backflow (LaRocca, 1993).

✎ **NOTE:** If the veins are fragile or if the patient is on anticoagulants, avoid using a tourniquet; constricted blood flow may overdistend fragile veins, causing vein damage, vessel hemorrhages, or subcutaneous bleeding.

SPECIAL PROBLEMS

Before initiating I.V. therapy, the nurse must know the patient's diagnosis and allergies. Conditions involving alterations in skin surface, hard sclerosed veins, obesity, and edema will affect the technique that the therapist will use for a successful venipuncture (Table 10–5).

Alterations in Skin Surfaces

Take precautions in patients with alterations in skin surfaces due to lesions, burns, or disease process. Patients with altered skin integrity are often photosensitive and

TABLE 10–5. **SPECIAL PROBLEMS**

Alterations in skin surfaces
    Systemic lupus erythematosus
    Dermatitis
    Skin lesions
    Burns
Hard sclerosed veins
    Renal failure
    Intravenous drug abuser
    Sickle cell patient
Obese patient
Edematous patient

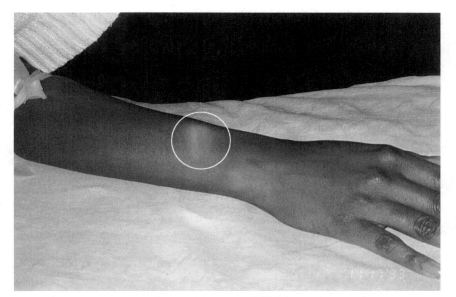

Figure 10–5. Tangential lighting.

need additional protection of already damaged tissue. Tangential lighting is recommended (Fig. 10–5). This indirect lighting does not flatten veins or cause damage to the skin. Use a light directed toward the side of the patient's extremity to illuminate the blue veins and provide a guide for venipuncture. This technique can also be used on dark-skinned patients.

Hard Sclerosed Vessels

If the peripheral vessels are hard and sclerosed because of a disease process, due to personal misuse, or frequent drug therapy, venous access will be difficult. The practitioner should assess for collateral circulation. To find collateral veins, the nurse can use the multiple tourniquet technique. By increasing the *oncotic* pressure inside the tissue, blood is forced into the small vessels of the periphery, Fig. 10–6). This technique helps the novice to learn the difference between collateral veins and sclerosed vessels. Usually, veins appear in the hand with this approach (Fabian, 1995).

Procedure
Place one tourniquet high on the arm for 2 minutes and leave in place. The arm should be stroked downward toward the hand.

After 2 minutes, place a second tourniquet at midarm just below the antecubital fossa for 2 minutes.

If soft collateral veins do not appear in the forearm, place a third tourniquet at the wrist.

✎ **NOTE:** Tourniquets must not be left on longer than 6 minutes.

335

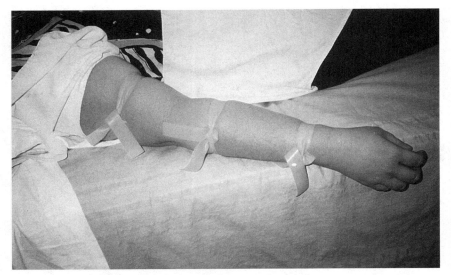

Figure 10–6. Multiple-tourniquet technique.

Obesity

In patients with excessive adipose tissue, the veins in the extremities react one of two ways to the subcutaneous fat:

1. The vessels will be buried deep in the tissue, thereby requiring a 2-inch catheter to access the vein.
2. The vasculature will be forced to the surface because the veins have been displaced by the adipose tissue. A vessel can usually be located below the antecubital site, on the lateral dorsum of the forearm.

Multiple tourniquet technique can be used to identify veins in obese patients. Place one tourniquet on the lower forearm and one tourniquet 2 minutes later at the wrist to visualize hand veins.

✎ **NOTE:** Use of a blood pressure cuff is not recommended on obese patients because increased pressure from the cuff can cause backflow of blood.

Edema

In locating accessible vasculature in the patient with edema, the nurse must displace tissue fluid with digital pressure. Often this will allow visualization of an accessible vein. Care must be taken not to contaminate the site once the area is prepared. Venipuncture must be done quickly after the area is prepped to prevent the edematous fluid from obscuring the site.

✎ **NOTE:** Edematous fluid causes an increase in oncotic pressure. Therefore, if the fluid is not infusing after the catheter is in place, suspect that the vein may have collapsed as a result of the oncotic pressure in the tissue (Fabian, 1995).

Nursing Plan of Care

THE PEDIATRIC CLIENT

Focus Assessment

Subjective
Interview parents for current health status

Objective
Measure height and weight for calculation of body surface area and drug dosage. Note developmental level.

Outcome Criteria
The patient will:
Maintain hydration status, with decreased edema
Demonstrate beneficial effects from I.V. therapy
Return to pre-illness weight
Have normal vital signs for age
Participate in activities appropriate to age
Demonstrate reduced fear behaviors
Participate in decision-making process about self-care when appropriate

Nursing Diagnoses
1. Impaired skin integrity related to I.V. infiltration, diarrhea, edema or dry skin
2. Alteration in comfort, pain, related to position of I.V.
3. Risk for infection related to invasive procedures
4. Potential anxiety related to the procedure of I.V. therapy
5. Altered body image related to placement of I.V. therapy equipment
6. Alteration in family process related to hospitalization of family member
7. Parental role conflict related to illness and/or hospitalization of a child
8. Sensory and perceptual alterations related to fluid imbalances
9. Ineffective thermoregulation related to newborn transition to extrauterine environment
10. Fear related to loss of control, autonomy, independence, competence, and self-esteem

Nursing Management: Critical Activities
Monitor intake and output.
Explain procedures and equipment.
Provide opportunities for nonnutritive sucking in infant.
Encourage parents to provide daily care of child.
Instruct parents in performing special care for child.
Inform parents about child's progress.
Explain rationale for treatment and procedures to parents and child when appropriate.
Comfort infant after painful procedure.
Maintain daily routine during hospitalization.
Provide quiet, uninterrupted environment during naptime and night-time as appropriate.
Immobilize when appropriate for venipuncture.
Use appropriate equipment for delivery of safe I.V. therapy.
Perform I.V. checks every 2 hours and document.
Monitor for fluid overload.
Monitor vital signs.
Maintain universal precautions.
Calculate drug dosage correctly and double check with another nurse before administration.

PATIENT EDUCATION

PEDIATRIC PATIENT

Provide age-appropriate instructions.

Infant: Encourage parents to keep in infant's line of vision and encourage parents to comfort child.

Toddler: Instruct to allow child to participate during instruction, give simple explanations, explain procedures in relation to what child sees, hears, tastes, smells, and feels; emphasize aspects of procedures that require cooperation (e.g., lying still).

Communicate using behaviors; use play-demonstrate with dolls and small replicas of equipment

Limit teaching sessions to 5–10 minutes.

Prepare immediately before procedure.

Preschool: Explain procedure in simple terms and in relation to how it affects the child.

Demonstrate use of and allow child to play with equipment.

Encourage "playing out" on a doll.

Avoid overestimating child's comprehension; encourage child to verbalize.

Limit each teaching session to 10–15 minutes.

Explain unfamiliar situations such as noises, light.

School age: Explain procedures using correct terminology; explain reasons for procedures using anatomic drawings.

Explain function and operation of equipment in clear terms.

Allow manipulation of and practice with equipment.

Allow for questions and discussion.

Limit teaching sessions to 20 minutes.

Instruct in advance of procedures.

Use small groups or encourage teaching of peers.

Instruct parents.

Provide ways to maintain control (e.g., deep breathing, counting, relaxation).

Adolescent: Involve client in all decisions.

Discuss how procedure may affect physical appearance.

Be aware of adolescent's difficulty with accepting authority.

Instruct in groups and encourage peer instruction.

Teaching session can be as along as 45 minutes.

Source:
From Wong, D.L. (1995). *Nursing care of infants and children,* 5th ed. St. Louis: Mosby–Year Book.

ELDERLY PATIENT

Speak slowly, clearly, and directly to the elder patient with sensory deficits.

Address the patient by his or her proper name.

Explain the steps of any procedure to increase cooperation and decrease anxiety.

Do not use terminology that is unfamiliar (Andersen, 1989; Weinstein, 1993).

HOME CARE ISSUES

PEDIATRIC PATIENT

Focus on psychosocial and developmental needs of child and family in planning home infusion therapy.

Because the child is more mobile and active in the home, use a portable infusion device that is easy for the child and family to operate.

Encourage parents to spend private time with each of their children.

Keep in mind that parents need support from a home care agency in case the hospital unit nurses are not available; this may increase anxiety and fear.

Identify alternate caregivers.

ELDERLY PATIENT

Specific challenges of the elderly patient in administration of home infusion therapy:

Patient may be less ready to adapt to environmental changes, especially relating to independence.

Teaching of complex drug admixtures, tubing connections, I.V. maintenance, I.V. pumps programming, and accessing and de-accessing devices requires patience and step-by-step approaches. All equipment should be user-friendly. Written teaching material, video programs, and demonstration with return demonstration can be helpful (Weinstein, 1993).

Evaluation of language or cultural differences can dramatically affect understanding of necessary health care concepts.

Sensory changes occur with aging (e.g., in vision, hearing, and manual dexterity). Observe the client working with various devices (the needleless system may eliminate the risk of needle-stick injuries) to ensure proficiency.

COMPETENCY CRITERIA

Competency Statement: The competent I.V. therapy nurse will be able to administer I.V. therapy to the pediatric patient.

COGNITIVE CRITERIA

	Skilled	*Needs Education*

PATIENT ASSESSMENT
1. Assesses psychosocial needs and developmental level.

2. Includes parent participation where appropriate.

PERFORMANCE CRITERIA
1. Chooses age-appropriate site for venous access:

   Scalp vein

   Dorsum of hand

   Dorsum of foot

2. Makes age-appropriate selection of venipuncture device.

3. Makes choice of equipment appropriate for safe infusion to pediatric patient:

   500-mL fluid container or less

   Use of volume control device

   Appropriate choice of electronic infusion device

   Appropriate choice of cannula length and gauge.

5. Documentation of site assessments:

   Every 2 hours

SUGGESTED EVALUATION CRITERIA

Written test for cognitive criteria

Demonstration of I.V. techniques on pediatric model

Demonstration of I.V. technique with supervision on pediatric patient.

KEY POINTS

Pediatric I.V. therapy
    Physiologic characteristics of the neonate
        Total body weight 90% water, high ratio of extracellular water to intracellular water
        Metabolic demand influenced by increased muscular activity, thermal stress, congenital abnormalities, and respiratory distress syndrome
        Heat production increases caloric expenditure by 7% per degree of temperature elevation
        Immature renal system
        Integumentary system important in regulation of fluid and electrolyte needs
    Physical assessment
        Risk factors
            Prematurity
            Catabolic disease states
            Hypothermia and hyperthermia
            Metabolic and respiratory acid-base imbalances
        Components
            Measurement of head circumference (up to 1 year)
            Height or length
            Vital signs
            Skin turgor
            Presence of tears
            Moistness and color of mucous membranes
            Urinary output
            Characteristics of fontanelles
            Level of child's activity
        Assessment of fluid needs
            Meter square method
            Weight method
            Caloric method
        Factors affecting fluid needs
            Temperature elevation
            Loss of gastrointestinal fluids
            Diarrhea
            Small intestinal drainage
    Site selection
        Peripheral routes
            Scalp veins (controversial)
                Frontal
                Preauricular
                Supraorbital
                Occipital
            Dorsum of hand and forearm
                Requires limb immobilization
            Dorsum of foot
                Contraindicated in child who is walking
    Selecting the equipment
        Administration equipment
            Safety of the child

341

Activity level
Age and size
Needle selection
Scalp vein—27- to 19-gauge
Over-the-needle catheter–preferred
26- to 24-gauge for neonates
24- to 22-gauge for children
Venipuncture techniques
Perform venipuncture in separate room.
Use pacifier for neonates and infants.
Use mummy and clove-hitch immobilizers.
Warm hands before applying gloves.
Use rubberband to dilate scalp veins.
Use surgical lubricating jelly under adhesive tape.
Stabilize cannula with padded tongue blade.
Use stickers or drawings as rewards.
Always have extra help.
Medication administration
Intermittent infusions
In-line calibrated chamber
Retrograde infusion
Syringe pump
Formulas for delivery of pediatric therapies
Body weight method
Body surface area
Bastedo's rule
Clark's rule
Cowling's rule
Fried's rule
Young's rule
Alternative administration routes
Intraosseous infusions
Good route in emergency situation for delivery of fluids and medications
Limited site for 24 hours
Sites: proximal tibia, distal tibia and femur
Used only in children under 6 years of age.
Contraindications
Cellulitis or infected burn
Fractured bone
Osteoporosis
Osteogenesis imperfecta
Umbilical vein and arteries
Emergency access in delivery room
Hemodynamic monitoring in neonatal ICU

Geriatric I.V. therapy
Physiologic changes
Homeostatic mechanisms less efficient
Immune system becomes hyporesponsive to foreign antigens
Cardiovascular: arteries chemically and anatomically changed, elastic fibers
fray and split, increased collagen fibers, and decrease elasticity of wall
Skin: loss of subcutaneous supporting tissue, thinning of skin
Fluid balance in the elderly

342

Renal structures: decreased glomerular filtration rate
  Total body weight water reduced by 6% leading to potential fluid volume
    deficit
  Assessment guidelines for fluid volume disturbances in the elderly
    Skin turgor
    Temperature
    Rate and filling of veins in hand or foot
    Daily weight
    Intake and output
    Center of tongue should be moist
    Postural blood pressure
    Swallowing ability
    Functional assessment of patient's ability to obtain fluids
Venipuncture techniques
  Device selection
    Consideration of skin and vein changes
    Softer catheter materials and small-gauge needles
    Microdrip administration set
  Vein selection
    Adequate tissue and skeletal support
    Adequate (side) lighting
    Light application of tourniquet

Special problems
  Alterations in skin surfaces
    Consider the patient's photosensitivity and potential for skin damage.
    Use tangential lighting.
  Hard sclerosed vessels
    Multiple tourniquet technique
    Palpation of hard sclerosed veins versus softer collateral circulation
  Obesity
    Use of 2-inch catheters
    Use of lateral veins displaced by adipose tissue
    Use of multiple tourniquet techniqe
  Edema
    Displace edema with digital pressure.

CRITICAL THINKING ACTIVITY

1. You are working on a pediatric ward and assigned a 6-month-old baby with meningitis. The I.V. is placed in the baby's scalp. You assess the baby and find the site covered with a white paper cup and lots of tape; the baby's eye beneath the cup is swollen. What is the problem? How do you remedy this situation?

2. You must start an I.V. on a 70-year-old obese person with a diagnosis of systemic lupus erythematosus. What do you need to consider before venipuncture, and what techniques should you use to be successful?

3. You must start an I.V. on a 10-year-old boy who has never been hospitalized. His diagnosis is osteomyelitis. How would you approach this patient?

4. You are working in an emergency room and a 2-year-old near-drowning victim is brought in and is in respiratory distress. Would you consider intraosseous infusion?

POST-TEST, CHAPTER 10

Fill in the missing term in the following sentences.

1. _____ infusion is the delivery of fluids and electrolytes into the medullary cavity in the bone.

2. The _____ method calculates the metabolic expenditure of energy in figuring fluid replacement.

3. The period of extrauterine life up to the first 28 days of life is called the _____ period.

4. The breakdown of chemical compounds into more elementary principles by the body is referred to as _____.

5. The _____ _____ _____ is determined through use of a nomogram.

6. List three of the six common reasons for I.V. therapy in an infant.

A. _____

B. _____

C. _____

7. The preferred choice for I.V. site in the young infant under age 9 months is the:
   A. Frontal vein in the scalp
   B. Dorsum of the foot
   C. Dorsum of the hand
   D. Occipital vein on the head

8. The weight method of estimating fluid requirements in a child is:
   A. Weighing diapers and estimating output to replace sensible losses
   B. Formula based on weight in kilograms to estimate fluid needs
   C. Calculation of metabolic expenditure of energy based on weight
   D. Determined by use of a nomogram

9. In a dark-skinned person the best method for locating an accessible vein is:
   A. Multiple tourniquets
   B. Tangential lighting
   C. Direct overhead lighting
   D. Light application of tourniquet

10. What is the most appropriate needle for use on a 2-month-old infant?
   A. 18 gauge over-the-needle catheter
   B. 23- to 25-gauge scalp vein needle
   C. 16-gauge scalp vein needle
   D. 22- to 24-gauge over-the-needle catheter

11. Intraosseous infusion is contraindicated in patients with:
   A. Fractures in the extremities
   B. Infected burns
   C. Osteoporosis
   D. All of the above

12. When performing an I.V. on a toddler, methods that can be used to assist the therapist in this invasive procedure based on developmental age, would include:
   A. Letting the child express feelings and scream
   B. Encouraging the child to hold a favorite toy or blanket
   C. Performing the procedure quickly with assistance from parents or other staff
   D. All of the above

13. When performing an I.V. on a school-age child, it is important to:
    A. Explain the procedure to the patient in simple terms
    B. Limit explanations and perform procedure quickly
    C. Demonstrate the procedure using a doll or stuffed animal
    D. None of the above

14. List six of the nine key points in assessment of fluid status in the elderly.

    A. _____

    B. _____

    C. _____

    D. _____

    E. _____

    F. _____

ANSWERS TO CHAPTER 10

PRE-TEST

1. C	6. F	11. D	16. A
2. D	7. E	12. E	17. C
3. E	8. B	13. D	18. T
4. B	9. A	14. A	19. T
5. A	10. A	15. C	20. T

POST-TEST

1. Intraosseous
2. Caloric
3. Neonatal
4. Catabolism
5. Body surface area
6. Fluid volume deficit, electrolyte imbalance, nutritional support, antibiotic therapy, and chemotherapy
7. C
8. B
9. B
10. D
11. D
12. D
13. A
14. Skin turgor, temperature, rate and filling of veins in hand or foot, intake and output, daily weight, center of tongue for moisture, postural changes affect blood pressure, swallowing ability, functional assessment of patient's ability to obtain fluids

REFERENCES

American Association of Retired Persons (AARP) (1985). *A Profile of Older Americans.* U.S. Department of Health & Human Services.

Andersen, P. (1989). A fresh look at assessing the elderly. *RN6*, 28–39.

Arthur, G.M. (1984). When your littlest patients need IVs. *RN, 7*, 30–34.

Blatz, S., & Paes, B.A. (1990). Intravenous infusion by superfical vein in the neonate. *Journal of Intravenous Nursing, 13* (2), 122–128.

Chameides, L. (1992). *Textbook of pediatric advanced life support.* Dallas: American Heart Association.

Coulter, K. (1992). Intravenous therapy for the elder patient: Implications for the intravenous nurse. *Journal of Intravenous Nursing (Supplement 15)* S18–S23.

Delaney, C.W., & Lauer, M.L. (1988). *Intravenous therapy: A guide to quality care.* Philadelphia: J.B. Lippincott.

Enrich, M. (1991). Performing venipuncture in elderly patients. *Nursing 91, 21.*

Fabian, B. (1991). *I.V. therapy across the generations.* Intravenous Nursing Society Annual Conference, Orlando, Florida.

Fabian, B. (1995). Intravenous therapy in the older adult. In Terry, J., Baranowski, L., Lonsway, R., & Hedrick, C., eds. *Intravenous therapy: Clinical principles and practice. Intravenous Nurses Society.* Philadelphia: W.B. Saunders.

Intravenous Nursing Society. (1996). *Standards of practice.* Philadelphia: J.B. Lippincott.

Gaukroger, P.B., Roberts, J.G., & Manners, T.A. (1988). Infusion thrombophlebitis: A prospective comparison of 645 vialon and teflon cannulae in anesthetic and postoperative use. *Anaesthesia Intensive Care, 16* (3), 265–271.

Hadaway, L. (1991). I.V. tips. *Geriatric Nursing, 2,* 78–81.

Hodge, D. (1985). Intraosseous infusions: A review. *Pediatric Emergency Care, 1* 215–218.

Jarmen, C. (1985). Vein trauma: Its complications and prevention. *Intravenous Theapy News,* (7), 4.

LaRocca, J. (1993). *Pocket guide to intravenous therapy,* 2nd ed. St Louis: Mosby–Year Book, 14–36.

Marlow, D.R., & Redding, B.A. (1988). *Textbook of pediatric nursing,* 6th ed. Philadelphia: W.B. Saunders.

Metheny, N.M. (1996). *Fluid and electrolyte balance: Nursing considerations,* 3rd ed. Philadelphia: J.B. Lippincott.

Peck, K.R., & Altieri, M. (1988). Intraosseous infusions: An old technique with modern applications. *Pediatric Nursing, 14* (4), 296–298.

Pflaum, S. (1979). Investigation of intake-output as a means of assessing body fluid balance. *Heart & Lung, 8,* 495.

Robinson, S., & Demuth, P. (1985). Diagnostic studies for the aged: What are the dangers? *Journal of Gerontological Nursing, 11* (6).

Rossetti, V.A., Thompson, B.M., & Miller, J. (1985). Intraosseous infusion: An alternative route of pediatric intravascular access. *Annals of Emergency Medicine, 14,* 885–888.

Smeltzer, S.C., & Bare, B.G. (1992). *Brunner and Suddarth's textbook of medical-surgical nursing,* 7th ed. Philadelphia: J.B. Lippincott, pp. 165–193.

Spivey, W.H. (1987). Intraosseous infusions. *Journal of Pediatrics, 111* (5), 639–643.

Stifter, J., & Shanahan, N. (1994). The IV bubbles and boards system. *Journal of Pediatric Nursing, 9* (6), 417–419.

Taylor, S. (1992). Lost in the system. *Journal of Intravenous Nursing (Supplement 15)* S2–S6.

Tietjen, S.D. (1990). Starting an infant's I.V. *American Journal of Nursing, 5,* 44–46.

Weinstein, S.M. (1990). Math calculations for intravenous nurses. *Journal of Intravenous Nursing, 13* (4), 231–236.

Weinstein, S.M. (1993). *Plumer's principles and practices of intravenous therapy,* 6th ed. Philadelphia: J.B. Lippincott.

Wheeler, C.A. (1989). Pediatric intraosseous infusion: An old technique in modern health care technology. *Journal of Intravenous Nursing, 12* (6), 371–376.

Wheeler, C.A., & Frey, A.M. (1995). Intravenous therapy in children. In Terry, J., Baranowski, L., Lonsway, R., & Hedrick, C. *Intravenous therapy: Clinical principles and practice. Intravenous Nurses Society.* (467–494) Philadelphia: W.B. Saunders.

Whitehouse, M.J. (1992). The physiology of aging. *Journal of Intravenous Nursing (Supplement 15)* S7–S13.

Wong, D.L. (1995). *Nursing care of infants and children,* 5th ed. St. Louis: Mosby–Year Book.

United States Department of Health and Human Services. (1990). *Healthy People 2000.* Washington: U.S. Government Printing Office.

UNIT THREE

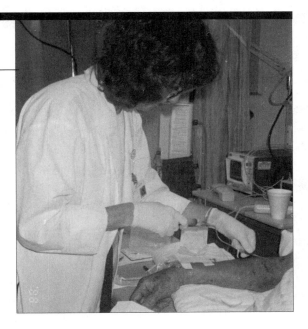

ADVANCED PRACTICE

CHAPTER 11
Administration of Intravenous Medications

CHAPTER 12
Central Venous Access Devices

CHAPTER 13
Transfusion Therapy

CHAPTER 14
Antineoplastic Therapy

CHAPTER 15
Nutritional Support

Administration of Intravenous Medications

CHAPTER CONTENTS

GLOSSARY
LEARNING OBJECTIVES
PRE-TEST, CHAPTER 11
ADVANTAGES OF INTRAVENOUS MEDICATION
DISADVANTAGES OF INTRAVENOUS
  MEDICATION
Drug Interactions
Adsorption
Errors in Mixing
Speed Shock
Extravasation
Chemical Phlebitis
DRUG COMPATIBILITY
Physical Incompatibility
Chemical Incompatibility
Therapeutic Incompatibility
METHODS OF INTRAVENOUS MEDICATION
  ADMINISTRATION
Continuous Infusion
Intermittent Infusion
Direct Injection (I.V. Push)
Continuous Subcutaneous Infusion
Intraspinal Medication Infusion

Arteriovenous Fistula
ANTI-INFECTIVE ADMINISTRATION
  CONSIDERATIONS
Antibiotics
Antifungal Agents
Antiviral Agents
NARCOTIC INFUSION CONSIDERATIONS
Patient-Controlled Analgesia
INVESTIGATIONAL DRUGS
NURSING PLAN OF CARE: ADMINISTRATION
  OF I.V. MEDICATIONS
PATIENT EDUCATION
HOME CARE ISSUES
Home Antibiotic Therapy
Home Pain Management
COMPETENCY CRITERIA
KEY POINTS
CRITICAL THINKING ACTIVITY
POST-TEST, CHAPTER 11
ANSWERS TO CHAPTER 11
Pre-Test
Post-Test
REFERENCES

GLOSSARY

Absorption   Process of movement of medication from drug administration sites to the vasculature
Adsorption   Attachment of one substance to the surface of another
Admixture   Combination of two or more medications
Ambulatory infusion device   An electronic infusion device specifically designed in size to be worn on the body to promote patient mobility and independence
Biotransformation   Metabolism; the enzymatic alteration of a drug molecule

Bolus Concentrated medication or solution given rapidly over a short period of time; may be given by direct I.V. injection or I.V. drip

Chemical incompatibility Change in the molecular structure or pharmacologic properties of a substance, which may or may not be visually observed

Clinical trial Planned experiment that involves patients and is designed to evoke an appropriate treatment of future patients with a given medical condition

Compatibility Capable of being mixed and administered without undergoing undesirable chemical or physical changes or loss of therapeutic action

Delivery system A product that allows for the administration of medication

Distribution Process of delivering a drug to the various tissues of the body

Drug interaction An interaction between two drugs; also, a drug that causes an increase or decrease in another drug's pharmacologic effects

Epidural Situated on or over the dura mater

Incompatibility Chemical or physical reaction that occurs among two or more drugs or between drug and delivery device

Intermittent drug infusion I.V. therapy administered at prescribed intervals

Intraspinal Spaces surrounding the spinal cord, including epidural and intrathecal

Intrathecal Within a sheath, surrounded by the epidural space and separated from it by the dura mater; contains cerebrospinal fluid

Intravenous push Manual administration of medication under pressure over 1 minute or as manufacturer of medication recommends

Multiple-dose vial Medication bottle that is hermetically sealed with a rubber stopper and designed to be entered more than once

Physical incompatibility An undesirable change that is visually observed

Single-dose vial Medication bottle that is hermetically sealed with a rubber stopper and is intended for one-time use

Therapeutic incompatibility Undesirable effect occurring within a patient as a result of two or more drugs being given concurrently

Vesicant I.V. medication that causes blisters and tissue injury when it escapes into surrounding tissue

LEARNING OBJECTIVES

Upon completion of this chapter, the reader will be able to:

- Define terminology related to administration of I.V. medications.
- Identify the advantages of I.V. medications.
- List the hazards associated with I.V. medications.
- Identify the methods through which medications may be delivered by the I.V. route.
- Identify three incompatibilities related to I.V. therapy.
- Describe the proper technique in delivery of I.V. bolus medication.
- Describe the treatment of adverse effects of I.V. medications.
- State the precautions to be followed when medication is infused via the epidural route.
- List the key steps in dressing management of an intraspinal catheter.
- Describe the method of delivery and nursing consideration for intraperitoneal therapy.
- Describe the special considerations when administering anti-infective therapy, chemotherapeutic agents, and narcotics via the I.V. route.
- List the key points in delivering medications intravenously for pain control.
- Describe the nurse's role in the delivery of investigational drugs.
- Develop a plan of care for the patient receiving I.V. medications using the nursing process.

PRE-TEST, CHAPTER 11

Match the definition in column II with the term in column I.

Column I

1. _____ adsorption
2. _____ biotransformation
3. _____ single-dose vial
4. _____ epidural
5. _____ therapeutic incompatibility
6. _____ chemical incompatibility
7. _____ physical incompatibility
8. _____ drug interaction
9. _____ clinical trial
10. _____ distribution

Column II

A. Planned experiment designed to evoke an appropriate treatment for a given medical condition

B. A change in the molecular structure or properties of a substance

C. An undesirable effect when two or more drugs are given concurrently

D. An interaction between a drug and another drug that result in increase or decrease in pharmacologic effects

E. A process of delivering a drug to the various tissues

F. Metabolism; enzymatic alteration of a drug molecule

G. An undesirable change that is visual

H. Medication that is hermetically sealed with a rubber stopper and intended for one-time use

I. Situated over the duramater

J. Attachment of one substance to the surface of another

11. Which of the following are advantages of I.V. medications?
    A. Route for irritating substances, instant drug action, and better control administration
    B. Speed shock, rapid onset of action, and allows for absorption of drugs in gastric juices
    C. Prevents errors in compounding of medication, low risk of infiltration, and low risk of phlebitis
    D. Allows for uninterrupted control of rate, low risk of side effects, and low risk of adsorption

12. Incompatibilities of drugs fall into three classes, which include:
    A. Physical, incompatible, and chemical
    B. Physical, chemical, and therapeutic
    C. Therapeutic, absorption, and distribution

Match the description of the catheter in column II with the term in column I.

Column I

13. _____ epidural
14. _____ intrathecal
15. _____ subcutaneous

Column II

A. Catheter is placed over the dura mater

B. Needle is inserted into the tissue spaces

C. Catheter is within a sheath, contains spinal fluid

351

16. **T F** I.V. bolus medication should be given slowly and according to manufacturer's recommendations.

17. **T F** Alcohol should not be used on epidural catheter dressing management because of the risk of migration of alcohol into the epidural space.

18. **T F** Hazards of I.V. medication include the risk of extravasation.

19. **T F** Intermittent infusions can be given by piggyback, by intermittent infusion, or by I.V. push.

20. The role of the registered nurse in investigational drugs would include:
    A. Communication with Institutional Review Board
    B. I.V. administration of investigational drug
    C. Assisting with final study report
    D. Participating in collection of data
    E. All of the above

In the future, which I shall not see, for I am old, may a better way be opened! May the methods by which every infant, every human being will have the best chance of health, the methods by which every sick person will have the best chance of recovery, be learned and practiced! Hospitals are only an intermediate state of civilization never intended, at all events, to take in the whole sick population.

FLORENCE NIGHTINGALE, 1860

ADVANTAGES OF INTRAVENOUS MEDICATION

The infusion of I.V. medication provides a direct access to the circulatory system, a route for administration of fluids and drugs to patients who cannot tolerate oral medications, a method of instant drug action, and a method of instant drug administration termination. This route offers pronounced advantages over subcutaneous, intramuscular, and oral routes (Table 11–1). Drugs that cannot be absorbed by other routes because of the large molecular size of the drug or destruction of the drug by gastric juices can be administered directly to the site of distribution, the circulatory system, via I.V. infusion. Drugs with irritating properties that cause pain and trauma when given by the intramuscular or subcutaneous route can be given intravenously. When a drug is administered intravenously, there is instant drug action, which is an advantage in emergency situations. The I.V. route also provides instant drug termination if sensitivity or adverse reactions occur. This route provides for control over the rate in which drugs are administered; prolonged action can be controlled by administering a dilute medication infusion intermittently over a prolonged time frame (Weinstein, 1993).

DISADVANTAGES OF INTRAVENOUS MEDICATION

Despite the many advantages of I.V. medication, there are disadvantages associated with this venous route, which are not found in other drug therapies (Table 11–2). The number of drug combinations, along with the ever-increasing production of drugs and parenteral fluids, has compounded these disadvantages. The disadvantages specific to the administration of I.V. drugs include drug interactions, drug loss via adsorption of I.V. containers and administration sets, errors in mixing techniques, the complications of speed shock, extravasation of vesicant drugs, and phlebitis (Todd, 1988).

TABLE 11–1. **ADVANTAGES OF INTRAVENOUS MEDICATION ADMINISTRATION**

1. Provides a direct access to the circulatory system
2. Provides a route for drugs that irritate the gastric mucosa
3. Provides a route for instant drug action
4. Provides a route for delivering high drug concentrations
5. Provides for instant drug termination if sensitivity or adverse reaction occurs
6. Provides for better control over rate of drug administration
7. Provides a route of administration in patients in whom use of the gastrointestinal tract is limited

353

TABLE 11–2. **DISADVANTAGES OF INTRAVENOUS MEDICATION**

1. Drug interaction due to incompatibilities
2. Adsorption of the drug impaired due to leaching into I.V. container or administration set
3. Errors in compounding (mixing) of medication
4. Speed shock
5. Estravasation of a vesicant drug
6. Chemical phlebitis

The nurse responsible for delivery of I.V. medications must have technical knowledge of the mechanism of drug delivery and an awareness of drug action and adverse effects to ensure safe delivery of the medication.

Drug Interactions

Drug interactions are not always clear-cut. Many factors affect drug interactions, including drug solubility and drug compatibility. The potential for incompatibilities is unique to the injectable drugs. Mixing of two incompatible drugs in a solution can cause an adverse interaction.

FACTORS AFFECTING DRUG SOLUBILITY AND COMPATIBILITY INCLUDE
1. Drug concentration
2. Brand of I.V. fluid or drug
3. Type of administration set
4. Preparation technique, duration of drug-drug, or drug-solution contact
5. pH value
6. Temperature of the room and light

Drugs can be compatible when mixed in certain solutions, but incompatible when mixed with others. Mixing two incompatible drugs in solution in a particular order may be enough to avoid a potentially adverse interaction (Gahart, 1995).

The pH of both solution and drug must be considered when compounding medication. Drugs that are widely dissimilar in pH values are unlikely to be compatible in solution. For example, dextrose solutions are slightly acidic, with a pH of 4.5 to 5.5. Several antibiotics on the market have an acidic pH that is stable in dextrose; however, alkaline antibiotics, such as carbenicillin, are unstable when mixed with dextrose. Dextrose, with a pH of 4.5 to 5.5, should be used as a base for acidic drugs; sodium chloride solution, with a pH value of 6.8 to 8.5, should be used for alkaline medication dilution.

✎ **NOTE:** When in doubt about I.V. drug compatibilities, a good practice is to flush the I.V. administration set with sodium chloride before and after medications are infused (Todd, 1988).

Adsorption

Adsorption is the attachment of one substance to the surface of another. Many drugs adsorb to glass or plastic. The disadvantage associated with adsorption is that the patient receives less drug than was actually intended. The amount of adsorption is difficult to predict and is affected by the following: drug concentration, solution of

TABLE 11–3. DRUGS THAT HAVE INCREASED ADSORPTION IN PVC CONTAINERS

Vitamin A acetate (not the palmitate form)
Insulin
Phenothiazine tranquilizers (Thorazine, Compazine)
Hydralazine (Apresoline)
Warfarin (Coumadin)

the drug, amount of surface contacted by the drug, and temperature changes (D'Arcy, 1983).

An example of adsorption is the binding of insulin to plastic and glass containers. The insulin rapidly adsorbs to I.V. containers and tubing until all potential adsorption sites are saturated. During the initial part of an infusion, very little insulin may reach the patient; later after adsorption sites are saturated, more of the insulin in solution is delivered to the patient. To prevent this from occurring, injecting the drug as close to the I.V. insertion site as possible will promote better therapeutic drug effects (Todd, 1988).

Polyvinylchloride (PVC) and plastic flexible I.V. bags promote drug adsorption. There are several drugs that have significant loss during infusion in PVC plastic solution containers (Table 11–3).

✎ **NOTE:** When mixing medications into glass or plastic systems, refer to manufacturers guidelines to prevent adsorption.

PVC containers of infusion solutions incorporate diethylhexyphthalate (DEHP) as a plasticizer to make the PVC soft and pliable. Some drug formulations leach this plasticizer out of the plastic matrix and into the solution. Because DEHP is fat-soluble, I.V. fat emulsion products extract the plasticizer from the PVC bags and tubing (Mazur, Stennett, & Egging, 1989).

DEHP is also leached from PVC bags by organic solvents and surfactants contained in some drugs, which may result in DEHP-induced toxicity. (DEHP has been found to be carcinogenic in rats [Harris, 1981].)

Many drug manufacturers recommend nonphthalate delivery systems in the package inserts. Two systems are being studied to reduce the risk of DEHP toxicities: PVC-plasticizer butyl-n-trihexy citrate (BTHC) in packaging of blood products (Snyder, Hedberg, & Hapychank, 1993) and ethylvinyl acetate (EVA) (Noah & Godin, 1994). The use of EVA administration sets decreases the risk of DEHP toxicity in adult patients and eliminates the risk in pregnant patients, neonates, and infants.

✎ **NOTE:** For fat emulsion products, total parenteral nutrient solutions, and drug formulations that leach DEHP, use non-PVC administration sets and containers (Pearson & Trissel, 1993).

Errors in Mixing

Drug toxicity, subtherapeutic infusion, or erratic therapeutic effects can result from inadequate mixing of a drug into the infusion container. Inadequate mixing can contribute to a bolus of medication delivered to the patient, which may cause adverse effects (Gong & King, 1983).

355

✎ **NOTE:** Burning at the I.V. site from a presumably dilute drug is a warning that the concentration of the drug is too high and needs to be further diluted. (See Chapter 9 for dilution guidelines.)

FACTORS THAT CONTRIBUTE TO INADEQUATE MIXING INCLUDE:
1. Length of time required to adequately mix drugs in flexible bags
2. Addition of a drug to a hanging flexible bag
3. Insufficient needle length or incomplete needle insertion through the injection port (use at least a 1-in. needle)
4. Additives injected at a slow rate into the primary bag (the turbulence of fast flow promotes mixing, especially in glass containers)
5. Inadequate movement of the additive from the injection port (e.g., the long, narrow sleeve-type additive ports on some flexible bags, as opposed to the button-type, hinder effective mixing)
6. Use of immiscible or very dense drugs
7. Nonexistent or improper mixing caused by human error (Gong & King, 1985)

10 KEY RECOMMENDATIONS FOR ADEQUATE MIXING OF I.V. MEDICATIONS
1. Gently invert the I.V. container several times to adequately mix the medication with the solution, taking care to avoid foaming the solution.
2. When inversion is impossible, gently swirl or rotate to mix, to prevent the drug from settling to the bottom of the container.
3. When agitating an intermittent infusion set, clamp off the air vent; if the vent becomes wet, the solution will not infuse properly after mixing.
4. Vacuum devices can facilitate mixing in plastic flexible bags by creating a vacuum and drawing any drug left in the port into the body of the bag.
5. When possible, use premixed solutions from the manufacturer; premixed heparin or potassium chloride solutions, for example, can save time and avoid dose errors as well as preclude mixing problems.
6. Add one drug at a time to the primary I.V. solution. Mix and examine thoroughly before adding the next drug.
7. Add the most concentrated or most soluble drug to the solution first, because some incompatibilities, such as precipitates, require a certain concentration or amount of time to develop. Mix well; then add the dilute drugs.
8. Add colored additives last to avoid masking possible precipitates or cloudiness.
9. Always visually inspect containers after adding and mixing drugs; hold the container against a light or a white surface and check for particulate matter, obvious layering, or foaming.
10. If you do not have a clear understanding of the compatibility or stability of the admixtures you are using, check the manufacturer's recommendation, or consult a pharmacist (Todd, 1988).

✎ **NOTE:** Because of the complexity of this function, many hospitals allow only registered pharmacists to prepare admixtures.

Speed Shock

The nurse must be aware that speed shock can be caused by too-rapid administration of a drug. Rapid onset of action is a double-edged sword: on one side, it is to the patient's advantage to have rapid action in certain clinical situations; on the other side, once infused, the rapid onset cannot be recalled. (See Chapter 9 for additional information on speed shock.)

Extravasation

The nurse must be aware of the patency of the I.V. cannula prior to initiating an infusion to prevent extravasation of a vesicant drug. (See Chapter 9 for additional information on extravasation.)

Chemical Phlebitis

Chemical phlebitis can occur from the pH of the medication; a pH greater than 11.0 or less than 4.3 is most irritating to the vein wall. Antibiotics, chemotherapeutic drugs, potassium chloride, and diazepam (Valium) are known to cause irritation to vein walls and promote chemical phlebitis. (See Chapter 9 for further information on phlebitis.)

DRUG COMPATIBILITY

Compatibility is required for a therapeutic response to prescribed therapy. Chemical, physical, and therapeutic compatibilities must be identified before admixing and administering I.V. medications.

An incompatibility results when two or more substances react or interact so as to change the normal activity of one or more components. Incompatibility may be manifested by harmful or undesirable effects and is likely to result in a loss of therapeutic effects.

Incompatibility may occur when:

1. Several drugs are added to a large volume of fluid to produce an admixture.
2. Drugs in separate solutions are administered concurrently or in close succession via the same I.V. line.
3. A single drug is reconstituted or diluted with the wrong solutions.
4. One drug reacts with another drug's preservative.

Specific incompatibilities fall into three categories: physical, chemical, and therapeutic.

Physical Incompatibility

A physical incompatibility is also called a pharmaceutical incompatibility. Physical incompatibilities occur when one drug is mixed with other drugs or solutions to produce a product unsafe for administration.

Insolubility and absorption are the two types of physical incompatibility. Insolubility occurs when a drug is added to an inappropriate fluid solution, creating an incomplete solution or a precipitate. This risk occurs more frequently with multiple additives, which may interact to form an insoluble product. Signs of insolubility include visible precipitation, haze, gas bubbles, and cloudiness. Some precipitations may be microcrystalline, smaller than 50 microns, and not apparent to the eye. The use of micropore filters is intended to prevent such particles from entering the vein. The use of a 0.22-micron inline filter reduces the amount of microcrystalline precipitates.

The presence of calcium in a drug or solution usually indicates that a precipitate might form if mixed with another drug. Ringer's solution preparations contain calcium, so check carefully for incompatibility before adding any drug to this solution.

Other physical incompatibilities caused by insolubility include the increased degradation of drugs added to sodium bicarbonate, and the formation of an insoluble precipitate when sodium bicarbonate is combined with other medications in emergency situations.

The following are important recommendations regarding physical drug incompatibilities:

- Never administer a drug that forms a precipitate.
- Do not mix drugs prepared in special diluents with other drugs.
- When administering a series of medications, prepare each drug in a separate syringe. This will lessen the possibility of precipitation. Insolubility may also result from the use of an incorrect solution to reconstitute a drug.
- Follow the manufacturer's directions for reconstituting drugs.

Chemical Incompatibility

A chemical incompatibility is defined as the reaction of a drug with other drugs or solutions, which results in alterations of the integrity and potency of the active ingredient. The most common cause of chemical incompatibility is the reaction between acidic and alkaline drugs or solutions, resulting in a pH that is unstable for one of the drugs. A specific pH or a narrow range of pH values is required for the solubility of a drug and for the maintenance of its stability, once it has been mixed.

Therapeutic Incompatibility

A therapeutic incompatibility is an undesirable effect occurring within a patient as a result of two or more drugs being given concurrently. An increased therapeutic or a decreased therapeutic response is produced.

This incompatibility often occurs when therapy dictates the use of two antibiotics. For example, in the use of chloramphenicol and penicillin, chloramphenicol has been reported to antagonize the bacterial activity of penicillin. If prescribed, penicillin should be administered at least 1 hour before the chloramphenicol to prevent therapeutic incompatibility.

Therapeutic incompatibility may go unnoticed until the patient fails to show the expected clinical response to the drug or until peak and trough levels of the drug show a lack of therapeutic levels. If an incompatibility is not suspected, the patient may be given increasingly higher doses of the drug to try to obtain the therapeutic effect (Lippincott Learning System, 1984).

A compatibility chart (Appendix B) identifies the physical and chemical incompatibilities of commonly prescribed drugs.

✎ NOTE: When more than one antibiotic is prescribed for intermittent infusion, stagger the time schedule so that each can be infused individually.

METHODS OF INTRAVENOUS MEDICATION ADMINISTRATION

There are many methods used to administer I.V. medications, including continuous, intermittent, intraspinal, and intraperitoneal infusions, or I.V. push. Other methods of medication administration include infusion through a ventricular reservoir and arteriovenous fistula.

358

NURSING RESPONSIBILITIES

To identify whether a prescribed route (continuous, intermittent, or push) is appropriate

To use aseptic technique in the preparation of an admixture

To identify the expiration date on solutions and medications

To follow manufacturer's guidelines for preparation and storage of medication

To be knowledgeable of the pharmacologic implications relative to patient clinical status and diagnosis

To verify that all solution containers are free of cracks, leaks, and punctures

To monitor the patient for therapeutic response to medication

Continuous Infusion

Continuous infusion is defined as large-volume parenteral solutions of 250 to 1000 mL of infusate administered over 2 to 24 hours. Medication added to these large-volume infusates are administered continuously. These infusions should be regulated by an I.V. pump or controller to ensure an accurate flow rate.

ADVANTAGES

Admixture and bag changes can be performed every 8 to 24 hours.

Constant serum levels of the drug are maintained.

DISADVANTAGES

Monitoring the drug rate can be erratic if not electronically controlled.

There is a higher risk of drug incompatibility problems.

Accidental bolus infusion can occur if medication is not adequately mixed with solution.

PROCEDURE FOR ADMINISTRATION OF CONTINUOUS INFUSIONS

(Verify the physician's order, educate the patient regarding purpose of therapy, and document the procedure and any teaching that you performed.)

1. Spike the I.V. container with an I.V. administration set.
2. Regulate the flow rate.
3. Based on the type of drug being administered, monitor the patient at the recommended time intervals for therapeutic and nontherapeutic effects of the drug.
4. Place time-tape on the bag, even when a pump or controller is used, to verify administration rate at a quick glance.

✎ **NOTE:** When adding medication to a infusion container, use single-dose medication vials instead of multiple-dose vials to decrease potential for infection, complications, and medication errors.

Intermittent Infusion

Intermittent infusion refers to any administration of a medication or an infusion that is not continuous. Technological advances have produced alternatives for the administration of intermittent doses. Types of intermittent infusions are piggyback through the established pathway of the primary solution, simultaneous infusion, use of volume control set, and intermittent infusions through a locking device.

359

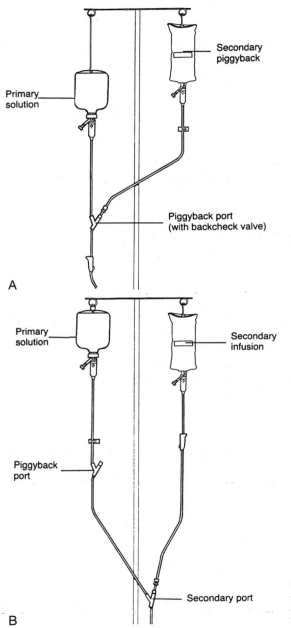

Primary
solution

Secondary
piggyback

Piggyback port
(with backcheck valve)

A

Primary
solution

Secondary
infusion

Piggyback
port

Secondary port

B

Figure 11–1. Methods of delivery of secondary infusions. (*A*) Secondary piggyback infusion. (*B*) Simultaneous infusion.

Piggyback Through Primary Pathway

Piggy infusion through an established pathway of the primary solution is the most common method for drug delivery by the intermittent route. The drug is diluted in 50 to 250 mL of 5% dextrose in water or 0.9% sodium chloride and administered over 15 to 90 minutes (Baldwin, 1995). When infusing medications via this method the secondary infusion is administered via the piggyback port with the backcheck valve (Fig. 11–1, A). This Y port is located on the upper third of the primary line. Although the primary infusion is interrupted during the piggyback infusion, the drug from the intermittent infusion container comes in contact with the primary solution below the piggyback injection port; therefore the drug and the primary solution should be compatible.

ADVANTAGES
Risk of incompatibilities is reduced.
Larger drug dose can be administered at a lower concentration per milliliter than with the I.V. push method.
Peak flow concentrations occur at periodic intervals.
There is a decreased risk of fluid overload.

DISADVANTAGES
Administration rate may not be accurate unless electronically monitored.
High concentration of drug in intermittent solution may cause venous irritation.
I.V. set changes can result in wasting a portion of the drug.
If the patient is not properly monitored, fluid overload or speed shock could result.
Drug incompatibility can occur if the administration set is not adequately flushed between medication administrations.

Simultaneous Infusion (Primary and Secondary)

Secondary infusions can be infused concurrently with the primary solution. Rather than connecting the intermittent infusion at the piggyback port, it is attached to the lower Y site (Fig. 11–1, B). Disadvantages of administration of secondary concurrent with primary solution include the tendency for blood to back up into the tubing once the secondary infusion has been completed, causing occlusion of venous access device and increased risk of drug incompatibility. Drug incompatibility is a greater risk with the simultaneous infusion method.

Volume Control

This method of intermittent delivery of medication is used most frequently with pediatric patients or when a small amount of a well-controlled drug needs to be administered to critical care patients. Medication is added to the volume control chamber and diluted with I.V. solution. The infusion is generally over 15 minutes to 1 hour. Volumes delivered vary from 25 mL to 150 mL per drug dose (Fig. 11–2).

ADVANTAGES
Runaway infusions are avoided without the use of electronic infusion devices.
Volume of fluid in which the drug is diluted can be adjusted.

361

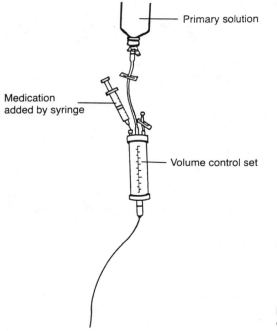

Primary solution

Medication
added by syringe

Volume control set

Figure 11–2. Administration of medication via a volume control chamber.

Medication must travel the length of the tubing before it reaches the patient, there is a significant time delay.
A portion of the medication can be left in the tubing after the chamber empties.
Incompatibilities may develop when the chamber, which is usually within the primary line, is used for multiple drug deliveries.
Labeling of the chamber must coincide with the drug being delivered; if multiple drugs are delivered, this could present a problem.

Intermittent Infusions Through a Locking Device

Medication administered by intermittent infusion is usually diluted in 1 to 50 mL of infusate and infused over a 1- to 15-minute period. An intermittent infusion is attached directly to an I.V. lock. Saline or heparinized saline is used to maintain patency of the lock.

ADVANTAGES
Incompatibilities are avoided.
A minimal amount of fluid is provided to the patient on restricted intake.
Minimal drug is wasted.

DISADVANTAGES
If the fluid container runs dry, blood backs into the cannula and tubing and could cause a clot (Weinstein, 1993).

After each infusion of medication, the lock must be flushed with heparinized saline or saline (depending on agency policy) to maintain patency.

PROCEDURE FOR ADMINISTRATION OF INTERMITTENT MEDICATION THROUGH LOCKING DEVICES
(Verify the physician's order, educate the patient regarding the purpose of therapy, and document the procedure and any teaching you may have performed.)

1. Wash hands.
2. Flush lock with 1 to 2 mL of 0.9% sodium chloride.
3. Infuse the drug at the prescribed rate.
4. Following the drug delivery, flush the lock with 0.9% sodium chloride or heparinized sodium chloride solution.

✎ **NOTE:** Exert a positive pressure on the syringe when withdrawing from the I.V. lock to prevent a backflow of blood into the I.V. catheter.

Volume Control Chamber

This method of intermittent delivery of medication is used most frequently with pediatric patients or when delivery of small amount of well-controlled drug needs to be administered to critical care patients. Medication is added to the volume control chamber and diluted with I.V. solution. The infusion is generally over 15 minutes to 1 hour. Volumes delivered vary from 25 to 150 mL per drug dose (Fig. 11–2).

ADVANTAGES
Runaway infusions are avoided without the use of electronic infusion devices.
Volume of fluid in which the drug is diluted can be adjusted.

DISADVANTAGES
Medication must travel the length of the tubing before it reaches the patient, so there is a significant time delay.
A portion of the medication can be left in the tubing after the chamber empties.
Incompatibilities may develop when the chamber, which is usually within the primary line, is used for multiple drug deliveries.
Labeling of the chamber must coincide with the drug being delivered. If multiple drugs are delivered this could present a problem.

Direct Injection (I.V. Push)

I.V. push administration of a medication provides a method of administering high concentrations of medication. Administration via this route can be accomplished by direct penetration of a vein, by penetration of vein using a syringe, and needle scalp vein infusion set or over-the-needle infusion device, or by access of low injection port of primary administration sets. The purpose is to achieve rapid serum concentrations.

Direct injection requires that the drug be drawn into a syringe prior to administration or that the drug be available in a prefilled syringe. Needle protector or needleless systems can be used connected to the venous access device or with administration sets to deliver the medication (Baldwin, 1995).

ADVANTAGES
Barriers of drug absorption are bypassed.
Drug response is rapid and usually predictable.
Patient is closely monitored during the full administration of the medication.

363

Adverse effects occur at the same time and rate as therapeutic effects.

The I.V. push method has the greatest risk of adverse effects and toxicity, because serum drug concentrations are sharply elevated.

Speed shock is possible from too rapid administration of medication.

Adverse effects that can occur during administration of a medication directly into a vein are: changes in level of consciousness, vital functions, and reflex activity (Burman & Berkowitz, 1986).

✎ **NOTE:** If adverse effects occur, supportive care is the basis for treatment of most symptoms because specific antidotes are available for only certain drugs.

PROCEDURE FOR DIRECT ADMINISTRATION

(Verify the physician's order, educate the patient regarding the purpose of therapy, and document the procedure and any patient teaching that you may have performed.)

1. Check compatibility of drug with primary solution.
2. Dilute opioid narcotics and follow recommendation of manufacturer for administration.
3. Swab lowest Y port with alcohol or betadine.
4. Insert syringe with medication into Y site.
5. Pinch tubing to primary solution.
6. Inject one fourth of medication into patient over a 15- to 20-second period.
7. Unpinch tubing allowing primary solution to flush. *Watch patient for any adverse effects.*
8. Repeat steps 5 to 7, delivering one fourth of drug each time for three more times.
9. When all the desired drug is delivered, remove syringe.

✎ **NOTE:** This process should take *at least* 1 minute; however, always follow recommendations of the manufacturer for delivery of the drug. For example, drugs such as phenytoin and diazepam must be delivered over a lengthy period of time; the manufacturer provides specific guidelines for administration.

Continuous Subcutaneous Infusion

Continuous subcutaneous infusion is a practical and simple approach to pain management. Pain affects approximately 65% to 85% of cancer patients (Murphy, 1990). Two factors that contribute to unsatisfactory pain management are (1) inadequate dosage and titration of available pain medications and (2) limited resources to properly educate and advise physicians and nurses on pain management. Patients who require parenteral narcotics are candidates for continuous subcutaneous infusion. This type of infusion therapy can be established for the following types of patients who require intermittent injection, usually longer than 48 hours (McLaughlin-Hagan, 1990):

- Patients unable to take medications by mouth.
- Patients who require subcutaneous injections for more than 48 hours.
- Patients who require parenteral narcotics but have poor venous access.

ADVANTAGES

Easy care for home management of pain

Decreased number of times tissue is traumatized by repeated injections

Better home management of pain, which decreases hospital time

Decrease in central nervous side effects associated with intermittent drug therapy, such as nausea, vomiting, and drowsiness

Decrease in pain breakthrough

DISADVANTAGES

Local irritation at infusion site

Rapidly escalating pain of dying patient requiring larger volumes of drug; this route is inappropriate for volumes larger than 1 mL/hour (Coyle, Mauskop, Maggard, & Foley, 1986).

PROCEDURE FOR ADMINISTRATION OF CONTINUOUS SUBCUTANEOUS INFUSION

(Verify the physician's order, educate the patient regarding the purpose of therapy, and document the procedure and any patient teaching you may have performed.)

1. Establish baseline vital signs.
2. Have patients rate their pain on a scale of 1 to 10.
3. Establish subcutaneous access per hospital policy and use continuous infusion guidelines.
4. Use a 24-gauge catheter, with a 26-gauge insertion needle. The Soft-set (MiniMed Technologies) also has a 42-inch microbore tubing attached to the infusion device, which can be then be attached to a patient-controlled analgesia (PCA) pump. This system has a Leur lock hub. The tubing is made of polyfin, which is compatible with most drug deliveries (Fig. 11–3).
5. Prime tubing if needed.
6. Administer prescribed bolus dose and immediately begin the continuous infusion.
7. Obtain vital signs, neurologic signs, and pain level assessment every 30 minutes (four times) and as needed.

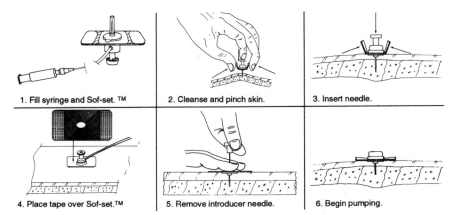

1. Fill syringe and Sof-set. ™   2. Cleanse and pinch skin.   3. Insert needle.

4. Place tape over Sof-set.™   5. Remove introducer needle.   6. Begin pumping.

Figure 11–3. Steps in subcutaneous infusion. (Courtesy of MiniMed Technologies, Sylmar, California.)

Intraspinal Medication Infusion

Spinal opiate receptor sites were discovered in 1973, and subsequently selective spinal opiate analgesia was developed—"selective" because only pain is alleviated (Bromage, 1980). The first controlled study describing intrathecal administration of morphine in humans was reported in the late 1970s (Wang, Nauss, & Thomas, 1979). The rationale for this method of drug administration is that it allows for direct delivery of narcotic or dilute anesthetic to the receptors in the brain and spinal column.

The spinal anatomy consists of two spaces, the epidural space and the intrathecal space. *Intraspinal* is the term used to encompass both the epidural and intrathecal spaces surrounding the spinal cord. *Intrathecal* space is surrounded by the epidural space and separated from it by the dura mater; the intrathecal space contains cerebrospinal fluid, which bathes the spinal cord. The epidural and intrathecal spaces share a common center, the spinal cord. *Epidural* space surrounds the spinal cord and intrathecal space and lies between the ligamentum flavum and the dura mater. This is a potential space, since the ligamentum flavum and the dura mater are not separated until medication or air is injected between them. This potential space contains a venous network of veins that are large and thin-walled and has a strong leukocytic activity to reduce the risk of infection. Dividing epidural and intrathecal spaces is a tough, fatty membrane called the dura. The dura's permeability is important in determining how fast epidural drugs cross into the intrathecal space and how long they remain there to be active (St. Marie, 1989). The epidural space also contains fat in proportion to a person's body fat. Opiate receptor sites are cells contained in the dorsal horn of the spinal cord, at which point opioids combine with their respective receptor site to generate analgesia (Bonica, 1990).

Intraspinal analgesia can provide relief to patients suffering from intractable pain. Intraspinal analgesia does not cause the central nervous system side effects that systemic narcotic delivery can cause. Multiple studies show that in the surgical and postsurgical settings, epidural morphine is superior to a systemic narcotic for abdominal, pelvic, thoracic, spinal surgery, and obstetrics (Slater, Zeitlin, & Edwards, 1985; Zola & McLeod, 1983).

Local anesthetic agents are frequently used with intraspinal narcotics and are instrumental in controlling pain and reducing postoperative complications. When a patient experiences acute pain, the sympathetic system (part of the autonomic nervous system) is activated, increasing the workload of the heart. When intraspinal local anesthetic agents are administered, a sympathetic block results, which produces a decrease in blood pressure, pulse, and respirations. The advantages of adding local anesthetic agents to an epidural narcotic are that it produces a sympathetic block, resulting in decreased workload on the heart, and decreases the incidence of thrombophlebitis and paralytic ileus.

A disadvantage to local anesthetics is the nurse's lack of understanding of such agents. Nurses must be educated to the use of these agents (St. Marie, 1991).

Epidural Administration

PATIENT SELECTION CRITERIA
Control of pain associated with cancer

Surgical patient who is to have extensive surgery performed, such as thoracic or abdominal surgery

Victims of trauma to the chest area or limbs who have no increased intracranial pressure and normal bleeding times

ADVANTAGES

Permits control or alleviation of severe pain without the sedative effects

Permits delivery of smaller doses of a narcotic to achieve desired level of analgesia

Prolongs the analgesia (average about 14 hours)

Allows for continuous infusion if needed

Allows terminal cancer patients treated with epidural narcotics to be more comfortable and mobile (Slater, Zeitlin, & Edwards, 1985)

Can be used for short-term or long-term therapy

Does not produce motor paralysis or hypotension

DISADVANTAGES

Only preservative-free narcotics can be used.

Complications such as paresthesia, urinary retention, and respiratory depression (greatest 6 to 10 hours after injection) can occur.

Catheter-related risks can occur (e.g., infection, dislodgment, and leaking).

Pruritus can occur on face, head, and neck or may be generalized.

✎ **NOTE:** Have naloxone (Narcan), 0.4 mg I.V., available to counteract respiratory depression.

Procedure for Insertion and Maintainance of Epidural Catheters

The insertion of the epidural catheter is a sterile procedure and is a function performed by a physician or anesthesiologist. Administration of medication by a nurse through an epidural catheter must be in accordance with each state's Nurse Practice Act.

1. Avoid the use of preservatives (mainly alcohol) in medication because they have a destructive effect on neural tissue (Lieb & Hurtig, 1985). The drug most frequently used is preservative-free morphine. Other preservatives are methylparaban, sodium bisulfite, sodium hydroxide, buffers, benzoalcohol, and phenol. Preservative-free morphine is available in 0.5 mg/mL and 1 mg/mL concentrations.
2. The physician uses an 18-gauge needle inserted between L2 and L3, or L3 and L4.
3. Lidocaine is injected subcutaneously. Insert the needle and thread the catheter through the needle so that the catheter tip is at approximately the dermatome level affected by the pain (Fig. 11–4).
4. After insertion, lay the exposed catheter length cephalad along the spine and over the shoulder. Tape the entire length of the exposed catheter in place to provide stability and protection. The end of the catheter and the filter are generally placed on the patient's chest wall and taped securely in a position that allows the patient or significant other to access the catheter for use.
5. Clearly label the epidural catheter after placement to prevent accidental infusion of fluids or medications.
6. Epidural catheters can be connected in one of three ways: implantable pump or an implantable port, or it can be threaded subcutaneously so it exits out the side of the body.
7. The medication infused via an epidural catheter should be administered via an electronic infusion device.

✎ **NOTE:** A 0.22-micron filter is recommended to prevent introduction of particulate matter or bacteria into the epidural space.

367

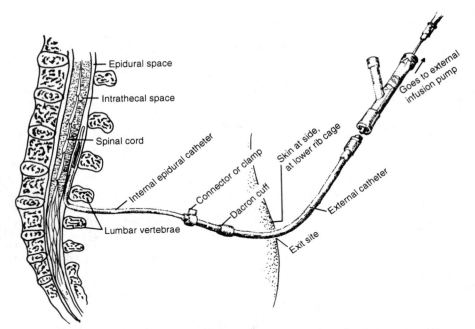

Figure 11–4. Epidural catheter for pain relief. (From St. Marie, B. [1989]. Administration of intraspinal analgesia in the home care setting. *National Intravenous Therapy Association, 12*[3], 166. Copyright 1989 by the National Intravenous Therapy Association. Reprinted by permission.)

NURSING RESPONSIBILITIES
Patient and family education
Site and dressing management
Medication administration
Evaluation of pain relief

✎ **NOTE:** Ineffective pain control should be reported to the physician or anesthesiologist who is managing care of the epidural catheter.

Nursing Care

Monitoring

A flow sheet should be used to monitor the patient's response to epidural medication. This allows tracking of the patient's analgesia and any side effects (Fig. 11–5). Included on the flow sheet are:

Evaluation of mental status
Respiratory status
Indication of numbness in the lower extremities
Signs of infection
Bowel function
Bladder function
Integrity of epidural system
Narcotic dose
Patient's pain rating

EPIDURAL FLOWSHEET
INTERMITTENT OR CONTINUOUS INFUSION

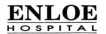

DATE _____ MEDICATION _____

EDUCATION: CHART ON BACK OF FLOW SHEET

1) INTERMITTENT INJECTIONS: VS Q 15" X 2 THEN Q 4 HOURS
2) CONTINUOUS INFUSION: VS Q 15" X THEN Q 4 HOURS
   A) RESP., SEDATION LEVEL, MOTOR RESPONSE, DERMATOMES (ANESTHETICS) Q 1 HOUR X 4, THEN Q 2 HOURS

FOR ANY INFUSION RATE INCREASE RETURN TO INITIAL ASSESSMENT FREQUENCIES

TIME															
TERMPERATURE															
BLOOD PRESSURE															
PULSE															
RESPIRATIONS															
SEDATION LEVEL															
PAIN SCALE															
SITE ASSESS .Q8°															
MOTOR RESPONSE NO DEFICIT															
DERMATOMES LEVEL/RESPONSE															
S/SX TOXICITY															
INITIALS															

ASSESS PAIN Q 4 HOURS FOR ALL TYPES OF EPIDURAL ANALGESIA

SEDATION LEVEL	**PAIN**	**DERMATOMES**
3 – Alert/Awake	0 – 10 scale	(Anesthetics only)
2– Occassionally drowsy, easy to awake	**0 –** no pain	
1 – Frequently drowsy, easy to arouse	**10** – worst pain	
0 – Somnolent, difficult to arouse		
S – Normal sleep, easy to arouse		

ANESTHETICS
S&SX TOXICITY
Circumoral tingling
Muscle twitching
"Metallic" taste/tinnitus

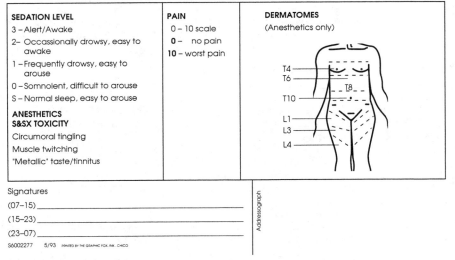

Signatures
(07–15) _____
(15–23) _____
(23–07) _____
S6002277   5/93   PRINTED BY THE GRAPHIC FOX. INK . CHICO

Addressograph

Figure 11–5. Example of continuous or intermittent epidural flow sheet. (Courtesy of N.T. Enloe Hospital, Chico, California, with permission.)

Site Care

Epidural catheters must be handled carefully during site care because they are easily dislodged (St. Marie, 1995). Dressing change in hospital or home care should be frequent and follow agency policy and procedure.

369

(Verify the physician's order, educate the patient regarding the purpose of therapy, and document the procedure, including any patient teaching you may have performed.)

1. Assemble equipment; wash hands thoroughly.
2. Inspect insertion site for signs of infection or drainage.
3. Verify with another nurse that a preservative-free narcotic is mixed in normal saline solution.
4. Assess patient for baseline data and vital signs.
5. Use sterile gloves. Scrub the injection cap with povidone-iodine and allow 2 minutes of contact time. Wipe with a sterile 2-in × 2-in gauze pad to remove any excess iodine.
6. Enter the injection cap using the 3-mL empty syringe and a 25-gauge $\frac{5}{8}$-inch needle. Gently aspirate to verify that the catheter tip is not in the subarachnoid space by observing that less than 1 mL of fluid returns. Discard any fluid withdrawn.
7. Rescrub injection cap with povidone-iodine.
8. Begin infusion via pump connected to extension tubing and filter or inject intermittent dose at approximately 5 mL per minute.
9. Check catheter cap for secureness; tighten as needed.
10. Document.
11. Assess patient every 15 minutes twice, then every 4 hours for vital signs. Check level of consciousness every hour for 24 hours, then every 4 hours.

✎ **NOTE:** Have naloxone (Narcan) available, 0.4 mg, to treat respiratory depression or increased sedation.

✎ **NOTE:** Never use alcohol for site preparation or for accessing the catheter because of the potential for alcohol migration into the epidural space.

Dressing Management of Epidural Catheter

This is a sterile procedure.

1. Wash hands with antimicrobial soap and water for at least 1 minute.
2. Remove old dressing. Use cottonball soaked in sterile water to assist in lifting the edge of dressing.
3. Wet cotton-tipped applicator in povidone-iodine solution; clean area starting at the catheter, working outward in a circular motion. Repeat two more times and allow area to dry. (Note whether any crusted areas are around the catheter; if so, remove them by using a swab dipped in hydrogen peroxide before using the povidone-iodine.)
4. Apply new transparent dressing.
5. Remove the tape holding the catheter end, clean skin under the tape, allow to dry, and retape for comfort and safety (St. Marie, 1995).

✎ **NOTE:** Do not use alcohol on skin or at dressing site because of the risk of migration of alcohol into the epidural space and the possibility of neural damage.

Intrathecal Administration

The intrathecal injection of a narcotic requires approximately 10 times less medication than is needed in the epidural space. The intrathecal space, however, is associated with a greater risk for infection. When intrathecal catheters are used for long-term applications, they are connected to an implantable pump to reduce the risk of infection.

370

ADVANTAGES

Useful for delivery of certain antineoplastic agents, antibiotics, analgesics, and anesthetic agents

Effective alternative to oral or parenteral therapy for abatement of pain associated with cancer because of direct delivery of narcotic to opiate receptors in the brain and spinal column

Allows for low doses of drug to produce the same degree of analgesia as high doses required systemically

DISADVANTAGES

Possible life-threatening side effects

Potential for spinal fluid leak

Potential infection (Akahoshi, Furuike-McLaughlin, & Enriquez, 1988)

PROCEDURE FOR ADMINISTRATION OF MEDICATION VIA
THE INTRATHECAL CATHETER

(Verify the physician's order, educate patient regarding the purpose of therapy, and document procedure including any patient teaching you may have performed.)

1. Use sterile gloves and mask.
2. Use noncoring needles to access ports and pumps.
3. Use preservative-free medications.
4. Avoid using alcohol for site preparation and for accessing the catheter because of the potential for alcohol migration into the intrathecal space.
5. A 0.22-micron filter without surfactant should be used for medication administration.
6. Assess for therapeutic response and complications.

✎ **NOTE:** When an intrathecal catheter is attached to an implanted pump, the manufacturer's guidelines regarding aspiration must be adhered to.

Side Effects of Intraspinal Narcotic Infusions

The goal of managing side effects with intraspinal narcotic infusions is early intervention. Side effects include nausea, vomiting, urinary retention, pruritus, and respiratory depression. (See Table 11–4 for a list of common medications used for intraspinal narcotic administration.) Nausea and vomiting can be controlled with antiemetics such as prochlorperazine (Compazine).

Excessive drowsiness or confusion can occur when too much narcotic is being administered. This is usually improved by decreasing the amount of epidural narcotic infusion. Titrating an opioid antagonist, such as naloxone (Narcan), 0.2 mg I.V., or an agonist/antagonist, such as nalbuphine (Nubain), 5 to 10 mg

TABLE 11–4. **MEDICATIONS USED FOR INTRASPINAL**
NARCOTIC ADMINISTRATION

Agonists	Antagonists	Anesthetics
Morphine	Butorphanol (Stadol)	Bupivacaine (Marcaine)
Meperidine (Demerol)	Nalbuphine (Nubain)	
Sublimaze (Fentanyl)	Pentazocine (Talwin)	
Hydromorphone (Dilaudid)		

subcutaneously, may reverse side effects without eliminating the analgesia (St. Marie, 1995).

Urinary retention is a common side effect and may occur 10 to 20 hours after the first injection of intraspinal narcotic. This may require either administration of be-thanecol (Urecholine) or intermittent catheterization.

Pruritus is caused by the opiate's interacting with the dorsal horn and not by a histamine release. This is best treated with an antagonist rather than with diphen-hydramine (Benadryl). After an epidural injection, 8.5% of all patients experience pruritus; after an intrathecal injection, 46% experience pruritus.

Complications Associated With Epidural Pain Management

Epidural pain management is not without risks and complications, including inade-quate pain relief, respiratory depression, infection, and catheter migration. The nurse must assess adequate pain control carefully. Inadequate pain relief can occur for three reasons: epidural catheter migration, insufficient dosages of narcotics and local anesthetics, and undetermined surgical complication.

Respiratory depression from epidural or intrathecal narcotic administration is a risk. Vital signs should be assessed and naloxone should be available to reverse de-pressant effects of a narcotic (Rosen, 1990).

Infections are rare from epidural catheters, but precautions should be instituted to keep the catheter insertion process and exit site sterile. If an infection develops elsewhere in the body, the patient should be evaluated for removal of the epidural catheter (St. Marie, 1995).

Catheter migration may occur in two ways:

The catheter may migrate through the dura mater into the intrathecal space, creating an overdose of narcotic.
The catheter may migrate into an epidural vein or subcutaneous space, creating inadequate pain relief.

✎ **NOTE:** If catheter migration is suspected, the physician should be notified and placement check verified by an anesthesiologist.

Arteriovenous Fistula

An arteriovenous (AV) fistula facilitates accessing of the vascular system. AV fistulas are used for administration of parenteral therapies.

PROCEDURE FOR DELIVERY OF ARTERIOVENOUS PARENTERAL THERAPY
Nurse must be knowledgeable regarding the type of fistula that is in place: syn-thetic, bovine graft, or anastamosis.
The integrity of the graft site must be determined before venipuncture by pal-pation and auscultation.
Use sterile technique; wear sterile gloves.
Arterial pressure within the AV fistula increases the potential for bleeding.
Potential complications include but are not limited to infection, occlusion, and thrombosis.

ANTI-INFECTIVE ADMINISTRATION CONSIDERATIONS

Before administering antibiotic, antifungal, and antiviral agents intravenously, it is essential to understand the pharmacotherapeutics related to these drugs. Manufacturer recommendations for administration should be followed carefully. Anti-infectives are administered to achieve therapeutic coverage based on culture and sensitivity reports.

KEY QUESTIONS IN DELIVERY OF ANTIMICROBIAL AGENTS
1. Has the infecting organism been identified (suspected or confirmed by culture)?
2. Is the organism resistant to any antimicrobials?
3. Is the site of infection identified?
4. What is the status of the host (patient) defenses?
5. Is the nurse familiar with the antimicrobial pharmacokinetics?
6. What is the status of the patient's renal and hepatic function?
7. Is monitoring the patient's blood levels necessary to avoid toxicity of dosage?
8. Does the patient have an allergy to the anti-infective agent? (Mathewson-Kuhn, 1994)

Antibiotics

Antibiotic's action is either bacteriostatic, inhibiting bacterial cell wall synthesis and producing a defective cell wall, or bactericidal, altering intracellular function of the bacteria. A knowledge of each antibiotic administered is essential for safe delivery of the medication.

GENERAL NURSING CONSIDERATIONS
1. Be knowledgeable of the antibiotic ordered, it's normal dosage, side effects and compatibilities and the purpose of the antibiotic in treatment of the patient's infection (Table 11–5).
2. Be sure the drug has not expired.
3. Be familiar with reconstitution, dilution, and storage information.
4. Correctly label the admixture with drug name, concentration, diluent, date, time, and initials.
5. Be familiar with potential adverse effects of the drug.
6. Use strict aseptic technique throughout administration.
7. Be aware that the drug must be delivered at specified times to ensure maintenance of the proper drug levels and to identify therapeutic, subtherapeutic, and toxic drug levels.
8. Use assessment skills to monitor functions of the organ or organs that metabolize the antibiotic.
9. Evaluate the patient every shift for sensitivity to the drug.
10. Be prepared to respond to anaphylaxis (Delaney & Lauer, 1988).

Antibiotic Compatibility Issues

Nurse's Drug Alert (1985) addressed the issue of infusing morphine, hydromorphone, or meperidine via the same administration set as used for infusing antibiotics. In this investigational study, it was found that the following incompatibilities occurred:

- Physical change in administration set (pale yellow to light green) when morphine, hydromorphone, or meperidine was added to minocycline or tetracycline
- Physical incompatability immediately when merperidine was infused into a line with nafcillin, cefoperazone, or mezlocillin (Nieves-Cordero, 1985)

373

TABLE 11–5. **CATEGORIES OF ANTIBIOTICS**

Antibiotic	Key Points in I.V. Administration
β-Lactamase agents	Can cause phlebitis.
	Never administer procaine penicillin by I.V. route.
	Interaction: Aspirin increases blood levels.
	Concomitant use of bacteriostatic agents decrease activity of penicillin.
Cephalosporin	Be aware of nephrotoxic effects.
	Do not administer if patient is penicillin-sensitive.
	Rotate sites often; high risk for phlebitis.
	Monitor renal function with blood urea nitrogen and creatinine.
	Use cautiously in pregnant and lactating women.
Aminoglycosides	Assess for muscle weakness.
	Assess blood urea nitrogen and serum creatinine levels.
	Assess balance and hearing functions for any damage to the eighth cranial nerve.
Chloramphenicol	Only administer intravenously.
	Assess for bone marrow suppression.
Erythromycin	High risk of phlebitis.
	One of the safest antibiotics.
Fluoroquinolones	Maintain fluid intake to prevent crystalluria.
	Can cause venous irritation; administer over 60 minutes.
Tetracycline	Do not administer to patients with liver dysfunction.
	Do not administer to patients with renal failure.
	Assess for superinfections.
	I.V. site must be rotated frequently owing to venous irritation and thrombophlebitis.

Sources: Data from Mathewson-Kuhn M. (1994). *Pharmacotherapeutics: A nursing process approach.* Philadelphia: F.A. Davis. Copyright 1994 by F.A. Davis; Deglin, J.H., & Vallerand, A.H. (1995). *Davis's drug guide for nurses,* 4th ed. Philadelphia: F.A. Davis. Copyright 1995 by F.A. Davis.

Antifungal Agents

The method of action of antifungal agents is injury to the cell wall of the fungi. The drugs in this classification are specifically targeted for fungi (Table 11–6); three fungal drugs can be given by the I.V. route: amphotericin B, fluconazole, and miconazole. The most frequently administered antifungal agent by I.V. route is amphotericin B. Key points in delivery of antifungal agents are (1) most are infused as a suspension; (2) these drugs should not be filtered; and (3) they should be administered slowly over 2 to 6 hours.

Antiviral Agents

Antiviral agents are selectively toxic to viruses. A safe, broad-spectrum antiviral drug has yet to be discovered. Most chemicals administered by the I.V. route to combat virus growth are antimetabolites or are related to the antimetabolites used in treating malignant tumors (Table 11–7). These drugs tend to be toxic and usefulness is limited. They are administered in selected situations. At present there are six antiviral agents infused by the I.V. route: acyclovir, ganciclovir, pentamidine isethionate, vidarabine, zidovudine, and foscarnet.

TABLE 11–6. **I.V. ANTIFUNGAL MEDICATION GUIDELINES**

Antifungal Agent	Key Points in Delivery
Amphotericin B	Light-sensitive, but protection is not necessary. Use on hospitalized patient only. Monitor vital signs, intake and output. During therapy, frequently test renal and liver function. To reduce nephrotoxic effects: Administer mannitol, 12.5 g before and after each dose. *Incompatibility:* Not compatible with any solution with a pH below 4.2. Do not mix with any drug unless absolutely necessary; there are many incompatibilities.
Fluconazole (Diflucan)	I.V. use only. Administered in a glass system. Inadequate treatment may lead to recurrent infection. Hepatotoxicity may occur. If any signs and symptoms of liver disease exist, laboratory analysis should be done and the drug discontinued. *Incompatibility:* Manufacturer states: "Do not add supplemental medication."
Miconazole (Monostat IV)	Hospitalize the patient for the first several days of initial treatment. Monitor blood counts, electrolytes, and lipids. Can be administered intrathecally and as bladder irrigant. Pruritus is a common side effect. *Incompatibility:* Considered incompatible in syringe or solutions with any other drug.

Sources: Data from Deglin, J.H., & Vallerand, A.H. (1995). *Davis's drug guide for nurses,* 4th ed. Philadelphia: F.A. Davis. Copyright by F.A. Davis; and Mathewson-Kuhn, M. (1994). *Pharmacotherapeutics: A nursing process approach,* 3rd ed. Philadelphia: F.A. Davis.

NARCOTIC INFUSION CONSIDERATIONS

Pain management begins with complete assessment of the patient's pain, including location, intensity, quality, frequency, onset, duration, aggravating and alleviating factors, associated symptoms, and coping mechanisms. Pain perception and tolerance are highly individual responses. According to McCafferty & Beebe (1989), the definition of pain is "whatever the experiencing person says it is, existing whenever he says it does."

Many therapeutic approaches are available for pain including behavioral approaches, application of heat and cold, massage, physical therapy, management with narcotics and nonnarcotics by oral, subcutaneous, or I.V. routes, neurosurgery, and anesthestics (Murphy, 1990).

Morphine is the narcotic most commonly used for continuous infusion for pain management (Table 11–8). Continuous infusions lead to a continuous level of pain control without the peaks of side effect development and the troughs of breakthrough pain. Generally less drug is needed to prevent the recurrence of the pain (Coyle et al, 1986).

375

TABLE 11–7. I.V. ANTIVIRAL ADMINISTRATION GUIDELINES

Antiviral Agent	Key Points in Administration
Acylovir (Zovirax) Treats: Herpes simplex virus (HSV-1, HSV-2)	Can cause renal tubular damage if too rapidly infused; make sure patient is adequately hydrated. *Incompatibility:* Blood products, dobutamine, protein solutions, or dopamine.
Ganciclovir (Cytovene) Treats: Cytomegalovirus (CMV), varicella zoster (I.V. only)	Follow guidelines for handling cytotoxic drugs. Maintain hydration. Assess renal (CMV) function. Do not use during pregnancy unless justified. *Incompatibility:* Any other drug or solution because of alkaline pH.
Pentamidine isethionate (Pentam 300) Treats: *Pneumocystis carinii* Investigational use: Hypoglycemia, cardiac arrhythmias, trypanosomiasis visceral	Specific use only. Has numerous side effects: severe hypotension. Monitor blood glucose levels. Before and after therapy: blood urea nitrogen, complete blood count. Has numerous side effects which may be life-threatening. *Incompatibility:* All drugs.
Adenine arabinoside (vidarabine) Treats: Herpes simplex encephalitis Investigational use: Immunocompromised patients	I.V. infusion only. Confirm diagnosis of encephalitis with brain biopsy. Use caution in cerebral edema or potential fluid overload. *Incompatibility:* Blood products and protein solutions.
Zidovudine (AZT) Treats: Symptomatic AIDS and advanced AIDS-related complex	Specific use only; only a cure. Frequent blood counts. Anemia is a side effect. Toxicity may be increased by nephrotoxic or cytotoxic drugs. Protect from light. *Incompatibility:* Blood products and protein solutions.
Foscarnet (Foscavir) Treats: Viral infections due to CMV, acylovir-resistant herpes	Monitor for renal impairment. Prehydration required prior to infusion.

Sources: Data from Deglin, J.H., & Vallerand, A.H. (1995). *Davis's drug guide for nurses,* 4th ed. Philadelphia: F.A. Davis. Copyright 1995 by F.A. Davis; and Mathewson-Kuhn, M. (1994). *Pharmacotherapeutics: A nursing process approach,* 3rd ed. Philadelphia: F.A. Davis. Copyright 1994 by F.A. Davis.

The World Health Organization and the American Pain Society (1989) have grouped analgesia into three types: opioids, nonnarcotic analgesics and nonsteroidal anti-inflammatory drugs (NSAIDs), and adjuvants.

Opioids include narcotic analgesics and narcotic agonists. Nonnarcotic analgesics, nonopioids, and NSAIDs provide relief of mild to moderate pain. Adjuvants include drugs to treat other signs and symptoms of pain, such as depression, anxiety, and nausea; often these are referred to as coanalgesics (McGuire, 1990).

Patient-Controlled Analgesia

The concept of patient-controlled analgesia (PCA) began in 1970. PCA is a pain management strategy that allows the patient to self-administer I.V. narcotic pain medi-

TABLE 11–8. I.V. NARCOTIC ADMINISTRATION GUIDELINES

Narcotic	Key Points in Administration
Agonist	
Meperidine 10–50 mg every 2–4 h	Avoid in patients with impaired renal function. *Must be diluted.* Shorter-acting than morphine. Not recommended I.V. in children. Caution in glaucoma, head injuries, chronic obstructive pulmonary disease. Cough reflex is suppressed.
Morphine 2.5–15 mg every 2–6 h	Caution in patient with impaired ventilation, bronchial asthma, increased intracranial pressure, liver failure. *Should be diluted.*
Hydromorphone 2–4 mg every 4–6 h	Caution in head injuries, respiratory depression, and increased intracranial pressure. Slightly shorter duration than morphine. *Should be diluted.*
Levorphanol 2–3 mg every 4–6 h	Accumulates on days 2–3, long plasma half-life. I.V. is usually not the route of choice. Subcutaneous is usual route.
Agonist/Antagonist Agents	
Pentazocine 5–10 mg every 3–4 h	May cause psychotomimetic effect. Contraindicated in myocardial infarction patient. Low addictive element. Contraindicated in children under 12. *May be given undiluted.*
Nalbuphine 10 mg every 3–6 h	Caution in head injury, pregnancy, lactation. *May be given undiluted.*
Butorphanol 1 mg every 3–4 h	Caution in respiratory depression, head injury, and impaired liver or kidney function. *May be given undiluted.*
Partial Agonist	
Buprenorphine 0.3 mg, repeat every 6 h	May produce withdrawal in narcotic-dependent patients. Caution in asthma, respiratory depression, or impaired renal or hepatic function. Contraindicated in children under 12. *May be given undiluted.*

Sources: Data from Deglin, J.H., & Vallerand, A.H. (1995). *Davis's drug guide for nurses,* 4th ed. Philadelphia: F.A. Davis. Copyright 1995 by F.A. Davis; and *Principles of analgesic use in the treatment of acute pain and chronic cancer pain: A concise guide to medical practice,* 2nd ed. Skokie, IL: American Pain Society. Copyright 1989 by the American Pain Society.

cation by pressing a button that is attached to a computerized pump (Panfilli, Brunchkorts, & Dundon, 1988). The goal of PCA is to provide the patient with a serum analgesia level for comfort with minimal sedation (Ryder, 1991). Putting patients in charge of their own pain management makes sense because only the patient knows how much he or she is suffering.

1. Define the types of patients to use the PCA device.
2. Develop teaching tools.
3. Select the appropriate equipment.
4. Select the medications used and establish consistency of use and dosage.
5. Define who will handle the side effects and provide an appropriate method of communication (St. Marie, 1991).

CANDIDATES FOR WHOM PCA SHOULD BE CONSIDERED
1. Patients who are anticipating pain that is severe yet intermittent (e.g., patients suffering from kidney stones)
2. Patients who have constant pain that worsens with activity
3. Pediatric patients who are older than 7 years of age and capable of being taught to manage the PCA machine
4. Patients who are capable of manipulating the dose button
5. Patients who are motivated to use PCA

KEY CONCEPTS OF PCA
1. In the first 24 hours after surgery, the patient has the greatest need for pain control.
2. Studies have shown that the best results for PCA occur when the patient can administer a bolus every 5 to 10 minutes.
3. When patients have control of their narcotic doses, they will keep the narcotic within therapeutic levels.
4. When patients are in control and know they can get more immediate pain relief by pushing a button, they are more relaxed (White, 1988).
5. Analgesia is most effective when a therapeutic serum level is consistently maintained.
6. Postoperative patients can easily titrate doses according to need and avoid peaks and troughs associated with conventional I.V. and intramuscular administration of narcotics.
7. Studies have found that orthopedic patients seemed more tolerant of repositioning when on PCA.
8. Patients with abdominal surgery ambulate sooner postoperatively.
9. PCA patients are better able to cough and deep breathe (Kleiman, Lipman, & Hare, 1987).

INVESTIGATIONAL DRUGS

Administration of investigational medications shall be in accordance with state and federal regulations. Signed informed patient consent is required prior to patient participation in the investigation.

Investigational drugs are defined as medications that are not approved for general use by the Food and Drug Administration (FDA). Many clinical trials are conducted as a form of planned experiment that evoke appropriate treatment of future patients with a given medical condition. Clinical trials are designed to discover a drug's efficacy in selected patient populations.

Following are the phases of FDA drug studies.

Phase I: Clinical pharmacology and therapeutics
  Evaluate drug safety.
  Determine an acceptable single drug dosage for levels of patient tolerance for acute multiple dosing.

Phase II: Initial clinical investigation for therapeutic effect
   Evaluate drug efficacy.
   Conduct a pilot study.
Phase III: Full-scale evaluation of treatment
   Evaluate the patient population for which drug is intended.
Phase IV: Postmarketing surveillance
   Provide additional information about the efficacy or safety profile.

The role of the registered nurse in investigational drugs is to assist the investigator (physician) in conducting the study.

KEY POINTS IN THE ROLE OF THE NURSE IN INVESTIGATIONAL DRUGS

1. Communicating with Institutional Review Board (IRB); familiarity with their policies and Federal regulations (copies of communication between the investigator and the IRB should be copied to the sponsor)
2. Writing informed consent, explaining to patient, and obtaining signature
3. Communicating with hospital's legal counsel and ethics committee to complete protocols
4. I.V. administration of the investigational drug
5. Participating in collection of data
6. When required, assisting with blood sampling
7. Assisting with final study report, which is a requirement of the US Federal regulations for the sponsor (Weinstein, 1987)

General ethical requirements of clinical research worldwide are outlined in the *Declaration of Helsinki,* issued by the World Medical Association in 1960 and revised in 1975. This document has been accepted internationally as the basis for ethical research (Popock, 1983).

Nursing Plan Of Care

ADMINISTRATION OF I.V. MEDICATIONS

Focus Assessment

Subjective

Review present illness
Review current drug therapy
Review previous drug therapy and side effects
Lifestyle for home care
Note any allergies prior to starting medication

Objective

Observe ability to ingest and retain fluids.
Monitor vital signs.
Weigh patient.
Assess patient-related factors that may alter patient's response to drug, such as age or renal, liver, and cardiovascular function.
Assess current medications for clues to drug interaction and incompatibility.

Patient Outcome Criteria

The patient will:
Respond therapeutically to the drug
Demonstrate improved fluid balance
Verbalize understanding of the purpose of the medication
Demonstrate absence of complications associated with I.V. therapy

Continued on following page

PATIENT EDUCATION

Instruct patient on expected actions and adverse effects of medication.
Instruct patient on administration of anti-infectives around the clock to maintain
   blood levels.

HOME CARE ISSUES

The rapidly growing home care infusion industry now provides many I.V. drugs.
Medications that are now being delivered in the home include:

Cardiovascular drugs
Antihypertensives
Heparin
Interferon
Colony-stimulating factors
Chelation therapy (deferoxamine)
Growth hormones
Gammaglobulin

380

Home Antibiotic Therapy

Computerized ambulatory infusion devices (drug pumps) have enabled antimicrobial therapy to be safely and effectively administered in the home with minimal disruption in the patient's life. When administering antimicrobials in the home, safety, effectiveness, acceptance, and cost need to be considered.

Safety. Patients who are able to care for themselves are the best candidates for using ambulatory pumps and usually make the adjustment quickly.

Effectiveness. To ensure effective treatment, coordination of care among the patient, nurse, physician, and pharmacist is essential.

Acceptance. Unless the patient understands the treatment, procedure, and administration regimen and accepts them into his or her lifestyle, home antimicrobial therapy will not be successful.

Cost. Delivering antimicrobial therapy at home is cost-effective as long as it *effectively* treats the problem. Medicare and third party payers have recognized financial savings using this method (Brown, 1988).

✎ **NOTE:** Clinical assessment of the patient on antibiotics is based on the same standards, regardless of treatment environment, including monitoring for adverse reactions, disease process and laboratory tests.

Home Pain Management

Advanced technology now allows continuous or intermittent self-administration of analgesics in the home, usually with a patient-controlled analgesia (PCA) pump or portable pump. I.V., intrathecal, epidural, or subcutaneous routes can be used (Weinstein, 1993).

✎ **NOTE:** As with any I.V. medication delivery, emergency drugs should be readily available and protocols established for their use.

COMPETENCY CRITERIA

Competency Statement: The competent nurse will demonstrate management of epidural catheter.

COGNITIVE CRITERIA

	Skilled	*Needs Education*

1. **Describes the spinal anatomy and physiology:** Intraspinal
    1. Intrathecal
    2. Epidural
 Opiate receptor sites		

2. **Discusses types, modes, and actions of epidural medications:** Preservative free medication Hydrophilic properties Lipophilic properties		
3. **Identifies side effects and nursing interventions for complications from epidural analgesia:** Spinal headache Urinary retention, pruritus, nausea, drowsiness, parathesia Respiratory depression Catheter migration		

PERFORMANCE CRITERIA

1. **Uses preservative-free medication.**

2. **Labels epidural catheter as designated line.**

3. **Demonstates dressing change for epidural catheter.**

4. **Uses 0.22 micron filter.**

5. **Uses electronic infusion device to administer medication.**

6. **Uses flow sheet to monitor patient's response to epidural medication.**

SUGGESTED EVALUATION CRITERIA

Cognitive:
Written test
Verbal discussion with preceptor

Performance:
Return demonstration with preceptor

KEY POINTS

Advantages of I.V. medications
1. Provides a direct access to the circulatory system
2. Provides a route for drugs that irritate the gastric mucosa
3. Provides a route for instant drug action
4. Provides a route for delivering high drug concentrations
5. Provides for instant drug termination if sensitivity or adverse reaction occurs
6. Provides a route of administration in patients in whom use of the gastrointestinal tract is limited

Disadvantages of I.V. medications
1. Drug interaction due to incompatibilities
2. Adsorption of the drug impaired due to leaching into I.V. container or administration set
3. Errors in compounding of medication
4. Speed shock
5. Extravasation of a vesicant drug
6. Chemical phlebitis

Drug interactions
Adsorption
Errors in mixing
Speed shock
Extravasation
Chemical phlebitis

Drug incompatibilities
Physical
Chemical
Therapeutic

Methods of I.V. medication administration
Continuous infusion
Intermittent infusion
  Piggyback
  Infusion using heparin or saline locking device
  Volumetric chamber
I.V. push
Continuous subcutaneous infusion
Intraspinal medication infusion
  Epidural
  Intrathecal
Arteriovenous fistula

383

Key questions in delivery of antimicrobial agents
Has the infecting organism been identified?
Is the organism resistant to any antimicrobials?
Is the site of the infection identified?
What is the status of the host defenses?
Is the nurse familiar with the antimicrobial pharmacokinetics?
Is the patient's renal and hepatic function known?
Is monitoring the patient's blood levels necessary?
Does the patient have an allergy to the anti-infective agent?
Antibiotics
  Categories
    β-Lactamase agents
    Cephalosporin
    Aminoglycosides
    Chloramphenicol
    Erythromycin
    Fluoroquinolones
    Tetracycline
Antifungal agents
  Amphotericin B
  Fluconazole
  Miconazole
Antiviral agents
  Acyclovir
  Ganciclovir
  Pentamidine
  Isethionate
  Vidarabine
  Zidovudine

Types of pain (according to WHO and American Pain Society)
Opioids
Nonnarcotic analgesics and nonsteroid anti-inflammatory drugs
  (NSAIDs)
Adjuvants

Investigational drugs
Administration of investigational medications in accordance with state and federal regulations
Phases of FDA drug studies
  Phase I—Clinical pharmacology and therapeutics
  Phase II—Initial clinical investigation
  Phase III—Full-scale evaluation and treatment
  Phase IV—Post-marketing surveillance

384

CRITICAL THINKING ACTIVITY

1. The patient requires pain medication and the order is for 2 mg of morphine I.V. every 2 hours as needed for pain. Discuss the key points to remember in delivering this medication by the I.V. push route.

2. You are working in a small rural outpatient clinic. A patient comes in in respiratory distress with electrolyte imbalance. The physician orders a primary solution of 5% dextrose and 0.45% normal saline with vitamins B and C and aminophyllin. Also ordered is 20 mEq of potassium chloride to be administered over 2 hours. No pharmacist is available to assist you with this admixture. How do you infuse these medications and how do you check for compatibility?

3. You are mixing two medications in one syringe for an I.V. push administration. The solution has turned a pale yellow. Can you safely administer this drug? If not, what type of incompatibility is this?

4. A patient complains of burning from the antibiotic that was just started. The antibiotic is diluted in 100 mL of 5% dextrose in water piggybacked to run 45 minutes. What alternatives do you have in dealing with this complaint?

POST-TEST, CHAPTER 11

1. List three of the five advantages of I.V. medication delivery.

   A. _____

   B. _____

   C. _____

2. Which of the following are incompatibilities of I.V. therapy?
   A. Intermittent, physical, and biotransformation
   B. Drug interaction, drug synergism, and drug tolerance
   C. Physical, chemical, and therapeutic

3. Methods by which a registered nurse can deliver medication via the I.V. route include all of the following EXCEPT:
   A. I.V. push (bolus)
   B. Continuous subcutaneous infusion
   C. Continuous infusion
   D. Piggyback
   E. Epidural

4. A key point in infusion of I.V. antifungal drugs is:
   A. Most are infused as a suspension.
   B. Drugs should not be filtered.
   C. Drugs should be administered slowly.
   D. All of the above.

5. WHO and the American Pain Society have grouped analgesics into three categories, which are:
   A. Opioids, nonnarcotic nonsteroid, and adjuvants
   B. Anesthetics, nonnarcotic, and cholinergics
   C. Adrenergics, opioids, and opiates

6. List the important steps in dressing change of an epidural catheter.

7. I.V. push medications should be administered according to manufacturer's recommendations but not faster than:
   A. 5 minutes
   B. 10 minutes
   C. 1 minute
   D. 30 seconds

8. The goal of patient-controlled analgesia is to provide the patient with:
   A. a serum analgesia level for comfort without sedation
   B. a serum analgesia level to achieve sedation
   C. a method of euthanasia
   D. limited control over pain management

9. The role of the nurse in investigational drugs is to:
   A. Conduct the study
   B. Administer the investigational drug under physician direction
   C. Take the role as investigator
   D. Has no role in the administration of investigational drugs

10. Which of the following are side effects of epidural pain medication?
    A. Urinary retention, pruritus, and respiratory depression
    B. Respiratory depression, peptic ulcer, and hemiparesis
    C. Pruritus, nausea, and urinary incontinence

Match the definition in column II to the term in column I.

Column I

11. _____ distribution
12. _____ absorption
13. _____ compatibility
14. _____ intrathecal
15. _____ therapeutic incompatibility
16. _____ chemical incompatibility
17. _____ physical incompatibility
18. _____ admixture
19. _____ delivery system

Column II

A. A product that allows for the administration of medication

B. Process of movement of medication from drug administration site to vasculature

C. Capable of being mixed and administered without undergoing undesirable changes

D. Process of delivering a drug to the various tissues of the body

E. Undesirable change that is visual

F. Undesirable effect occuring within a patient as a result of two or more drugs being given concurrently

G. Change in molecular structure of a substance

H. Combination of two or more medications

I. Inside the spinal cord

ANSWERS TO CHAPTER 11

PRE-TEST

1. J	6. B	11. A	16. T
2. F	7. G	12. B	17. T
3. H	8. D	13. A	18. T
4. I	9. A	14. C	19. T
5. C	10. E	15. B	20. E

POST-TEST

1. Allows for absorption of drugs unstable in gastric juices
Provides a route for drug with irritating properties
Provides a route for instant drug action
Permits termination of infusion if sensitivity occurs
Provides better control over rate of administration of drug
2. C
3. E

4. D
5. A
6. Wash hands with antimicrobial soap.
Remove old dressing.
Wet cotton-tipped applicator in povidone-iodine solution and clean area, starting at catheter and working outward.
Let dry.
Apply new transparent dressing.
Do not used alcohol on skin or dressing site.

7. C
8. A
9. B
10. A
11. D
12. B
13. C

14. I
15. F
16. G
17. E
18. H
19. A

REFERENCES

Akahoshi, M.P., Furuike-McLaughlin, T., & Enriquez, N.C. (1988). Patient controlled analgesia via intrathecal catheter in outpatient oncology patient. *Journal of Intravenous Nursing, 11* (5), 289–292.

American Pain Society. (1989). *Principles of analgesic use in the treatment of acute pain and chronic cancer pain. A concise guide to medical practice* (2nd ed). Skokie, IL: American Pain Society.

Baldwin, D.R. (1995). Pharmacology. In Terry, J., Baranowski, L., Lonsway, R., & Hedrick, C., eds. *Intravenous therapy: Clinical principles and practice.* (192–195). Philadelphia: W.B. Saunders.

Bonica, J.J. (1990). *The management of pain* (2nd ed). Philadelphia: Lea & Febiger.

Bromage, P.R. (1980). State of art: Extradural and intrathecal narcotics. *Anesthesia and Analgesia, 59,* 473–480.

Brown, J.M. (1988). Innovative antibiotic therapy at home. *Journal of Intravenous Nursing, 11* (6), 397–401.

Burman, R., & Berkowitz, H. (1986). IV bolus: Effective, but potentially hazardous. *Critical Care Nurse, 6* (1), 22–27.

Coyle, N., Mauskop, A., Maggard, J., & Foley, K.M. (1986). Continuous subcutaneous infusions of opiates in cancer patients with pain. *Oncology Nursing Forum, 13* (4), 53–57.

D'Arcy, P.F. (1983). Drug interactions with medical plastics. *Drug Intelligence Clinical Pharmacy, 17,* 726–731.

Delaney, C.W., & Lauer, M.L. (1988). *Intravenous therapy: A guide to quality care.* Philadelphia: J.B. Lippincott.

Gahart, B.L. (1996). *Intravenous medications,* 12th ed. St. Louis: Mosby–Year Book.

Gong, H., & King, C.Y. (1983). Inadequate drug mixing: A potential hazard in continuous intravenous admixture. *Heart & Lung, 12* (5), 528–532.

Harris, G.W. (1981). *Conference on phthalates.* Washington, DC: US Department of Health and Human Services, 189–192.

Kleiman, A.G., Lipman, B.D., & Hare, S. (1987). PCA vs. regular IM injections for severe post-op pain. *American Journal of Nursing, 11,* 1491–1492.

Lieb, R.A., & Hurtig, J.B. (1985). Epidural and intrathecal narcotics for pain management. *Heart and Lung, 14* (2), 164–171.

Lippincott Learning System (1984). *Incompatibilities: I.V. Therapy study guide and workbook.* Philadelphia: J.B. Lippincott.

Lonsway, R.A. (1988). Care of the patient with an epidural catheter: An infection control challenge. *Journal of Intravenous Nursing, 11* (1), 52–54.

Mathewson-Kuhn, M. (1994). *Pharmacotherapeutics: A nursing process approach* (3rd ed). Philadelphia: F.A. Davis.

May, G., & Lukacsko, P.K. (1985). *A guide to parenteral analgesia using the CADD-PCA infusion pump.* NJ: Pharmacia, Inc.

Mazur, H.I., Stennett, D.J., & Egging, P.K. (1989). Extraction of diethylhexyphthalate from total nutrient-containing polyvinylchloride bags. *Journal of Parenteral Enteral Nutrition, 13,* 59–62.

McCaffery, M., & Beebe, A. (1989). *Pain: Clinical manual for nursing practice.* St. Louis: Mosby–Year Book.

McGuire, L. (1990). Administering analgesics: Which drugs are right for your patient. *Nursing 90, 4,* 34–41.

McLaughlin-Hagan, M. (1990). Continuous subcutaneous infusion of narcotics. *Journal of Intravenous Therapy, 13* (2), 119–124.

Murphy, D. (1990). Home pain management continuous infusion narcotics. *Journal of Intravenous Nursing, 13* (6), 355–358.

Nieves-Cordero, A. (1985). Compatibility of narcotic analgesic solutions with various antibiotics during simulated Y-site injections. *American Journal of Hospital Pharmacy, 42,* 1108–1109.

Nightingale, F (1860). Notes on Nursing. New York: Appleton & Co.

Noah, V.A., & Godin, M. (1994). A perspective on di-20ethyl-hexyphthalate in intravenous therapy. *Journal of Intravenous Therapy,* (4) 210–211.

Nurses Drug Alert. (1985). Compatibility of antibiotics and narcotics given intravenously. *American Journal of Nursing, 85* (5), 59–60.

Panfilli, R., Brunchkorst, L., & Dundon, R. (1988). Nursing implications of patient-controlled analgesia. *Journal of Intravenous Nursing, 11* (2), 75–77.

Pearson, S.D., & Trissel, L.A. (1993). Leeching of diethylhexylphalate for polyvinylchloride containers by selected drugs and formulation components. *American Journal of Hospital Pharmacy, 50,* 1405–1409.

Popock, S.J. (1983). *Clinical trials: A practical approach.* Chichester England: John Wiley & Sons.

Rosen, H. (1990). An epidural analgesia program: Balancing risks and benefits. *Critical Care Nurse, 10* (8), 32–41.

Ryder, E. (1991). All about patient-controlled analgesia. *Journal of Intravenous Nursing, 14* (6), 372–379.

Slater, E.M., Zeitlin, G.L., & Edwards, M.G. (1985). Experience with epidural morphine for post-surgical pain in a community setting. *Anesthesiology Review, 12* (3).

Snyder, E.L., Hedber, S.L., & Napychank, P.A. (1993). Stability of red cell antigens and plasma coagulation factors stored in a nondiethylhexyl phthalate-plasticized container. *Transfusion 33,* 515–519.

St. Marie, B. (1989). Administration of intraspinal analgesia in the home care setting. *Journal of Intravenous Nursing, 12* (3), 164–168.

St. Marie, B. (1991). Narcotic infusions: A changing scene. *Journal of Intravenous Nursing, 14* (5), 334–343.

St. Marie, B. (1995). Pain management. Terry, J., Baranowski, L., Lonsway, R., & Hedrick, C. *Intravenous Therapy Clinical Principles and Practices.* Philadelphia: W. B. Saunders, 277–297.

Todd, B. (1988). Intravenous drug hazards: Interactions, absorption, inadequate mixing. *Geriatric Nursing, 1,* 20–22.

Wang, J.K., Nauss, L.F., & Thomas, J.E. (1979). Pain relief by intrathecally applied morphine in man. *Anesthesiology, 50* (2), 149–151.

Weinstein, S.M. (1987). Use of investigational drugs. *National Intravenous Therapy Association, 10* (5), 336–347.

Weinstein, S.M. (1993). *Plumer's principles and practices of intravenous therapy.* Philadelphia: J.B. Lippincott, pp 407–419.

White, P. (1988). Patient-controlled analgesia. *Anesthesiology, 2* (3), 339–350.

Zola, E., & McLeod, D. (1983). Comparative effects and analgesic efficacy of the agonist-antagonist opioids. *Drug Intelligence Clinical Pharmacy, 17.*

CHAPTER 12

Central Venous Access Devices

CHAPTER CONTENTS

GLOSSARY
LEARNING OBJECTIVES
PRE-TEST, CHAPTER 12
ANATOMY OF THE VASCULAR SYSTEM
Venous Structures of the Arm
Venous Structures of the Chest
CENTRAL VENOUS CATHETER MATERIALS
Silicone Elastomers (Silastic)
Polyurethane
Elastomeric Hydrogel
Coatings
Lumens
SHORT-TERM AND LONG-TERM ACCESS
    DEVICES
Short-Term Devices
Long-Term Devices
Tunneled Catheter with Groshong Valve
Implanted Ports

Insertion
Nursing Management of Implanted Ports
OCCLUDED CENTRAL VENOUS DEVICES
Mechanical Occlusion
Thrombotic Occlusion
Nonthrombotic Occlusion
NURSING PLAN OF CARE: MANAGEMENT OF
    CENTRAL VENOUS ACCESS DEVICES
PATIENT EDUCATION
HOME CARE ISSUES
COMPETENCY CRITERIA
KEY POINTS
CRITICAL THINKING ACTIVITY
POST-TEST, CHAPTER 12
ANSWERS TO CHAPTER 12
Pre-Test
Post-Test
REFERENCES

GLOSSARY

Anatomic measurement   Determination of body dimension

Broviac catheter   Tunneled venous catheter with one Dacron cuff with an outer diameter of 1.0; useful for infusion of nutrient solutions

CVC   Central venous catheter

CVTC   Central venous tunneled catheter

Cutdown   Surgical procedure for exposure and cannulation of a vein

Distal   Farthest from the heart; farthest from the point of attachment; below previous site of cannulation

Extravascular malpositioning   Introducer of the central venous percutaneous catheter is passed out of the vessel and into the pleural space or the mediastinum

Groshong catheter   Surgically implanted, long-term tunneled Silastic catheter; unique in that it has a two-way valve adjacent to the closed tip, which prevents backflow of blood

Hickman catheter   Long-term tunneled Silastic catheter inserted surgically

Implanted port   Catheter surgically placed into a vessel, body cavity, or organ and attached to a reservoir, which is placed under the skin

Infraclavicular Situated below a clavicle

Intravascular malpositioning Catheter tip of a percutaneous, tunneled or implanted port coils in the vessel, which advances into a venous tributary other than the superior vena cava, or does not reach the superior vena cava

Lymphedema Swelling of an extremity caused by obstruction of lymphatic vessels

Midclavicular Long (20- to 24-in) intravenous access device made of a soft flexible material inserted into one of the superficial veins of the peripheral vascular system and *advanced to proximal axillary or subclavian veins*

Peripherally inserted central venous catheter (PICC) Long (20- to 24-in) I.V. access device made of a soft flexible material (silicone or a polymer); the PICC is usually inserted into one of the superficial veins of the peripheral vascular system and advanced into the central system

Silicone Material containing silicone carbon bond, used as lubricants, insulating resins, and waterproofing materials

Thrombogenicity Generating or production of thrombosis

Trendelenburg position Position in which the head is lower than the feet; used to increase venous distention

Tunneled catheter Catheter designed to have a portion lie within a subcutaneous passage before exiting the body

VAD Vascular access device

LEARNING OBJECTIVES

Upon completion of this chapter, the reader will be able to:

- Define the glossary of terms as related to central venous devices.
- Discuss the hazard associated with percutaneous insertion of central lines: intravascular malpositioning and extravascular malpositioning.
- Differentiate between short-term and long-term access devices.
- Identify the advantages of peripherally inserted central catheters (PICCs).
- Identify candidates for PICC.
- Discuss the procedure for insertion of a PICC.
- List the steps in dressing management of a PICC.
- Identify the complications associated with PICCs.
- Identify the advantages of tunneled Silastic catheters.
- State the advantages of the implanted port.
- Compare the advantages and disadvantages of tunneled catheters with the advantages and disadvantages of implanted ports.
- Discuss the nursing management of tunneled catheters and implanted ports.
- Identify the potential complications associated with central venous tunneled catheters and implanted ports.
- Use the nursing process in providing nursing care to the patient with a central venous access device.

PRE-TEST, CHAPTER 12

Match the definition in column II to the abbreviation in column I.

Column I

1. _____ CVC

2. _____ CVTC

3. _____ VAD

4. _____ PICC

Column II

A. Intravenous device inserted into superior vena cava via the peripheral vasculature

B. Vascular access device

C. Central venous access device

D. Central venous catheter

5. Advantages of the peripherally inserted catheters include:
   A. Decreases risk of pneumothorax and air embolism on insertion
   B. Preserves peripheral vascular system in the upper extremity
   C. Eliminates the pain of frequent venipunctures
   D. Decreases cost and is time-efficient
   E. All of the above

6. The best site selection for a peripherally inserted central catheter would include:
   A. Basilic vein
   B. Innominate vein
   C. Jugular vein

7. Key points in dressing management of peripherally inserted central catheters would include:
   A. Change dressing after the first 24 hours.
   B. Use sterile technique.
   C. Inspect the catheter insertion site for redness, swelling, and drainage.
   D. Use care not to dislodge the catheter during the dressing change.
   E. Transparent dressing is recommended after the first 24 hours.
   F. All of the above.

8. Complications related to the insertion of peripherally inserted central catheters include:
   A. Bleeding, malposition of the catheter, and nerve damage
   B. Phlebitis, infection, and air embolism
   C. Bleeding, cardiac arrhythmias, and infection

9. Advantages of central venous tunneled catheters include:
   A. Can be repaired if catheter breaks or leaks
   B. Is useful for all I.V. therapies
   C. Eliminates multiple venipunctures
   D. All of the above

True-False

10. **T F** Luer-locking connectors should be used on all centrally placed catheters.

11. **T F** The Hickman catheter should be flushed with 10 mL of sodium chloride and heparin after each blood drawing.

12. **T F** Groshong catheters must be flushed with heparinized saline.

As long as the beginner pilot, language learner, chess player, or driver is
following rules, his performance is halting, rigid, and mediocre. But with the
mastery of the activity comes the transformation of the skill which is like the
transformation that occurs when a blind person learns to use a cane. The
beginner feels pressure in the palm of the hand which can be used to detect the
presence of distinct objects such as curbs. But, with mastery the blind person
no longer feels pressure in the palm of the hand, but simply feels the curb. The
cane has become an extension of the body.

Expert Performance, DREYFUS AND DREYFUS, 1997

A similar transformation occurs with the expert nurse clinician's tools.

ANATOMY OF THE VASCULAR SYSTEM

To understand the placement of central venous catheters (CVCs), it is important to understand the anatomy of the upper extremity venous system, arm, and axilla. The veins of importance include basilic, cephalic, axillary, subclavian, internal and external jugular, right and left innominate (brachiocephalic) veins, and superior vena cava. It is also imperative that the registered nurse be fully aware of the anatomic position and structures of the arm and axilla venous system when insertion of peripherally inserted central catheters are desired.

Venous Structures of the Arm

The venous structures of the arm include the cephalic and the basilic veins. The cephalic vein ascends along the outer border of the biceps muscle to the upper third of the arm. It passes in the space between the pectoralis major and deltoid muscles. The vein decreases in size just a few inches above the antecubital fossa and may terminate in the axillary vein or pass above or through the clavicle in a descending curve. Normally, the cephalic vein turns sharply (90 degrees) as it pierces the clavipectoral fascia and passes beneath the clavicle. Near its termination, the cephalic vein may bifurcate into two small veins—one joining the external jugular and one joining the axillary vein. Valves are located along the cephalic vein's course (Gray, 1977). The basilic vein is larger than the cephalic vein. It passes upward in a smooth path along the inner side of the biceps muscle and terminates in the axillary vein. A catheter threaded in the basilic vein may have a tendency to enter the jugular vein (Bridges, Carden, & Takac, 1979). If the patient's head is turned toward the side of insertion during catheter placement, this malposition may be avoided (Fig. 12–1).

Venous Structures of the Chest

The venous structures of the chest include the subclavian, the internal and external jugular, and innominate veins, and the superior vena cava. The subclavian vein extends from the outer border of the first rib to the sternal end of the clavicle and measures about 4 to 5 cm in length; the right brachiocephalic vein measures about 2.5 cm, and the left brachiocephalic vein measures about 6 to 6.5 cm. The external

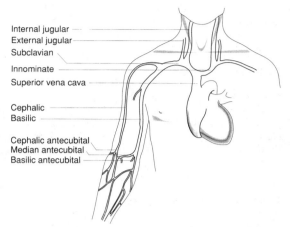

Figure 12–1. Anatomic venous structures of the arm and chest. (Source: Markel, S., & Reynan, K. [1990]). Impact on patient care: 2652 PIC catheter days. *Journal of Intravenous Nursing, 13*(6), 349. Copyright 1990 by the *Journal of Intravenous Nursing.*)

jugular lies on the side of the neck and follows a descending inward path to join the subclavian vein along the middle of the clavicle. The internal jugular vein descends first behind and then to the outer side of the internal and common carotid arteries; it joins the subclavian vein at the root of the neck. Valves are present in the venous system until approximately 1 in before the formation of the innominate vein. The right innominate vein is about 1 in long and passes almost vertically downward to join the left innominate vein just below the cartilage of the first rib. The left innominate vein is about 2.5 in long and larger than the right innominate vein. It passes from left to right in a downward slant across the upper front of the chest. It joins the right innominate vein to form the superior vena cava. The superior vena cava receives all blood from the upper half of the body. It is composed of a short trunk 2.5 to 3 in long. It begins below the first rib close to the sternum on the right side, descends vertically slightly to the right, and empties into the right atrium of the heart (Speer, 1990). The right atrium receives blood from the upper body via the superior vena cava and from the lower body via the inferior vena cava. The venae cavae are referred to as the great veins. The right atrium is larger than the left atrium, and its walls are thin (Weinstein, 1993).

CENTRAL VENOUS CATHETER MATERIALS

Most vascular access devices (VADs) are made of biocompatible materials including polyurethane, elastomeric hydrogel, and silicone elastomers. The composition and biocompatibility of the catheter material may influence the development of several CVC-related complications such as catheter-related sepsis (Baranowski, 1993).

All catheters—whether used for short-term or long-term access—should have a radiopaque lateral strip or a radiopaque distal end for visualization on x-ray (Speer, 1990).

Silicone Elastomers (Silastic)

Silastic is soft and pliable and cannot be inserted by the conventional over-the-needle technique. Catheters made of Silastic require special insertion procedures with or without guidewires. Because of its soft, flexible nature, silicone is less likely to dam-

395

age the intima of the vein wall and is reported to be less thrombogenic. Most long-term CVCs and peripherally inserted central catheters (PICCs) are made of Silastic (Baranowski, 1993).

Polyurethane

Polyurethane is a commonly used material for short-term percutaneously placed CVCs and is more frequently being used in long-term CVCs and PICCs. Polyurethane is stiffer than silicone and softens after insertion, making threading of the catheter easier. Polyurethane catheters have thinner walls owing to greater tensile strength than silicone catheters. Polyurethane is similar to silicone in biocompatibility and is thrombus-resistant.

Elastomeric Hydrogel

Elastomeric hydrogel is a newer catheter materials. This material is available for CVCs. A proposed advantage of the material is the stiffness it provides during insertion and subsequent softening following insertion.

Coatings

To further decrease the risk of complications inherent with even the most biocompatible materials, catheters coated or bonded with hydrophilic materials, antiseptic substances, antibiotics, or heparin are available (Baranowski, 1993). The quest for bacteria resistant materials has led to studies in which antibiotics were bonded to the catheter insertion site (Trooskin, Donetz, & Harvey, 1985). A study using CVCs impregnated with silver sulfadiazine and chlorhexidine compared with standard catheters suggests that patients with the impregnated catheters had a reduced incidence of catheter infections (Maki, Wheeler, & Stoltz, 1991). Use of CVCs bonded with antibiotics or antimicrobial agents appears to be of promise in the future in reducing catheter-related septicemias.

Lumens

Catheters are available in single, double, triple, and recently quadruple lumens. The diameter of each lumen varies because of the need for larger diameters for administration of hypertonic or viscous solutions. Refer to manufacturer information to ascertain which lumen is the largest if you are administering vesicant or hypertonic solution through one lumen. See Fig. 12–2 for lumen sizes.

For most solutions and medications, any lumen may be selected for infusion. It is recommended that the distal lumen be used for administration of vesicant solutions. The proximal lumen should be used for blood withdrawal, when possible, to avoid contamination of the specimen from solutions infusing into the other lumens (Fig. 12–3).

SHORT-TERM AND LONG-TERM ACCESS DEVICES

Several factors must be considered when selecting the appropriate CVC, including the duration and type of therapy, evaluation of the patient's venous access, medical history, current diagnosis, and patient's activity level. For long-term devices, the

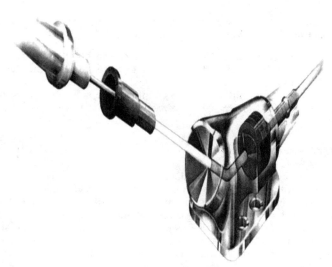

Figure 12–2. Single, double, and triple lumens. (Courtesy of Bard Access Systems, Salt Lake City, Utah.)

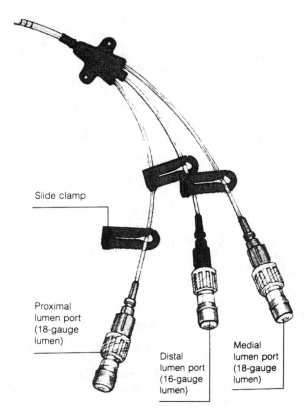

Slide clamp

Proximal
lumen port
(18-gauge
lumen)

Distal
lumen port
(16-gauge
lumen)

Medial
lumen port
(18-gauge
lumen)

Figure 12–3. Injection parts of the triple-lumen catheter include the proximal lumen port, distal lumen port, and medial lumen port. The distal port (*middle line*) is usually the largest of the three lines.

397

patient's and caregiver's ability to perform or assist with catheter care as well as the financial impact need to be considered (Baranowski, 1993).

✎ **NOTE:** After insertion of the catheter, verification by chest x-ray must be obtained before any infusion. After placement of the catheter, the devices can be closed with an injection cap and heparinized while catheter tip location is verified by radiologic examination. Do not infuse any solution but isotonic fluids without additives if the physician desires an x-ray with free-flowing solution.

Short-Term Devices

Short-term devices are intended to be used for days to weeks. These devices can be single-lumen or multiple-lumen catheters made of several materials. They are inserted by a percutaneous venipuncture and are not tunneled under the skin. The infraclavicular, jugular, or femoral veins are the sites used if performed by a physician, and the veins of the antecubital area are used if performed by a registered nurse specially trained for peripheral central venous access. See Table 12–1 for a summary of features, advantages, and disadvantages of short-term percutaneous devices.

Percutaneous Catheters

In 1961, the first I.V. catheter for accessing the central circulation was introduced (Stewart & Sanislow, 1961). Subclavian catheterization was initially inserted using surgical cutdown technique such as advocated by Heimback and Ivey (1976). However, percutaneous introduction into the subclavian vein using the Seldinger through-the-needle guidewire technique is now generally preferred. The percutaneous short-term catheter is secured by suturing, and the catheter is not tunneled. This catheter may remain in place for 7 days.

The most common site for insertion of the percutaneous catheter is the infraclavicular approach to the subclavian vein.

The patient is placed in the Trendelenburg position with a rolled bath blanket or towel between the shoulders. The patient should be instructed to perform a Valsalva maneuver during the venipuncture procedure to increase the size of the veins. This exit site on the upper chest is well suited for many types of dressings, and care of the site is not complex (Fig. 12–4).

✎ **NOTE:** The infraclavicular approach site requires a well-hydrated patient.

The internal jugular vein is an accessible site for the physician; however, care of this site is more difficult. The motion of the neck, a beard on males, long hair, and close proximity of respiratory secretions prevent the adequate use of transparent occlusive dressings. The femoral veins are not recommended for this type of therapy because of the difficulty of placement of the catheter tip. It is also impossible to maintain an occlusive dressing on the femoral exit site (Hadaway, 1990).

Dressing Management

The percutaneous catheter can be dressed in one of two ways, depending on agency policy. An occlusive gauze or tape or a transparent semipermeable membrane (TSM) dressing may be used. In today's practice the TSM dressing has gained popularity because of its occlusive nature and ability to visualize the site.

Most protocols for frequency of dressing changes are based on empirical success and range from every other day to weekly changes, depending on the type of dressing and the patient population.

398

TABLE 12–1. COMPARING CENTRAL VENOUS CATHETERS

Type/Use	Features	Advantages	Disadvantages
		Short-Term Catheters	
Percutaneous Up to several weeks Intended for days to several weeks.	*Material:* polyurethane, Silastic, Aquavene *Length:* 6–30 cm *Gauge:* 14–27F *Available Features:* Heparin, hydromere, antibiotic and antiseptic coatings, and antimicrobial cuff available Preattached extensions with clamps Multiple lumens	Inserted at bedside; cost-effective, easy to remove, easy to exchange over guidewire	Placement time limited (usually 7 days) Requires sterile dressing changes; requires daily heparin flushes; catheter may break; requires activity restrictions
Peripherally inserted central catheters Up to several months	*Material:* polyurethane, Silastic, Aquavene *Length:* 33.5–60 cm *Gauge:* 14–25F *Lumen:* double Groshong valve Insertion trays, spare needles, spare catheters, and repair kits available Preattached extension with clamps	Inserted at bedside by specially trained RN; cost-effective, easy to remove, reliable for long-term use; eliminates risks associated with chest or neck insertion; preserves integrity of peripheral vascular system	Requires sterile dressing changes; requires routine heparin flushes except with Groshong valve in place; catheter may break; requires activity restrictions; may not be possible to withdraw blood for sampling
		Long-Term Catheters	
Tunneled Long-term intermittent continuous or daily I.V. access	*Material:* polyurethane *Length:* 55–90 cm *Gauge:* 2.7–19.2F *Lumen:* multiple Groshong valve Detachable hub Antimicrobial collagen cuff	Inserted at bedside; can remain in place indefinitely; requires aseptic dressing changes; clean when site is healed; can be repaired externally; self-care possible	May require routine heparin flushes, except with Groshong valve; catheter may break; daily to weekly site care; may be difficult to remove

TABLE 12–1. COMPARING CENTRAL VENOUS CATHETERS (*Continued*)

Type/Use	Features	Advantages	Disadvantages
		Long-Term Catheters	
Implanted ports Long-term intermittent, continuous or daily I.V. access	*Material:* *Catheter*—Silastic, polyurethane *Port*—titanium, stainless steel, plastic *Height:* 9.8–17 mm *Width of base:* 24–50 mm *Lumen:* dual Groshong valve Can access dome port from any angle Preattached catheter/port or 2-piece system Several catheter/port locking devices available	No dressing changes required, monthly heparin flushes, no activity restrictions, reduced risk of infection	Requires needle to access, expensive; requires minor surgery to remove

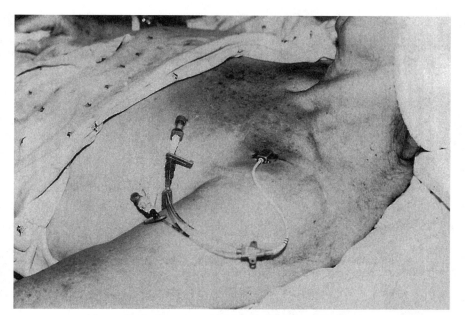

Figure 12–4. Placement of infraclavicular percutaneous catheter.

Sterile Gauze and Tape or TSM Dressings

The gauze dressing should be changed every 48 hours or according to agency policy. The entire surface and all edges must be secured with tape to ensure that the dressing is closed and intact (Perrucca, 1995).

EQUIPMENT
Dressing kit
One pair gloves
One pair sterile gloves
Three alcohol swab sticks
Three povidone-iodine swab sticks
Two 2 × 2 gauze sponges
Two 3 × 3 gauze sponges
One benzoin tincture swab stick
One 4 × 7 Elastoplast dressing
One pair sterile scissors
Tape

PROCEDURE
1. Determine any patient allergies.
2. Explain procedure to patient.
3. Wash hands.
4. Prepare equipment.
5. Place patient in supine position.
6. Instruct patient to turn head away from insertion site.
7. Put on mask and unsterile gloves.
8. Remove old dressing.
9. Open dressing kit.

401

10. Put on sterile gloves.
11. Inspect catheter insertion site for redness, tenderness, swelling, and drainage (culture site if needed).
12. Cleanse area with 70% isopropyl alcohol swab sticks, beginning at the insertion site and moving in a circular motion out to the former adhesive border. Repeat three times.
13. In the same manner cleanse area with povidone-iodine swab sticks and let dry for 1 to 2 minutes. (Check for iodine allergy before the using of povidone-iodine.) (Fig. 12–5)
14. Apply TSM or sterile gauze dressing with tape over entire gauze dressing. Secure all edges.
15. Place a split piece of 1-in tape under the exposed catheter hub and onto the dressing to eliminate air pocket surrounding hub.
16. Label dressing with date and time of procedure and initial.
17. Chart time dressing changed, condition of site, and sign.

✎ **NOTE:** The optimum frequency for changing TSM dressings is unknown, but dressings should be changed at established intervals (generally every 2 to 7 days) or immediately if the integrity of the dressing is compromised. Consider changing this type of dressing every 48 hours, particularly with high-risk patients (INS, 1990).

Peripherally Inserted Central Catheters

The peripherally inserted central catheter (PICC) is designed for 6 weeks to several months. PICCs are inserted by trained I.V. nurses and can be inserted at the bedside. Initially, the PICC was developed for use in neonates because of the catheter's small

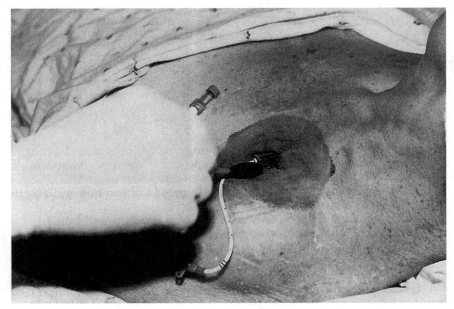

Figure 12–5. Cleansing the central line site with povidone-iodine solution.

diameter and the material's flexibility. The PICC is available as a single-lumen or a multiple-lumen device.

Indications for PICC Use

The following indications for PICC use include therapy-based, clinical use, and diagnostic purposes.

THERAPY-BASED	CLINICAL	DIAGNOSTICS
Antibiotics	Chest injuries	AIDS
Blood sampling	Coagulopathies	Cancer
Chemotherapy	Immunocompromise	Cystic fibrosis
Central venous pressure	Mechanical ventilation	Dehydration
measurements	Radical neck dissection	Endocarditis
I.V. fluids	Respiratory compromise	Malnutrition
Pain management	Inability to cooperate during	Orthopedics
Parenteral drugs	subclavian insertion	Infectious
Parenteral nutrition	Inability to undergo surgical	diseases
	procedure for access	
	Neurologic conditions	
	contraindicating changes in	
	head position	
	Physical disability for	
	positioning, such as kyphosis	

(Source: From Ryder, M.A. [1993]. Peripherally inserted central venous catheters. *Nursing Clinics of North America, 8*(1), 29–35.)

ADVANTAGES
1. Because of peripheral insertion, eliminates potential complication of pneumothorax or hemothorax
2. Decreases risk of air embolism owing to the ease of maintaining the insertion site below the heart
3. Decreases pain and discomfort associated with frequent venipuncture
4. Preserves peripheral vascular system of upper extremities
5. Is cost- and time-efficient
6. Appropriate for home placement and home I.V. therapy
7. Reliable vascular access throughout the course of antibiotic or chemotherapy

DISADVANTAGES
1. Special training required to perform procedure
2. Forty-five minutes to 1 hour needed to complete procedure
3. Daily care required
4. Strict catheter maintenance guidelines necessary to prevent clotting of catheter
5. Small-lumen PICCs not recommended for obtaining blood samples because of possible collapse of catheter on aspiration

VEIN SELECTION
Basilic vein
Cephalic vein
Median-cephalic vein
Median-basilic vein

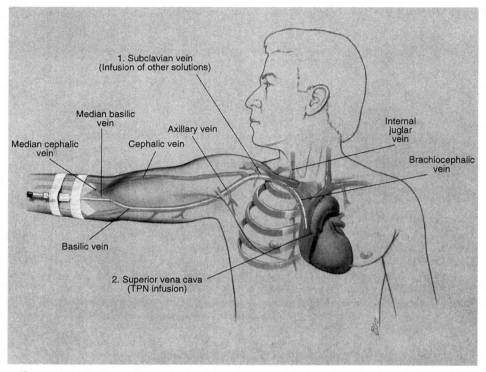

Figure 12–6. Anatomic placement of peripherally placed central catheter. (Courtesy of Medi-visuals, Dallas, Texas.)

✎ **NOTE:** All these sites are acceptable; however, the basilic vein and the median antecubital are the preferred insertion sites. Each should be assessed immediately below the antecubital space (Fig. 12–6).

Placement

According to the recommendations of the Food and Drug Administration (FDA) Central Venous Catheter Working Group (1989), the Intravenous Nursing Society Standards of Practice 1990, and the AACN *Policy and Procedure Manual for Critical Care* (1993), catheterization should be performed with full aseptic technique.

PICCs are placed in patients under sterile conditions by a specially trained registered nurse in settings such as a patient's room, outpatient area, or the patient's home. PICCs are placed in the superior vena cava. Various PICC designs are available for insertion including the breakaway needle introducer, the peel-away sheath, the guidewire, or a slotted needle on a drum cartridge (Markel & Reynen, 1990). A midclavicular approach is used in some settings, and these catheters should be referred to as midclavicular catheters.

The actual procedure varies with different manufacturer's products, the following procedure is suggested for insertion of a PICC.

1. Place patient in dorsal recumbent position and obtain allergy history.
2. Scrub hands using antiseptic soap for 60 seconds.
3. Don mask and prepare work area.

4. Position protective covering under patient's arm.
5. Place tourniquet on mid-upper arm for final vein assesment.
6. Measure arm with sterile tape. For PICC placement in the superior vein cava, measure from the anticubital insertion site up the arm to the shoulder and across the shoulder. Continue to sternal notch and down to the third intercostal space.
7. Select vein and release tourniquet.
8. Apply nonpowdered sterile gloves.
9. Prepare site with 70% isopropyl alcohol, starting at insertion site and cleaning outward in a circular motion in an 8 to 10 in diameter. Repeat 3 times.
10. Repeat cleansing with povidone-iodine.
11. Remove and discard gloves.
12. Apply tourniquet snugly.
13. Don second pair of sterile gloves.
14. Drape arm with sterile towels, creating a sterile field.
15. Inject subcutaneously 0.5 mL or less of 1% lidocaine to anesthetize the insertion site.
16. Make venipuncture.
17. Pull back stylet and slowly advance introducer.
18. Remove stylet.
19. Slowly advance catheter to prevent damage to the vein.
20. Release tourniquet.
21. Continue to advance catheter slowly over 5 to 10 minutes. Have patient turn head toward the insertion site with the chin placed downward on the clavicle.
22. Remove the introducer.
23. Slowly advance the remaining catheter to the measured length.
24. Gently remove guidewire from catheter.
25. Prime and attach extension tubing and injection cap.
26. Flush with 0.5 mL of 0.9% sodium chloride solution.
27. Aspirate with 0.9% sodium chloride to check for blood return.
28. Assess blood for type of flow, color, consistency, and pulsation.
29. Flush vigorously with remaining sodium chloride, followed by heparinized saline.
30. Tape with Steri-Strips or suture in place.
31. Cover with 4 × 4 gauze and sterile wrap for 24 hours.
32. Obtain chest x-ray for catheter tip placement.
33. Document (Brown, 1989; Roundtree, 1991; Perucca, 1995).

✎ **NOTE:** Some PICCs are designed for suture placement to stabilize the catheter, or Steri-Strip skin closure is used to close the exit site.

✎ **NOTE:** Centers for Disease Control and Prevention (CDC, 1995) recommends changing the PICC catheter every 6 weeks with no recommendation for frequency of change when duration of therapy is expected to exceed 6 weeks.

Nursing Management of PICCs

Dressing Management

A small amount of bleeding from the insertion site occurs for the first 24 hours after insertion. After 24 hours, the original dressing must be replaced with one that can remain in place up to 7 days. *Dressing change is a sterile procedure.*

1. Wear gloves for the dressing removal.
2. Remove the transparent dressing gently, being careful not to dislodge or pull on the catheter.

405

3. Assess the insertion site, the arm, and the track of the vein for redness, tenderness, edema, and drainage.
4. Remove gloves and put on a new pair of sterile gloves to clean the skin around the insertion site.
5. Use three alcohol swab sticks followed by three povidone-iodine swab sticks.
6. Slide a 2 × 2 gauze pad under the catheter just below the insertion site if drainage is present.
7. If catheter is not sutured, place Steri-Strips over the insertion site to prevent migration of the catheter.
8. Apply a new transparent dressing over the gauze and exposed catheter including the hub.
9. Initial and date your dressing (Masoorli & Angeles, 1990).

✎ **NOTE:** Avoid stretching the catheter during dressing changes and catheter removal. Stretching or excessive pressure can cause the catheter to rupture.

✎ **NOTE:** PICC dressing should be changed at intervals similar to those for other central line dressings. Patients who are very active or perspire profusely will need more frequent dressing changes (Brown, 1990) (Fig. 12–7).

Flushing Procedure

As with many venous access devices, flushing the PICC involves the saline–administration of medication–saline–heparin method (SASH). This flushing procedure is recommended to eliminate problems with incompatible drugs. The amount of heparin necessary to flush the device should be double the internal lumen (INS, 1990) volume. (Table 12–2). A concentration of 10 to 100 U/mL can be used; however, 100 U/mL tends to be the recommendation (Roundtree, 1991). Flushing procedures vary from agency to agency.

Use heparin 10 to 100 U/mL, 2 to 3 mL every 24 hours to maintain patency (Ryder, 1993).

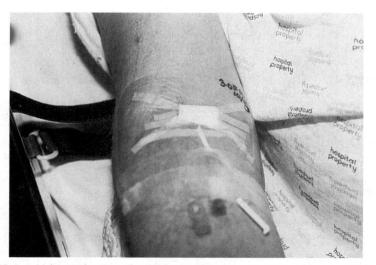

Figure 12–7. Initial PICC dressing. The newly placed PICC has Steri-Strips to secure the line and a gauze pad under the transparent dressing for the first 24 hours.

TABLE 12–2. **CARE OF CENTRAL VENOUS CATHETERS**

Type	Flushing	Tubing Change	Dressing Change
		Short-Term Catheters	
Percutaneous	1:10 to 1:00 unit heparin in volume equal to twice the volume capacity of tubing (1–5 mL) plus any extensions daily to weekly	Primary and secondary sets—every 48 hours; every 24 hours with TPN Luer-lock tubing	Change every 48 hours for gauze dressing or PRN; every 2–7 days or PRN for TSM dressing. Use 3 swabs of 70% isopropyl alcohol and 3 swabs of povidone-iodine from site outward to cleanse site. No antimicrobial ointments are recommended.
PICCs	1:10 to 1:00 U heparin in volume equal to twice the volume capacity of tubing (1 mL) plus any extensions daily	Same as above	Same as above. Remove dressing by pulling upward to avoid dislodging the catheter.
		Long-Term Catheters	
Tunneled catheters	1:10 to 1:00 U heparin in volume equal to twice the volume capacity of tubing (4 mL) plus any extensions daily to weekly With Groshong catheter, use 5 mL of 0.9% sodium chloride flush weekly	Same as above	Same as above Hydrogen peroxide may be used to remove crusting. Soap and water cleansing with no dressing is sufficient after exit site is healed.
Implanted ports	1:10 to 1:00 U heparin in volume equal to twice the volume capacity of tubing (3 mL) plus any extensions	Same as above	Same as above. No dressing is needed once incision is healed. Stabilize device with Steri-Strips. Change noncoring needle at least weekly.

PRN = as needed; TPN = total parenteral nutrition; TSM = transparent semipermeable membrane.

✎ **NOTE:** Do not use a tuberculin syringe for flushing because it can cause too much pressure; a 10-mL syringe may be used safely.

Use of Infusion Pump

The PICC line has been used successfully with all types of infusion pumps. With 3.0F and smaller PICCs, an infusion pump may be necessary to maintain the infusion and patency of the line.

Blood Sampling

If blood sampling is needed from the PICC, a 2.8F or larger catheter may be required. (All companies manufacture a 2.8F or larger catheter.) Because the walls of the PICC line are soft, they collapse easily when a strong vacuum is applied. A gentle touch with a syringe rather than a Vacutainer will yield a successful sample.

Blood Administration

Blood products may be administered through a 3.8F or larger PICC. Care should be taken to flush the line thoroughly after administration of a blood product.

Repair

The PICC can be repaired in one of two ways: use of manufacturer-specific hub repair kit or replacement of catheter over a guidewire. PICCs can be temporarily repaired with a coated blunt needle inserted into the trimmed end of the broken catheter. If the peripherally inserted central line is damaged, another catheter can be placed. An exchange-over-wire procedure can be used as a last resort for salvage of the line. The guidewires used for this procedure can be extremely long; therefore, strict sterile technique with gowning is recommended.

The guidewire is inserted into the catheter to be removed, and the catheter is pulled out over the wire. A new catheter is then threaded back over the wire. After the new catheter is in place, the guidewire can be removed. A chest x-ray should be done to verify placement of the new catheter tip. This procedure should be performed only by experienced I.V. nurses certified to insert a PICC (INS, 1990). There are specific manufacturer recommendations for this procedure.

Insertion Complications

Bleeding

Bleeding is a common complication associated with any nontunneled catheter. Slight oozing may be observed within the first few hours secondary to movement of the arm. In patients with thrombocytopenia or in situations in which multiple venipunctures have occurred, careful observation following insertion is required. Excessive bleeding beyond 24 hours after insertion is unusual. Mild pressure dressing may be required to control bleeding. Signs and symptoms include hematoma, severe pain, swelling, numbness, and tingling, cool, and mottled skin (Ryder, 1993).

Tendon or Nerve Damage

The median nerve lies parallel and medial to the brachial artery in the antecubital space. On the lateral side, the lateral cutaneous nerve is proximal to the cephalic vein. Because of the close proximity to these nerves, damage is a risk (Ryder, 1993). Signs and symptoms are numbness, tingling, or weakness of the area innervated by the nerves.

Cardiac Arrhythmias

This complication is related to irritation of the myocardial wall by an overinserted guidewire or catheter (Lowell & Boothe, 1991). Some institutions require the patient to be placed on a cardiac monitor during placement of a PICC in the superior vena cava. Catheters positioned in the heart are at risk of causing myocardial erosion, perforation, cardiac tamponade, and endocardial abscess (Ellis, Vogel, & Copeland, 1989).

Malposition of Catheter

Central venous catheter tip migration can occur during insertion. However, postinsertion migration can occur in:

- Patients who frequently experience nausea and vomiting during the course of therapy
- Respiratory patients who have bouts of severe coughing, causing the catheter tip to migrate
- Physically active patients

✎ **NOTE:** If the patient complains of pain in the shoulder, neck, or arm at insertion site, catheter placement should be checked by x-ray examination at any time during the course of therapy.

Both intravascular and extravascular malpositioning of all types of short-term devices have been reported. Extravascular malpositioning can occur when the introducer slips out of the vein and the catheter is passed into the pleural space or the mediastinum (primarily during a subclavian catheterization). Intravascular malpositions are more common and can be seen with all approaches to the central vascular system. The catheter may coil in the vessel, advance into the right atrium or one of the smaller venous tributaries, or not be advanced far enough to reach the superior vena cava from the antecubital site. The catheter must be repositioned if malpositioning occurs (Ryan & Gough, 1984; Vasquez, 1980).

✎ **NOTE:** A way to avoid intravascular malpositioning of the catheter in the jugular vein is by having the patient turn the head toward the side of the venipuncture. This changes the angle of the catheter to move downward toward the superior vena cava.

Catheter Embolism

Care should be taken to remove the break-away needle (introducer) before threading the catheter. Catheter shearing is the most common cause of catheter embolism, but it can also result from retraction of the catheter into the arm after external breakage, or rupture of the catheter with forceful irrigation, or from the "pinch-off" syndrome (Ryder, 1993). Managing catheter embolism involves retaining the fragment in the arm and preventing migration into the central veins, heart, pulmonary artery, or lung periphery. If the potential of catheter embolization occurs, immediately apply local pressure or a tourniquet proximal to the site. Obtain an x-ray to determine the location of the embolus. X-ray visualization may be difficult if the segment is short (Dunbar, Mitchell, & Lavine, 1981).

Postinsertion Complications

Phlebitis and Cellulitis

Mechanical phlebitis is the most common complication seen with the PICC line, usually occurring in the first 48 to 72 hours after insertion. This complication occurs more frequently in women than men and with left-sided insertions. To treat phlebitis, apply warm, moist compresses to the upper arm between the insertion site and the shoulder for 20 minutes four times a day. Elevation of the extremity and mild exercise can be effective in resolving or controlling the phlebitis (Brown, 1989).

Cellulitis is usually caused by *Staphylococcus epidermidis* or *S aureus*. Signs and symptoms are pain, tenderness, and redness at the catheter site spreading in a diffuse circular pattern into the surrounding subcutaneous tissue. Cellulitis responds well to oral antibiotics and may not require catheter removal.

Infection (Catheter Sepsis)

Infection rates with PICC lines have been extremely low compared with other types of central lines. An estimated 50,000 to 100,000 patients in U.S. hospitals develop a nosocomial intravascular device-related bloodstream infection, 90% of which originate from CVCs of various types (Maki, 1992). Low infection rates have been documented with studies of PICCs (Brown, 1989; Kyle & Meyers, 1990). Pemberton (1986) states that patients requiring multiple-lumen catheters are usually more acutely ill and therefore at higher risk for developing sepsis related to multiple lumens.

Thrombosis and Thrombophlebitis (Occlusion of Catheter)

Deep vein thrombosis of the subclavian vein is rare. Causes are injury to the intima of the vein wall, obstructed blood flow, and changes in composition of the blood. The use of biocompatible catheter material has decreased this complication. Occlusions of the catheter can be avoided by routine flushing, not using excess force, flushing vigorously after viscous solution administration, and not mixing incompatible drugs.

Air Embolism

Air embolism is rare with PICCs because the catheter exit site is below the level of the heart, which helps to maintain adequate pressure within the system. The innominate veins and the superior vena cava lie within the thoracic cavity where intrathoracic pressure remains negative. When the external end of a central catheter is open to atmospheric pressure, air moves inward toward the negative pressure.

✎ **NOTE:** A 14-gauge needle with an internal diameter of 0.072 in can transmit 100 mL of air per second. In humans, the average lethal rate of injection has been calculated at 70 to 159 mL/s (Ordway, 1973), but as little as 100 mL of air forced rapidly into the venous system can be fatal (Peters & Armstrong, 1978).

Twiddler's Syndrome (Dislodgment of the Catheter)

Twiddler's syndrome results in dislodgment of the catheter owing to patient manipulation of the dressing and catheter. Signs and symptoms include edema or drainage at the exit site and palpable cord. Assess the catheter length frequently. Inform the patient that the catheter may become dislodged if it is manipulated (Camp-Sorrell, 1995). To prevent this, (1) loop and tape the catheter securely, (2) use occlusive dressing, (3) use a flexnet stocking to cover the PICC, (4) avoid pulling on the vascular access device, and (5) avoid manipulation of the catheter by hand.

410

Declotting the Line

The PICC line may be cleared by using urokinase according to the manufacturer's recommendation. When attempting to declot the catheter with urokinase, the small volume of the PICC line must be taken into consideration as well as catheter rupture strengths.

✎ **NOTE:** The drugs phenytoin (Dilantin) and diazepam (Valium) have been documented as causing problems when infused through a PICC line. When either of these drugs is given, crystals form inside the lumen, resulting in occlusion of the catheter. It is not known whether there is an interaction between the drug and the catheter material or another drug that may have been inside the lumen (Hadaway, 1989).

Long-Term Devices

Devices designed for long-term use can be divided into two categories: tunneled catheters and implanted ports. These catheters are made of Silastic or polyurethane and are available in single or multiple lumens. They require a surgical procedure for insertion.

Central Venous Tunneled Catheters

Central venous tunneled catheters (CVTCs) have been available since 1975, when Broviac catheters were introduced for long-term total parenteral nutrition. The Broviac catheter was followed by a modified version, the Hickman catheter, which could accommodate the delivery of therapies to bone marrow transplant patients. CVTCs became the prototype for a variety of tunneled catheters currently on the market for various therapies. Inserted through a subcutaneous tunnel, these catheters are often referred to as indwelling catheters, tunneled central venous catheters, or right atrial catheters (see Table 12–1).

CVTCs are intended to be used for months to years to provide long-term venous access for obtaining blood samples and for administering drugs, blood products, and total parenteral nutrition.

CVTCs are composed of polymeric silicone with a Dacron polyester cuff that anchors the catheter in place subcutaneously. This cuff is about 2 in from the catheter's exit site, which becomes embedded with fibroblasts within 1 week to 10 days after insertion, reducing the chances for accidental removal and minimizing the risk of ascending bacterial infection. CVTCs are available with single, double, or triple lumens. They vary in size from pediatric to adult with most internal lumens ranging from 0.5 to 1.6 mm.

One of the advantages of CVTCs is that a break or tear in the catheter is easy to repair without adhesive. Depending on the type of catheter and the type of repair needed, adhesive may be required.

✎ **NOTE:** CVTCs are easily maintained in the home setting.

An attachable cuff (Vita-Cuff) is available for CVTCs. This cuff is made of biodegradable collagen impregnated with silver ion. Subcutaneous tissue grows to the cuff providing a mechanical barrier, and the silver ion provides a chemical barrier against organisms. This cuff has proved to be cost-effective in decreasing catheter-related septicemia (Maki, 1988).

Insertion of Tunneled Catheter

CVTCs are inserted with the patient under local or general anesthesia by surgical cutdown of a centrally located superficial vein—usually the external jugular or ce-

411

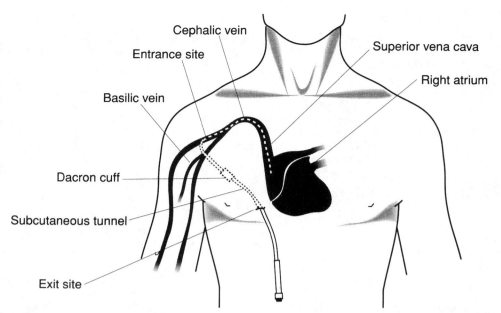

Cephalic vein

Entrance site

Basilic vein

Superior vena cava

Right atrium

Dacron cuff

Subcutaneous tunnel

Exit site

Figure 12–8. Anatomic placement of tunneled catheter. (Courtesy of Bard Access Systems, Salt Lake City, Utah.)

phalic vein. A separate proximal incision is made on the chest or abdominal wall, and the catheter is directed through a subcutaneous tunnel between the two incisions. The catheter is open at the distal and proximal ends and trimmed to the approximate estimated length and threaded through the subclavian vein into the superior vena cava. The position is confirmed by fluoroscopy, adjusted if needed, and then sutured to the skin or the incision is closed with Steri-Strips. These remain in place for 10 to 14 days (Fig. 12–8).

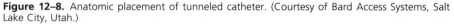

ADVANTAGES
1. Can be repaired if it breaks or tears
2. Can be used for many purposes including:
   Blood samples
   Monitoring central venous pressure
   Administration of total parenteral nutrition
   Drug administration
3. Can be used for the patient with chronic need for I.V. therapy

DISADVANTAGES
1. Daily to weekly site care
2. Cost of maintenance supplies (dressings, materials, and changes; frequency of flushing and cap changing)
3. Surgical catheter insertion procedure that requires maintenance
4. Can affect the patient's body image (Camp-Sorrell, 1990)

Flushing Procedure

Flushing procedures vary according to the agency. Generally it is accepted practice to flush the CVTCs (except the Groshong) with twice the catheter volume of

412

heparinized saline (volumes range from 0.8 to 1.6 mL). After medication administration or daily maintenance, flush the catheter with saline; then follow with heparinized saline.

✎ **NOTE:** Various care settings recommend using anywhere from 1 to 10 mL with concentrations ranging from 10 to 1000 U/mL. The frequency of flushing also varies from 2 days to once per week (Freedman & Bosserman, 1993).

Repair of the Catheter

The CVTC can tear during reinsertion of the introducer needle, during intermittent therapy when I.V. push therapy is performed, or when using scissors near the catheter site. When this happens, blood usually backs up and fluid leaks from the site (except Groshong valve catheters). Air can enter the catheter through the tear, causing an air embolism.

Keeping up to date on repair methods can be difficult. Several types of repair kits are available. CVTCs can be repaired without a kit, but this requires a certain amount of creativity and knowledge. Types of repair include blunt-end needle repair, splicing sleeve with adhesive, manufacturer-specific hub or body repair kit, and the plastic catheter method.

To repair the catheter, you will need: sterile gloves, mask, sterile drapes, sterile scissors, povidone-iodine solution, extension set and the appropriate repair kit.

✎ **NOTE:** Avoid serrated clamps on the catheter.

STEPS IN CATHETER REPAIR
1. Clamp the catheter immediately between the chest wall and the tear (Fig. 12–9).
2. Cleanse the end of the catheter with povidone-iodine if the patient is not allergic to iodine.
3. Cut off and discard the damaged portion of the catheter with sterile scissors.
4. Insert a blunt-end needle with the appropriate gauge into the end of the remaining length of catheter.
5. Place an injection cap in the hub of the needle and heparinize the catheter.
6. Tie a silk suture around the needle and catheter to secure.

The catheter is then ready to use until permanent repair is done. Many of the long-term devices have permanent repair kits, which involves splicing a new section of catheter with an end connector to the rest of the catheter.

Nursing Management of Tunneled Catheters

1. Be sure the catheter is capped at all times. If it becomes uncapped, follow the steps for flushing the catheter. Note: The catheter should be clamped if malfunction is suspected or when catheter breakage occurs.
2. Keep all sharp objects away from the catheter. Never use scissors or pins on or near the catheter.
3. If the catheter leaks or breaks, take a nonserrated clamp and clamp the catheter between the broken area and the exit site. Cover the broken part with a sterile gauze bandage and tape it securely. Do not use the catheter. Notify the physician.
4. Protect the catheter when showering or bathing by covering the entire catheter with transparent dressing or clear plastic wrap.
5. Flush after a blood drawing with 10 mL of 0.9% sodium chloride.
6. Heparin is used to maintain patency of the catheter.

413

Connector Instructions

1. *Transfer white sleeve (A) onto catheter from connector.*

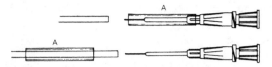

2. *Firmly push catheter onto adapter to Position B.*

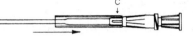

3. *Slide white sleeve onto colored hub to Position C.*

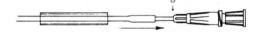

4. *Remove and discard stylet.*

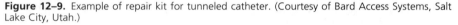

Figure 12–9. Example of repair kit for tunneled catheter. (Courtesy of Bard Access Systems, Salt Lake City, Utah.)

Tunneled Catheter with Groshong Valve

A development in CVTCs is the application of the Groshong valve feature, which has been marketed since 1984. This catheter has a few unique features that set it apart from other CVTCs. The Groshong catheter is made of soft, flexible, Silastic. The outer diameter dimensions are small. The catheter is available in single, double, or triple lumens. The Silastic material has a recoil memory that returns it to its original configuration if accidentally pulled. Another unique feature of the Groshong catheter is the two-way valve placed near the distal end, which restricts backflow of blood, but can be purposefully overridden to obtain venous blood samples. This valve eliminates the need for flushing with heparin. The valve is open inward, minimizing the risks of blood backing up the catheter lumen (Fig. 12–10). The Groshing valve feature is now available on a variety of CVCs, including PICCs and ports.

✎ **NOTE:** External clamps should not be used; they are unnecessary and could damage the catheter (Camp, 1988).

Insertion of Tunneled Catheter with Groshong Valve

Other catheters are tunneled up from the exit site, the Groshong placement is reversed. After the Groshong catheter is at the desired site, the catheter length is

414

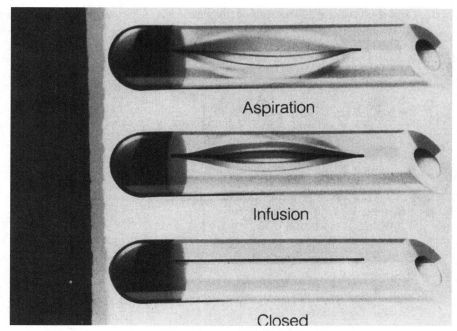

Aspiration

Infusion

Closed

Figure 12–10. Three-position Groshong valve. (Courtesy of Bard Access Systems, Salt Lake City, Utah.)

adjusted before the connector is placed into the proximal end. The Groshong distal end is closed, soft, rounded, and flexible.

Flushing Procedure

Policies and procedures vary from institution to institution. The Groshong catheter should be flushed every 7 days with 0.9% sodium chloride when not in use. Maintain aseptic technique. After administration of medications, the catheter should be flushed with 5 mL of sodium chloride. After the administration of viscous solutions such as lipids, flush briskly with 20 mL of sodium chloride to prevent crystallization of the catheter tip. Manufacturers recommend that the catheter be irrigated with a syringe attached directly to the connection hub of the Groshong.

Blood Sampling

1. Withdraw and discard 5 mL of blood.
2. Draw blood sample.
3. Flush catheter briskly with 20 mL of 0.9% sodium chloride.

✎ **NOTE:** Brisk flushing creates a swirling effect at the distal end of the catheter. If flushing is not performed briskly, a blood clot may form. Raising the arms and repositioning the bed may assist in obtaining a blood sample.

415

Tunneled Catheter Management with Groshong Valve

1. *Do not clamp the catheter:* Clamping is not necessary because of the special valve, and clamping can cause damage, such as leak or tearing of the catheter.
2. Never use acetone such as nail polish remover or tape remover on or near the catheter, because it can dissolve the catheter.
3. Protect the catheter when showering or bathing by covering the entire catheter with transparent tape or clear plastic wrap.
4. Straining or heavy lifting can cause a small amount of blood to back up into the catheter. If blood is evident in the catheter line, flush.
5. After blood sample is obtained, flush briskly with 20 mL of 0.9% sodium chloride.
6. Keep all sharp objects away from the catheter. Never use scissors or pins on or near the catheter.

Dressing Management of all Tunneled Catheters

This is a sterile procedure. To change the dressings, follow these steps:

1. Wash hands.
2. Put on mask if patient is neutropenic; then put on sterile gloves.
3. Remove dressing from site.
4. Inspect site for redness, swelling, and drainage.
5. Remove gloves and put on a second pair of sterile gloves.
6. Using 3 alcohol swab sticks, cleanse exit site, rotating in a circular method from inside outward.
7. Using 3 povidone-iodine swab sticks, cleanse site rotating in a circular method from inside outward; let dry 1 to 2 minutes. (Check for patient allergy to iodine prior to use of povidone-iodine.)
8. Use TSM dressing over site.
9. Tape catheter to the dressing, and coil remaining tubing using a chevron technique.

Injection Cap Change of all Tunneled Catheters

To change the injection cap, follow this sterile procedure:

1. Wear gloves.
2. Swab connection of cap with povidone-iodine.
3. Remove old cap.
4. Screw on new cap.
5. Wipe off excess povidone-iodine with alcohol swab.

Complications Associated with all Tunneled Catheters

1. **Exit site infection.** Proper dressing technique minimizes the risk of exit site infection. Temperature elevation, redness, swelling, or drainage at the site must be reported immediately to the nurse or physician.
2. **Sepsis.** All elevated temperatures must be reported. If bacteria ascend the catheter and enter the patient's circulation, the patient may become septic. Secondary catheter sepsis may result from an infection in another body system such as urinary tract infection or upper respiratory infection.
3. **Thrombosis.** Thrombosis can develop in the vessel in which the catheter is situated. Signs of thrombosis such as tenderness and swelling of the arms, neck, and shoulder on the catheter side of the body must be reported immediately (Handy, 1989).
4. **Catheter migration.** It is good practice to infuse normal saline before and after administering medications. This clears the heparin from the catheter; also

swelling or a subcutaneous burning sensation can be detected with the sodium chloride before injection of a medication. Dye studies can confirm tip placement.

5. **Clot formation.** A clot can form in a catheter because of improper flushing technique or lack of flushing procedure with the right atrial catheter. Difficulty in or total inability to flush the catheter must be reported immediately to the physician. Attempt to declot the catheter using urokinase following hospital protocol (Bjeletich, 1987).

6. **Torn or leaking catheter.** A catheter can tear or develop a leak from improper use. Always use a smooth or padded clamp on the catheter when changing the injection cap. Rotate the clamping sites. Tape catheter up when not in use to prevent tugging. Never put anything sharp next to the catheter. If a tear or leak is detected, the nurse or patient must immediately place the clamp between the tear or leak and the entry site. Call the physician.

7. **Air embolism.** If the cap is removed when the catheter is not clamped or a tear develops, an air embolism can enter the system. Use only Luer-locking devices. Secure all connections during an infusion.

✎ **NOTE:** If an air embolism occurs at home, treatment consists of closing off the open end of the catheter, placing the patient in Trendelenburg position on the left side, and obtaining immediate emergency assistance.

Implanted Ports

Implanted ports have been available for venous access since 1983. Implanted ports are another form of CVC. Originally, implanted ports were targeted to the oncology patient who required frequent intermittent venous access. Ports consist of a reservoir, silicone catheter, and central septum (Fig. 12–11). The self-sealing septum can usually withstand 1000 to 2000 needle punctures. Ports have raised edges to facilitate puncture with a noncoring needle. The port is made of stainless steel or titanium. The septum is connected to a silicone catheter (Riser, 1988). Many types of implanted vascular access devices are available today, but all are inserted in the same location and have the same use (see Table 12–1).

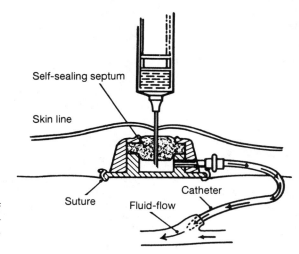

Self-sealing septum

Skin line

Suture

Fluid-flow

Catheter

Figure 12–11. Cross-section of subcutaneous port showing fluid injection. (Courtesy of Sims Deltech, St. Paul, Minnesota.)

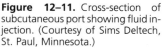

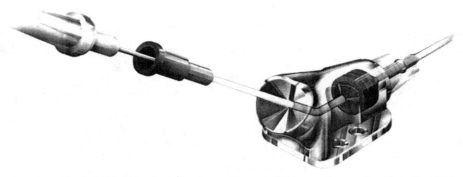

Figure 12–12. CathLink 20 implanted port uses 20-gauge 1¾-in over-the-needle catheter to access the port. (Courtesy Bard Access Systems, Salt Lake City, Utah.)

A new line of implanted ports is the CathLink 20 (Bard Access Systems), which is available in three sizes: standard profile, low profile, and ultra-low profile, allowing for placement approaches ranging from chest wall to lower arm. The CathLink 20 is designed for use with standard 20-gauge 1¾-in. over-the needle I.V. catheter, rather than noncoring Huber needle. The CathLink 20 port eliminates angles and large reservoirs with a layered silicone septum, which increases the septum longevity. The port is flushed with 5 mL of heparinized sodium chloride once every 4 weeks when not in use (Fig. 12–12).

ADVANTAGES
Less risk of infection when used intermittently
Less interference with daily activities
Little site care
Needs minimal flushing
Easy access for fluids, blood products, or medication administration
Less body image disturbance owing to lack of external catheter device
Few limitations on patient activity

DISADVANTAGES
Cost of insertion (considerably higher than with other vascular access devices)
Postoperative care is 7 to 10 days
Discomfort of repeated needle sticks
Minor surgical procedure necessary to remove device

✎ **NOTE:** Placement is not recommended in the obese patient, after chest-radiation, or at mastectomy sites (Camp-Sorrel, 1990).

Insertion

The port is inserted after a local anesthetic is administered; the entire procedure takes from 30 minutes to 1 hour. An incision is made in the upper to middle chest, usually near the collarbone, to form a pocket to house the port. The Silastic catheter is inserted via cutdown into the superior vena cava; the port is then placed in the subcutaneous fascia pocket. The port contains a reservoir leading to the catheter. The incision for the port pocket is sutured closed, and a sterile dressing is applied. The dressing may be removed after the first 24 hours. This area should be cleaned daily with a povidone-iodine solution and a sterile gauze pad until the incision has healed, about 10 days to 2 weeks after insertion.

The subcutaneous port system catheter can be placed in any of the following: superior vena cava, hepatic artery, peritoneal space for intraperitoneal therapy, and epidural space.

✎ **NOTE:** Implanted ports are available in one or two septum chambers. Ports designed for peripheral access are also available.

Nursing Management of Implanted Ports

Accessing the Port

This is a sterile procedure.

1. Wearing nonsterile gloves, palpate the port to find the entry septum.
2. Put on sterile gloves.
3. Using an alcohol swabstick (3) cleanse exit site, rotating in a circular method from inside outward, repeat 3 times.
4. Using povidone-iodine swabstick (3) cleanse site, rotating in a circular method from inside outward, repeat 3 times, then let dry 1 to 2 minutes. (Check for patient allergy to iodine prior to use of povidone-iodine.)
5. Attach a 6-mL syringe of heparin solution to the stopcock at the end of the extension tubing.
6. *Connect the appropriate gauge noncoring right angle needle* to the Luer lock at the other end and prime the tubing.
7. Palpate the port to find the center of the septum.
8. Insert the noncoring right-angle needle into the center, pushing until the needle stops.
9. Aspirate a small amount of blood to check for patency and position.
10. Using firm steady pressure, flush the port with approximately 10 mL of sodium chloride at the rate of less than 5 mL/minute. If swelling occurs or the patient complains of pain or burning sensation, the needle is improperly positioned.
11. Disconnect syringe and discard.
12. **Injecting a bolus**
    Attach the syringe containing the prescribed drug.
    Carefully disconnect the syringe to prevent any of the drug from dripping on the patient's skin.
    Attach the second 10-mL syringe of saline solution and flush the injection port and catheter.
    Disconnect the syringe and discard.
    Attach the 5-mL syringe of heparin solution and inject all 5 mL to prevent occlusion at the catheter tip.
    Withdraw the needle, being careful not to twist or tilt.
    Observe the injection site for signs of extravasation.
    Use alcohol swabs, moving in a circular motion from the center of the port out to remove the povidone-iodine from the skin.
13. **Injection of a continuous infusion**
    Prepare site and access as for bolus.
    Roll a sterile 2 × 2 gauze pad and place under the needle hub and Luer lock to support the needle.
    Apply tincture of benzoin to the gauze to help the Steri-Strips adhere.
    Secure the needle hub and tubing by applying Steri-Strips across the hub, using a chevron taping technique.

419

Apply transparent dressing over the entire system.

Attach the extension to the I.V. line from the infusion pump.

Tape all connections unless using Luer-lock connections.

✎ **NOTE:** I.V. tubing must be changed every 24 hours. The dressing and extension tubing must be changed every 4 to 7 days.

14. When infusion is concluded, inject the saline and disconnect the syringe. Then, attach a 10-mL syringe of heparin solution to the stopcock and flush the port.
15. Withdraw the noncoring needle without twisting or tilting.
16. Remove the tincture of benzoin with alcohol, and apply a small bandage if necessary. (Viall, 1990; Sims Deltec, 1990.)

Flushing Procedure

Flushing procedures vary from institution to institution. Flush the system with 5 mL of heparinized saline in a 10-mL syringe. If the port is not being used, flush with heparinized saline every 4 weeks. If the port is used for medication administration or blood component therapy flush after every infusion (Sims Deltec, 1990).

Blood Sampling

1. Insert noncoring needle attached to extension tubing and secure needle with tape.
2. Release clamp and flush with 5 mL 0.9% sodium chloride in a 10 mL syringe to confirm that fluid flows through the system.
3. Withdraw at least 3 mL of blood, clamp tubing, and discard syringe and blood.
4. Attach syringe and release clamp. Withdraw desired amount of blood for sampling.
5. Clamp tube and attach syringe with 2 mL heparinized saline in a 10 mL syringe. Release clamp and flush system.
6. Clamp tube and attach syringe with 20 mL of 0.9% sodium chloride. Release clamp and flush system.
7. Clamp tube and attach syringe with 5 mL heparinized saline in a 10 mL syringe. Release clamp and flush system, leaving a heparin lock (Sims Deltec, 1990).

Complications

The same complications associated with CVTCs can occur with the implanted port.

Site infection or skin breakdown. The port site must be regularly assessed for redness, swelling, drainage, or breaks in skin integrity; promptly report significant findings to the physician. Instruct caregivers how to assess site and what to report.

Sepsis. This is a potential problem; any temperature elevations need to be reported.

Thrombosis. Any pain and tenderness in the neck, shoulder, or arm on the port side of the body must be reported, since these signs and symptoms could indicate thrombosis.

Clot formation. The catheter portion and port of this system constitute a potential site for clot formation, especially if used for blood withdrawal. Any difficulty in flushing can indicate a clot and must be reported to the physician or nurse as soon as detected.

Air embolism. When the implanted port is not in use, risk of air embolism does not exist. However, when the port has been accessed there is a direct route from the outside to the patient's central circulation. The risks during access are the same as for other CVCs.

Port migration. The port is sutured in place but it can move out of position if one or more sutures becomes loose. The patient and family are advised to report any difficulty in accessing the port.

Extravasation. If the special needle is not in place through the septum of the port and the position is not confirmed, fluid can extravasate and collect subcutaneously resulting in burning or swelling around the port during infusion. Patients and nurses must always verify placement, secure needle before initiating the infusion, and observe for signs of swelling or burning.

Dislodgment or Twiddler's syndrome. This syndrome results from malposition of the port owing to patient hand manipulation of port. The setup placement should be assessed prior to assessing the port. Inform the patient of the possible dislodgment of the port (Camp-Sorrell, 1990).

KEY POINTS IN CARE OF THE IMPLANTED PORT

Use non-coring needle with appropriate port.

Change needle and extension tubing every 7 days.

Flush port with 0.9% sodium chloride and heparin every 4 weeks if port is not in use or after every infusion, following procedure outlined.

For continuous infusion, change dressing every 72 hours.

For continuous infusion, change tubing every 24 hours.

OCCLUDED CENTRAL VENOUS DEVICES

Vascular access devices (VADs) can become occluded as a result of mechanical obstruction, thrombotic occlusion, or drug precipitation (nonthrombotic). The treatment must begin promptly; therefore, systematic evaluation of the catheter patency needs to be ongoing. If a VAD occlusion is left untreated, secondary complications can occur, such as loss of venous access, morbidity of recannulation, and risk of catheter infection due to a fibrin sheath for bacterial or fungal colonization (Bagnall-Reeb, Ryder, & Anglim, 1994).

Preventive care of clot formation and subsequent occlusion include careful catheter insertion; routine assessment of dressings, exit sites, tubing, pumps, infusion bags, and clamps; meticulous technique in blood sampling; and avoiding potential drug or solution incompatibilities (Bagnall-Reeb, Ryder, & Anglim, 1994).

Mechanical Occlusion

External causes of occlusion are a kinked or closed clamp. External occlusion of flow may be caused by clogged injection cap, clogged I.V. filter, infusion pump that has been turned off, or an empty I.V. bag. Occlusion can also occur at the catheter exit site or vein entry if the suture used to secure the line constricts the catheter. The catheter can be pinched closed as a result of the patient's position by pressure of the clavicle against the first rib (pinch-off) or it can be obstructed by lodging the catheter tip against the vein wall (Hinke, Zandt-Stastny, & Goodman, 1990). Malposition of the catheter on insertion or catheter tip migration after placement may result in catheter kinking.

Management

When I.V. flow is occluded, first determine whether the cause is external. Examine the I.V. setup for kinked tubing, closed clamps, empty infusion bag, and readjustment

421

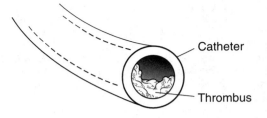

Figure 12–13. Intraluminal occlusion. (Source: Bagnall-Reeb, Ryder, & Anglim [1994]. Venous Access Device Occlusions Independent Study Module. Illinois: Abbott Laboratories.)

of the I.V. delivery system. Having the patient change positions may correct the problem. Finally, chest radiography may be helpful to confirm catheter tip placement and rule out migration (Bagnall-Reeb, Ryder, & Anglim, 1994).

Thrombotic Occlusion

An occlusion by a thrombus may occur in as many as 25% of VADs (Bagnall, Gomperts, & Atkinson, 1989). Thrombus formation can occur within the first 24 hours following insertion. A variety of thrombotic events can result in catheter occlusion.

Intraluminal Occlusion

Intraluminal occlusion occurs when the lumen of the catheter is obstructed by either clotted blood or an accumulation of fibrin. Frequently, the cause is blood remaining in the catheter following inadequate irrigation or retrograde flow (Fig. 12–13). Also, poor flushing technique after blood sampling may allow layers of fibrin to accumulate over time, narrowing or obstructing the lumen.

Fibrin Sleeve and Fibrin Tail

Platelet aggregation and fibrin deposition may completely encase the surface of the catheter and form a sac around the distal end of the catheter (Fig. 12–14). The sac causes retrograde flow of infusate up the catheter. The infusate may be observed on the skin (in nontunneled catheters), in the skin tunnel (in tunneled catheters), or in the subcutaneous pocket of implanted ports (Bagnall-Reeb, Ryder, & Anglim, 1994). A "tail" of fibrin extending off the catheter tip can occur owing to platelet aggregation and fibrin accumulation. The tail usually does not interfere with infusion but may occlude the catheter on aspiration. This is commonly known as the "ball valve effect."

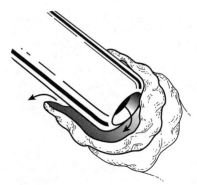

Figure 12–14. Fibrin sleeve. (Source: Bagnall-Reeb, Ryder, & Anglim [1994]. Venous Access Device, Independent Study Module. Illinois: Abbott Laboratories.)

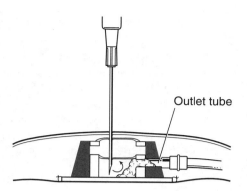

Outlet tube

Figure 12–15. Portal reservoir occlusion. (Source: Bagnall-Reeb, Ryder, & Anglim [1994]. Venous Access Device, Independent Study Module. Illinois: Abbott Laboratories.)

Venous Thrombosis

Endothelial damage to a blood vessel can result in fibrin deposition at the point of cellular damage. If the thrombus occurs along the wall of the vein, it is a *mural thrombus*. If the thrombus completely occludes the vein, it is called a *venous thrombosis*.

Portal Reservoir Occlusion

Fluid viscosity or improper flushing technique can produce fibrin or precipitate deposits within the reservoir of the port (Fig. 12–15). Accumulation of deposits leads to obstruction of the tube.

Management

Gentle aspiration may dislodge the occlusive material from within the catheter lumen. Thrombolytic agents are the only available drugs to lyse existing clots. They convert plasminogen to plasmin, which acts directly on the clot to dissolve the fibrin matrix.

✎ **NOTE:** Forceful flushing of the catheter to push the clot into the circulation is *not* recommended. The use of a guidewire or snare to manipulate the clot out of the catheter is also *not* recommended.

Urokinase

Urokinase (Abbokinase Open Cath by Abbott Laboratories pH 6.0–7.5) is an enzyme, a potent direct activator of the endogenous fibrinolytic system, which converts plasminogen to the proteolytic enzyme plasmin. Plasmin degrades fibrin clots, as well as fibrinogen and other plasma proteins associated with clotting. The effects of fibrinolytic activity decreases within a few hours after discontinuation of the drug. Urokinase will not dissolve drug precipitate or anything other than blood products.

Use

For I.V. catheter clearance, inject urokinase, 5000 IU (1 mL specifically diluted). The amount should be equal to the volume in the catheter. Dilute with sterile water for injection without preservatives.

TECHNIQUE AND RATE OF ADMINISTRATION
Confirm occlusion with 10-mL syringe.
Obtain patient consent and physician order.

423

Slowly and gently inject specifically diluted and premeasured urokinase into catheter.

Wait 5 minutes.

Gently aspirate to remove clot.

Repeat every 5 minutes until clot clears for 30 minutes.

If unsuccessful, cap catheter for 1 hour and reattempt to declot.

✎ **NOTE:** Avoid force while attempting to clear catheter, because the catheter may rupture or dislodge the clot into the circulation.

Studies have supported that residence time of urokinase ranged from 30 minutes to 3 hours before full use of the port was successfully established (Lawson, 1991).

Contraindications

Patients who have active internal bleeding, intracranial neoplasm, hypersensitivity to urokinase, liver disease, subacute bacterial endocarditis, or visceral malignancy or who have had a cerebrovascular accident within the past 2 months, or intracranial or intraspinal surgery, should not receive urokinase.

Drug Incompatibilities

Do not mix with any other medication in any manner.

Complications

Bleeding. Bleeding may occur in two general forms: surface bleeding from invaded or disturbed sites (punctures, incision) or internal bleeding from the gastrointestinal tract, genitourinary tract, vagina, or intramuscular, retroperitoneal, or intracerebral sites. *Fatalities due to cerebral or retroperitoneal hemorrhage have occurred.* The antidote is administration of plasma volume expanders such as fresh plasma fluids, along with whole blood if hemorrhage is unresponsive to blood replacement. Aminocaproic acid can be used.

Allergic Reactions. These reactions are rare and are usually in the form of rash, bronchospasm, or anaphylaxis.

Fever. Fever can occur and should be symptomatically controlled with acetaminophen rather than aspirin (Gahart & Nazareno, 1996).

NURSING CONSIDERATIONS
Observe patient continuously.

Do not use force when instilling urokinase into catheter.

Work with declotting the catheter every 15 minutes.

If necessary, obtain thrombin time, prothrombin time, or activated partial thromboplastin time to monitor.

Keep physician informed.

Nonthrombotic Occlusion

Nonthrombotic occlusions are caused by mineral precipitates. Precipitates results from poorly soluble I.V. fluid components or the interaction of the infusate with other solutions. Hydrochloric acid (HCL) and sodium bicarbonate ($NaHCO_3$) have been used successfully to clear central lines of precipitates caused by minerals, such as calcium and phosphate, or by medications with a high pH.

HCL is indicated when there is a precipitate in the catheter of the infusate. It is not effective for declotting fat globules (lipid emulsions) (Testerman, 1991). The action of HCL is to lower the pH and therefore increase the precipitation solubility, which results in dissolution and return of catheter patency.

When infusing medications with a high pH such as phenytoin (pH 11–12), the CVC can become occluded. NaHCO$_3$ (pH 8) has successfully restored patency (Goodwin, 1991). Check with agency protocols for the actual steps in clearing an occluded line with HCL or NaHCO$_3$.

It is important to initiate nursing interventions as soon as an occlusion is suspected. Refer to the guidelines for treating a totally obstructed VAD (Fig. 12–16). Keep in mind that instillation and indwelling time vary among institutions.

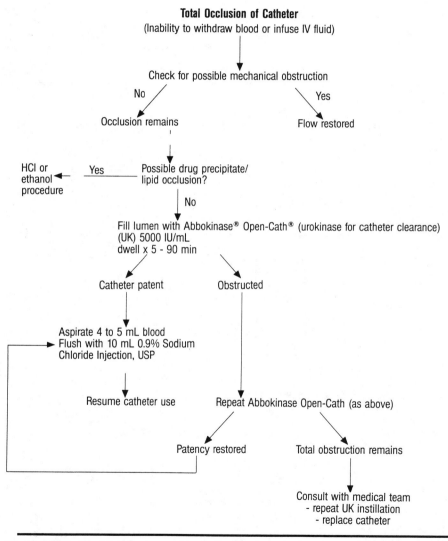

Figure 12–16. Algorithm for therapy for totally obstructed venous access device. (Source: Bagnall-Reeb, Ryder, & Anglim [1994]. Venous Access Device Occlusions Independent Study Module. Illinois: Abbott Laboratories.)

MANAGEMENT OF CENTRAL VENOUS ACCESS DEVICES

Focus Assessment

Objective

Interview regarding present knowledge of illness, vascular access device (VAD).
Identify learning need and ability.

Subjective

Assess competency and dexterity of patient in managing VAD.
Inspect site for signs of infection.
Inspect dressing for integrity.
Examine peripheral I.V. central catheter (PICC) and tunneled catheters for integrity.
Obtain baseline vital signs.

Patient Outcome Criteria

The patient will:
1. Be free of complications associated with insertion and postinsertion of central venous catheters (CVCs)
2. Describe anxiety and coping patterns
3. Demonstrate progressive healing of tissue
4. Demonstrate a willingness and ability to resume self-care and role responsibilities.
5. Verbalize and demonstrate acceptance of appearance
6. Verbalize deficiency in knowledge or skill related to central venous access device

Nursing Diagnoses

Anxiety (mild, moderate, severe), related to threat to change in health status, misconceptions regarding therapy
Altered tissue perfusion (cardiopulmonary), related to infiltration of vesicant medication
Body image disturbance related to perceptions of VAD
Decreased cardiac output related to sepsis, contamination
Fear related to insertion of catheter; fear of "needles"
Impaired gas exchange related to ventilation-perfusion imbalance; dislodged VAD
Impaired skin integrity related to VAD; irritation from I.V. solution; inflammation; infection
Impaired physical mobility related to pain or discomfort resulting from placement and maintenance of VAD
Knowledge deficit (VAD and maintenance of I.V. solution) relating to lack of exposure
Risk of infection related to broken skin or traumatized tissue from the VAD

Nursing Management: Critical Activities

Assist with insertion of central line.
Insert PICC according to agency protocol.
Maintain central line patency and dressing according to agency protocol.
Perform I.V. site care according to agency protocol.
Monitor for fluid overload.
Maintain occlusive dressing.
Monitor for infiltration and infection.
Maintain sterile technique.
Use an infusion pump for delivery of solutions when appropriate.
Monitor vital signs.
Monitor daily weight.
Monitor intake and output ratios.

PATIENT EDUCATION

Instruct on type of central venous access device, purpose and length of catheter or port that will be inserted.

Instruct on signs and symptoms to report, such as increased temperature, discomfort, pain, and difficult breathing.

Instruct on site care of PICC, CVTC, or implanted port.

Teach emergency measures for clamping the catheter if it breaks.

Instruct on flushing protocol.

Instruct on access line for administration of medication, total parenteral nutrition, or fluids.

HOME CARE ISSUES

Central venous access devices are frequently used in the home for administering total parenteral nutrition, chemotherapy or biologic therapy, blood component therapy, and pain control, and for frequent blood sampling. Home infusion is comprehensive, beginning with principles of asepsis, handwashing, and universal precautions. It is essential to assess whether the patient being considered for using a central venous line at home is interested in and motivated to learn self-care. This procedure requires a certain level of intellectual, emotional, and physical capacity and commitment to comply. If the patient is not physically or emotionally able to self-administer or monitor care, a reliable caregiver must be available. Pretreatment assessment includes:

1. Taking a health history, including issues relevant to planned therapy
2. Verifying the medication and dosage that the patient is to receive
3. Reviewing complications and side effects of drug therapy and central line management
4. Reviewing patient's history and past experience, if appropriate, with central lines
5. Assessing patient's current knowledge of managing central lines
6. Providing written instruction and diagrams of accessing line, site care, and flushing protocol

COMPETENCY CRITERIA

Competency Statement: Demonstrate skill in nursing management of CVAD access, dressing care, blood drawing, and vascular access device.

COGNITIVE CRITERIA

	Knowledgeable	Needs Education
1. Identifies correct catheter tip placement:		
Superior vena cava		
Radiology confirmation		
Catheter stabilization		
2. Identifies complications of CVC:		
Air, or catheter embolism		
Pneumothorax, hemothorax		
Pulmonary embolism		
Local infection/septicemia		
Twiddlers syndrome		
3. States interventions for catheter problems:		
Declotting techniques		
Severed catheter management		
Ruptured catheter repair		
4. Identifies types and advantages of CVC:		
Catheter materials		
Tunneled catheters		
Implanted ports		
Multilumen catheters		

PERFORMANCE CRITERIA

	Skilled	Needs Education
1. Performs baseline assessment of catheter patency:		
Checks all clamps		
Checks catheter for kinds		

428

Determines proper needle position with subcutaneous infusion ports

Has patient change position

Gently aspirates and irrigates the catheter

2. **Demonstrates agency protocol in using thrombolytic agent to declot line:**

Gathers apropriate equipment

Reviews drug allergy history

Dons sterile gloves

Administers urokinase according to procedure

Maintains sterility throughout procedure

Stays with patient for 15 min after urokinase instillation and observes for complications

Documents procedure

3. **Demonstrates blood withdrawal from CVC:**

Follows agency procedure

Discards 5–10 mL of blood

4. **Uses appropriate flushing procedure for each catheter:**

PICC

Tunneled catheters

Groshong valve catheters

Implanted ports

5. **Accesses implant port using appropriate needle:**

Implanted ports with septum (noncoring Huber needle)

CathLink implanted port (20-gauge 1¾-in. over-the-needle catheter)

10. **Demonstrates injection cap changes using sterile technique**

SUGGESTED EVALUATION CRITERIA

Preceptor observation of technique

Written test for cognitive criteria

Return demonstration on model

KEY POINTS

Anatomy of the vascular system
 Venous structures of the arm
  Cephalic vein
  Basilic vein
 Venous structures of the chest
  Subclavian vein
  Right and left brachiocephalic
  External jugular vein
  Internal jugular vein
  Right and left innominate veins
  Superior vena cava (which receive all blood from upper half of body)

CVC materials
 Silicone elastomers
 Polyurethane
 Elastomeric hydrogel and Vialon
 Lumens
 Coatings
  Hydrophilic materials
  Antiseptic substances
  Antibiotics
  Heparin
 Single, double, triple, and quadruple gauge

Short-term and long-term access devices
 Short-term devices
  Percutaneous catheters
   Dressing management
    Gauze or tape dressing (change every 48 to 72 hours)
    TSM (change every 4 to 7 days)
  PICCs
   Placement by trained I.V. nurse
   Site: Peripheral, preferably basilic vein
   Advantages
    Decrease in risk factors associated with subclavian placements such as hemothorax, pneumothorax, air embolism
    Decrease in pain associated with frequent venipunctures
    Cost-effective
    Appropriate for home care
   Disadvantages
    Special training required
    Time to complete procedure (45 minutes to 1 hour)
    Daily care required
    Catheter maintenance guidelines
    Nursing management of PICCs
   Dressing management
    Change initial dressing after 24 hours. Thereafter, apply transparent dressing the same as any TSM central dressing.

Flushing procedure
    Follow SASH using 10 to 100 U heparin.
    Use 2 mL of saline followed by 1 mL heparinized saline
    Flush after every medication administration, blood drawing, or blood administration (these catheters can clot easily).
Blood sampling
    Maintain integrity of the catheter.
Blood administration
    Administer through a 3.8F or larger PICC.
Repair
    Use manufacture-specific repair kit.
    Replace catheter over a guidewire.
Declotting the line
    Use urokinase following consent from patient, physician's order, and a clear policy and procedure.
Insertion and postinsertion complications

Insertion	Postinsertion
Bleeding at site	Phlebitis and cellulitis
Tendon or nerve damage	Infection
Cardiac arrhythmias	Thrombosis (clot formation)
Malposition of catheter	Air embolism
Catheter embolism	

Long-term devices
CVTCs
    Uses: Blood sample drawing, administration of medications, blood products, and parenteral nutrition
    Material: Polymeric silicone with a Dacron cuff that anchors the catheter in the subcutaneous tissue
    Lumen: Single, double, and triple
    Advantages: Repairable if torn or catheter breaks; eliminates multiple needle sticks; multipurpose
    Disadvantages: Daily to weekly site care; cost of maintenance and supplies; surgical procedure; body image may possibly be affected
        Repair of the catheter
        Complications
            Site infection
            Sepsis
            Thrombosis
            Catheter migration
            Clot formation
            Torn or leaking catheter
            Air embolism
        Key points in care of CVTCs
            Be sure catheter is capped at all times.
            Keep all sharp objects away from catheter.
            If the catheter leaks or breaks, take a nonserrated clamp and clamp catheter between broken area and exit site.
            Protect catheter when showering or bathing.
        Flush after a blood draw with 10 mL 0.9% sodium chloride and correct amount of heparin (heparin is used to maintain patency).
Groshong valve
    Key points in care of Groshong valve catheter
    Do not clamp catheter.
    Keep sharp objects away from catheter.

If catheter leaks or breaks, cover the broken part with a sterile gauze bandage and tape securely.

Protect catheter when showering or bathing.

Straining or heavy lifting can cause a small amount of blood to back up into the catheter.

After blood sampling, flush with 20 mL of normal saline.

Implanted ports

Material: Silicone catheter with a central septum made of titanium or steel

Uses: Blood sampling, administration of medication, blood products, and parenteral nutrition

Available: Single or double septum

Advantages: Less risk of infection, less interference with daily activities, little site care, needs minimal flushing, less body image disturbance, few limitations on patient activity

Disadvantages: Cost of insertion, postoperative care is 7 to 10 days, discomfort of repeated needle sticks, minor surgical procedure necessary to remove device

Complications: Site infection or breakdown, sepsis, thrombosis, clot formation, air embolism, port migration, extravasation

Key points in care of implanted ports

Use noncoring needle for access with appropriate port. Use 20-gauge 1¾-in. over-the-needle catheter for the CathLink.

Change needle and extension tubing every 7 days.

Flush port with normal saline and heparin every 4 weeks if port is not in use or after every infusion.

Tubing and dressing management are necessary only with continuous use.

Occluded CVCs

Mechanical occlusion

Causes: Kinked or closed clamp; clogged cap or filter, infusion pump turned off, empty I.V. bag

Management

Thrombotic occlusion

Causes: Intraluminal thrombus or clot, fibrin sleeve, fibrin tail, mural thrombus or total venous thrombosis, portal reservoir obstruction

Urokinase: 5000 IU in 1 ml specifically diluted solution

Technique: Insert drug into catheter, attempt every 5 minutes for 30 minutes to withdraw the clot. Reattempt after 1 hour. (Clots can usually be removed in 30 minutes to 3 hours)

Contraindications to urokinase: Internal bleeding cerebrovascular accident (within 2 months), intracranial neoplasm, hypersensitivity to urokinase, liver disease, subacute bacterial endocarditis or visceral malignancy, intracranial or intraspinal surgery

Complications of urokinase administration: Bleeding, allergic reactions, fever

Nonthrombotic occlusion

Cause: Mineral precipitate

Management: HCL and $NaHCO_3$

CRITICAL THINKING ACTIVITY

1. As a new graduate, you have been asked to change a complicated abdominal dressing on a patient postoperatively. This patient is receiving chemotherapy via a Hickman tunneled catheter. As you are cutting the dressing off you accidently puncture the catheter. What do you do? How could this have been avoided?

2. Check the flushing of central lines policy and procedure at the agency in which you are working. Does the procedure clearly give steps in the flushing of a Hickman, Groshong, and the implanted port?

3. You attempt to flush the recently inserted PICC line to administer the next dose of antibiotics. The line does not flush; resistance is felt. What do you do?

4. You are the charge nurse and a newly employed nurse assertively states that she will insert the new PICC on her patient because she has put in many PICCs in her former job as a home care I.V. nurse. How do you handle this situation?

433

POST-TEST, CHAPTER 12

Match the following definitions in column II to the terms in column I.

Column I

1. _____ extravascular malpositioning
2. _____ intravascular malpositioning
3. _____ lymphedema
4. _____ distal
5. _____ cutdown

Column II

A. Swelling of extremity

B. Farthest from the heart

C. Passage of introducer into the pleural cavity

D. Surgical procedure for exposure of a vein for cannulation

E. Catheter tip advanced into venous tributary other than superior vena cava

True-False

6. **T F** The term central venous catheter refers to catheters placed in the central chest vasculature, usually the superior vena cava.

7. **T F** The basilic vein is an appropriate choice for cannulation of the PICC.

8. **T F** Ideal material for CVC should include biocompatibility, thromboresistance, and nonhemolytic properties.

9. **T F** Vascular access devices are only available as single lumens.

10. **T F** Short-term access devices are appropriate for therapy lasting longer than 7 days to weeks.

11. Implanted ports, when not in use, can be flushed every:
    A. Week
    B. 2 weeks
    C. 3 weeks
    D. 4 weeks

12. Major complications of short-term central venous access devices would include:
    A. Phlebitis or cellulitis
    B. Intravascular and extravascular malpositioning
    C. Air embolism
    D. All of the above

13. When tunneled catheters are used, the advantages to the patient include:
    A. Remains patent without flushing procedures
    B. Can be replaced easily
    C. Can be used for multiple purposes
    D. Minimal body image change associated

14. The drug of choice for declotting a clotted short-term or long-term device is:
    A. Wydase
    B. Urokinase
    C. Monoamine oxidase
    D. Acetylcholinesterase

15. Identify three of the seven complications of tunneled catheters.

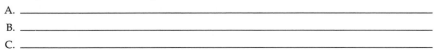

   A. _____

   B. _____

   C. _____

434

16. List the six nursing management points of tunneled catheters.

    A. _____
    B. _____
    C. _____
    D. _____
    E. _____
    F. _____

17. List the six key points in care of the Groshong valve.

    A. _____
    B. _____
    C. _____
    D. _____
    E. _____
    F. _____

18. Describe the procedure of accessing an implanted port for injecting a bolus.

    A. _____
    B. _____
    C. _____
    D. _____
    E. _____
    F. _____
    G. _____
    H. _____
    I. _____

ANSWERS TO CHAPTER 12

PRE-TEST

1. D	4. A	7. F	10. T
2. C	5. E	8. A	11. T
3. B	6. A	9. D	12. F

POST-TEST

1. C
2. E
3. A
4. B
5. D
6. T
7. T
8. T
9. F
10. T
11. D
12. D
13. C
14. B
15. Skin infection, sepsis, thrombosis, catheter migration, clot formation, torn or leaking catheter, air embolism
16. A. Be sure catheter is clamped at all times.
    B. Keep sharp objects away from catheter.
    C. If the catheter leaks or breaks, clamp immediately between broken area and the exit site; cover with sterile gauze.
    D. Protect the catheter when showering or bathing.
    E. Use 10 mL of saline and heparin after drawing blood.
    F. Heparin must be used to keep catheter free of clots.

17. A. Do not clamp the catheter.
    B. Keep all sharp objects away from the catheter.
    C. If the catheter leaks or breaks, cover with sterile gauze and tape securely.
    D. Protect the catheter when showering or bathing.
    E. Straining or heavy lifting can cause a small amount of blood to back up into the catheter. If blood is evident in the catheter line, flush.
    F. After blood sample is obtained, flush briskly with 20 mL of saline.
18. A. Use sterile procedure.
    B. Palpate port with sterile gloves.
    C. Use povidone-iodine swabs to clean injection site. Start at septum and swab outward to 6 in. Repeat three times.
    D. Attach a 6-mL syringe of heparin solution to the stopcock at the end of the extension tubing.
    E. Connect the appropriate noncoring needle to the Luer lock at the other end and prime the tubing.
    F. Put on a fresh pair of sterile gloves.
    G. Palpate the port to find the center of the septum.
    H. Insert noncoring needle.
    I. Aspirate a small amount of blood to check for patency and position.

REFERENCES

Bagnall, H., Gompers, E., & Atkinson, J. (1989). Continuous infusion of low-dose urokinase in the treatment of central venous catheter thrombosis in infants and children. *Pediatrics, 83,* 963–966.

Bagnall-Reeb, H., Ryder, M., & Anglim, M.A. (1994). *Venous access device occlusions: Independent study module.* Illinois: Oncology Nursing Society, Abbott Laboratories Pharmaceutical Products Division.

Baranowski, L. (1993). Central venous access devices: Current technologies, uses, and management strategies. *Journal of Intravenous Therapy, 16*(3), 167–194.

Bjeletich, J. (1987). Declotting central venous catheters with urokinase in the home by nurse clinicians. *National Intravenous Therapy Association, 10*(6), 428–430.

Bridges, B.B., Carden, E., & Takac, F.A. (1979). Introduction to central venous pressure catheters through arm veins with a high success rate. *Can Anaesthesia Society Journal, 26,* 128–131.

Brown, J.M. (1989). Peripherally inserted central catheter use in home care. *Journal of Intravenous Nursing, 12*(3), 144–150.

Camp, D.L. (1988). Care of the Groshong catheter. *Oncology Nursing Forum, 15*(6), 745–748.

Camp-Sorrell, D.L. (1990). Advanced central venous access selection of catheters, devices and nursing management. *Journal of Intravenous Nursing, 13*(6), 361–368.

Camp-Sorrell, D.L. (1995). Advances in tunneled and nontunneled catheters: Nursing management strategies. In Conners R., & Winters R.W. (eds.) *Home infusion: Current status and future trends* (pp. 55–70). American Hospital Publishing Company.

Department of Health and Human Services. (1995). *Intravascular device-related infection prevention guideline availability: Notice—Federal Register.* Atlanta: Centers for Disease Control and Prevention.

Dreyfus, H.L., & Dreyfus, S.E. (1977). *Uses and abuses of multiattribute and multiaspect model of decision making.* Unpublished manuscript, Department of Industrial Engineering and Operations Research, University of California, Berkeley.

Dunbar, R.D., Mitchell, R., & Lavine, M. (1981). Aberrant location of central venous catheters. *Lancet, 1,* 711.

Ellis, L.M., Vogel, S.B., & Copeland, E.M. (1989). Central venous catheters vascular erosions: Diagnosis and clinical course. *Annuals of Surgery, 209,* 475.

Freedman, S.E., & Bosserman, G. (1993). Tunneled catheters. *Nursing Clinics of North America, 28*(4), 851–858.

Gahart, B.L., & Nazareno, A.R. (1996). *Intravenous medications* (12th ed.). St. Louis: Mosby-Year Book.

Gray, H. (1977). Anatomy, descriptive and surgical. New York: Crown.

Hadaway, L.C. (1989). Evaluation and use of advanced I.V. technology. Part I: Central venous access devices. *Journal of Intravenous Nursing, 12*(2), 73–81.

Hadaway, L.C. (1990). An overview of vascular access devices inserted via the antecubital area. *Journal of Intravenous Nursing, 13*(5), 297–306.

Handy, C.M. (1989). Vascular access devices hospital to home care. *Journal of Intravenous Nursing, 12*(1), 10–18.

Heimbach, D., & Ivey, T.D. (1976). Technique for placement of a permanent home hyperalimentation catheter. *Gynecology Obstetrics, 143,* 634–646.

Hinke, D.H., Zandt-Stastny, D.A., & Goodman, L.R. (1990). Pinch-off signs: A complication of implantable subclavian vascular access devices. *Radiology, 177*(2), 353–356.

Hohal, V.L., & Ause, R.G. (1971). Fibrin-sleeve formation on indwelling subclavian central venous catheters. *Archives of Surgery, 102,* 253–258.

Intravenous Nursing Society. (1990). *Standards of practice.* Philadelphia: J.B. Lippincott.

I.V. Management Services. (1990). *PICC: Care, use and maintenance.* Salinas, CA: I.V. Management Services.

Lowell, J.A., & Boothe, A. (1991). Venous access: Preoperative, operative, and postoperative dilemmas. *Surgical Clinics of North America, 71,* 1231.

Lum, P.S., & Soski, M. (1989). Management of malpositioned central venous catheters. *Journal of Intravenous Nursing, 12*(6), 356–365.

Maki, D.G. (1988). An attachable silver-impregnated cuff for prevention of infection with central venous catheters: A prospective randomized multicenter trial. *American Journal of Medicine, 85,* 307–314.

Maki, D.G. (1992). Infections due to infusion therapy. In Bennett, J.V., & Brachman, P.S. (eds.). *Hospital infections* (p. 849) Boston: Little, Brown.

Maki, D.G., Wheeler, S.J., & Stoltz, S.M. (1991). (Abstract). *American Society for Microbiology.*

Masoorli, S., & Angeles, T. (1990). PICC lines: The latest home care challenge. *RN, 1,* 44–50.

May, G.S., & Davis, C. (1988). Percutaneous catheters and totally implantable access systems: A review of reported infection rates. *Journal of Intravenous Nursing, 11*(2), 97–103.

Ordway, C.B. (1973). Air embolism via CVP catheter without positive pressure. *Annuals of Surgery, 179,* 479.

Pemberton, L.B. (1986). Sepis for triple-use single lumen catheter during total parenteral nutrition in surgical or critically ill patients. *Archives of Surgery, 12*(5), 591–593.

Perrucca, R. (1995). Intravenous monitoring and catheter care. In Terry, J., Baranowski, L., Lonsway, R., & Hedrick, C. *Intravenous therapy: Clinical principles and practice* (pp. 392–399). Philadelphia: W.B. Saunders.

Peters, J.L., & Armstrong, R. (1978). Air embolism occurring as a complication of central venous catheterization. *Annuals of Surgery, 187,* 375.

Plumer, A.L., & Cosentino, F. (1987). *Principles and practices of intravenous therapy.* Philadelphia: J.B. Lippincott.

Riser, S. (1988). Patient care manual for implanted vascular access devices. *Journal of Intravenous Nursing, 11*(3), 166–168.

Roundtree, D. (1991). The PIC catheters: A different approach. *American Journal of Nursing, 91*(8), 22–27.

Ryan, J.A., & Gough, J. (1984). Complication of central venous catheterization for total parenteral nutrition: The role of the nurse. *National Intravenous Therapy Association, 8*(1), 29–35.

Ryder, M.A. (1993). Peripherally inserted central venous catheters. *Nursing Clinics of North America, 28*(4), 937–970.

Sims Deltec. (1990). Clinical information—PORT-A-CATH and P.A.S.PORT implantable access devices. St. Paul, MN: Sims Deltec.

437

Speer, E.W. (1990). Central venous catheterization: Issues associated with the use of single-multiple lumen catheters. *Journal of Intravenous Nursing, 13*(1), 30–39.

Stewart, R.D., & Sanislow, G.A. (1961). Silastic intravenous catheter. *New England Journal of Medicine, 265,* 1238–1285.

Testerman, E.J. (1991). Restoring patency of central venous cathets obstructed by mineral precipitation using hydrochloric acid. *Journal of Vascular Access Networks, 1*(2), 22–23.

Trooskin, S.Z., Donetz, A.P., & Harvey, R.A. (1985). Prevention of catheter sepsis by antibiotic bonding. *Surgery, 97,* 547–551.

Vasquez, R.M. (1980). Subclavian catheterization. *American Journal of Intravenous Therapy & Clinical Nutrition, 80*(5), 11–29.

Viall, C.D. (1990). Daily access of implanted venous ports: Implications for patient education. *Journal of Intravenous Nursing, 13*(5), 294–296.

Viall, C.D. (1990). Your complete guide to central venous catheters. *Nursing 90, 2,* 34–41.

Weinstein, S.M. (1993). *Plumer's principles and practice of I.V. therapy.* Philadelphia: J.B. Lippincott.

CHAPTER 13

Transfusion Therapy

CHAPTER CONTENTS

GLOSSARY
LEARNING OBJECTIVES
PRE-TEST, CHAPTER 13
BASIC IMMUNOHEMATOLOGY
Antigens (Agglutinogens)
Antibodies (Agglutinins)
Testing of Donor Blood
Compatibility Testing
Blood Preservatives
BLOOD DONOR COLLECTION METHODS
Homologous
Autologous
Designated
BLOOD COMPONENT THERAPY
Whole Blood
Packed RBCs
Washed RBCs
Deglycerolized RBCs
Granulocytes
Platelets
Fresh Frozen Plasma
Cryoprecipitate
COLLOID VOLUME EXPANDERS
Albumin and Plasma Protein Fraction
ALTERNATIVE PHARMACOLOGIC THERAPIES
Blood Substitutes
ADMINISTRATION OF BLOOD COMPONENTS
Step 1: Physician's Order

Step 2: Equipment Selection and Preparation
Step 3: Patient Preparation
Step 4: Obtaining Blood Product from the
    Blood Bank
Step 5: Preparation for Administration
Step 6: Initiation of Transfusion
Step 7: Monitoring the Transfusion
Step 8: Discontinuation of Transfusion
SUMMARY WORKSHEET
COMPLICATIONS ASSOCIATED WITH BLOOD
    COMPONENT THERAPY
Transfusion Reactions
Other Complications
Risks of Transfusion Therapy
NURSING PLAN OF CARE: DELIVERY OF BLOOD
    COMPONENT THERAPY
PATIENT EDUCATION
HOME CARE ISSUES
COMPETENCY CRITERIA: BLOOD
    ADMINISTRATION
KEY POINTS
CRITICAL THINKING ACTIVITY
POST-TEST, CHAPTER 13
ANSWERS TO CHAPTER 13
Pre-Test
Post-Test
REFERENCES

GLOSSARY

ABO system   Human blood groups that are inherited; groups determined according to which antigens are present on the surfaces of red blood cells and which antibodies are present in the plasma

Agglutinin   An antibody that causes particulate antigens, such as other cells, to adhere to one another, forming clumps

Agglutinogen   An antigenic substance that stimulates the formation of a particular antibody

Allergic reaction   Reaction from exposure to an antigen to which the person has become sensitized

439

Alloimmunization   Development of an immune response to alloantigens; occurs during pregnancy, blood transfusions, and organ transplantation

Antibody   Protein produced by the immune system that destroys or inactivates a particular antigen

Antigen   Any substance eliciting an immunologic response, such as the production of antibody specific for that substance

Autologous donation   Blood donated before needed, to be used only by donor

Blood component   Product made from a unit of whole blood such as platelet concentrate, red blood cells, fresh frozen plasma, cryoprecipitate

CPD   Citrate-phosphate-dextrose; a preservative for collected blood

CPDA-1   Citrate-phosphate-dextrose-adenine; a preservative that extends the shelf life of stored blood to 35 days

Delayed transfusion reaction   Adverse effect occurring after 48 hours and up to 180 days after transfusion

Designated donation   Transfer of blood directly from one donor to specified recipient

Febrile reaction   Nonhemolytic reaction to antibodies formed against leukocytes

Hemoglobin   Respiratory pigment of red blood cell having the reversible property of taking up oxygen or of releasing oxygen

Hemolysis   Rupture of red blood cells, with the release of hemoglobin

Hemolytic transfusion reaction   Blood transfusion reaction in which an antigen-antibody reaction in the recipient is due to incompatibility between red cell antigens and antibodies

HLA   Human leukocyte antigen; used for tissue typing and relevant for transplant histocompatibility

Homologous donation   Donation of blood in similar structure from a volunteer donor

Hypothermia   Abnormally low body temperature

Immediate reaction   Adverse effect occurring immediately or up to 48 hours after infusion

Immunohematology   Study of blood and blood reactions

Microaggregate   Microscopic collection of particles such as platelets, leukocytes, and fibrin, which occurs in stored blood

Pheresis   Derived from the Greek word *aphairesis*, meaning "to take away"; used to denote the removal of blood, the separation into component parts, the retention of only the parts needed, and the return of the rest to the donor (e.g., removal of plasma is plasmapheresis)

Phlebotomy   Withdrawal of blood from a vein

Plasma   Fluid portion of the blood, composed of a mixture of proteins in solution

Reaction   Term that denotes the clinical symptoms caused when the red cells of either the recipient or the donor are destroyed in the recipient during a transfusion

Refractory   Not responsive or readily yielding to treatment

Rh system   Second most important system; Rh antigens are inherited and found on the surface of red blood cells; classified as positive or negative based on whether D antigen is present

Serum   The cells and fibrinogen-free amber-colored fluid after blood or plasma clots

Thrombocytopenia   Abnormally small number of platelets in the blood

LEARNING OBJECTIVES

Upon completion of this chapter, the reader will be able to:

- State the antigens of the ABO system.
- Define the terms related to basic immunohematology.
- State the definition of HLA.
- Identify the universal blood donor type.
- Identify the presence of antibodies in the ABO system.
- Identify the Rh antigens located on the red blood cells.
- Identify the preservatives used in donor blood storage.
- Summarize the tests used to screen donor blood.

- Distinguish among homologous, autologous, and designated blood.
- Define the terminology related to transfusion therapy.
- Describe each of the blood components.
- List the indications for use of each blood component.
- State the key points in the administration of red cells, platelets, granulocytes, fresh frozen plasma, and cryoprecipitate.
- Describe the procedure for administration of blood components.
- List the symptoms of hemolytic transfusion reaction, both acute and delayed.
- State the signs and symptoms of febrile transfusion reaction and allergic transfusion reaction.
- Differentiate between febrile and allergic transfusion reactions.
- Use nursing process to deliver safe transfusion therapy.

PRE-TEST, CHAPTER 13

Match the definition in column II to the term in column I.

Column I

1. _____ agglutinin
2. _____ antigen
3. _____ alloimmunization
4. _____ agglutinogen
5. _____ designated donor
6. _____ autologous donor
7. _____ HLA
8. _____ immunohematology
9. _____ ABO
10. _____ Rh

Column II

A. Dantigen found on the surface of red blood cells, positive or negative

B. An antigenic substance that stimulates the formation of an antibody

C. Substance eliciting an immunologic response

D. Study of blood and blood reactions

E. Antigens present on the surface of red blood cells

F. Human leukocyte antigen

G. Development of immune response to alloantigens

H. Antibody that causes particulate antigens to adhere to one another

I. Donation of one's own blood prior to transfusion

J. Transfer of blood directly from one donor to a specified recipient

11. The preservative CPDA-1 extends the life of collected cells to:
    A. 25 days
    B. 30 days
    C. 35 days
    D. 42 days

12. The universal plasma donor type is:
    A. A
    B. O
    C. AB
    D. B

13. Transfusions are screened for all of the following *except*:
    A. Syphilis
    B. Human immunodeficiency virus (HIV)

441

C. Surface hepatitis B
D. Mononucleosis
E. Hepatitis C

14. The antigens in the blood system would include all of the following *except:*
    A. ABO
    B. Rh
    C. HLA
    D. IgM

Match the definition in column II to the term in column I.

Column I

15. _____ blood component
16. _____ microaggregate
17. _____ plasma
18. _____ delayed reaction
19. _____ hemolytic transfusion reaction
20. _____ pheresis
21. _____ immediate reaction
22. _____ hemoglobin
23. _____ refractory
24. _____ hemolysis

Column II

A. Respiratory pigment of red blood cell
B. Fluid portion of blood
C. Removal of blood, separation into component parts, and retention of part
D. Adverse effect occurring immediately or up to 48 hours after transfusion
E. Not responsive nor readily yielding to treatment
F. Adverse effect occurring 48 hours up to 180 after transfusion
G. Rupture of red cells
H. Product made from a unit of whole blood
I. Microscopic collection of particles, which occurs in stored blood
J. Red cells destroyed in the recipient during a transfusion

25. Cryoprecipitate is the component used to treat:
    A. Bleeding disorders related to factor VIII deficiency
    B. Acute massive blood loss
    C. Chronic anemia
    D. Bleeding disorders related to factor IX deficiency

26. Platelets are used to provide:
    A. Protein
    B. Clotting factors
    C. Red blood cells
    D. Granulocytes

27. Whole blood is used to treat:
    A. Chronic anemia
    B. Deficiency in factor VIII
    C. Massive blood loss
    D. White blood cell deficiency

28. The recommended rate of infusion for 1 U of packed red blood cells is no longer than
    A. 1 hour
    B. 2 hours
    C. 4 hours
    D. 6 hours

To ensure delivery of safe transfusion therapy, the nurse must possess a knowledge and understanding of the blood system as well as basic immunohematology. He or she must also be knowledgeable about the theory and practical management of blood component therapy. The first part of this chapter introduces the reader to fundamental concepts of immunohematology, blood grouping, and the criteria for donor blood, including homologous, designated autologous, donation. Fundamental concepts of blood component therapy, administration equipment, administration techniques for each blood component, and management of transfusion reactions are presented in the second part of the chapter.

BASIC IMMUNOHEMATOLOGY

Immunohematology is the science that deals with antigens of the blood and their antibodies. The antigens and antibodies are genetically inherited and determine the blood group. An antigen is a substance capable of stimulating the production of an antibody and then reacting with that antibody in a specific way. Antigens of the blood are called agglutinogens. Any substance that can elicit an immunologic response is AB antigen. They are located on the cells. The three antigens on the red blood cells (RBCs) that cause problems and are routinely tested for are A, B, and Rh D. The human leukocyte antigen (HLA) is located on most cells in the body except mature erythrocytes. Antibodies are found in the plasma or serum.

Antigens (Agglutinogens)

ABO System

The most important antigens in the blood are the surface antigens, A and B, which are located on the RBC membranes in the ABO system (Table 13–1). The name of the blood type is determined by the name of the antigen on the RBC. Individuals who have A antigen on the RBC membrane are classified as group A; B antigens, group B; A and B surface antigens, group AB; and neither A or B antigens, group O. This ABO system was discovered in 1901 by Dr. Karl Landsteiner. See Table 13–2 for an ABO compatibility chart.

Rh System

After A and B, the most important RBC antigen is the D antigen, which was discovered in 1940 by Drs. Landsteiner and Wiener. The Rh system is so called because of its relationship to the substance in the RBCs of the Rhesus monkey. There are ap-

TABLE 13–1. **ABO BLOOD GROUPING CHART**

Blood Groupings	Recipient Antigens on RBCs	Antibodies Present in Plasma
A	A	Anti-B
B	B	Anti-A
AB	A and B	None
O	None	Anti-A and Anti-B

443

TABLE 13–2. **ABO COMPATIBILITY CHART**

Blood Type	Compatible RBC	Compatible Plasma
A	A, O	A, AB
B	B, O	B, AB
AB	AB, O	AB
O	O	O, AB, A, B

Universal plasma donor is **AB:** AB has no anti-A or anti-B antibodies in the plasma. Universal blood donor is **O-negative.**

Note: When giving O-negative to an uncrossmatched patient, administer packed cells so that the anti-A and anti-B antibodies within the serum are removed.

proximately 50 Rh-related antigens; the five principal antigens are D, C, E, c, e. A person who has D antigen is classified as Rh-positive; one lacking D is Rh-negative. Eighty-five percent of the population is classified as D-Rh-positive (Walker, 1993). D antibodies build up easily; therefore, typing is done to ensure that D-negative recipients receive D-negative blood. Rh-negative recipients should receive Rh-negative whole blood and RBC components.

HLA System

The HLA antigen was originally identified on the leukocytes, but it has been established that HLA is present on most cells in the body. It is located on the surface of white blood cells (WBCs), platelets, and most tissue cells. HLA typing or tissue typing, is important in patients with transplants or multiple transfusions and for paternity testing. The HLA system is very complex and is involved in immune regulation and cellular differentiation.

The HLA system is important in transfusion therapy because HLA antigens of the donor unit can induce alloimmunization in the recipient. This alloimmunization has been found to be a major factor in the onset of refractoriness to random donor platelet support. HLA incompatibility is a possible cause of hemolytic transfusion reactions, and HLA antibodies as well as granulocyte- and platelet-specific antibodies have been implicated in the development of nonhemolytic transfusion reactions.

Methods used to decrease HLA alloimmunization include HLA matching and leukocyte depletion of the donor unit (Walker, 1993).

A standard unit of blood that has not been depleted of leukocytes contains 5×10^9 leukocytes. The American Association of Blood Banks has designated that an RBC product may be labeled leukocyte-depleted if it retains 80% of the original RBC concentration, but only 5×10^6 of leukocytes. Blood may be depleted of leukocytes during three periods: (1) immediately after collection, (2) 6 to 24 hours after collection, and (3) at the time of infusion (Walker, 1993).

Third-generation leukocyte-depleting filters used at the bedside remove all but an insignificant number of leukocytes from a unit of blood (Cook, 1995).

✎ **NOTE:** Patients receiving multiple transfusions are at particular risk for developing complications related to leukocytes, such as sensitization to leukocyte antigens, nonhemolytic febrile reactions, transmission of leukocyte-mediated viruses and graft-versus-host disease (Walker, 1993).

Antibodies (Agglutinins)

Antibodies within the blood system are proteins that react with a specific antigen. Antigens are agglutinins in that particulate antigens, such as other cells, adhere to

444

one another in response to a specific antigen. The antibodies anti-A and anti-B are produced spontaneously in the plasma after birth and usually form in the first 3 months of life. An antibody has the same name as the antigen with which it reacts. For example, anti-A reacts to antigen A.

Naturally occurring antibodies, like those in the ABO system, are blood group antibodies that agglutinate erythrocytes containing corresponding antigens in a saline solution and are called *saline antibodies*. The naturally occurring antibody in the blood, which occurs within the inherited blood group, is called immunoglobulin mu (IgM). *Complete antibodies* is the term for naturally occurring antibodies. Intravascular hemolysis may occur in vivo with naturally occurring antibodies (IgM).

Immunoglobulins or immune antibodies are a group of glycoproteins (complex molecules containing protein and sugar molecules) in the serum and tissues of mammals that possess antibody activity. Immunoglobulin molecules are divided into five classes: IgG, IgA, IgM, IgD, and IgE. These antibodies are produced by the immune system in response to previous exposure to the antigen via prior transfusion or pregnancy; they are not genetically inherited. When these antibodies meet with their corresponding antigen, the cells are affected but not destroyed in the intravascular system. The sensitized cells are removed intact by the reticuloendothelial system, primarily the spleen and liver (Suez, 1995).

Other Blood Group Systems

In addition to the ABO and Rh blood group antigens, over 500 other antigens can be found on human RBCs (Walker, 1993). There are 24 known systems associated with RBCs (Weir, 1995).

The following are the most common groups identified.

ABO	Lewis
Rh	MNS
Kell	P
Duffy	Lutheran
Kidd	

Corresponding antibodies to all but ABO and Rh systems are found so infrequently that they do not usually cause common problems in transfusion therapy.

Testing of Donor Blood

At the time of donation, every unit of blood intended for homologous donation must undergo the following tests by the blood bank; Table 13–3 summarizes testing of donor blood.

1. The ABO group must be determined by testing the RBCs with anti-A and anti-B serums and by testing the serum or plasma with A and B cells.
2. The Rh type must be determined with anti-D serum. *Units that are D-positive must be labeled Rh-positive.*
3. Most blood banks test all donor blood for clinically significant antibodies. If all donors are not tested, then at least blood from donors with a history of prior transfusion or pregnancy should be tested for unexpected antibodies before the crossmatch.
4. All donor blood must be tested to detect transmissible disease. The blood component must not be used for transfusion unless the tests are nonreactive, negative, or within the normal range (see Table 13–3).
5. Each unit must be appropriately labeled. The label must include the following information: name of the component, type, and amount of anticoagulant, vol-

445

TABLE 13–3. **SUMMARY OF TESTING DONOR BLOOD**

Routine Tests

ABO blood typing
Rh blood typing
Activated partial thromboplastin time (APTT)
Complete blood count (CBC with differential)
Crossmatching of packed cells and whole blood
Factor VIII (antihemophilic factor) assay
HLA-A, -B, -C tissue typing
HLA antibody identification
HLA disease association antigen testing
HLA-DR tissue typing
HLA lymphocytotoxic
   Antibody testing
   Crossmatching/organ
   Transplantation
Platelet count
Platelet antibody testing
Platelet crossmatching (as a supplement to HLA matching)
Prothrombin time (PT)
Red cell antigen typing (other than ABO/Rh)

Tests for Transmissible Disease

Hepatitis B surface antigen testing (HBsAg)
Hepatitis B core antibody testing (Anti-HBc)
Hepatitis B surface antibody testing (Anti-HBs)
Human immunodeficiency virus* (anti-HIV, formerly anti-HTLV-III, anti-LAV)-ELISA and
   Western blot
Human immunodeficiency virus (anti-HIV2) (since 1992)
Human T-cell lymphotropic virus type I antibody testing (anti-HTLV-1)
Serologic test for syphilis (RPR)
Hepatitis C antibody testing (anti-HCV)

*As of 1996, HIV antigen testing is licensed by the FDA and also used to test donated blood.
Source: From California Department of Health and Human Services, Food and Drug Administration, American Association of Blood Banks, 1996.

ume of unit, required storage temperature, name and address of collecting facility, a reference to the circular of information, type of donor (volunteer, autologous, or paid), expiration date, and donor number (Fig. 13–1).

✎ **NOTE:** The label should also include statements indicating "this product may transmit infectious agents" and "properly identify intended recipient."

6. The facility performing the compatibility testing must do ABO and Rh grouping confirmation tests on a sample obtained from the originally attached segment of all units of whole or red cells (Walker, 1993).

Compatibility Testing

Recipients of transfusions must be tested for ABO and Rh grouping. In addition, antibody screening and a compatibility test must be performed. Previous exposure to an antigen by pregnancy or transfusion may have caused the patient to develop an antibody against an antigen.

446

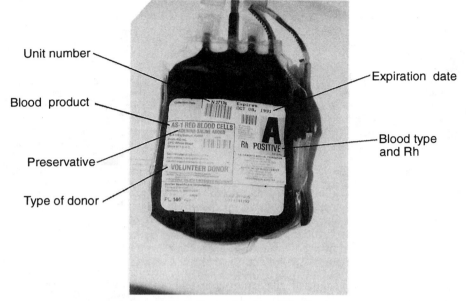

Unit number

Expiration date

Blood product

Preservative

Blood type
and Rh

Type of donor

Figure 13–1. Correct labeling of blood unit.

Compatibility testing is performed between the recipient's plasma and the donor's RBCs to ensure that the specific unit intended for transfusion to the recipient is not incompatible. Blood from the donor and recipient are mixed and incubated under a variety of conditions and suspending media. If the cells do not agglutinate, the donor's blood indicates compatibility. Blood bank personnel are responsible for providing serologic compatible blood for transfusion.

When testing is complete, transfusion therapy can begin. The blood bank has two objectives: (1) to prevent antigen-antibody reactions in the body and to identify antibody that the recipient may have and (2) to supply blood from a donation that lacks the corresponding antigen. The testing of donor blood and recipient blood is intended to prevent adverse effects of transfusion therapy.

Blood Preservatives

One donation of blood amounts to approximately 450 mL, and the volume of anticoagulant preservative is about 65 mL. There are several available RBC preservatives. Understanding of the RBC preservative is necessary because adverse reactions may occur in some patients because of chemicals in the anticoagulant-preservative solution.

The solutions in the blood collection bag have a dual function: as anticoagulant and as RBC preservative. Citrate is used in all blood preservatives as an anticoagulant. Citrate binds with free calcium in the donor's plasma. Blood will not clot in the absence of free or ionized calcium. Citrate prevents coagulation by inhibiting the calcium-dependent steps of the coagulation cascade. Preservatives provide proper nutrients to maintain RBC viability, function, and metabolism. In addition, refrigeration at 1° to 6°C preserves RBCs and minimizes proliferation of bacteria (Walker, 1993).

447

In 1971, CPD became a common preservative for blood. Compared with ACD, it offers a higher pH to prevent acid buildup in stored RBCs. Phosphate is added to buffer the decrease in pH. The compound in the RBC that facilitates the transport of oxygen is 2,3-diphosphoglycerate (2,3-DPG). When the pH of the blood drops, there is a decrease in 2,3-DPG and therefore a lowering of the oxygen carrying capacity of the blood. The 2,3-DPG levels remain higher in blood stored in CPD compared with ACD preservative. The expiration of RBCs preserved in CPD is 21 days stored at 1° to 6°C.

CPD-adenine (CPDA-1) was licensed in 1978. This preservative contains adenine, which helps the RBCs synthesize ATP during storage. Cells have improved viability in this anticoagulant preservative because ATP is better preserved than in ACD or plain CPD. This preservative lengthens the shelf life of the blood to 35 days at 1° to 6°C.

Newer additive systems that contain CPDA-1 plus various preservative combinations of substances such as saline or mannitol are now available. These additives are used only with packed RBCs and extend their expiration to 42 days after day of collection. FDA-approved additives include AS-1 (ADSOL), AS-3 (Nutrice) and AS-5 (Optisol) (Walker, 1993).

✎ **NOTE:** RBCs prepared with AS-1, AS-3, and AS-5 have better flow rates and do not require dilution with saline.

✎ **NOTE:** Hypocalcemia is an adverse reaction that can occur when large amounts of citrated blood are infused in a person with impaired liver function.

BLOOD DONOR COLLECTION METHODS

Homologous

The term homologous donation describes transfusion of any blood component that was donated by someone other than the intended recipient. Most transfusions depend on homologous sources and are provided by volunteer donors.

Guidelines for Homologous Donor

Donor selection for homologous collection is based on a limited physical examination and a medical history to determine the safety of the donated unit.

Strict criteria have been established for selection of prospective donors:

1. Brief health history, including illnesses, surgeries, drugs and medications, and immunization information
2. Screening for diseases
3. Stable vital signs
4. Age
5. Weight (smaller volumes should be drawn from donors weighing less than 110 lbs)
6. No evidence of skin lesions at site of venipuncture
7. Adequate venous access for venipuncture
8. Donation of blood or plasma within last 8 weeks or 48 hours since hemapheresis
9. Hemoglobin and hematocrit of at least 12.5 g/dL and 38% in males and 12.0 g/dL and 36% in females

448

Autologous

Autologous donation refers to the collection, storage, and delivery of a patient's own blood. This option is considered for patients who are likely to receive a transfusion during elective surgery (Gerber, 1994). Patients may be able to donate their own blood before the operation. The use of autologous blood avoids the possibility of alloimmunization because it does not contain foreign RBCs, platelets, and leukocyte antigens. The risk of exposure and disease transmission is also eliminated. Because of this the use of autologous blood is regarded as safer than homologous transfusion. However, risks associated with labeling and documentation are still present. The same precautions used for preparing and administering a homologous blood component must be observed (Poposvsky, 1986).

ADVANTAGES
Eliminates the risk of isoimmunization (sensitization to RBC, platelet, and leukocyte antigens)
Eliminates the risk of exposure to blood-borne infectious agents
Expands the blood resources
Reduces the need for homologous blood (decreases dependence on the volunteer donor supply)
Option for patients who find homologous transfusion unacceptable on religious grounds
Has a physiologic pH and higher levels of 2,3-DPG than does banked blood (2,3-DPG increases the oxygen carrying capacity of hemoglobin)
Contains more viable RBCs than banked blood

DISADVANTAGE
A unit of predeposited autologous blood costs approximately $120.00 because of increased paperwork and special handling.

Guidelines for Autologous Donor

Autologous transfusion can be accomplished through preoperative collection or from intraoperative or postoperative blood salvage. For preoperative collection, blood is collected into an anticoagulant/preservative solution and stored. The 42-day shelf life of RBCs needs to be considered. If necessary, RBCs can be stored frozen. However, frozen storage is not routinely recommended because of the considerable expense and the limitation of some blood banks.

The criteria for patient selection for autologous donation is not as restrictive as with homologous donations. There are no age limits, and underweight patients can have proportionately smaller units withdrawn. Typically, autologous blood is not drawn more often than once a week. The last donation should be at least 72 hours and preferably 1 week before an operation to avoid hypovolemia during surgery. It is best to collect blood as far in advance of the intended date of surgery as is feasible. Except in special circumstances, the hemoglobin should be 11 g/dL and the hematocrit 33% or greater before each donation.

Oral iron supplementation should be considered to replenish bone marrow iron reserves for autologous donors (Walker, 1993).

Types

There are five types of autologous blood currently in use: (1) predeposit, (2) posttraumatic salvage, (3) perioperative salvage or intraoperative deposit, (4) intraoperative salvage, and (5) postoperative salvage.

449

Predeposit

Predeposit autologous blood donation is the collection and storage of the patient's own blood for reinfusion during or following a later operation. This blood is held for use for elective surgery. Predeposit requires the approval of the donor patient's physician and the blood bank physician (Peterson, 1992).

Post-Traumatic Salvage

Post-traumatic salvage is the immediate reinfusion of blood collected from a site of injury. Hemothorax has been studied most extensively.

Perioperative Salvage

Perioperative salvage or intraoperative deposit involves withdrawal of blood early in a procedure for use as a volume replacement later in the same procedures. Typically, 2 U of blood are collected early in the surgery. The collected volume is replaced with physiologic solution, and the units are then ready if volume replacement becomes necessary (Peterson, 1992).

Intraoperative Salvage

Intraoperative salvage is the most widely used form of autologous transfusion. Blood shed from the operative field is collected via suction and processed in a cell-washing device for immediate reinfusion.

Postoperative Salvage

Postoperative salvage involves the salvage of blood from the surgical field in a single-use, self-contained reservoir for immediate return and reinfusion to the patient. This technique is used most often following cardiac surgeries and, recently, with orthopedic surgeries.

✎ **NOTE:** Any autologous blood must be filtered during reinfusion to eliminate the possibility of microclots or debris being infused into the patient (Peterson, 1992).

Designated

Designated donation refers to the donation of blood from selected friends or relatives of the patient. Most blood centers and hospitals provide this service. Designated donations have been requested more frequently because of the concern over the risk of transfusion-transmitted diseases. However, there is no evidence that designated donations are safer than blood provided by transfusion service (Walker, 1993). Relatives or friends who may be members of a risk group may feel forced into donating and hesitate to identify themselves as a risk group member (Fig. 13–2).

Guidelines for Designated Donor

The selection and screening of designated donors are the same as for other homologous donors, except that the units collected are labeled for a specific recipient. The

450

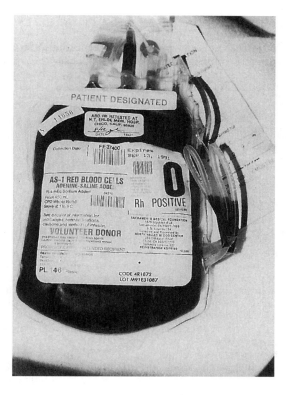

Figure 13–2. Designated donor unit.

designated donor must pass all the history and screening tests required, and the unit must be compatible with the intended recipient (Walker, 1993).

BLOOD COMPONENT THERAPY

Blood is the fluid tissue that circulates through the heart, arteries, capillaries, and veins. It supplies oxygen and food to the other tissues of the body and removes carbon dioxide and the waste products of metabolism from the tissues. Blood is a "liquid organ" with functions as extraordinary and unique as those of any other body organ. Fifty-five percent of blood is plasma (fluid); the remaining cellular portion (45%) is made up of solids: RBCs, WBCs, and platelets.

In the last decade, heightened awareness of the risks and benefits of transfusion therapy has dramatically affected transfusion practices. New methods of testing have improved the risk of infection transmission; however, the association of blood product administration with virus activation, immunosuppression, increased tumor recurrence, and the increased incidence of bacterial infection has demanded serious consideration. As a result, the administration of allogeneic blood components is carefully evaluated. Autologous blood donations have increased substantially and as an alternative to blood component administration are evaluated and applied when appropriate.

451

Whole Blood

Whole blood is composed of RBCs, plasma, WBCs, and platelets. The volume of each unit is approximately 500 mL and consists of 200 mL of RBCs and 300 mL of plasma. Advances in the use of blood components have made the administration of whole blood rarely necessary.

Uses

Most whole blood units are now used to prepare valuable separate RBC and plasma components to meet specific clinical needs. A whole blood unit can be centrifuged and separated into three components: RBCs, plasma, and platelet concentrates. By transfusing the patient with the specific component needed rather than with whole blood, the patient is not exposed to unnecessary portions of the blood product, and valuable blood resources are conserved (Fig. 13–3).

Few conditions require transfusion of whole blood. A unit of whole blood increases RBC mass, which provides oxygen carrying capacity and provides plasma for blood volume expansion. The primary indication for use is for patients experiencing acute massive blood loss of greater than 30% of their blood volume. This type of patient requires both increased oxygen carrying capacity and restoration of blood volume, or hemorrhagic shock could develop. Infusions of crystalloid or colloid solutions should be started immediately to restore intravascular volume.

When whole blood has been stored for over 24 hours, degeneration of some of its components occurs, resulting in nonviable platelets and granulocytes. In addition, levels of factor V and factor VIII decrease with storage. Therefore, a whole blood transfusion would not provide a therapeutic platelet transfusion or replace several clotting factors. Stable coagulation factors II, VII, IX, X, and fibrinogen are well maintained throughout the storage period for whole blood units.

✎ **NOTE:** In an adult, 1 U of whole blood increases the hemoglobin by about 1 g/dL or the hematocrit by about 3% to 4% (Walker, 1993).

Unless a patient who receives whole blood needs volume replacement, in addition to oxygen carrying capacity, fluid overload may occur. Plasma contained in whole blood provides an unnecessary volume load to patients who do not require or cannot tolerate excessive volume expansion.

Whole blood should not be given to patients with chronic anemia who are normovolemic and require only an increase in RBC mass. The administration of whole blood is also indicated for neonatal exchange transfusion.

Administration

Amount: 500 mL
Cannula size: 20-gauge or larger preferred for rapid flow rates
Usual rate: 2 to 4 hours
Administration set: Straight or Y type with filter or microaggregate recipient set

Compatibility

Whole blood requires type and crossmatching and must be ABO-identical.

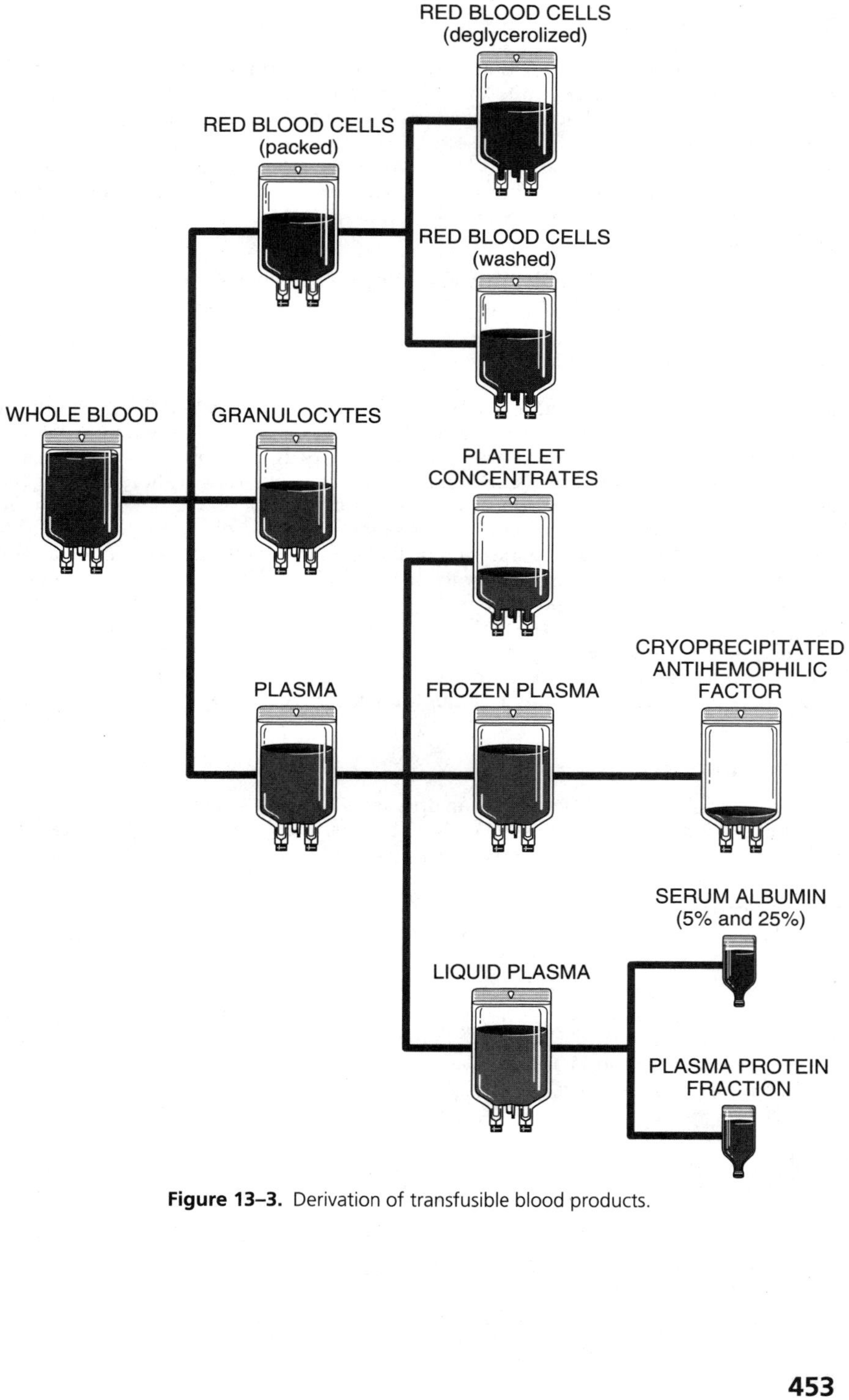

Figure 13–3. Derivation of transfusible blood products.

Packed RBCs

Packed red blood cell (PRBC) units are prepared by removing 200 to 250 mL of plasma from a whole blood unit. The remaining PRBC concentrate has a volume of approximately 300 mL. Each unit contains the same RBC mass as whole blood, as well as 20% to 30% of the original plasma, leukocytes, and some platelets. The advantages of PRBCs over whole blood are decreased plasma volume in an RBC unit and decreased risk of circulatory overload. Another advantage is that since most of the plasma has been removed, less citrate, potassium, ammonia, and other metabolic byproducts are transfused.

✎ **NOTE:** In a normal adult patient, 1 U of PRBCs should raise the hemoglobin level approximately 1 g/dL and the hematocrit 3% (Walker, 1993).

Uses

PRBCs are used to improve the oxygen carrying capacity in patients with symptomatic anemia. The administration of PRBCs should be considered only if improvement of the RBC count cannot be achieved by nutrition, drug therapy, or treatment of the underlying disease. A definitive hemoglobin and hematocrit threshold has not been established for when transfusion of PRBCs is indicated or above which transfusion would be inappropriate. Criteria for transfusion are based on multiple variables including hemoglobin and hematocrit levels, patient symptoms, amount and time frame of blood loss, and surgical procedures (Walker, 1993). Patients with chronic anemia should be transfused only if they are symptomatic owing to a decrease in oxygen carrying capacity because they usually adjust to the lower hemoglobin level and should not be exposed to transfusion-associated risks unless necessary. Even if large volumes of blood are lost, other components such as platelets and plasma coagulation factors can be provided, rather than using whole blood (Baranowski, 1993).

Administration

Administration of PRBCs is used for an operative blood loss of over 1200 mL of blood. An operative blood loss of less than 1000 to 1200 mL of blood can be replaced by crystalloid or colloid solutions rather than with PRBCs (Walker, 1993).

TRANSFUSE RBCS
To increase oxygen carrying capacity in anemic patient

DO NOT TRANSFUSE RBCS
For volume expansion
In place of a hematinic
To enhance wound healing
To improve general well being
(NIH, 1993)

Administration Summary

Amount: 250 mL
Cannula size: 20- to 18-gauge preferred, since use of a 22-gauge does not always allow free flow and may require an infusion pump
Usual rate: $1\frac{1}{2}$ to 2 hours
Administration set: Straight or Y type with 170-μ filter microaggregate or leukocyte-depleting fitter (Fig. 13–4)

454

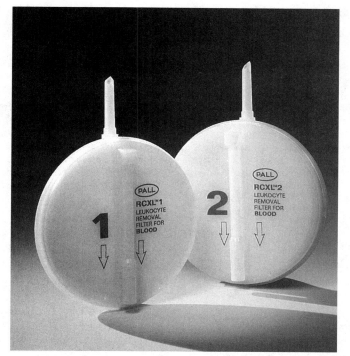

Figure 13–4. Leukocyte filters, such as the ones pictured here, are added to standard blood administration set to additionally filter red blood cells of leukocytes. (Courtesy of Pall Biomedical Products Corporation, New York, with permission.)

Compatibility

PRBCs require typing and crossmatching before being transfused into a patient.

✎ **NOTE:** If the plasma has been removed, the unit of PRBC does not have to be ABO-identical but it must be ABO-compatible.

Washed RBCs

PRBCs can be "washed" with sterile saline using machines specially designed for this purpose. Saline washing removes most of the plasma, reduces the concentration of leukocytes, and removes platelets, along with cellular debris. Some RBC loss also occurs in the washing process, resulting in a reduced hematocrit. Washing may be performed at any time during the shelf life of a unit of blood.

✎ **NOTE:** The washing procedure is an open system process. Therefore, once a unit of blood has been washed, it must be used within 24 hours following preparation because of the risk of bacterial contamination (AABB, 1989).

Uses

Washed cells are used for patients with severe or recurrent allergic reactions because washing removes plasma proteins, which may induce the allergic reaction. Washed cells are also used for neonatal and intrauterine transfusions.

455

Compatibility

Type and crossmatch are required, and the unit must be ABO-compatible.

Deglycerolized RBCs

Deglycerolized RBCs are prepared to allow for freezing of cells for long-term storage to preserve rare units of RBCs and autologous donor units. The RBCs are frozen after removal of the plasma by adding glycerol, a cryoprotective agent. Glycerol enters the cell and protects the cell from damage due to cell dehydration and mechanical injury from ice formation. Before transfusion, glycerol is removed by washing to prevent osmotic hemolysis. This washing process also has the advantage of removing leukocytes, platelets, and plasma.

Uses

Use and applications are the same as for washed cells.

✎ **NOTE:** Deglycerolization of RBCs extends storage to 3 years or more; a thawed unit is stored at 4°C and must be used within 24 hours.

Granulocytes

Granulocyte concentrations are prepared by leukapheresis from a single donor. Each unit contains granulocytes, variable amounts of lymphocytes, platelets, and RBCs suspended in 200 to 300 mL of plasma.

Uses

Prophylactic use of granulocyte transfusion is of questionable therapeutic value, and this transfusion is given infrequently. Indications are limited and the goals of therapy should be clearly defined (Walker, 1993). The use of granulocytes is indicated for patients with neutropenia who have been febrile for 24 to 48 hours and have evidence of significant infection that is unresponsive to appropriate antibiotic therapy or other modes of therapy. The patient should have a reasonable chance of recovering from the episode of neutropenia with an expected eventual chance for recovery of bone marrow function. Granulocyte transfusion has not proved effective in patients with localized infections or infections with agents other than bacteria. Septicemia should be documented by cultures to identify the infecting organism and sensitivities.

The patient is expected to experience chills, fever, and allergic reactions to the transfusion. These side effects can be managed with the use of diphenhydramine or meperidine, steroids, and nonaspirin antipyretics and by slowing of the transfusion rate. The transfusion should not be discontinued unless severe respiratory distress occurs. The concentrate must be infused within 24 hours after collection; to achieve maximal clinical effect it should be delivered as soon as possible (Walker, 1993).

Administration Summary

> Amount: 300 to 400 mL suspended in 200 to 300 mL of plasma
> Cannula size: 20- to 18-gauge preferred
> Usual rate: 1 to 2 hours; slower if reaction occurs
> Administration set: Straight or Y type with filter; microaggregate filter contraindicated

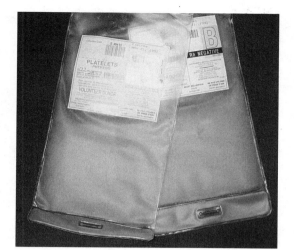

Figure 13–5. Platelets.

Compatibility

Donor blood must be ABO- and Rh-compatible, because a unit of granulocytes is usually heavily contaminated with RBCs. There is no set standard regarding the amount or duration of granulocyte therapy, but generally transfusion therapy is delivered for at least 4 consecutive days.

Platelets

Platelets can be supplied as either random-donor concentrates or single-donor concentrates. Platelet concentrates (random donor) are prepared from individual units of whole blood by centrifugation. The platelets are stored at room temperature (20° to 24°C) with constant, gentle agitation to maintain viability of the platelets. Platelets can be stored for up to 5 days, depending on the plastic formation of the storage bag. Single-donor platelet pheresis products are collected from a single donor, and all unneeded portions of the donor's blood are returned back to the donor. A single pheresis unit is equivalent to 6 to 8 U of random donor platelets (Fig. 13–5). The use of a single-donor unit has the obvious advantage of exposing the recipient to fewer donors and is ideal for treating patients who have developed HLA antibodies from previous transfusions and have become refractory (unresponsive) to random donor platelets. HLA typing may be indicated when patients become refractory to platelets after multiple transfusion. Platelet crossmatch procedures are also being evaluated for their usefulness with refractory patients.

✎ **NOTE:** One platelet concentrate should raise the recipient's platelet count 5000 to 10,000. The usual dose is 6 to 10 U of concentrate (Walker, 1993).

Uses

Platelets are administered to control or prevent bleeding from platelet deficiencies resulting in thrombocytopenia or for the presence of functionally abnormal platelets. Indications for platelet transfusion include:

- Hemorrhage with platelet count less than $50,000/\mu L$
- Surgery with platelet count less than $100,000/\mu L$

457

- Nonbleeding patients with rapidly dropping counts, less than 15,000 to 20,000/μL

Indications for platelet transfusion therapy should be based on the individual patient, since patients do not carry the same risk of bleeding at all times. For instance, many stable thrombocytopenic patients can tolerate platelet counts below 5000/μL with evidence of minor hemorrhage but without serious bleeding (Walker, 1993). Platelet transfusions at higher platelet counts may be required for patients with systemic bleeding and for patients at high risk for bleeding because of additional coagulation defects, sepsis, or platelet dysfunctions related to medication or disease. Significant spontaneous bleeding with platelet counts above 20,000/μL are rare. Platelet transfusions are usually not effective in patients with conditions in which rapid platelet destruction occurs, such as idiopathic autoimmune thrombocytopenia purpura (ITP) and untreated disseminated intravascular coagulation (DIC). With these conditions, platelet transfusions should be used only in the presence of active bleeding (Rutman & Miller, 1985).

Administration

TRANSFUSE PLATELETS
To control or prevent bleeding associated with deficiencies in platelet number or function

DO NOT TRANSFUSE PLATELETS
To patients with ITP (unless there is life-threatening bleeding)
Prophylactically with massive blood transfusions
Prophylactically following cardiopulmonary bypass
(NIH, 1993)

The half-life of platelets is 3 to 4 days; transfusions may be repeated every 1 to 3 days. The platelets may be infused as rapidly as the patient tolerates, with infusion rates ranging from 1 to 2 mL/min up to 5 min/bag. Platelets should be delivered to infants by means of a syringe-type device and can be transfused at a rate of 1 mL/min.

The effectiveness of platelet transfusions may be altered if fever, infection, or active bleeding is present. To determine the effectiveness of a transfusion, platelet counts may be checked at 1 hour and 24 hours after transfusion. Poor platelet count recovery may also indicate that the patient may be refractory to random donor platelets.

Administration Summary

Amount: 30 to 50 mL/U; usual dose 6 to 8 U
Cannula size: 20- to 22-gauge
Usual rate: 1 U in 5 to 10 minutes as tolerated
Administration set: Component syringe or Y drip set; tubing should be rubber-free to prevent platelets from sticking; use saline as primer

Platelet concentrates may be pooled before administration or infused individually. If pooled, platelets should be transfused within 6 hours.

Compatibility

Preferably, platelets should be ABO-compatible; but, when unavailable, mismatched platelets may be given. Crossmatching is not required. Rh matching is also preferred. Standard pretransfusion compatibility testing is not done for platelets.

458

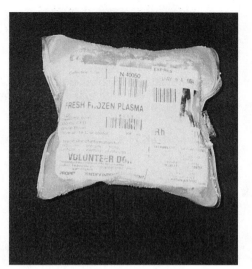

Figure 13–6. Plasma.

Fresh Frozen Plasma

Fresh frozen plasma (FFP) is prepared from whole blood by separating and freezing the plasma within 6 hours of collection. FFP may be stored for up to 1 year at −18°C or lower. The volume of a typical unit is 200 to 250 mL. FFP does not provide platelets, and loss of factors V and VIII, the labile clotting factors, is minimal (Fig. 13–6).

Uses

FFP is primarily used to provide replacement coagulation factors. It is indicated for patients with multiple coagulation factor deficiencies secondary to liver disease, DIC, and the dilutional coagulopathy resulting from massive volume load or volume replacement. FFP is indicated for patients with demonstrated factor deficiencies for which there is no coagulation concentrate available, such as deficiencies of factor V or XI. FFP may also be used for coumarin drug reversal when time does not permit reversal by stopping the drug or administering vitamin K. Patients with other rare deficiencies such as antithrombin III deficiency and thrombotic thrombocytopenia purpura may also benefit from FFP.

✎ **NOTE:** FFP contains optimal levels of all plasma clotting factors with approximately 200 U factor activity per bag and 200 to 400 mg fibrinogen per bag (AABB, 1986).

Administration

Before being transfused, FFP must be thawed in a 30° to 37°C waterbath with gentle agitation or kneading. The thawing process takes up to 30 minutes, and the FFP should be transfused as soon as possible after thawing or within 6 hours. FFP must be delivered through a standard blood filter. It can be infused as fast as the patient tolerates or condition indicates. Rates of 4 to 10 mL/min have been suggested, and most units are generally completed within 1 to 2 hours.

To increase the level of clotting factors in patient with a demonstrated deficiency

DO NOT TRANSFUSE FFP
For volume expansion
As a nutritional supplement
Prophylactically with massive blood transfusion
(NIH, 1993)

Administration Summary

Amount: 200 to 300 mL
Cannula size: 20- to 22-gauge
Usual rate: 1 to 2 hours
Administration set: Straight or Y type with filter

Compatibility

Compatibility testing is not required; however, the patient's ABO group must be known before product selection to make sure A or B antibodies present in the plasma are compatible with the patient's RBCs. The small amount of antibodies possibly present in plasma are not considered clinically important. If the patient's blood type is not known, group AB can be safely given. Rh match is not required.

Cryoprecipitate

Cryoprecipitate is the insoluble portion of plasma that remains as a white precipitate after FFP is thawed at 4°C under special conditions. Cryoprecipitate is separated from plasma and refrozen. Cryoprecipitate has a shelf life of 1 year and contains concentrated factor VIII: C, factor VIII: vWF (von Willebrand factor), fibrinogen, and factor XIII. It is the only concentrated source of fibrinogen.

Uses

Cryoprecipitate is primarily used to control bleeding associated with a deficiency or defect in one of the coagulation factors. Its use is indicated for the treatment of hemophilia A, von Willebrand's disease, hypofibrinogenemia, factor VIII deficiency, and obstetric complications or other situations associated with consumption of fibrinogen, such as DIC.

Administration

Cryoprecipitate is thawed before being transfused and must be used within 6 hours. The inside of the bag should be rinsed with a small amount of saline to maximize recovery. Cryoprecipitate should be administered through a standard blood filter, and, as with platelets administration sets, small priming volumes are recommended to decrease loss of the product in the set. The cryoprecipitate units are usually pooled to simplify administration. Cryoprecipitate should be transfused as rapidly as the patient can tolerate.

Administration Summary

Amount: 10 to 15 mL of diluent added to precipitate unit; usual dose 6 to 10 U
Cannula size: 20- to 22-gauge

Usual rate: As rapidly as possible; approximately 10 mL/min
Administration set: Component syringe or Y drip set

Compatibility

Compatibility testing is not done, but the cryoprecipitate should be ABO-compatible with the patient's RBCs, because a very small volume of plasma is present. If the patient's blood group is not known, group AB is preferred, but any group can be given in an emergency because the plasma volume is small. Rh matching is not required.

COLLOID VOLUME EXPANDERS

Products are available that do not require screening techniques. These products are colloid volume expanders. These include albumin, plasma protein fraction (PPF), dextran, and hetastarch (HES).

Normal human serum albumin is the most widely used colloid solution. It is heat-treated for viral inactivation and free from hepatitis risk. PPF is also a hepatitis-free plasma derivative and is less expensive than albumin. Dextran is a branched polysaccharide available in low molecular weights: 40,000 (dextran 40) and 70,000 (dextran 70). It is dissolved in either 0.9% sodium chloride or 5% dextrose. Dextran's use as a volume expander is limited by two factors. It can interfere with coagulation and platelet adhesion, and it has been associated with rare anaphylactic reactions (Phillips & Kuhn, 1995).

HES is an amylopectin derivative marketed in a 6% sodium chloride solution. Because of its structural similarity to glycogen, HES is less likely to cause anaphylaxis than dextran (Gridley, 1986).

Albumin and Plasma Protein Fraction

Albumin is a plasma protein that supplies 80% of plasma's osmotic activity and is the principal product of fractionation. Administered as PPF and as more purified albumin, albumin and PPF are derived from donor plasma and prepared by the cold alcohol fractionation process and then subsequently heated. Both products do not transmit viral diseases because of the extended heating process. Normal serum albumin is composed of 96% albumin and 4% globulin and other proteins. It is available as a 5% or 25% solution. PPF is a similar product except that it is subjected to fewer purification steps in the fractionation process and contains about 83% albumin and 17% globulins. PPF is available only in a 5% solution.

Uses

PPF and 5% albumin are isotonic solutions and therefore are osmotically equivalent to an equal volume of plasma. They cause a plasma volume increase and are used interchangeably and share the same clinical uses. Both are used primarily to increase plasma volume resulting from sudden loss of intravascular volume as seen in patients with hypovolemic shock from trauma or surgery. Their use may also be indicated in individual cases to support blood pressure during hypotensive episodes or induce diuresis in fluid overload to assist in mobilization of fluid. The plasma derivatives lack clotting factors and other plasma proteins and therefore should not be considered plasma substitutes. Neither component will correct nutritional deficits or chronic hypoalbuminemia.

461

The 25% albumin is hypertonic and is five times more concentrated than 5% albumin. The 25% albumin is used to draw fluids out of tissues and body cavities into intravascular spaces. *This solution must be given with caution.* Principal uses for 25% albumin include, plasma volume expansion, hypovolemic shock, burns, and prevention and treatment of cerebral edema.

✎ **NOTE:** Albumin 25% must not be used in dehydrated patients without supplemental fluids or in patients at risk of circulatory overload.

Administration

Albumin and PPF are supplied in glass bottles. Albumin in 5% concentrations is available in 250 mL and 500 mL of saline, and concentrations of 25% are supplied in units of 50 mL and 100 mL of saline. Manufacturers recommend that the solution be used within 4 hours of opening. Depending on the manufacturer, the solutions are sometimes supplied with an infusion set. Blood transfusion sets and filters are not required for infusion of albumin.

Albumin, 5% and 25%, may be given as rapidly as the patient tolerates for reduced blood volumes. When the blood volume is normal or only slightly reduced, rates of 2 to 4 mL/min have been suggested for 5% albumin, and 1 mL/min for 25% albumin. More caution is used when infusing PPF, since hypotension may occur with a rate greater than 10 mL/min (AABB, 1986).

Administration Summary

Amount: 5% solution 250 mL, 25% solution 50 to 100 mL
Cannula size: 20- to 22-gauge
Usual rate: 5% solution 2 to 4 mL/min; 25% solution 1 mL/min
Administration set: Comes with administration set in package

Compatibility

ABO or Rh matching and compatibility testing are not necessary for these components because antigens and antibodies are not present in these products. A summary of blood components is listed in Table 13–4.

ALTERNATIVE PHARMACOLOGIC THERAPIES

Alternatives for homologous blood continue. This issue has been addressed by alternative therapies to blood components, such as hematopoietic growth factor erythropoietin and desmopressin acetate (DDAVP). Erythropoietin is used for management of chronic anemia in dialysis patients. DDAVP is a synthetic analogue of L-arginine vasopressin and is used for increasing factor VIII and vWF and for management of patients with hemorrhagic disorders related to thrombocytopenia. Theses drugs decrease blood loss and the risk of bleeding, resulting in a reduced need for blood components (Baranowski, 1993).

Blood Substitutes

Efforts continue in the search to develop a practical RBC substitute. However, it may be several years before one is available for commercial use. Several products continue to be evaluated for their ability to serve as oxygen carriers as a substitute for RBCs. One is a synthetic material, a perfluorocarbon emulsion, which was found not to carry enough oxygen under practical conditions (Baranowski, 1993). Other prepara-

TABLE 13–4. SUMMARY OF BLOOD COMPONENTS

Blood Component	Volume	Action and Use	Infusion Guide	Special Considerations
Whole blood	200 mL RBCs 300 mL plasma Total = 500 mL	For acute, massive blood loss	0.9% sodium chloride primer; transfuse within 4 hours. Standard Blood filter; straight or Y-type set	Always ABO- and Rh-identical; 1 U whole blood raises hemoglobin 1 g and hematocrit 3% to 4%
PRBCs	250–350 mL	Improve oxygen carrying capacity in patient with symptomatic anemia, aplastic anemia, bone marrow failure due to malignancy, or chemotherapy	Same as for whole blood; transfuse within 4 hours Standard blood filter; leukocyte reduction filter when ordered	ABO-/Rh-compatible; 1 U raises the hemoglobin 1 g and hematocrit 3–4%
Washed RBCs	200–250 mL	Reduce incidence of allergic reactions (washing removes plasma proteins)	Same as for whole blood; 24-hour expiration date	Lab needs advanced notice to prepare cells Washing is an open system procedure; unit must be given within 24 hours of washing
Irradiated PRBCs	200–250 mL	Prevent graft-versus-host disease in immunocompromised patients	Same as for RBCs	Same as for RBCs
Deglycerolized RBCs (frozen)	200–250 mL	Prolonged storage of blood for rare blood types and autologous donations; minimizes allergic reactions	Same as for whole blood; infuse within 4 hours	Must be used within 24 hours of being thawed and deglycerolized
Granulocytes (Leukapheresis)	300–400 mL **Note:** Suspended in 200–250 mL of plasma	For neutropenia, fever, or significant infection unresponsive to antibiotics	Usually administered for 4 consecutive days Standard blood filter; administer slowly over 2–4 hours as soon as collected or at least within 24 hours	ABO-/Rh-compatible; reactions common Check vital signs every 15 min **Note:** Febrile reactions occur in about two thirds of patients; chills, fever, and allergic reactions common Requires premedication to control reactions

TABLE 13–4. SUMMARY OF BLOOD COMPONENTS (*Continued*)

Blood Component	Volume	Action and Use	Infusion Guide	Special Considerations
Platelets, random donor	50–70 mL/U Usual dose: 6–10 U	Control or prevent bleeding associated with platelet deficiencies	Administer as rapidly as patient can tolerate: 1 U/10 min or less Use blood filter, syringe push, or standard Y administration set; leukocyte depletion filter for platelets as ordered **Note:** RBC leukocyte filters cannot be used with platelets	1 U increases platelet count of 70-kg adult by 5000/μL Infuse individually or may be pooled; requires 20 minutes pooling time by laboratory; ABO/Rh preferred but not necessary Prophylactic medication with antihistamines; antipyretics may be needed to decrease incidence of chills, fever, and allergic reactions
Platelets, pheresis	Equivalent to 6 U from random donors	Same as for random donor; consider for patients anticipated to receive multiple long-term transfusions to limit exposure to multiple donors and reduce incidence of refractoriness	Same as for random-donor platelets	Same as for random-donor platelets
Fresh frozen plasma	200–250 mL	Replacement of clotting factors in patients with a demonstrated deficiency or for single-factor deficiency when concentrate not available	Storage is at 18°C for 1 year Standard blood filter; may be infused rapidly: 20 mL over 3 minutes or more slowly within 4 hours	Does not provide platelets 1 mL of raises the level of clotting factor 2–3%; requires 20 minutes defrosting time by lab Must be AB-compatible

Cryoprecipitate	Each unit contains factor VIII, von Willebrand's factor, factor XIII, fibrinogen 15 mL plasma (5–10 mL U). Usual order is for 6–10 U	Controls bleeding associated with deficiency in coagulation factors; treatment of hemophilia A, von Willebrand's disease, hypofibrinogenemia, factor VIII deficiency, DIC associated with obstetric complications	Standard blood filter; administer as fast as patient tolerates	ABO-compatible with patient's RBCs; if blood group unknown, use AB blood; Rh match not required. Infuse within 6 hours of thawing; saline may be added to bag to facilitate recovery of product
Albumin (5% = 12.5 g/250 mL; 25% = 12.5 g/ 50 mL)	5% solution is in concentration of 250 mL or 500 mL; 25% solution is in 50–100 mL concentration	Plasma volume expander. For hypovolemic shock. Support blood pressure during hypotensive episodes; induces diuresis in fluid overload	May be administered as rapidly as tolerated for reduced blood volume. Normal rates: 2–4 mL/min for 5% solution; 1 mL/min for 25% solution. Supplied in glass bottles with tubing for administration	25% albumin is hypertonic and is 5 times more concentrated than 5% solutions. Give with extreme caution; can cause circulatory overload. No type and crossmatch necessary; store at room temperature
Plasma protein fraction	Glass bottle with tubing 250 mL	Same as for albumin	Equivalent to 5% albumin	Has fewer purification steps than albumin; no type and crossmatch necessary; has high sodium content

TABLE 13–5. STEPS IN ADMINISTRATION OF A BLOOD COMPONENT

Step 1: Physician's order
Step 2: Equipment selection and preparation
Step 3: Patient preparation
Step 4: Obtaining blood product from blood bank
Step 5: Preparation for administration
Step 6: Initiation of transfusion
Step 7: Monitoring the transfusion
Step 8: Discontinuation of transfusion

tions being developed include intramolecular cross-linked or polymerized hemoglobin and products containing hemoglobin encapsulated in phospholipid liposomes (Pisiotto, 1989). Recombinant human hemoglobin is a cell-free hemoglobin-based blood substitute being investigated for perioperative blood replacement (Anon, 1994).

ADMINISTRATION OF BLOOD COMPONENTS

The procedure for obtaining a blood component from the hospital blood bank varies from institution to institution. Regardless of the specific institutional procedure, certain essential guidelines must be adhered to (Table 13–5).

Step 1: Physician's Order

A physician's order for the blood component is required. The order should specify which component to transfuse and the duration of the transfusion (up to 4 hours). When transfusing multiple types of components, the order should specify the sequence in which they are to be transfused and should specify any required modifications to the component (e.g., leukocyte filtration, irradiation, washing, HLA matching). Orders must specify premedications that are to be given before transfusion (Harovas & Anthony, 1993).

Step 2: Equipment Selection and Preparation

Selecting the proper equipment involves cannula selection, solution selection, obtaining administration sets, special filters, blood warmers, and electronic monitoring devices.

Cannula

An I.V. line should be started, according to institution protocol, using the gauge size recommended for the component to be administered. Usually a 18- or 20-gauge catheter is used to provide adequate flow rates. Free flow through a 22-gauge catheter is sometimes difficult with RBC units and may require the use of a pump. A 22-gauge catheter is appropriate for delivery of plasma products.

✎ NOTE: If the patient requires medication or solution administration while the blood component is being administered, a second I.V. site should be initiated.

466

Solution

No solution other than 0.9% sodium chloride shall be added to blood or blood components (INS, 1990). The use of dextrose in water can cause RBC hemolysis, and lactated Ringer's solution is not recommended because it contains enough ionized calcium to overcome the anticoagulant effect of CPDA-1 and allows small clots to develop.

Administration Sets

Blood administration sets are available as a two lead Y-type tubing or as single-lead tubing. Y-type administration sets allow for infusion of 0.9% saline before and after each blood component. A T-type set also allows for dilution of PRBCs that are too viscous to be transfused at an appropriate rate. Platelets and cryoprecipitate should be infused through a filter similar to the standard blood filter but with a smaller drip chamber and shorter tubing so that less priming volume is needed. A syringe device designed specifically for platelets and cryoprecipitate may also be used to administer these products.

All blood components that are appropriate for the component or specifically requested by physician order must be filtered. Blood administration sets come with an inline filter. Most routine blood filters have a pore size of 170 microns designed to remove the debris that accumulates in stored blood. It is necessary to fill the filter chamber completely to use all the surface area. One filter can usually be used for 2 to 4 U, depending on the manufacturer, the type of filter, the type of blood product, and the age of the cells. As debris in the filter accumulates, the rate of flow through the filter is slowed. In addition, because of the hazard of hemolysis and bacterial contamination, the filter should not be left hanging in place for extended periods and then reused.

✎ **NOTE:** The maximum time for use of a blood filter is 4 hours.

Special Filters

Microaggregate filters and leukocyte-depleting filters are also available for use. These filters are designed to be added to a standard administration set or come already incorporated into the tubing. Microaggregate filters are designed to remove 20- to 40-micron particles, filtering out the microaggregates that develop in stored blood. Microaggregates consist primarily of degenerated platelets, leukocytes, and strands of fibrin. Leukocyte-depleting filters are used for the delivery of PRBCs and platelets (Figs. 13–7). The filters may be used for leukocyte depletion after blood collection in the blood bank or at the time of administration. Human leukocyte antigen immunization (alloimmunization) is directly linked to the number of leukocytes present in a blood product (Cook, 1995). These filters are capable of removing more than 99.9% of the leukocytes present in the unit. These new-generation filters were developed in response to data supporting clinical benefits associated with the administration of leukocyte-poor blood products. The benefits include prevention of nonhemolytic transfusion reactions, HLA alloimmunization, and leukocyte-mediated viral transmission. These filters are more expensive than the standard blood filter and therefore are generally used only per physician order. When using microaggregate or leukocyte-removal filters, follow manufacturer recommendations regarding the number of units that can be filtered through one filter (Baranowski, 1991).

Blood Warmers

Specific equipment is also available to warm blood if needed. Most transfusions do not require the use of a blood warmer. Warming of blood toward body temperature

467

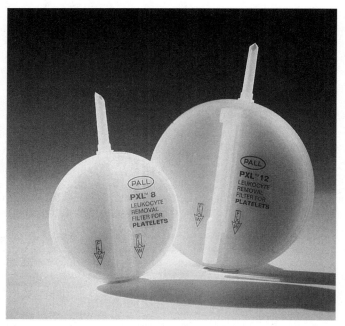

Figure 13–7. High-efficiency leukocyte-removal filter for platelet transfusion. (Courtesy of Pall Biomedical Products Corporation, New York, with permission.)

is indicated for rapid or massive transfusions, in neonatal exchange transfusions, or for patients with potent cold agglutinins.

✎ **NOTE:** Only temperature devices specifically designed to warm blood should be used. Blood components should not be placed in microwave ovens because damage to RBCs occurs.

Electronic Monitoring Devices

Some transfusions may require an electronic monitoring device to control the flow. Only pumps designed for the infusion of whole blood and PRBCs may be used because other types of infusion pumps may cause hemolysis. Pumps require the use of special tubing and filters. Little if any increased hemolysis occurs secondary to use of most infusion pumps. A specific manufacturer should be consulted for detailed information on the suitability of any particular infusion pump for transfusing blood components.

A pressure bag is a commonly used device for increasing flow rates during transfusion, usually in an emergency or during surgery. This device has a sleeve into which the blood bag is inserted, and the sleeve is inflated by filling it with air from a pressure manometer. As the unit of blood empties, the pressure of the sleeve decreases; therefore, it should be observed frequently and reinflated when necessary. (See Chapter 7 for further information and an illustration of blood administration equipment.)

Step 3: Patient Preparation

Patient preparation begins when the transfusion of a blood component is anticipated. Urgency factors related to the transfusion may affect the amount of time available to prepare the patient for the transfusion. The steps of the nursing process are activated, including assessment and the establishment of new goals and interventions related to the transfusion.

The patient's and the patient's family's understanding of the need for blood, procedure, and related concerns need to be assessed. Concerns are typically expressed regarding the risks of disease transmission, and these need to be addressed.

✎ **NOTE:** As required by institution-specific protocols, informed consents should be done and a written consent form signed.

The patient should be instructed regarding the length of time for the procedure and the need for monitoring of physical condition and vital signs. Signs and symptoms that may be associated with a complication of the component to be given should be explained to the patient and family. It is not necessary to offer graphic explanations regarding symptoms; rather, the patient should be asked to report any different sensations after the transfusion has been started along with a brief description of possible symptoms. Since transfusions typically take several hours, preparation also includes making the patient physically comfortable.

The final step of patient preparation includes a thorough assessment of the patient. Baseline vital signs should be taken. Consult with the physician before initiating the transfusion if the vital signs are abnormal. Premedication with diuretics, antihistamines, or antipyretics may be necessary to help keep the vital signs at an acceptable level. The patient should also be questioned regarding any symptoms they may be experiencing that could be confused with a transfusion reaction.

✎ **NOTE:** The patient teaching and assessment should be documented in the chart.

Step 4: Obtaining Blood Product from the Blood Bank

As a rule, except in emergency situations, no more than one blood component per patient should be picked up at one time. The blood component should not be obtained until the patient is ready to receive the component. The transfusion must be initiated within 30 minutes from the time the component is released from the blood bank. If the transfusion is delayed more than 30 minutes, the component should be returned to the blood bank for proper storage. Whole blood and PRBCs must be refrigerated at a temperature between 1° and 6°C. Special refrigerators are available in the blood bank to maintain these temperatures and are equipped with an alarm that sounds if the temperature is outside the appropriate range.

✎ **NOTE:** Refrigerators on the units may not be used to store blood products.

Proper identification of the blood component and the recipient are essential. Several items must always be verified and recorded before the transfusion is initiated:

- The physician's order should always be verified before picking up the component.
- When the blood is issued, verification should include *name and identification number* of the recipient, which must be recorded on the blood request form.

469

✎ **NOTE:** The transfusion form becomes part of the patient's permanent record.

- *The notation of ABO group and Rh type* must be the same on the primary blood bag label and on the transfusion form. This information is to be recorded on the attached compatibility tag or label.
- *The donor number* must be identically recorded on the label of the blood bag, the transfusion form, and the attached compatibility tag.
- The color, appearance, and *expiration date* of the component must be checked.
- *The name of the person issuing the blood, the name of the person to whom the blood is issued, and the date and time of issue must be recorded.* Often this is in a book in the laboratory.

Step 5: Preparation for Administration

Before obtaining the blood component (step 4), the correct tubing, 0.9% sodium chloride, and appropriate catheter should be in place. It is vitally important that the site be checked to ensure that the I.V. line is patent.

Baseline vital signs should be obtained, including temperature, blood pressure, pulse, and respirations. The patient should also be assessed for any symptoms that could later be confused as a transfusion reaction (e.g., rash, fever, shortness of breath, and lower back pain) (Harovas & Anthony, 1993). A transfusion record and report form is helpful for recording component specifics, vital signs, administration specifics, and reactions (Fig. 13–8).

- At the time of infusion, *verification* should include checking the component against the physician's order. The blood component should be verified with another registered nurse or a state-certified licensed vocational or practical nurse or physician.
- *Compare donor numbers and the ABO group and Rh type* on the transfusion record with the information on the blood component. The information on the label and compatibility tag should be identical.

✎ **NOTE:** It is helpful if one nurse reads the information for verification to the other nurse; errors can be made if both nurses look at the tags together.

- *Check the expiration date and time.*

✎ **NOTE:** Unless the exact time is given, the component expires at midnight on the expiration date.

- At the bedside, *compare the full name and hospital identification number on the patient's identification wristband with the name and number that is on the form attached to the blood component.*

✎ **NOTE:** Watch for any discrepancies during any part of the identification process; the transfusion should not be initiated until the blood bank is notified and any discrepancies are resolved.

Step 6: Initiation of Transfusion

To administer whole blood or PRBCs, spike the blood container with the Y set and hang. Turn off the 0.9% sodium chloride and turn on the blood component. It is recommended that transfusions be started at 2 mL/min or no more than 50 mL over the first 5 to 15 minutes of the transfusion. If the patient shows signs or has symptoms of an adverse reaction, the transfusion can be stopped immediately and only a small amount of blood product will have been infused. Once the first 15 minutes is safely over, the rate of flow can be increased to complete the transfusion within the amount

TRANSFUSION PROCEDURE CHECKLIST

INITIAL

- [ ] Record Donor Number(s) and Component
- [ ] Information verified at bedside
- [ ] Normal Saline used with transfusion
- [ ] Record time started
- [ ] Record amount given
- [ ] Record time stopped
- [ ] Record reactions (if any)
- [ ] Vital Signs at 0, 15, 30, and every 30 minutes thereafter
- [ ] Infusion completed within 4 hours
- [ ] Copy of completed form and empty bag to laboratory - DO NOT REMOVE LABEL FROM BLOOD BAG

VITAL SIGNS

TIME	BLOOD PRESSURE	PULSE	RESPIRATION	TEMP
0				
15				
30				
60				
90				
120				
150				
180				
210				
240				

AT THE TIME OF TRANSFUSION PLEASE VERIFY:

I have verified the name, medical record number, transfusion arm-band number, blood group and type for the donor and recipient as recorded on labels and forms for the following units (one unit of WB, PC, FFP or maximum of 10 units platelet concentrate, or cryoprecipitate per transfusion procedure and report form). I have further verified the identification of the recipient.

DONOR NUMBER   COMPONENT

_____   _____

_____   _____

_____   _____

_____   _____

_____   _____

Signature of person   Signature of verifier
initiating transfusion

TRANSFUSION RECORD:

Date and Time Started: _____

Date and Time Stopped: _____

Record Amount Given if Less Than Full Unit(s): _____

Record Initials if Blood Warmer Used: _____

Transfusion Armband Number: _____

REPORT OF SUSPECTED TRANSFUSION REACTION:

- [ ] Increased Pulse Rate
- [ ] Chills
- [ ] Elevation of temperature >2° F
- [ ] Headaches
- [ ] Nausea or Vomiting
- [ ] Flushing of skin
- [ ] Backpain/Muscle aching
- [ ] Darkening of urine (hemoglobinuria)
- [ ] Petechiae
- [ ] Hypotension
- [ ] Dyspnea
- [ ] Chest pain

If any of the above signs or symptoms are observed during or following the transfusion:

- [ ] (initial) Stop the transfusion immediately, keep the IV open with normal saline
- [ ] Notify physician immediately _____ physician contacted
- [ ] Notify Transfusion Service immediately (x1187)

Technologist Notified

- [ ] Recheck the patient identification, crossmatch tag, and blood bag to determine if the patient received the correct unit.
- [ ] Send unit with administration set to the Transfusion Service.

Signature of Person Reporting Suspected Transfusion Reaction

Comments: _____
_____
_____

Figure 13–8. Transfusion procedure checklist.

of time indicated by the physician or by policy. The rate of infusion should be based on the patient's blood volume, hemodynamic condition, and cardiac status. *Gloves should be worn to handle blood products* (Fig. 13–9).

✎ **NOTE:** Blood should be infused within a 4-hour period. When a longer transfusion time is clinically indicated, the unit may be divided by the blood bank and the portion not being transfused can be properly refrigerated.

Step 7: Monitoring the Transfusion

The patient's vital signs should be monitored at the end of the first 15 minutes and then periodically throughout the transfusion. Careful observation of the patient during and after a blood transfusion is necessary to provide a more reliable assessment.

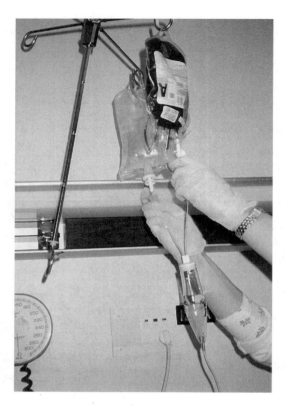

Figure 13–9. Hanging PRBCs with Y administration set. Always wear gloves when handling blood products.

✎ **NOTE:** The patient should be observed for at least 5 minutes after initiation of a blood component (INS, 1990).

✎ **NOTE:** Patient education is required for conscious patients. They should be instructed to call if any unusual symptoms or sensations occur during a transfusion. Inform the patient that a nurse will be checking the transfusion and vital signs at least every 30 minutes.

Step 8: Discontinuation of Transfusion

When the unit is complete, flush the tubing with 0.9% sodium chloride. Because of the sodium and chloride content, a minimal amount should be used to complete the transfusion. At this point, another unit may be infused, the unit and line may be discontinued, the line can be capped with a prn adaptor, or a new infusion line and solution container may be administered.

✎ **NOTE:** Do not save previous solutions and tubing, which were interrupted to give the blood component; they are considered contaminated. Restart with a fresh set and solution (Walker, 1993).

When the unit of blood has been infused, the time, volume given, and patient's condition should be documented. Some transfusion service departments require that a copy of the completed transfusion form be returned to them. Returning the blood component after an uncomplicated transfusion is not required in all facilities. If disposal is allowed on the unit, use hospital standards in disposing the blood bag in contaminated trash.

A Note on Medications

Drugs should never be mixed with the blood component to be administered. One reason is the indeterminate effect the medication may have on the blood component. Also, if a reaction occurs, it would be difficult to ascertain whether it was the drug or the blood component that was responsible for the adverse effect. Another reason is that if the transfusion needs to be interrupted, it would be impossible to calculate the amount of drug that the patient received. If a patient required I.V. medications during the course of the transfusion, a separate I.V. site should be started for the blood.

✎ **NOTE:** Absolutely no medications or solutions other than 0.9% sodium chloride shall be added to blood or blood components (INS, 1990; Walker, 1993).

SUMMARY WORKSHEET

STEPS IN INITIATING A TRANSFUSION

Step 1:

Step 2: Catheter:
        Solution:
        Administration set:

Step 3:

Step 4: Criteria

Step 5: Prior:
        Criteria:

Step 6:

Step 7: Guidelines:

Step 8:

COMPLICATIONS ASSOCIATED WITH BLOOD COMPONENT THERAPY

Despite the numerous and obvious benefits, there are complications associated with blood component therapy. These include transfusion reactions, circulatory overload, potassium toxicity, hypothermia, and hypocalcemia.

Transfusion Reactions

INS Standards of Practice (1990) dictate that a transfusion reaction requires immediate intervention. Interventions include but are not limited to:

- Terminating the transfusion
- Maintaining patency of the cannula with 0.9% sodium chloride
- Notifying the physician and hospital blood bank or transfusion services
- Implementing other interventions as indicated

Hemolytic Reactions

Acute

The most serious and potentially life-threatening reaction is acute hemolytic transfusion reaction. This type of reaction occurs after infusion of incompatible RBCs. There are two types of RBC destruction. First, intravascular hemolysis, in which the RBCs are destroyed with hemolysis directly in the bloodstream, is usually seen with ABO-incompatible RBCs. Second, extravascular hemolysis, in which the cells are coated with the antibody and subsequently removed by the reticuloendothelial system, is seen in Rh incompatibility. These incompatibilities may lead to an activation of the coagulation system and release of vasoactive enzymes, which can result in vasomotor instability, cardiorespiratory collapse, or DIC. Intravascular hemolysis is the most serious and is usually fatal (National Blood Resource Group, 1991).

Incompatibilities involving other RBC antigens and IgG antibodies can result in fever, anemia, hyperbilirubinemia, and a positive direct antibody test. The severity

474

of the reaction can be dose-related, but can occur with less than 30 mL of blood administered. Most hemolytic reactions are a result of clerical errors, such as incorrect labeling of the blood specimen or errors in identifying the patient.

Signs and Symptoms

The first symptoms include a burning sensation along the vein in which the blood is being infused. This symptom is quickly followed by lumbar pain, flank pain, flushing of the face, and chest pain.

If infusion is allowed to continue, symptoms include fever, chills, hemoglobinemia, oozing of blood at the injection site, shock, and DIC.

Interventions

Stop the transfusion. Disconnect the tubing from the I.V. catheter and infuse fresh saline not contaminated by the blood.

✎ **NOTE:** In acute hemolytic transfusion reaction, you *must not* give the patient another drop of donor blood.

Notify the physician and blood bank or transfusion service *immediately*. Monitor vital signs and maintain intravascular volume with fluids to prevent renal constriction. In addition, diuretics, mannitol, and dopamine can support the renal and vascular systems. This is an emergency situation. The patient's respiratory status may have to be supported.

Prevention

Extreme care during the entire identification process is the first step in prevention. The transfusion must be started slowly, and the nurse must remain with the patient during the first 5 to 15 minutes of the transfusion.

Delayed

Delayed transfusion reaction is a result of RBC antigen incompatibility other than the ABO group. Rapid production of RBC antibody occurs shortly after transfusion of the corresponding antigen as a result of sensitization during previous transfusions or pregnancies. Destruction of the transfused RBCs gradually occurs over 2 or more days or up to several weeks after the transfusion. Most reactions of this type go unnoticed and are common.

Signs and Symptoms

A decrease in hemoglobin and hematocrit levels, persistent low-grade fever, malaise, and indirect hyerbilirubinemia are symptoms that occur with delayed transfusion reaction.

Interventions

No acute treatment is usually required. Monitor hematocrit, renal function, and coagulation profile routinely for all patients receiving transfusions. Notify physician and transfusion services if delayed reaction is suspected.

Prevention

Avoid clerical errors.

Nonhemolytic Febrile Reactions

Nonhemolytic febrile reactions are defined as a temperature rise of 1°C or more occurring in association with transfusion and not having any other explanation. These are usually reactions to antibodies directed against leukocytes or platelets. Febrile reactions occur in only 1% of transfusions; repeat reactions are uncommon. It can occur immediately or within 1 to 2 hours after transfusion is completed. Fever is the symptom associated with this type of transfusion reaction.

Signs and Symptoms

Signs and symptoms of a nonhemolytic febrile reaction are *fever*, chills, headache, nausea and vomiting, hypotension, chest pain, dyspnea and nonproductive cough, and malaise.

Interventions

Stop transfusion.
Keep the vein open with normal saline.
Notify the physician.
Monitor vitals signs.
Physician might order antipyretics.

✎ **NOTE:** In a nonhemolytic febrile reaction, you may turn off the blood and turn on the sodium chloride primer and infuse slowly. Do not take the blood down until notified by the physician. Leave the blood hanging but clamp the Y connector to the blood unit.

Prevention

This type of reaction can be prevented or reduced by the use of leukocyte-poor blood components. HLA-compatible products may also be indicated.

Allergic Reactions

In its mild form, allergic reactions constitute the second most common type of reaction and are probably caused by antibodies against plasma proteins. The patient may experience mild localized urticaria or full systemic anaphylactic reaction. This can occur immediately or within 1 hour after infusion. Most reactions are mild and respond to antihistamines.

Signs and Symptoms

Signs and symptoms of allergic reactions include itching, hives (local erythema), rash, urticaria, runny eyes, anxiety, dyspnea, wheezing, decreased blood pressure, shock, gastrointestinal distress, and cardiac arrest and death.

Intervention

Stop transfusion. Keep the vein open with normal saline. Notify the physician. Monitor the vital signs. For mild reaction, administer antihistamines per physician order, and continue transfusion if symptoms subside. For severe anaphylactic reactions, administer epinephrine, steroids, and dopamine, and maintain intravascular volume with fluids as ordered by the physician.

Prevention

For mild reactions, the patient may receive antihistamines, such as diphenhydramine (Benadryl), before the transfusion. Transfuse patients who have a history of anaphylaxis with IgA-deficient blood products, washed RBCs, or deglycerolized RBCs. With mild reaction, the transfusion may be continued after antihistamines are administered and the symptoms have subsided. Severe reactions may require discontinuation of the transfusion and drug therapy to support the vascular system.

Other Complications

Other complications of blood component therapy include circulatory overload, potassium toxicity, hypothermia, and hypercalcemia.

Circulatory Overload

Circulatory overload can occur when rapid or excessive blood is infused over a short period of time. Be aware of the amount of sodium chloride being administered to the patient in conjunction with the transfusion.

Signs and Symptoms

Dyspnea, enlarged neck veins, congestive heart failure, and pulmonary edema occur during circulatory overload.

Interventions

Stop the transfusion.
Elevate the patient's head.
Notify the physician.
Phlebotomize, if necessary.
Administer diuretics, if necessary.

Prevention

Minimize the risk of overload by using PRBCs instead of whole blood, infusing at a reduced rate for the high-risk patient, and administering a diuretic when beginning the transfusion in high-risk patients.

Potassium Toxicity

Potassium toxicity is a rare complication. As the blood ages during storage, potassium is released from the cell into the plasma during RBC lysis. This increases the amount of potassium that the patient receives and depends on the number of units the patient receives along with the age of the blood when administered. Patients at risk for this complication are those with renal failure and those who receive massive transfusions of aged blood.

Signs and Symptoms

Signs and symptoms of potassium toxicity include immediate onset of hyperkalemia, slow, irregular heartbeat, nausea and muscle weakness, and electrocardiographic changes.

Hypothermia

When large volumes of blood are administered, hypothermia can occur owing to the consistently cool temperature of the blood. This risk brings about decreased temperature and chills. Treatment is to warm the patient with blankets. Use of a blood warmer during transfusions can be helpful to minimize this risk.

Hypocalcemia

A reaction to toxic proportions of citrate, which is used as a preservative in blood, can cause hypocalcemia. The citrate ion can combine with calcium, causing a calcium deficiency, or normal citrate metabolism is hindered by the presence of liver disease.

Signs and Symptoms

Signs and symptoms of hypocalcemia include tingling sensation in fingers, muscle cramps, hypotension, and tetany. Calcium levels should be carefully monitored in patients with liver disease. The use of washed RBCs helps to prevent this risk.

Risks of Transfusion Therapy

Despite dynamic advances in blood banking and transfusion medicine, there are still risks to blood component therapy. The patient should be told of alternatives to transfusion, including those risks to the patient if transfusion is not undertaken. Further, patients need to know about the blood center's autologous transfusion and patient-designated donor programs, without implication that there is added safety to the latter.

There are a number of potential risks surrounding transfusions (Table 13–6). Fevers, chills, and urticaria are among the most common adverse effects of transfusion but are usually not a major concern. A hemolytic transfusion reaction may occur with 1 of every 100 transfusions and result in a fatality in 1 of every 100,000 transfusion recipients.

Viral hepatitis is still a serious risk of transfusion. With the current screening procedures, a patient's chance is 1 in 30,000 that a pint of blood may result in a non-A or non-B viral hepatitis.

Currently the risk of a transfusion-associated HIV infection is remote, no more than 1 in 450,000. However, because AIDS may follow HIV infection, patients should be warned of the potential risk of this dreadful and usually fatal disease (Sacramento Medical Foundation Blood Center, 1995).

TABLE 13–6. **RISKS OF TRANSFUSION THERAPY**

Adverse Effects	Chance of Occurrence per Unit
Fever, chills, urticaria	1:100
Hemolytic transfusion reaction	1:11,000
Fatal hemolytic transfusion reaction	1:150,000
Viral hepatitis	1:30,000
HIV infection (and thus AIDS)	1:450,000

Source: Sacramento Blood Bank (1995). Transfusion risks and benefits. Sacramento, CA: Sacramento Medical Foundation.

NURSING PLAN OF CARE

DELIVERY OF BLOOD COMPONENT THERAPY

Focus Assessment

Subjective

Interview regarding understanding of need for blood component

Determine patient's understanding of options: autologous, homologous, and directed donations

Objective

Vital signs (blood pressure, pulse, respiration)

Temperature

Assessment of renal and cardiovascular systems

Assessment and evaluation of I.V. site prior to administration of blood component

Body weight

Level of consciousness

Review laboratory test

Current intake and output

Patient Outcome Criteria

The patient will:

1. Receive blood product without untoward effect or complications.
2. Display improvement of hemodynamic parameters and urine output of >1/2 m/kg/h.
3. Verbalize understanding of reasons for use of blood component.
4. Verbalize awareness of anxiety.

Nursing Diagnoses

Anxiety (mild, moderate, severe) related to threat to or change in health status; misconceptions regarding therapy

Decreased cardiac output related to sepsis, contamination

Fear related to homologous blood transfusion and the transmission of disease; fear of "needles"

Hyperthermia related to increased metabolic rate; illness; dehydration

Hypothermia related to exposure to cool or cold blood

Impaired physical mobility related to pain or discomfort resulting from placement and maintenance of I.V. catheter

Impaired skin integrity related to I.V. catheter; irritating I.V. solution; inflammation; infection; infiltration

Impaired tissue integrity related to altered circulation; fluid deficit or excess; irritating solution; inflammation; infection; infiltration

Impaired gas exchange related to ventilation perfusion imbalance; decreased oxygen-carrying capacity of the blood

Knowledge deficit related to purpose of blood component therapy; signs and symptoms of complications.

Risk for infection related to broken skin or traumatized tissue.

Nursing Management: Critical Activities

Verify physician orders

Obtain patient's informed consent

Monitor patient's immunologic status

Verify that blood product matches patient's blood type

Administer blood products as appropriate

Prime administration system with 0.9% sodium chloride

Prepare an I.V. pump is indicated

Continued on following page

479

PATIENT EDUCATION

Inform about signs and symptoms of transfusion reactions.
Instruct on need and physiologic benefit of blood product.
Inform on options: autologous, homologous, or designated donation.
Instruct on current statistics on transfusion risks.

HOME CARE ISSUES

Transfusion services can be delivered safely and efficiently in the home setting. It is an appropriate alternative for patients who require frequent transfusions but for whom hospitalization is not otherwise indicated. Usually the patient has physical limitations that make travel outside the home difficult (Grace & Tomaselli, 1995). For non–home-bound patients who require transfusions, administration in an outpatient infusion clinic may be a more cost-effective alternative.

Guidelines and standards need to be set with the patient's best interest in mind. The American Association of Blood Banks is creating standards for the home transfusion procedure, and the INS standards should be considered in the formulation of home transfusion therapy. Transfusions in the home setting include:

1. Packed red blood cells (PRBCs)
2. Modified PRBCs
3. Platelets
4. Cryoprecipitate
5. Plasma
6. Plasma derivatives
7. Factor VIII concentrate

✎ **NOTE:** Whole blood is not an alternative in the home setting (Monks, 1988).

Guidelines for Home Transfusion Therapy

1. Written physician's order is required.
2. The patient should be:
   In stable cardiopulmonary status and medical condition

480

Alert, cooperative, and able to respond appropriately to body reactions and communicate information to the nurse

3. The following also must be evaluated:
   Conducive home environment
   Capable adult present during transfusion
   Telephone access available
   Ready access to emergency medical service and primary physician during transfusion (Grace & Tomaselli, 1995)

4. Blood component should be transported to the home setting using blood bank standards.

5. Proper blood and patient identification should be carried out.

6. Baseline assessments should be made according to INS standards for monitoring the infusion.

7. Appropriate blood filter should be used.

8. Electromechanical devices may be used, but the product information should be checked to ensure that the pump is indicated for transfusion delivery and will not cause hemolysis of RBCs.

9. Use only 0.9% sodium chloride solutions to prime the administration set.

10. The nurse administering the transfusion must remain in the home setting throughout the transfusion and for an appropriate time after transfusion to check for complications.

11. Blood warming should not be considered for home transfusion because no more than 2 U of blood should be administered at one time in the home setting.

12. A biohazard bag should be brought to the home and all contaminated equipment disposed of according to state regulations.

13. Leave post-transfusion instructions that include but are not limited to:
    Emergency telephone numbers
    Information regarding signs and symptoms of delayed reactions
    Schedule of the post-transfusion assessment visit

14. Notify physician of the transfusion completion and the patient's response to therapy.

15. Charting must include but not be limited to:
    Type of I.V. solution and time started
    Type of blood product
    Vital signs, skin condition, and appearance
    Any patient symptoms or complaints
    The time blood product is discontinued
    Volume infused
    Reason for discontinuing the transfusion if done before completion of the infusion
    Patient reactions to the procedure

COMPETENCY CRITERIA: Blood Administration

Competency Statement: The competent nurse will demonstrate safe delivery of blood components.

COGNITIVE CRITERIA

	Knowledgeable	Needs Education
1. Identifies types and indications for use of blood or blood product:		
a. Red cells		
b. Platelets		
c. Granulocytes		
d. Cryoprecipitate/Factor VIII		
e. Fresh frozen plasma		
f. Albumin		

PERFORMANCE CRITERIA

	Skilled	Needs Education
1. Administers blood products according to AABB and institutional policy:		
a. Infuse no longer than 4 hours		
b. Only one administration set used per unit		
c. Only 0.9% sodium chloride as primer		
d. Minimum pore size filter 170 micron		
2. Monitors patient for adverse reactions to blood administration:		
a. Acute hemolytic reaction		
b. Delayed reaction		
c. Allergic reaction		
d. Nonhemolytic febrile reaction		
3. Monitors for complications associated with blood administration:		
a. Circulatory overload		
b. Hypocalcemia		
c. Hyperkalemia		
4. Demonstrates use of blood warmers.		

482

SUGGESTED EVALUATION CRITERIA

Cognitive Criteria: Written test

Performance Criteria: Return demonstration on model

Clinical observation of bedside skills

KEY POINTS

Basic Immunohematology

Immunohematology is the science that deals with antigens of the blood and their antibodies.

    Antigens (Agglutinogens)

        ABO system

        Rh system

        HLA system

    Antibodies (Agglutinins)

    Testing of Donor and Recipient Blood

        ABO and Rh grouping

        Crossmatching of the donor's blood

        Antibody screening and a compatibility test

        Tests for transmissible disease

Universal RBC donor is O-negative. Universal plasma donor is AB.

    Blood Preservatives

        CPD (citrate-phosphate-dextrose)—extends life of cells to 21 days

        CPDA-1 (citrate-phosphate-dextrose adenine)—extends life of cells to 35 days

        CPDA-1 plus additives (e.g., ADSOL)—extends life to 42 days

Blood Donor Collection Methods

    Homologous—blood donated by someone other than the intended recipient

    Autologous—patient's own blood

    Designated—blood donated from selected friends or relatives of the patient or recipient

Blood Component Therapy

    The administration of blood components allows for no margin of error. Component therapy refers to the delivery of components obtained from a unit of whole blood. Whole blood is composed of RBCs, plasma, WBCs, and platelets.

COMPONENT	INDICATIONS
PRBCs	Symptomatic acute and chronic anemia
Washed RBCs	Provides leukocyte poor RBC's for patients with recurrent allergic or febrile reactions
Deglycerolized RBCs	Long-term storage of RBCs to minimize febrile and allergic reactions
Granulocytes	Febrile patients with neutropenia unresponsive to antibiotic therapy
Platelets	Control bleeding in platelet deficiencies
Fresh frozen plasma	Replacement of coagulation factors
Cryoprecipitate	Deficiency of factor VIII, factor XIII, fibrinogen, Von Willenbrand's disease

483

Colloid Volume Expanders
 Albumin
 Plasma protein fraction
 Dextran
 Hetastarch

Administration of Blood Products
 Step 1: Physician's order
 Step 2: Equipment selection and preparation
 Step 3: Patient preparation
 Step 4: Obtaining blood product from the blood bank
 Step 5: Preparation for administration
 Step 6: Initiation of transfusion
 Step 7: Monitoring the transfusion
 Step 8: Discontinuation of transfusion

Complications of Transfusion Therapy
 Transfusion Reactions
  Acute hemolytic reactions
  Delayed hemolytic reactions
  Nonhemolytic febrile reactions
  Allergic reactions
 Other Complications
  Circulatory overload
  Potassium toxicity
  Hypothermia
  Hypocalemia
 Risks of Transfusion Therapy
  Fever, chills, urticaria
  Hemolytic transfusion reaction
  Viral hepatitis
  HIV infection

CRITICAL THINKING ACTIVITY

1. A friend wants to know if she can donate blood to be directly designated for her father. What do you tell her?

2. While caring for a patient who is to receive a unit of PRBCs, the patient expresses a fear of contracting AIDS from the transfusion. What do you tell the patient? Are there risks?

3. As a new graduate, what resources are available to you for providing patient teaching related to the donation of blood?

4. Review the policy and procedure for blood transfusion at the facility in which you work. Does the policy designate who should pick up the blood from the laboratory? Is the procedure clear about how to check blood out from the laboratory and how to administer the component safely?

5. If you were unclear on how to administer cryoprecipitate, what would you do?

6. Your patient develops an increase in temperature during a transfusion of PRBCs, the pulse rate is 120 and the patient is slightly short of breath. You discover baseline vital signs had not been taken, as you directed a nurse's aide to do prior to administering the transfusion. What would you do? Also, who is at fault?

7. At the beginning of your shift, you check on a unit of blood that had been hung before your shift. The unit of PRBCs is infusing slowly, with approximately 100 mL left. You agitate the bag slightly and discover a pinhole at the top of the bag. What do you do?

POST-TEST, CHAPTER 13

Match the definition in column II to the term in column I.

Column I

1. _____ HLA
2. _____ antibody
3. _____ CPD
4. _____ antigen
5. _____ ABO system
6. _____ homologous donation
7. _____ designated donation
8. _____ autologous donation
9. _____ Rh system

Column II

A. Preservative used for collected blood

B. Antigen used for tissue typing and relevant for transplant

C. Substance eliciting immunologic response

D. Protein produced by the immune system that destroys or inactivates an antigen

E. The most important antigen system in the blood

F. Concept of donating one's own blood before transfusion

G. D antigens found on the surface of RBCs—positive or negative

H. Transfer of blood directly from one donor to a specified recipient

I. Donation of blood in similar structure from volunteer donor

10. The universal blood donor is:
    A. O-positive
    B. O-negative
    C. AB-positive
    D. AB-negative

11. All the following statements related to the HLA system are true *except:*
    A. HLA is located on the surface of WBCs.
    B. Alloimmunization to HLA antigens is a factor in refractoriness to platelets.
    C. The use of type and crossmatch reduces the alloimmunization to the HLA antigen.
    D. The use of leukocyte-depleted blood can reduce the sensitization to HLA antigens.

12. Antibodies are found in:
    A. RBCs
    B. WBCs
    C. Plasma
    D. Antigens

13. Previous exposure to an antigen by pregnancy or previous transfusion may cause the patient to develop:
    A. An antibody to the antigen
    B. More antigens
    C. Alloimmunization to the antibody
    D. A tolerance to the transfusion

14. A chemical added to donor units to preserve the blood is:
    A. Sodium heparin
    B. Sodium citrate
    C. Sodium phosphate
    D. Dextrose aluminum

15. Blood bank testing for donor blood includes tests for the following diseases except:
    A. HBsAg
    B. Anti–HIV-1
    C. Anti–HTLV-1
    D. EBV (Ebstein-Barr virus)

Match the definition in column II to the term in column I.

Column I

16. _____ thrombocytopenia
17. _____ delayed reaction
18. _____ febrile reaction
19. _____ allergic reaction
20. _____ hemolytic transfusion
21. _____ blood component
22. _____ hemolysis
23. _____ plasma
24. _____ hypothermia
25. _____ immediate reaction

Column II

A. Adverse effect occurring immediately or up to 48 hours later

B. Adverse effect occurring after 48 up to 180 days after transfusion

C. A product made from a unit of blood

D. Rupture of RBC with release of hemoglobin

E. Fluid portion of blood

F. Abnormally low body temperature

G. Exposure to antigen to which the person has become sensitized

H. Abnormally small number of platelets in the blood

I. Destruction of RBCs by antibodies present in the blood of either donor or recipient

J. Nonhemolytic reaction to antibodies formed against leukocytes

26. Whole blood is indicated for:
    A. Treatment of anemia
    B. To provide RBCs and platelets
    C. Acute massive blood loss

27. Washed RBCs are used to:
    A. Provide leukocyte-poor RBCs
    B. Prevent or delay febrile transfusion reactions
    C. Prevent or delay allergic reactions
    D. All of the above

28. Indications for platelet transfusion include:
    A. Hemorrhage with a platelet count less than 50,000
    B. Nonbleeding patients with a platelet count of 80,000
    C. Preoperative patient with a platelet count of 150,000

29. Which of the following is a symptoms of a febrile transfusion reaction?
    A. Itching
    B. Hives
    C. Rash
    D. Chills and fever

30. The nursing interventions for an acute hemolytic reaction would be to:
    A. Slow the transfusion and call the physician
    B. Stop the transfusion and turn on the saline side of the administration set
    C. Stop the transfusion, disconnect the tubing from the I.V. catheter, and initiate new saline and tubing to keep the vein open

487

31. The component albumin 25% is hypertonic. Caution should be used by the nurse when infusing 25% albumin because this product can:
    A. Cause circulatory overload
    B. Cause clotting disorders
    C. Increase RBC hemoglobin
    D. Lower the blood pressure
32. The component FFP is used:
    A. For patients with hemophilia A
    B. For patients who have developed HLA antibodies
    C. To expand the plasma volume
    D. All of the above
33. The nurse must check all of the following with another nurse before initiating the transfusion except:
    A. ABO and Rh
    B. Patient name
    C. Unit number
    D. Expiration date
    E. Preservative

True-False

34. **T F** Lactated Ringer's solution is an acceptable solution to use with blood components.
35. **T F** Platelets may be given through unfiltered tubing.
36. **T F** Pressure bag sleeves may be used to increase flow rates when transfusing PRBCs.
37. **T F** Blood warmers may be used as an adjunct to transfusion when the patient is hypothermic.
38. List the eight steps in initiation of a transfusion.

Step 1 _____

Step 2 _____

Step 3 _____

Step 4 _____

Step 5 _____

Step 6 _____

Step 7 _____

Step 8 _____

ANSWERS TO CHAPTER 13

PRE-TEST

1. H	8. D	15. H	22. A
2. B	9. E	16. I	23. E
3. G	10. A	17. B	24. G
4. C	11. C	18. F	25. A
5. J	12. C	19. J	26. B
6. I	13. D	20. C	27. C
7. F	14. D	21. D	28. C

POST-TEST

1. B	24. F
2. D	25. A
3. A	26. C
4. C	27. D
5. E	28. A
6. I	29. D
7. H	30. C
8. F	31. A
9. G	32. D
10. B	33. E
11. C	34. F
12. C	35. F
13. A	36. T
14. B	37. T
15. D	38. Step 1: Physician's order
16. H	Step 2: Equipment selection preparation
17. B	Step 3: Patient preparation
18. J	Step 4: Obtaining blood product from
19. G	blood bank
20. I	Step 5: Preparation for administration
21. C	Step 6: Initiation of transfusion
22. D	Step 7: Monitoring transfusion
23. E	Step 8: Discontinuation of transfusion

REFERENCES

Anon. (1994). FDC reports: Prescription and OTC pharmaceuticals. *The Pink Sheet, 56,* 5–6.

American Association of Blood Banks. (1986). *Practical aspects of blood administration,* Philadelphia: J.B. Lippincott.

American Association of Blood Banks. (1989). *Blood transfusion therapy: A physician's handbook* (3rd ed.). Philadelphia: J.B. Lippincott.

Baranowski, L. (1991). Filtering out the confusion about leukocyte-poor blood components. *Journal of Intravenous Nursing, 14* (5), 298–305.

Baranowski, L. (1993). Current trends in blood component therapy: The evolution of safer, more effective product. *Journal of Intravenous Therapy, 15* (3), 136–149.

Cook, L.S. (1995). An overview of leukocyte depletion in blood transfusion. *Journal of Intravenous Therapy, 18* (1), 11–15.

Gerber, L. (1994). Autologous blood transfusion: Why and how. *Journal of Intravenous Nursing, 17* (2), 65–69.

Gridley, J.H. (1986). Blood component therapy. *Trauma Quarterly, 2* (3), 45–54.

Harovas, J., & Anthony, H. (1993). Your guide to trouble-free transfusions. *RN 93* (1), 28–35.

Intravenous Nursing Society. (1996). *Standards of practice.* Philadelphia: J.B. Lippincott.

McCloskey, J.C., & Bulechek, G.M. (1992). Iowa intervention project: Nursing interventions classification (NIC). (143). St Louis: Mosby-Year Book.

Monks, M.L. (1988). Home transfusion therapy. *Journal of Intravenous Nursing, 11* (6), 389–396.

National Institute of Health. (1993). Transfusion alert: Indications for use of red blood cells, platelets and fresh frozen plasma. No. 93-2974a. Bethesda, MD: U.S. Department of Health and Human Services.

Peterson, K.J. (1992). Nursing management of autologous blood transfusion. *Journal of Intravenous Nursing, 15* (3), 128–134.

Phillips, L.D., & Kuhn, M. (1995). Manual of IV medication IV meds fact finder. Boston: Little, Browning Nursing.

Pisciotto P.T. (1989). *Blood transfusion therapy: A physician's handbook,* 3rd ed. Arlington, VA: American Association of Blood Banks.

Popovsky. M.A. (1986). Autologous transfusion: Present practice and future trends. *National Intravenous Therapy Association, 9* (5), 292–294.

Suez, D. (1995). Intravenous immunoglobulin therapy: Indications, potential side effects and treatment guidelines. *Journal of Intravenous Nursing, 18* (4), 178–188.

Walker, R.H. (1993). *American Association of Blood Banks technical manual.* Bethesda, MD: American Association of Blood Banks.

Weir, J. (1995). Blood component therapy. In Terry, J., Baranowski, L., Lonsway, R., & Hedrick, C. (eds.). *Intravenous therapy: Clinical principles and practices.* (165–187). Philadelphia: W.B. Saunders.

CHAPTER 14

Antineoplastic Therapy

CHAPTER CONTENTS

GLOSSARY
LEARNING OBJECTIVES
PRE-TEST, CHAPTER 14
ROLE OF CLINICIAN
Patient Assessment and History
Treatment Objectives
CELLULAR KINETICS
Cell Cycle
Normal and Malignant Tissue Growth
Tumor Cell Kill
Drug Resistance
ANTINEOPLASTIC AGENTS
Classifications
Chemotherapy Dosing
Classes of Drugs
COMMON SIDE EFFECTS OF CHEMOTHERAPY
Short-Term Complications
Acute Reactions
Toxicities
ROUTES OF ADMINISTRATION
Systemic Routes
Regional Routes

Infusion Pumps
NURSING PLAN OF CARE: ANTINEOPLASTIC
  THERAPY
PATIENT EDUCATION
HOME CARE ISSUES
Patient and Family Education
Admixture
Transport of Drug
Administration
Disposal
Monitoring
Disposal of Excreta
COMPETENCY CRITERIA: ADMINISTRATION OF
  ANTINEOPLASTIC THERAPY
KEY POINTS
CRITICAL THINKING ACTIVITY
POST-TEST, CHAPTER 14
ANSWERS TO CHAPTER 14
Pre-Test
Post-Test
REFERENCES

GLOSSARY

Adjuvant Addition to primary treatment
AGC Absolute granulocyte count
Alopecia Loss of hair (scalp, facial, axillary, pubic, and body)
Antineoplastic Medication used for the treatment of cancer
Biologic response modifiers Agents that mimic, stimulate, enhance, inhibit, or alter the
  modifiers hosts responses to cancer.
BSA Body surface area
Cellular kinetics Study of mechanisms and rates of cellular changes; provides the basis
  for an understanding of action and side effects of anticancer agents
Chemotherapy Treatment of disease with chemical reagents that have a specific and
  toxic effect on the disease-causing microorganisms
Curative Successful treatment of a disease
Cytotoxic The degree to which an agent possesses a specific destructive action on certain
  cells or the possession of such action; antineoplastic agents that selectively kill dividing
  cells
Desquamation Shedding of the epidermis

Extravasation Leakage of a vesicant or irritant drug into the subcutaneous tissue that is capable of causing pain, necrosis, or sloughing of tissue

Hyperuricemia Enhanced blood concentrations of uric acid

Integumentary Cutaneous, dermal

Intraperitoneal (IP) Within the peritoneal cavity

Irritant A cancer chemotherapeutic agent capable of producing venous pain at the site and along the vein, with or without an inflammatory reaction

Leukopenia Any situation in which the total number of leukocytes in the circulating blood is less than normal, the limit of which is generally regarded as $5000/\mu L$

Mitosis Indirect cell division involving indirect nuclear division and division of the cell body; the process by which all somatic cells of multicellular organisms multiply

Myelosuppression Decrease in function of bone marrow resulting in decrease in fully functioning blood cells

Nadir count Point at which the blood counts are the lowest; usually 7 to 14 days after day 1 of chemotherapy

Neutropenia Diminished number of neutrophils in the blood

Nonstem cells Cells that differentiate

Oncologist Physician involved in the study and treatment of tumors

Palliative Use of procedures to promote client comfort and quality of life without the goal of cure of disease

Peripheral neuropathy Dysfunction of postganglionic nerves ranging from paresthesia to paralysis

Pruritus Itching

Stem cells Mother cells, having the capacity for both replication and differentiation

Synergistic Joint action of agents so that their combined effect is greater than the sum of their individual parts

Thrombocytopenia A condition in which there are abnormally small number of platelets in the circulating blood

Vesicant A drug capable of causing or forming a blister or causing tissue necrosis upon skin contact

LEARNING OBJECTIVES

Upon completion of this chapter, the reader will be able to:

- Define terminology related to administration of antineoplastic agents.
- Discuss the principles of cellular kinetics.
- Identify the phases of the cell cycle.
- Identify the goals of cancer antineoplastic therapy.
- Define the terms "cell cycle–specific" and "cell cycle–nonspecific."
- Identify the role of the clinician in administration of chemotherapy.
- State the action, drug specificity, and major side effects and specific nursing interventions with alkylating agents, antimetabolites, vinca alkaloids, hormones and hormone antagonists, and biologic response modifiers.
- State specific nursing interventions that are useful in helping patients deal with alopecia.
- List the medications available for treating nausea and vomiting.
- Identify the general procedure for extravasation.
- Identify agents available for oral care for patients receiving chemotherapy to prevent and treat stomatitis.
- Identify the major toxicities that can occur with antineoplastic therapy.
- Identify the common routes used for antineoplastic therapy.
- Use the nursing process in planning care for a patient receiving antineoplastic therapy.
- List the key areas of patient education for patients receiving chemotherapy.

PRE-TEST, CHAPTER 14

Match the following definitions in column II to the terms in column I.

Column I

1. _____ adjuvant
2. _____ curative
3. _____ palliative
4. _____ stem cell
5. _____ synergistic
6. _____ non-stem cell

Column II

A. Joint action of agent when combined effect is greater than the sum of individual agents

B. An addition to primary treatment

C. The successful treatment of disease

D. A mother cell, having capacity for both replication and differentiation

E. Use of procedures to promote comfort and quality of life without the goal of cure of disease

F. Cells that differentiate

7. List the phases of the cell cycle.

A. _____

B. _____

C. _____

D. _____

E. _____

8. Antineoplastic drugs that are cell cycle–dependent include:
A. Folic acid analogues
B. Nitrogen mustards
C. Nitrosureas
D. Platinum complexes

9. When a patient is receiving a chemotherapeutic agent that is nephrotoxic, which laboratory value should the nurse monitor?
A. Alkaline phosphatase
B. BUN/creatinine
C. Uric acid
D. Serum sodium

10. A drug commonly prescribed on a scheduled basis before and after chemotherapy to prevent nausea and vomiting is:
A. Diazepam
B. Haloperidol
C. Ondansetron
D. Ranitidine

11. Before administration of antimetabolite antineoplastic agent, it is important that the patient:
A. Has antiemetic medication
B. Is well hydrated
C. Receives an antacid
D. Receives a sedative

12. Agents given to increase hematopoiesis are:
   A. Colony-stimulating factors
   B. Interferons
   C. Interleukins
   D. Monoclonal antibodies

13. Agents given to enhance the body's immune system are:
   A. Antiestrogenic compounds
   B. Biologic response modifiers
   C. Hormones
   D. Alkylating agents

14. A patient receiving paclitaxel who has symptoms of peripheral neuropathy is most likely to be:
   A. Cardiotoxic
   B. Neurotoxic
   C. Nephrotoxic
   D. Hepatotoxic

15. A vesicant antineoplastic agent is infusing and the nurse checks the infusion and suspects infiltration. The first nursing action would be to:
   A. Remove the cannula
   B. Photograph the suspected site
   C. Apply warm compresses and continue administration of medication
   D. Stop the administration of the medication

16. The protocol for holding the antineoplastic agent until discussion with the physician would be when the patient presents with a white blood cell count of:
   A. 6000/μL
   B. 4000/μL
   C. 3000/μL
   D. 2000/μL

17. All the following are common nursing diagnoses associated with delivery of chemotherapeutic agents *except:*
   A. Altered nutrition
   B. Altered oral mucous membrane
   C. Fear and anxiety
   D. Impaired gas exchange

18. A patient considered neutropenic from bone marrow suppression is at risk for:
   A. Dehydration
   B. Infection
   C. Seizures
   D. Disseminated intravascular coagulation

These seasons of surviving are like the changing seasons of the year. We delight in the fragrant smell of spring, bask in the hot days of summer, then welcome the cool, crisp days of fall.

Lest we get too used to it all, the frosty chill of winter is upon us, and when we despair of ever seeing those spring daffodils, violets and tulips again, up they blossom once again to delight us, only in a different way.

Enduring seasons in survival give us renewed opportunities to learn more clearly the meaning of living and dying.

KAREN HASSEY DOW, RN, MS, *Cancer Survivor*

The nurse participating in administration of antineoplastic agents has a tremendous responsibility. The emphasis of this chapter is on the role of the nurse in understanding cellular kinetics, pharmacology of antineoplastic agents, routes of administration, and common side effects of chemotherapy.

ROLE OF CLINICIAN

Administering antineoplastic agents and caring for the client with cancer requires specific educational preparation and practical experience. The Oncology Nursing Society (ONS) has developed credentialing for the oncology nurse.

The nurse practicing in this specialty area is required to be knowledgeable about the biology of cancer, the pharmacology and principles of cancer chemotherapy, specific antineoplastic agents, major principles governing the administration of chemotherapy, and patient assessment and management (Weinstein, 1993).

Patient Assessment and History

Assessment begins by first determining the patient's knowledge base of the classification of their cancer and the symptoms and course of the disease. This is the first step in gathering a history from the client. The information gathered provides a framework for patient education. Included in the history should also be the patient's past medical history, prior organ impairment, or any secondary diagnosis that might influence the toxicities, side effects, and treatment modalities. A record of the total chemotherapeutic agents administered, doses, and any radiation (number of rads) is necessary to complete a cancer history (Groenwald, Frogge, Goodman, & Yarbro, 1990; Table 14–1).

Physical assessment includes the patient's laboratory and diagnostic imaging studies, nutritional status, and psychosocial and spiritual state. Appropriate nursing interventions are based on a complete history and physical assessment.

Treatment Objectives

The role of the clinician also includes an understanding of treatment goals and their rationale. The treatment goal of chemotherapy is situation-dependent. Chemotherapy can be curative when given as primary treatment. The therapeutic goal is also curative when chemotherapy is given as an adjuvant for tumors. Knowledge of the chemotherapy treatment, long-term and short-term side effects, symptom management, and

495

TABLE 14–1. ONCOLOGY PATIENT ASSESSMENT

Interview: Cancer History
Knowledge of classification of cancer
Symptoms
Course of disease
Past medical history
Prior organ impairment
Secondary diagnosis

Physical Assessment
Nutritional status
Laboratory tests
Diagnostic imaging studies: computed tomography, magnetic resonance imaging, x-ray
Psychological state
Spiritual state

lifestyle effects are important because two out of three cancer patients are candidates for chemotherapy at some point in their disease process (Dollinger, Rosenbaum, & Cable, 1991).

Chemotherapy can also be given to control the disease when cure is not realistic. The goal of palliative treatment is pain control. It can decrease pain caused by a tumor by relieving pressure on nerves, decreasing lymphatic congestion, and relieving organ obstruction (Doyle, 1995).

There are few absolute rules related to antineoplastic therapy; however, there are certain basic considerations in chemotherapy treatment.

1. The smaller the tumor burden, the easier the tumor is to treat.
2. Surgical debulking decreases the tumor burden and recruits resting malignant cells to start dividing, thereby increasing the sensitivity to chemotherapy.
3. The higher the chemotherapy dose, the better the chance for a tumor response.
4. Doses of chemotherapeutic agents are altered based on the degree of toxicity that the patient experiences.
5. The *therapeutic margin* is the difference between the dose producing the desired benefit and the dose resulting in unacceptable toxicity.
6. The therapeutic margin of antineoplastic agents is narrow compared with that of other types of drugs.
7. If the efficacy of the chemotherapeutic agents can be increased, there is better tumor response with a lower chemotherapy dose.

CELLULAR KINETICS

Cellular kinetics is the study of mechanisms and rates of cellular changes. This study is becoming more and more useful in planning treatment regimens and scheduling drug administration.

Cell Cycle

Antineoplastic agents act primarily on proliferating cells; therefore, it is important to examine the cell cycle and the growth of normal and malignant cells to understand the rationale for and effects of drug therapy (Fig. 14–1).

496

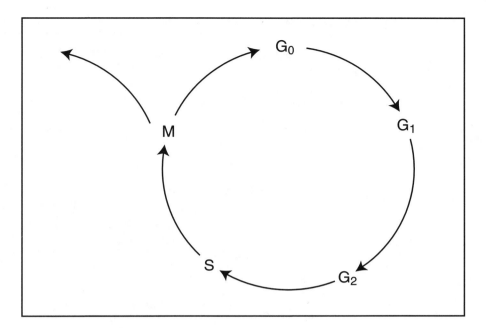

G_0	Nonproliferative resting phase
G_1	Presynthetic stage
G_2	Interval after synthesis of DNA
S	Synthesis of DNA
M	Mitosis (G_2 cell divides into two cells)

Figure 14–1. Cell cycle.

Four classic phases complete the cell growth cycle: G_1, S, G_2, and M. Some cells move out of the cell cycle after mitosis into G_0, becoming resting and nondividing cells. Other cells enter the first phase, G_1, which is the period between mitosis and the beginning of DNA synthesis when active RNA and protein synthesis occurs.

The G_1 phase is the most variable of all phases, and its length influences the rate of cell proliferation. Cells that are growing slowly have many cells in the G_1 phase, whereas cells that are growing rapidly have few cells in the G_1 phase. The cells then emerge from G_1 and enter the S phase, in which enzymes necessary for DNA synthesis increase in activity. This phase is finished when the cells DNA content has doubled. After the S phase, a resting period, called G_2 occurs. During this phase, the RNA and protein necessary for mitosis are synthesized. This phase extends from the end of DNA synthesis to the beginning of mitosis. The last phase of the cell cycle is the M phase, in which mitosis takes place. The formation of the spindle, separation of chromosomes, and the division of the cell into two cells occur (Baserga, 1981; Table 14–2).

Normal and Malignant Tissue Growth

In both normal and malignant tissues, three different cell populations affect growth: cycling cells, nondividing cells, and resting cells called G_0 cells. The cells that are

497

TABLE 14–2. **TIMING OF THE CELL CYCLE**

Phase	Description	Duration
G_1 (first)	Period between mitosis and beginning of DNA synthesis	8–48 hours
S (second)	Increase in activity of enzymes for DNA synthesis (concluded when DNA content doubles)	10–30 hours
G_2 (third)	Resting period during which RNA and protein necessary for mitosis are synthesized	1–12 hours
M (fourth)	Period during which mitosis takes place—division into two cells	1 hour

dividing continuously are the *cycling cells*. The group of cells that divide for a time and then complete their life cycle without dividing again are called *nondividing cells*. The third group is composed of G_0, or resting cells, which leave the cell cycle and remain dormant until conditions stimulate them to reenter the cell cycle and divide. Cycling cells and G_0, or resting cells, are further divided into stem cells and nonstem cells. Stem cells replenish the stem cell pool, and nonstem cells differentiate and enter the maturing groups of cells. As long as G_0 stem cells remain, a damaged cell population can be renewed.

Four interrelated factors must be considered during assessment of normal or tumor cells: the cell cycle time, the growth fraction, the total number of cells in the population, and the rate of cell loss (Skeel, 1995). The first factor, the cell cycle time, is the amount of time required for the cell to move from one mitosis to the next. Second, the growth fraction is the percentage of cycling cells in the entire cell population. The third factor is the total number of cells in the population determined at some point in time, which indicates how advanced the cancer is and provides a basis for growth measurement. As the total number of cells increases, so does the number of resistant cells. The fourth factor is the rate of cell loss or the number of cells that die or leave the cell population. Growth depends on the number of cells produced and the number of cells that die. Rate of growth depends on the cell cycle time, the growth fraction, and the rate of cell loss.

In tumor growth, there is a theory that as the tissue mass increases in size, the doubling time slows (Carter, Bakowski, & Hellman, 1987). Another factor that affects tumor growth is the decrease in nutrients available for each cell as the total mass increases and blood supply is outgrown. It has been found that some normal cells cycle faster than tumor cells in human beings. Overall, tumor cell cycling times range from 24 to 120 hours. The doubling time of most tumor cells ranges from 5 days to 2 years, with a mean of 1 to 3 months (Turbiana & Malaise, 1976). This longer doubling time is due to several factors. First, the growth fraction of human tumors varies from 0% to 100%. Second, many tumor cells die spontaneously. Turbiana, Richard, & Malaise (1975) found that about 48% of tumor cells die every day and their calculations have indicated that at least 5% to 97% of all tumor cells die spontaneously. Spontaneous death occurs from inadequate nutrition, cumulative genetic damage in tumor cells, and cell differentiation into nondividing cells.

Tumor Cell Kill

The goal of modern chemotherapy is to prevent cancer cells from multiplying, invading, metastasizing, and ultimately killing the host (Skeel, 1995). Most active cytotoxic agents are selectively toxic to rapidly proliferating cells; many G_0 or resting cells remain untouched. Resting stem cells can regenerate the tumor cell population.

The tumor mass increases in size, and the cells cycle at a slower rate; therefore, the growth fraction decreases and the cytotoxic effects of the drug diminish. The drugs are not only specific to cancer cells but are also toxic to normal proliferating cells. Normal cells most affected by chemotherapeutic drugs include hematopoietic or bone marrow cells, gastrointestinal epithelial cells, hair follicle cells, germinal cells, and embryonic cells.

The ability of antineoplastic agents to kill tumor cells comes from research that shows that these drugs kill tumor cells according to first-order kinetics. Certain drug doses destroy a constant fraction of tumor cells in the body, rather than a constant number of cells. Also, these drugs follow an exponential, or "log-kill," model. Therefore, cell kill may be expressed as a log-kill of two, meaning that the body's tumor burdens decreased from 10^8 to 10^6 cells (from 100,000,000 to 1,000,000). The maximum cell kill from a single drug dose has been found to be 2 to 5 logs. Treatment must be repeated many times to decrease the number of tumor cells in the body. Because a single dose always kills a fraction of the tumor cells, this hypothesis suggests that chemotherapy can never destroy all malignant cells in the body (Skeel, 1995).

The second hypothesis proposes that cell kill caused by antineoplastic drugs is related to relative growth fraction of the tumor at the time of treatment. Thus, the greatest tumor cell kill occurs when the growth fraction is greatest. The growth fraction is greatest when tumors are of intermediate size or less when they are very small or very large (ONS, 1989).

The biologic control of normal cells and tumor growth at the modular level has not yet led to improved therapy for cancer; however, it has helped to explain differences in response among populations of patients. Further work in this area may provide a powerful selective means of controlling neoplastic cell growth and lead to effective cancer treatment in the next decade. This is further discussed under biologic control modifiers.

Drug Resistance

Resistance to antineoplastic therapy is a combined characteristic whereby the drug is ineffective in controlling the tumor without excessive toxicity. Factors that influence resistance include the specific drug, the specific tumor, and the specific host.

The first dose of a drug is usually very effective in treating tumor cells, but successive doses at times decreases the effectiveness until no effect is seen. Many malignant cells develop drug resistance. There appears to be a similarity between cancer cell resistance to drugs and bacterial resistance to antibiotics. Thus, similar approaches such as large initial doses, combination drugs, alternating combinations of drugs, and earliest possible treatment of disease are used to overcome resistance and eventual tumor recurrence (ONS, 1989).

Cell resistance to antineoplastic drugs can be natural or acquired. Natural resistance results from the initial unresponsiveness of a tumor to a given drug. Acquired resistance refers to the unresponsiveness that emerges after initially successful treatment (Skeel, 1995).

ANTINEOPLASTIC AGENTS

Antineoplastic agents used in chemotherapy are classified according to their relationship to the cell cycle activity, their pharmacologic or chemical structure, their potential to cause necrosis if extravasated, and their emetic potential (Doyle, 1995).

Classifications

Antineoplastic agents are classified according to the cell life cycle. This classification has two categories: (1) cell cycle-specific drugs and (2) non–cell cycle-specific drugs. The chemical structure also provides a category by which the drugs can be classified; these are alkylating agents, antimetabolites, natural products, hormones and hormone antagonists, and biologic response modifiers.

Chemotherapeutic agents can also be classified according to their potential to cause local tissue reactions. The potential for alteration in skin and tissue integrity ranges from transient local discomfort during administration to severe tissue necrosis. Classification includes irritants and vesicants.

✎ NOTE: Many drugs are listed as both vesicants and irritants owing to lack of uniformity in the literature (Holleb, Fink, & Murphy, 1991).

Chemotherapy Dosing

Doses of antineoplastic agents used in chemotherapy are calculated according to body surface area (BSA). Clinical trials have provided a formula to determine the amount of each drug to be used in a particular regimen.

A nomogram chart is used to calculate the log of the height and weight (see Appendix A). Many institutions have computers that are programmed to determine the BSA. The oncologist uses weight changes to determine whether an adjustment in the total dosage is necessary to avoid overdosing or underdosing the patient.

✎ NOTE: It is important to weigh the patient before each course of chemotherapy.

The basic formula for determining the chemotherapy dosage is as follows:

$$BSA \times mg/m^2 = total\ dose$$

✎ NOTE: It is important to note whether the BSA was determined from ideal body weight or actual weight.

Classes of Drugs

Chemotherapeutic agents are divided into several classes. For two of the classes—alkylating agents and antimetabolites—the names indicate the mechanism of cytotoxic action. The hormonal agents refer to the physiologic type of drug, and the natural products reflect the source of the drugs. Biologic response modifiers mimic, stimulate, enhance, inhibit, or otherwise alter the host responses to the cancer (Table 14–3; Skeel, 1995).

Alkylating Agents

Alkylating agents were the first antineoplastic drugs and were developed as a result of government studies of biologic warfare (Doyle, 1995). These agents are a diverse group of chemical compounds capable of forming molecular bonds with nucleic acids, proteins, and many molecules of low molecular weight. The basis for their therapeutic use against cancers is the process of alkylation by which they cause interstrand and intrastrand cross-linkages in DNA, thereby blocking replication (Table 14–4).

500

TABLE 14–3. CLASSES OF ANTINEOPLASTIC DRUGS AND BIOLOGIC RESPONSE MODIFIERS

Class	Type
Alkylating agents	Nitrogen mustard
	Ethylenimine derivative
	Alkylsulfonate
	Nitrosourea
	Triazine
	Metal salt
Antimetabolites	Folic acid analogue
	Pyrimidine analogue
	Purine analogue
Natural products	Vinca alkaloids
	Antibiotics
	Enzymes
Hormones and hormone antagonists	Androgen
	Corticosteroid
	Estrogen
	Progestin
	Estrogen antagonist
	Androgen antagonist
Biologic response modifiers	Cytokines
	Colony-stimulating factors
	Monoclonal antibodies

Action

The alkylating agents are cell cycle-independent because they act on cells at any phase of the cycle. Most of the agents in this group are considered polyfunctional alkylating agents because they contain more than one alkylating group. The nitrosoureas are unique under the class of alkylating agents with respect to being non–cross-resistant with other alkylating agents, being highly lipid-soluble, and having delayed myelosuppressive effects. These agents can cross the blood-brain barrier.

The alkylating agents used as antineoplastic agents are nitrogen mustards, ethylenimines, alkyl sulfonate, nitrosoureas, triazine, and metal salts.

Major Side Effects

Alkylating agents have serious adverse reactions. Major side effects include toxicities to the hematopoietic, gastrointestinal, and reproductive systems, and all alkylating agents can be carcinogenic. These agents as a class share common side effects of alopecia, bone marrow depression, nausea and vomiting, and diarrhea.

TABLE 14–4. ALKYLATING AGENTS

Chlorambucil	Carmustine
Cyclophosphamide	Lomustine
Ifosfamide	Semustine*
Estramustine	Streptozocin
Mechlorethamine	Dacarbazine
Melphalan	Cisplatin
Thiotepa (triethylenethriophosphoramide)	Carboplatin
Busulfan	

*Investigational agent not yet approved by the FDA.

501

KEY NURSING INTERVENTIONS AND ASSESSMENT

1. Monitor I.V. sites for infiltration; many alkylating agents cause tissue necrosis with infiltration.
2. Monitor complete blood count (CBC) and platelets and liver enzymes.
3. Administer antiemetics.
4. Assess respiratory status and blood pressure with cyclophosphamide and carmustine; monitor for hypotension with busulfan melphalan.
5. Prehydrate for cisplatin and carboplatin.
6. Assess oral cavity for stomatitis.

Antimetabolites

The antimetabolites are a group of low molecular weight compounds that exert their effect because of similarity to naturally occurring metabolites involved in nucleic acid synthesis (Table 14–5). They are structurally similar to vitamins, coenzymes or normal cell products needed for growth and division of both normal and neoplastic cells.

Action

They interfere with the metabolic pathways of dividing cells and exert their greatest effect in the S phase of the cell cycle. A drug-induced block of DNA synthesis occurs when the antimetabolic agent is taken into the cell rather than the necessary nutrient or enzyme. This is the major cause of cell death from antimetabolite therapy (Mathewson-Kuhn, 1994).

Categories

Folic Acid Analogues

Folic acid and its derivatives are critical for the metabolism of proliferating cells. These drugs are potentially nephrotoxic. Methotrexate is an example of a folic acid analog. Side effects include pancytopenia, gastrointestinal toxicity, skin rash, headache, hepatotoxicity, and pulmonary toxic effects. Methotrexate is used as an immunosuppressive agent to prevent graft-versus host disease after allogeneic bone marrow transplantation.

Pyrimidine Analogues

These agents inhibit critical enzymes necessary for nucleic acid synthesis and may become incorporated into the DNA and RNA. Common side effects with pyrimidine agents include gastrointestinal disturbances, cardiac toxicity, and ataxia.

TABLE 14–5. **ANTIMETABOLITE AGENTS**

Methotrexate	Mercaptopurine
Azacitidine*	Thioguanine
Cytarabine	Pentostatin
Floxuridine	Cladribine
Fluorouracil	Fludarabine

*Investigational agent, not yet approved by FDA.

502

Purine Analogues

Purine agents interfere with normal purine interconversions and thus with DNA and RNA synthesis. These agents can cause bone marrow suppression, hyperuricemia, and acute hepatic toxicity.

Major Side Effects

The common side effects of antimetabolites are myelosuppression and gastrointestinal disturbances. Other side effects are stomatitis, esophagitis, elevation in liver function tests, photosensitivity, and severe nausea and vomiting.

KEY NURSING INTERVENTIONS AND ASSESSMENT
1. Assess oral mucosa for stomatitis.
2. Monitor CBC, platelets, and liver and renal enzymes.
   Stop drug if white blood cell (WBC) count drops below $3000/\mu L$.
   Administer antiemetics especially with cytarabine and mercaptopurine.
   High-dose methotrexate requires leucovorin rescue.

Natural Products

The natural products include vinca alkaloids, antibiotics, and enzymes (Table 14–6). Their modes of action differ significantly. These products are unlike the alkylating and antimetabolite agents, which are classified by mode of action. Natural products are classified together because of their sources are naturally occurring. Although they are classified together their action differ significantly (Mathewson-Kuhn, 1994).

Vinca Alkaloids

Action

The vinca alkaloids, vinblastine, vincristine, and vindesine, are derivatives of the plant vinca rosea (periwinkle). These agents are cell cycle-specific, active only when the cell is in the mitotic (M) phase of division. Vinca alkaloids interfere with the microtubule assembly in the mitotic spindle formation.

Major Side Effects

Adverse effects common with plant alkaloids are numbness and tingling of the extremities, loss of deep tendon reflexes, and ataxia. Vinca alkaloids can produce tissue necrosis if I.V. infusions containing these agents are allowed to extravasate.

TABLE 14–6. **NATURAL PRODUCTS**

Vinblastine	Paclitaxel (Taxol)
Vincristine	Docetraxel
Vindesine*	Etoposide
Vinorelbine	Teniposide

*Investigational use, not approved by FDA.

503

Anthracycline Antibiotics

Action

Anthracycline agents are derived from fermented products of different *Streptomyces* species. They are called anthracyclines because the anthracycline portion of their molecules produces the antineoplastic effect. These drugs act by reacting with DNA to form complexes that block DNA-directed RNA and DNA transcription. Current evidence suggests that both drugs are probably effective during all phases of the cell cycle and therefore are cell cycle-nonspecific.

Major Side Effects

The major side effects are leukopenia, thrombocytopenia, cardiac toxicity, arrhythmias, cardiomyopathy, nausea, vomiting, stomatitis, hyperpigmentation of skin, hepatotoxicity, and enhancement of cyclophosphamide-induced bladder injury. Some agents in this class can cause tissue necrosis if infiltration into subcutaneous tissues occurs (Mathewson-Kuhn, 1994).

✎ **NOTE:** The drug dextrazoxane (Zinecard) can now be used after doxorubicin to protect the heart from cardiotoxicity. It is not advised to use dextrazoxane for preventing cardiotoxicity at this time.

Enzymes

The agent L-asparaginase represents a unique development in the field of cancer chemotherapy. This enzyme was first isolated from *Escherichia coli* and is primarily used in the treatment of acute lymphoblastic leukemia.

Action

L-asparaginase destroys the amino acid asparagine, which is needed for protein synthesis, and thus leads to cell death. Many normal cells are not sensitive to the effects of this drug enzyme because they can synthesize their own supply of asparagine, which tumor cells cannot do. Antitumor effects of this drug are primarily in the G_1 phase of the cell cycle.

Major Side Effects

Because L-asparaginase is a foreign protein, it can produce hypersensitivity and anaphylactic reactions. Fever, anorexia, nausea, and vomiting all are signs of acute toxic reaction. Elevated blood urea nitrogen (BUN) and ammonia levels can result from the enzyme action of this agent. Liver function is often impaired and can increase the toxicity of other drugs.

✎ **NOTE:** Standard pretreatment options include (1) dexamethasone 20 mg I.V. or orally 12 hours and 6 hours before treatment or (2) diphenhydramine 50 mg orally and cimetidine or ranitidine 30 to 60 minutes before paclitaxel.

KEY NURSING INTERVENTIONS AND ASSESSMENT
1. Monitor patient closely during infusion for possible hypersensitivity reaction.
2. Premedicate with dexamethasone, diphendhydramine, or cimetidine before administration of paclitaxel.

504

3. Assess oral mucosa.
4. Assess infusion site frequently for infiltration; *avoid extravasation.*
5. Monitor CBC and platelets, cardiac enzymes, and electrocardiogram (ECG).
6. Make neurologic assessment to monitor for deviation and severity of peripheral neuropathy.
7. Administer antiemetics.
8. Monitor renal function.

Hormones and Hormone Antagonists

The hormones and hormone antagonists include steroidal estrogens, progestins, androgens, corticosteroids and their synthetic derivatives, nonsteroidal synthetic compounds with steroid or steroid-antagonist activity hypothalamic-pituitary analogues, and thyroid hormones. Each agent has diverse effects (Table 14–7).

Androgens

Action

Androgens exert their antineoplastic effect by altering pituitary function or directly affecting the neoplastic cells.

Major Side Effects

Nausea, vomiting, anorexia, myalgia, fluid retention, libido changes, and sterilization can result from use of androgens. Synthetic substances exert little or no masculinizing effects.

Corticosteroids

Action

Corticosteroids can cause lysis of lymphoid tumors that are rich in specific cytoplasmic receptors and may have other indirect effects as well. Anti-inflammatory effects help reduce sequelae of neoplastic activity and nausea and help to reduce cerebral edema secondary to cranial tumor growth or radiation.

Major Side Effects

Corticosteroids can cause muscle weakness, diarrhea, nausea, increased appetite, euphoria, pancreatitis, and thrombophlebitis. Changes in body fat distribution, increased risk of infection, potassium loss and rarely psychosis may also result.

TABLE 14–7. **HORMONES AND HORMONE ANTAGONISTS**

Hormone	Antagonist
Androgen	Fluoxymesterone
Corticosteroid	Prednisone, dexamethasone
Estrogen	Diethylstilbestrol
Progestin	Megestrol acetate, medroxyprogesterone acetate
Estrogen antagonist	Tamoxifen

Estrogens

Action

Estrogens suppress testosterone production in males and alter breast cancer cell response to prolactin.

Major Side Effects

Headache, nausea, weight changes, thromboembolism, and feminization in males can result from use of estrogens.

Progestins

Action

Progestins act directly at the level of the malignant cell receptor to promote differentiation.

Major Side Effects

Edema, pulmonary embolism, breast tenderness, hyperglycemia, and increased appetite can result from use of progestins.

Estrogen Antagonist

Action

Estrogen antagonist acts by competing with estrogen for binding on the cytosol estrogen receptor protein in cancer cells and affects the natural growth factors.

Major Side Effects

Anorexia, nausea, vaginal discharge, bleeding, hot flashes, and a temporary drop in WBCs can result from use of estrogen protagonist.

KEY NURSING INTERVENTIONS AND ASSESSMENT
1. Assess for mood swings, changes in psychological state.
2. For those taking steroids, monitor electrolytes.
3. Monitor blood pressure.
4. Assess males for signs of feminization with estrogens.
5. Assess for signs of phlebitis at I.V. site.
6. Assess females for masculinizing effects with androgens.
7. Encourage low-salt diet.
8. Monitor weight.

Biologic Response Modifiers

The term "biologic therapy" describes a variety of agents and therapeutic approaches derived from the biology of the immune system, the nature of tumor cells, and the relation between them (Parkinson, 1995). The goals of biologic response modifying agents are to (1) stimulate immunocompetence by active or passive means, (2) promote tumor-specific immunity, and (3) serve as an adjunct to other treatments to produce tumor regression.

506

A series of proteins are responsible for the growth and development of cells of the blood and lymphatic systems. These include the cytokines, colony-stimulating factors, and monoclonal antibodies.

Cytokines

A cytokine is a protein produced and secreted by a cell. Several central regulatory cytokines have been isolated, and some are now in general clinical use.

Interleukin-1 (IL-1)

IL-1 binds to a common receptor; this agent plays an important role in inflammation, inducing fever and acute-phase reactant release, and may play a role in tissue repair after injury. IL-1 has immunostimulatory properties that help to activate T lymphocytes and to induce the production of other cytokines. It is both a chemoprotector and a radioprotector, protecting against lethal myelosuppressive doses of cytotoxic agents. This biologic response modifier is investigational for wound healing and has chemoprotective and radioprotective properties.

Interleukin-2 (IL-2)

Originally termed T-cell growth factors, IL-2 is a lymphokine that binds to a specific cell surface receptor on activated T lymphocytes. It has powerful immunostimulatory properties and antitumor effects. This cytokine has significant toxicity and should be administered only by physicians experienced in its use. IL-2 is used as single-agent activity in metastatic renal cell carcinoma (FDA-approved) and malignant melanoma.

Interleukin-4 (IL-4)

IL-4 is stimulatory for B cells and is used with IL-2. It is currently investigational as an immunostimulatory agent.

Interleukin-6 (IL-6)

IL-6 has a central role in induction of the acute-phase response, it is important in B-cell growth.

Interleukin-7 (IL-7) and Interleukin-12 (IL-12)

IL-7 and IL-12 are important in T-cell activation; IL-12 will be studied as a cancer vaccine adjuvant. They are investigational and are currently in clinical trials as potential T-cell–enhancing agents.

Interferon-alpha and Interferon-beta

Initially studied for antiviral properties, the alpha and beta interferons have wide biologic effects; some have proved useful in cancer therapy. Interferon-alpha is FDA-approved for hairy-cell leukemia and AIDS-related Kaposi's sarcoma. This evokes response in chronic myelogeneous leukemia, low-grade non-Hodgkin's lymphoma, and cutaneous T-cell lymphomas. Interferon-alpha is under investigation in combination with 5-fluorouracil (5-FU), cisplatin, and other cytotoxic agents. Interferon-beta is still under investigation for use in cancer but is approved in therapy of multiple sclerosis.

Interferon-gamma

This cytokine is a weaker antiviral agent than the other interferon agents, but it has a wider range of immunobiologic properties. It is now being studied in combination with other biologic agents as an antitumor agent. It is FDA-approved for use in decreasing infections in chronic granulomatous disease.

Colony-Stimulating Factors

Colony-stimulating factors include the hematopoietic growth factors of erythropoietin, granulocyte colony-stimulating factor (G-CSF), interleukin-3, macrophage colony-stimulating factor (CSF-1), and thrombopoietin (TPO).

Erythropoietin

This colony-stimulating factor promotes the proliferation and differentiation of committed erythroid precursors. Erythropoietin may decrease transfusion requirements during chemotherapy and may be studied together with other factors in bone marrow failure states.

Granulocyte Colony-Stimulating Factor

G-CSF is a growth factor with proliferative activity for bone marrow progenitors. It stimulates the production of neutrophils and is FDA-approved. G-CSF decreases the length of myelosuppression following cytotoxic agents and reduces the duration of neutropenia and the incidence of febrile episodes during cytotoxic chemotherapy.

Interleukin-3 (IL-3)

Also known as "multi-CSF," IL-3 stimulates early multipotent marrow stem cells, Its status is investigational, and it is under study for myelorestorative properties.

Macrophage Colony-Stimulating Factor

CSF-1 is relatively lineage-specific. It is responsible for the proliferation and activation of monocytes. It is currently under investigation and has potential uses in infections and cancer.

Thrombopoietin

TPO, a recently isolated factor, enhances megakaryocyte development and will enter clinical trials for prevention and treatment of thrombocytopenia.

Monoclonal Antibodies

Antibodies binding to tumor-associated cell surface antigens can result in the destruction of tumor cells through a number of possible mechanisms, such as activation of complement and antibody-dependent, cell-mediated cytotoxicity. These antibodies may be useful as means of targeting cytotoxic radioisotopes, toxins, or drugs to tumors. Monoclonal antibody technology has made important contributions to cancer medicine.

508

Murine Monoclonal Antibody

The first monoclonal antibodies used, murine antibodies are weak activators of the human immune system. This agent it is approved for treatment of allograft rejection; other antibodies remain investigational for therapeutic purposes.

Human Monoclonal Antibody

This type of monoclonal antibody is difficult to generate in pharmacologic quantities (Parkinson, 1995).

TOXICITIES OF BIOLOGIC RESPONSE THERAPY

The toxicities of biologic agents are dose- and schedule-related. Administration of interferons on a daily basis is associated with systemic symptoms, fever, fatigue, and myalgia. The toxicities associated with IL-2 are dose-dependent and involve significant cardiovascular complications including hypotension and the development of capillary leak syndrome. Also, with IL-2 some patients develop an erythematous rash that may progress to desquamation (Parkinson, 1995).

KEY NURSING INTERVENTIONS AND ASSESSMENT

1. Assess emotional status.
2. Assess for flu-like symptoms.
3. Assess CBC, differential, platelets, electrolytes, and liver function before initiating therapy.
4. Assess for presence of infection.
5. Assess cardiac and pulmonary function.

COMMON SIDE EFFECTS OF CHEMOTHERAPY

Common side effects associated with chemotherapy include short-term complications, acute side effects, and toxicities (Table 14–8).

TABLE 14–8. **COMMON ADVERSE EFFECTS OF CHEMOTHERAPY**

Short-Term Complications
Venous fragility
Alopecia
Diarrhea
Altered nutritional status
Anorexia/taste alteration

Acute Side Effects
Hypersensitivity/anaphylaxis
Extravasation
Stomatitis and mucositis
Nausea and vomiting
Myelosuppression

Toxicities
Cardiac
Neurologic
Renal
Pulmonary

Short-Term Complications

Venous Fragility

Fragile veins are present in the elderly, poorly nourished, and debilitated patient. However, the patient receiving cytotoxic agents has an increased risk of vein fragility. If a patient has fragile veins, the nurse should attempt to cannulate the vein without the use of a tourniquet (Weinstein, 1993; see Chapter 10).

It is imperative that patients with fragile veins be assessed carefully before placement of a cannula for delivery of chemotherapy. Such patients are at higher risk for developing irritation from the antineoplastic agent. Patients receiving corticosteroid therapy have increased vascular fragility, and bleeding and bruising can occur around I.V. sites. Patients receiving chemotherapy and radiation therapy may have thrombocytopenia and therefore depression of platelet production, which increases vascular fragility (Smith, 1995).

Alopecia

The hair follicles are a group of rapidly dividing normal cells that are affected by the nonspecific action of some chemotherapeutic drugs (ONS, 1992). Chemotherapy-induced hair loss (alopecia) is reported to occur by two mechanisms, depending on the drug and dosage received. Atrophy of the hair bulb occurs from drug insult, and the hair falls out spontaneously or in response to a mechanical action such as combing. If the insult is minimal, a marked constriction of the hair shaft occurs, and the hair breaks off (ONS, 1992).

✎ **NOTE:** Hair loss from chemotherapy is not permanent, and regrowth is clinically evident in 4 to 6 weeks after the last dose of antineoplastic agent. Patient education should include information about loss of body hair in addition to scalp hair.

NURSING INTERVENTIONS FOR ALOPECIA
1. Provide information about hair loss.
2. Provide information about hair and scalp care.
3. Provide information about when to expect hair loss.
4. Provide information about obtaining a wig if the patient desires. Some sources recommend purchase of a wig after therapy because of weight loss and the possibility of poor fit if purchased before therapy.
5. Recommend keeping hair cut short because it is easier to manage.
6. Protect the scalp from sun and cold. (Jordan, 1993; ONS, 1992)

Theoretically, scalp hypothermia works to decrease blood circulation by causing vasoconstriction of the superficial blood vessels from the subcutaneous tissues and the external carotid arteries. The FDA approved the use of commercially marketed scalp hypothermia device in 1970. However, in 1990, because of the risks of scalp metastases, the commercial sale of all scalp cooling devices has been suspended. There are inconclusive and conflicting results in the literature, so presently there are no commercial products available. Informed consent should be obtained when using any method for scalp cooling (ONS, 1991).

Diarrhea

Diarrhea and abdominal cramping most often result from antimetabolites. There are many possible causes of diarrhea, such as *Clostridium difficile*, other intestinal infections, malabsorption syndrome, cancer-related treatments of chemotherapy, and radiation and biologic therapy (Doyle, 1995). Diarrhea can lead to discomfort, severe electrolyte abnormalities, altered social life, and poor quality of life.

510

TABLE 14-9. PHARMACOLOGIC MANAGEMENT OF DIARRHEA

Agent	Recommendation
Kaopectate	30–60 mL orally after each loose stool
Loperamide (Imodium)	2 capsules (4 mg) orally every 4 hours initially; then add 1 capsule (2 mg) after each loose stool; do not exceed 16 capsules per day
Diphenoxylate and atropine (Lomotil)	1–2 tablets orally every 4 hours as needed; should not exceed 8 tablets per day
Paregoric	1 tsp orally 4 × per day
Phenobarbital, hyoscyamine, atropine, scopolamine (Donnatal)	Anticholinergic, antispasmodic; may help relieve cramping Dose: 1–2 tablets orally every 4 hours as needed
Octreotide	May be useful for 5-FU-induced diarrhea Dose: 0.05–0.1 mg subcutaneously 3 times per day

Source: From Tipton, J.M., & Skeel, R.T. (1995). Management of acute side effects of cancer chemotherapy. In Skeel, R.T., & Lanchant, N.A. (eds.). *Handbook of cancer chemotherapy*, 4th ed. Boston: Little, Brown, 585, with permission.

Treatment of diarrhea is often symptomatic and usually requires no alteration in cancer therapy, although this side effect can be a dose-limiting factor with 5-FU. Agents that decrease bowel motility should not be used for longer than 24 hours, unless significant infections have been excluded. Medications commonly used to treat diarrhea are loperamide hydrochloride and diphenoxylate hydrochloride with atropine sulfate (Table 14–9).

Nursing management of diarrhea includes teaching patients the importance of early intervention to avoid complications related to diarrhea. Increasing intake of constipating foods such as cheese and eggs, using caution with dairy products, and eating food high in pectin, bulk, and fiber help to slow down peristalsis. Patients should avoid spicy, fatty, and greasy foods. Other foods to avoid include raw fruits and vegetables, nuts, caffeine, seeds, popcorn, and alcohol.

Constipation

Management of constipation in the oncology patient is not the same as that for the medical surgical patient. Enemas should be used with caution in the myelosuppressed patient, because they can be irritating to the mucous membranes and cause microscopic tears that can result in additional complications. In a patient with a low platelet count, bleeding can occur; in the patient with neutropenia, infection can result.

There are many causes of constipation; along with specific chemotherapeutic agents, narcotics, dietary deficiencies, and tumor involvement can result in intrinsic or extrinsic compression. Interventions depend on the underlying cause.

✎ **NOTE:** Patients on narcotics and those receiving vincristine or vinblastine require prophylactic stool softeners.

NURSING INTERVENTIONS FOR CONSTIPATION

1. Unless contraindicated, the patient should have 2 to 3 L of fluids per day.
2. Advise the patient to avoid foods known to be constipating (e.g., cheeses, eggs, refined starches, chocolate, candy).
3. Advise the patient to eat at the same time each day.
4. Encourage the patient to respond to the urge to defecate immediately and not wait.

511

5. Use stool softeners, laxatives, cathartics, and lubricants when appropriate; bulk laxatives keep the stool soft and have been found to be gentle (Doyle, 1995).

Altered Nutritional Status

Malnutrition is reported to occur in 50% to 80% of patients with advanced disease. Nutritional management of the patient with cancer involves early intervention using a supportive health care team. Patients with cancer often experience progressive loss of appetite and sometimes severe malnutrition. This side effect can be a result of therapy or a direct effect of the cancer. Malnutrition can result in a poorer response to therapy, an increased incidence of infections, and an overall worsening of the patient's well being (Tipton & Skeel, 1995).

NURSING INTERVENTIONS FOR ALTERED NUTRITIONAL STATUS
1. Nutritional assessment: Diet history, nutritional intake, anthropometric measurements, laboratory tests for anemia and serum albumin
2. Nutritional intervention: Diet, symptomatic treatment of nausea and vomiting, stomatitis and other gastrointestinal effects of chemotherapy, and supplemental nutrition, which can include creative high-protein and calorie supplements, enteral nutrition, or total parenteral nutrition.
3. Pharmacologic interventions: Pharmacologic appetite stimulation, which promote increased weight gain in some patients and decrease rate of weight loss in others. Currently being investigated to increase appetite are megestrol acetate 40 to 80 mg four times per day, cyproheptadine 8 mg three times per day, hydrazine sulfate, and pentoxifylline (Tipton & Skeel, 1995).

Anorexia and Alteration in Taste

Many treatments that patients receive result in taste alterations. Familiar foods may taste different when the gustatory sense is impaired. Patients receiving cisplatin, cyclophosphamide, or vincristine frequently complain that nothing tastes right. Some patient experience a bitter or metallic taste.

NURSING INTERVENTIONS FOR ANOREXIA AND ALTERATION IN TASTE
1. Serve foods on glass dishes.
2. Use plastic utensils rather than metal.
3. Use good oral hygiene before meals.
4. Arrange foods attractively on the plate.
5. Provide pleasant, relaxed environment for eating meals.
6. Use pleasant odors, such as cloves.
7. Avoid noxious odors.
8. Serve cold foods rather than hot foods.
9. Provide small, frequent meals.
10. Administer antiemetics before meals.
11. Add salt or sugar to foods to increase palatability (Doyle, 1995).

Acute Reactions

Hypersensitivity and Anaphylaxis

Some chemotherapeutic agents have a potential for causing hypersensitivity with or without an anaphylactic response. The nurse should be knowledgeable about chemotherapy and which agents are prone to evoke hypersensitivity. An allergy history should be documented. The following are agents for which hypersensitivity reactions may occur:

Arthracycline antibiotics   Mephalan (IV)
L-asparaginase   Paclitaxel
Bleomycin   Procarbazine
Cisplatin   Teniposide
Mechlorethamine (topical)

If a drug is known to cause hypersensitivity reactions, a test dose should be administered. A patient also can be premedicated prophylactically with corticosteroids, histamine antagonists, or both to prevent reactions. Emergency equipment should be immediately accessible, including oxygen, AMBU respiratory assist bag, intubation equipment, and medications (i.e., epinephrine, 1:10,000 solution; diphenhydramine [Benadryl], 25 to 50 mg; methylprednisolone (Solu-Medrol), 30 to 60 mg; hydrocrotisone (Solu-Cortef), 100 to 500 mg; dexamethasone, 10 to 20 mg; aminophylline; and dopamine (Tipton & Skeel, 1995).

Extravasation

Extravasation of a vesicant agent is a major complication of an antineoplastic drug administration. As the vesicant escapes the vein, the patient may experience a burning sensation at the insertion site, redness, or swelling. In the days to weeks that follow, the site may become reddened, firm, and necrotic, leading to infection prolonged illness, and functional as well as cosmetic problems (Tipton & Skeel, 1995). Irritant drugs cause inflammation or pain at the site of insertion.

Vesicant agents that are commonly used include:

Dactinomycin (Actinomycin D)   Mechlorethamine (nitrogen mustard)
Daunorubicin (Daunomycin)   Vinblastine (Velban)
Doxorubicin (Adriamycin)   Vincristine (Oncovin)
Idarubicin (Idamycin)   Vindesine (Eldisine)
Plicamycin (Mithramycin, Mithracin)   Vinorelbine (Navelbine)
Mitomycin (Mutamycin)

Irritant agents include:

Carmustine (BCNUO)   Mitoxantrone (Novantrone)
Dacarbazine (DTIC)   Paclitaxel (Taxol)
Etoposide (VP-16)   Teniposide (VM-26)

Large extravasations of concentrated solutions of cisplatin and 5-FU may be considered irritants (Tipton & Skeel, 1995; see Chapter 9).

Management

The management of patients with extravasated vesicants is controversial, with disagreements in the literature on antidotes. See Table 14–10 for general procedure if extravasation is suspected.

✎ NOTE: *The most effective management of extravasation is prevention.*

A complaint of pain or burning should be considered a symptom of extravasation until proved otherwise. Extravasation kits with the necessary drug antidotes and supplies are helpful (Table 14–11).

513

TABLE 14–10. GENERAL PROCEDURE FOR EXTRAVASATION

1. Stop administration of chemotherapeutic agent.
2. Leave needle in place and immobilize the extremity.
3. Aspirate any residual drug left in the tubing, the needle, or the suspected extravasation site; infiltrate the antidote, if ordered.
4. Remove the needle.
5. Avoid applying pressure to the extravasation site.
6. Photograph the suspected area.
7. Apply warm or cold compresses as indicated.
8. Elevate the arm.
9. Notify the physician.
10. Document the condition of site and treatment of extravasation thoroughly.

Stomatitis and Mucositis

The oral mucosa is vulnerable to the effects of chemotherapy. The likelihood of developing stomatitis from a drug depends on the agent, the dose, and the schedule of administration. Continuous rather than intermittent administration is more likely to cause stomatitis with antimetabolites (Tipton & Skeel, 1995).

Specific antineoplastic agents that may cause stomatitis include plant alkaloids (vincristine, vinblastine, etoposide), antimetabolites (methotrexate 5-FU, cytarabine), antitumor antibiotics (doxorubicin, dactinomycin, mitoxantrone, mitomycin, bleomycin), miscellaneous agents (hydroxyurea), and biologic agents (interleukins, lymphokine-activated killer [LAK] cell therapy).

Management of Oral Complications

It is important to implement good oral hygiene before initiating chemotherapy. The primary goal is prevention; however, when oral complications develop, the focus of care should be treatment of symptoms and continued good oral care. Patients with poor dental hygiene are more likely to develop stomatitis. Predisposing factors for stomatitis include poor oral hygiene, poor nutritional status, head and neck radiation, concurrent corticosteroid therapy, and high doses of chemotherapy (Doyle, 1995).

TABLE 14–11. RECOMMENDED EXTRAVASTION KIT CONTENTS

3-mL disposable syringe
5-mL disposable syringe
10-mL disposable syringe
1-mL disposable tuberculin syringe
Several disposable needles: 25-gauge × 5/8 inch (need separate one for each subcutaneous injection)
Luer-lock caps
Alcohol wipes
Cold and warm packs
Sterile surgical latex gloves
Sterile water for injection in 10-mL vial
Hyaluronidase 150 U/vial
Sodium thiosulfate (25%) for 50-mL vial
Other antidotes per protocol

Source: From Angel, F.S. (1995). Current controversies in chemotherapy administration. *Journal of Intravenous Nursing, 18* (1). 16–23, with permission.

TABLE 14–12. **AGENTS FOR ORAL CARE**

Oral Agent	Effects
Cleansing Agents	
Normal saline solution (1/2 tsp salt in 8 oz of water)	Economical, nondamaging
Hydrogen peroxide	Dilute with normal saline or tap water; germicidal, debriding
Sodium bicarbonate	Nonirritating, neutralizing acid in mouth
Lubricating Agents	
Saliva substitutes	Decrease dryness, similar to human saliva
Water- or oil-based lubricants	Useful emollient; oil-based lubricants should not be used in mouth owing to danger of aspiration
Analgesic Agents	
Healing/coating agents	
Sucralfate	Binds to mucosa, forms protective coating
Vitamin E	Protection to mucosa has healing properties
Tannic acid (Zilactin Medicated Gel)	Reduces discomfort by coating; is safe
Topical anesthetics	
Lidocaine viscous	Transient pain relief, absorbed systematically
Dyclonine	Transient pain relief, minimal systemic absorption
Benzocaine	Transient pain relief, minimal systemic absorption

Source: From Tipton, J.M. & Skeel, R.T. (1995). Management of acute side effects of cancer chemotherapy. In Skeel, R.T., & Lanchant, N.A. (eds.). *Handbook of cancer chemotherapy*, 4th ed. Boston: Little, Brown, 583, with permission.

✎ **NOTE:** Commercial mouthwashes and lemon glycerin swabs are not recommended for use because of their irritating and drying effects (Tipton & Skeel, 1995).

Patients should be instructed to eat soft foods with a smooth consistency. Cold, wet foods are soothing to irritated mucous membranes. Keeping the lips moistened with lip balm, aloe vera, or a petroleum-based gel promotes comfort and healing for dry, cracked lips (Table 14–12).

Nausea and Vomiting

Over the past 10 years, there have been many improvements in the prevention and control of nausea and vomiting. Nausea and vomiting are major complications of chemotherapy administration. For many patients it is the most distressing symptom that interferes with quality of life. Studies have shown that approximately 70% of all cancer patients receiving chemotherapy experience nausea and vomiting (Goodman, 1987). Uncontrolled nausea and vomiting can lead to severe fatigue and discomfort, fluid and electrolyte imbalances, nutritional problems, and gastroesophageal tears, and it may affect patient compliance with therapy (Angel, 1993).

Assessment

Patients with a history of motion sickness or morning sickness are more prone to chemotherapy-induced nausea and vomiting. Prior exposure to chemotherapy may stimulate anticipatory nausea and vomiting, especially in younger women. En-

515

tering the outpatient waiting room or hearing the sound of an I.V. pole may result in the patient's experiencing nausea. Multiple assessment scales have been used to measure nausea. Because of the subjective element, measurement is not always clear-cut (Doyle, 1995). The goal of therapy is to prevent the three phases of nausea and vomiting: (1) anticipatory (occurring prior to treatment), (2) acute (occurring the first 24 hours after treatment), and (3) delayed (occurring more than 24 hours after treatment).

NURSING INTERVENTIONS FOR NAUSEA AND VOMITING

Interventions such as hard candy and sour or tart foods such as lemons are helpful in controlling nausea. Avoiding fatty foods or foods with strong odor can decrease nausea and vomiting.

Acupressure in the form of bracelets positioned on the wrist over the acupressure point that controls nausea is a noninvasive, nontoxic intervention and is helpful for the patient who is only slightly nauseated or who is reluctant to take antiemetics (Dundee, Ghaly, Bill, et al., 1990).

Pharmacologic interventions include administration of antiemetics such as anticholinergics, antihistamines, barbiturates, benzodiazepines, benzoquinolizines, butyrophenones, cannabinoids, phenothiazines, corticosteroids, and substituted benzamides (Angel, 1993; Table 14–13). Most of these antiemetics cause sedation or extrapyramidal symptoms. A new class of antiemetics that is selective for serotonin antagonist receptors, ondansetron (Zofran), given orally or I.V., has demonstrated its efficacy in alleviating nausea and vomiting without the undesirable side effects of extrapyramidal symptoms (Evans, Harvey, & Mak, 1991).

✎ **NOTE:** Ondansetron (Zofran), I.V. or oral, is used frequently to control nausea.

Myelosuppression

Myelosuppression is the most common dose-limiting factor in administration of antineoplastic therapy. All antineoplastic agents have some effect on blood counts, but certain drugs or dose escalations can result in severe myelosupression. Doses of chemotherapeutic agents are escalated until myelosuppression is achieved. Patients at risk for prolonged myelosuppression include elderly patients with aplastic marrow, patients with bone marrow involvement, patients with prior radiation to the flat bones, patients heavily pretreated with chemotherapy, and patients with neoplastic infiltrates.

Neutropenia

Neutropenia (diminished number of neutrophils in the blood) predisposes the patient to infection, an absolute granulocyte count (AGC) of 1500 to 2000/μL puts the patient at a moderate risk for infection. An AGC lower than 500/μL places the patient at a severe risk for infection. Such patients should be started on broad-spectrum antibiotics within 12 hours of a drop in WBC count. Leukopenia is a drop in WBC count below 5000/μL. With the neutropenic patient, the only sign of infection may be an elevated temperature.

✎ **NOTE:** Antipyretic agents should be used with caution in patients with leukopenia so as not to mask infection.

Although major medical advances have resulted in improved survival rate, serious infections continue to place the immunocompromised patient at risk. Infection, together with neutropenia, is regarded as an emergency situation.

TABLE 14–13. ANTIEMETICS COMMONLY USED FOR PREVENTION AND TREATMENT OF CHEMOTHERAPY-INDUCED NAUSEA AND VOMITING

Agent	Route of Administration	Dosage (Adult)	Comments
Phenothiazines			
Prochlorperazine (Compazine)	PO PO sustained-release IV (slow) PR	10–20 mg q4–6h 10–30 mg q12h 2–10 mg q4h 25 mg q8–12h	Some extrapyramidal reactions; potential for severe postural hypotension when the agent is given I.V.; closely observe the patient and assist when getting out of bed or sitting up
Thiethylperazine (Torecan)	PO or PR IM	10 mg q4–6h 2 mg q4–6h	Some extrapyramidal reactions
Trimethobenzamide (Tigan)	PO IM or PR	250 mg q4–6h 200 mg q4–6h	Some extrapyramidal reactions
Butyrophenones			
Haloperidol (Haldol)	IV	1–3 mg q2–4h for 2–3 doses	Some extrapyramidal reactions
Substituted benzamide			
Metoclopramide (Reglan)	PO IV over 20 minutes	10–40 mg q6h 1–2 mg/kg at 2-hour intervals	Extrapyramidal reactions common particularly at higher doses; worse in younger patients; diarrhea may occur
Benzodiazepines			
Lorazepam (Ativan)	IM, IV, or PO	1–2 mg q4–6h	Sedation frequent; patients advised not to drive for 24 hours after taking

TABLE 14–13. ANTIEMETICS COMMONLY USED FOR PREVENTION AND TREATMENT OF CHEMOTHERAPY-INDUCED NAUSEA AND VOMITING (*Continued*)

Agent	Route of Administration	Dosage (Adult)	Comments
Steroids			
Dexamethasone (Decadron, Hexadrol)	IV or PO	10–20 mg to start, then 4 mg PO q6h in tapering doses	Potential for agitation, delirium, gastrointestinal bleeding
5-HT3 antagonists			
Ondansetron (Zofran)	IV over 15 minutes	6 mg/m^2 (0.15 mg/kg) prior to and at 4 and 8 hours after chemotherapy *or* 10–30 mg prior to chemotherapy	For highly emetogenic therapy; may be a mild headache and mild transient transaminase elevations; lower doses effective for less emetogenic regimens
	PO	8 mg 2–3 times in 24 hours	For moderately emetogenic therapy
Granisetron (Kytril)	IV	0.4 mg/m^2 (10 μg/kg) prior to chemotherapy	Similar to ondansetron, for highly emetogenic therapy
	PO	2 mg prior to *or* 1 mg q12h on days of chemotherapy	For moderately emetogenic therapy
Cannabinoids			
Dronabinol (Marinol)	PO	2.5–10.0 mg PO q6h	May be habit-forming; a controlled substance

IM = intramuscularly; PO = orally; PR = per rectum
Source: From Tipton, J.M., & Skeel, R.T. (1995). Management of acute side effects of cancer chemotherapy. In Skeel, R.T., & Lachant, N.A. (eds.). *Handbook of cancer chemotherapy*, 4th ed. Boston: Little, Brown, with permission.

Precautions are usually initiated when the patient's AGC is less than 1000/μL. The AGC can be calculated by the following formula.

$$AGC = total\ WBC \times (\%\ of\ segs\ +\ \%\ of\ bands)$$

PRECAUTIONS FOR NEUTROPENIC PATIENT

Place the patient in a private room with door closed at all times.

Place "Neutropenic Precaution" sign on door.

Place patient on low microbial neutropenic diet (serve only cooked food; avoid unpared fresh fruits, raw vegetables, and garnishes).

Upon entering and leaving the patient's room, *all persons must consistently and thoroughly wash hands.*

Prohibit patient contact by staff and visitors with transmissible illness.

Avoid contact with persons who have recently been vaccinated with live or attenuated virus vaccines.

Avoid exposure to stagnant water (e.g., denture cups, soap dishes, flower vases, water pitchers, respiratory equipment, and irrigation containers); stagnant water provides medium for *Pseudomonas aeruginosa.*

Prohibit fresh flowers, plants, or fresh fruit baskets (soil is source of *Staphylococcus marcescens*)

Assess patient's oral mucosa every 12 hours for stomatitis and skin for infection breakdown, lesions, and rashes.

Prevent rectal trauma by avoiding suppositories and enemas.

Assess for changes in neurologic function every 4 hours; central nervous system changes are often the first indicator of sepsis).

Avoid insertion of indwelling urinary catheters.

Assess I.V. site at least once per shift for signs of phlebitis.

Monitor patient's vital signs every 4 hours around the clock.

Use strict sterile technique when performing invasive procedures.

✎ **NOTE:** Notify the physician immediately of any indicators of impending infection; sepsis progresses rapidly in the immunocompromised patient.

Thrombocytopenia

A normal platelet count ranges from 150,000 to 400,000/μL. When the count is below 50,000/μL, there is a concern for the potential of bleeding. Values of 20,000 to 30,000/μL warrant closer watching. Presenting signs of a problem include bleeding gums, petechiae, nosebleeds, and multiple bruises. If the platelet count is below 20,000/μL, spontaneous frank bleeding can occur. Thrombocytopenia places the patient at risk for central nervous system bleeding, as well as gastrointestinal bleeding. The use of platelet transfusions for a nonbleeding patient is controversial. Some authorities recommend holding transfusions until the patient shows signs of bleeding, whereas others transfuse a patient when the platelet count is below 20,000/μL (Goodman, 1989; Rostad, 1991). Interventions include protecting the patient from unnecessary bleeding risks.

NURSING INTERVENTIONS FOR THROMBOCYTOPENIA

Encourage shaving with an electric razor.

Advise patient to avoid use of tampons.

Advise patient to avoid hazardous activity that may cause injury (contact sports and working with sharp instruments).

Avoid invasive procedures such as enemas and taking rectal temperatures.

Avoid use of aspirin-containing products and products with ibuprofen and indomethacin.

519

Anemia

A patient is considered anemic if the hemoglobin level is lower than 8 g/dL. Anemic patients may be asymptomatic or may present with headache, dizziness, light-headedness, shortness of breath, fatigue, pallor, hypothermia, and pale nailbeds and conjunctiva.

When fatigue is a factor, patients should be instructed to plan rest periods around activities. Weekly CBCs are needed to adjust dosage of a chemotherapeutic agent, depending on the nadir. The nadir count is usually the point at which the blood counts are the lowest and this is usually 7 to 14 days after the first day of chemotherapy (but is drug-specific). Refer to individual drug literature for specific information on nadirs of chemotherapeutic drugs (Phillips & Kuhn, 1996).

It is important to obtain blood counts just before administration of chemotherapy because of bone marrow depression. That is, chemotherapy affects the stem cells in the bone marrow, which are rapidly dividing, rather than the cells in the circulation, which have reached maturity. Most protocols require the WBC count to be at least $3000/\mu L$ with an AGC of $1500/\mu L$ (Doyle, 1995).

Toxicities

Neurotoxicity

Neurotoxicity can be an acute or chronic encephalopathy of the central nervous system or a peripheral degeneration. Peripheral neuropathy can cause considerable sensory and motor disability. The most common agents that cause neurotoxicity are paclitaxel (Taxol), cisplatin, carboplatin, and vinca alkaloids.

Patients usually complain of numbness and tingling of the hands and feet as beginning symptoms. As toxicity increases, patients complain of muscle pain, weakness, and disturbances in depth perception. Other symptoms are decreased sensation, constipation, and paralytic ileus. The symptoms, depending on severity, usually disappear in a few weeks (Lundquist & Holmes, 1993).

Because of decreased sensation, the patient with neurotoxicity and the family must be aware of safety issues. The decrease in sensation causes concern for caution with temperature changes (e.g., hot water, heating pads, electric blankets, hot stoves, and radiators). Exposure to cold is also a concern because these patients are less likely to realize the severity of the temperature.

Cardiac Toxicity (Congestive Cardiomyopathy)

The anthracyclines, especially doxorubicin or daunorubicin, can cause cardiotoxicity. Certain other chemotherapeutic agents, such as pacitaxel, mitoxantrone, idarubicin, cyclophosphamide, 5-FU, and 5-FU deoxyribonucleoside (FUDR) have also shown potential for cardiac toxicity. Early signs of cardiotoxicity include decrease in voltage of QRS complex and nonspecific ST- or T-wave change. The heart muscle becomes weakened, resulting in a decreased cardiac output with progression to congestive heart failure. These symptoms are difficult to diagnose. Frequent ECG monitoring to detect changes in voltage of the QRS helps to identify early signs of toxicity. Also, a baseline MUGA scan or an echocardiogram with an ejection fraction prior to known cardiotoxic chemotherapeutic agents administration and then repeat these tests at the halfway point of the total accumulated lifetime dose of drug monitors for cardiac toxicities.

Risk factors for cardiac damage are hypertension, arteriosclerosis, coronary artery disease, and prior radiation to mediastinum. (Rowinsky, McGuire, & Guarnieri, et al., 1991).

✎ **NOTE:** Because of the large number of women with breast cancer who are treated with doxorubicin as part of an adjuvant chemotherapy regimen, this group is of special concern and warrants ongoing clinical follow-up (Skeel & Ganz, 1995).

✎ **NOTE:** Dexrazoxane (Zinecard) for injection, a drug, is being used as a cardio-protective agent after administration of cumulative doses of doxorubicin. Since this drug is always given with cytotoxic drugs, the patients should be monitored closely. Dextrazoxane may add to the myelosuppression caused by chemotherapeutic agents and should not be used with chemotherapy regimens that do not contain an anthracycline (Pharmacia, 1995).

Pulmonary Toxicity

Toxicity to the pulmonary tissue damages the endothelial cells of the lung and results in pneumonitis and interstitial fibrosis. The agents that predispose the patient to pulmonary toxicity are bleomycin in doses exceeding 250 U/m^2 or 400 U total dose and carmustine in total doses of 1500 mg/m^2. Other antineoplastic agents known to be responsible for pulmonary toxicity are mitomycin, methotrexate, melphalan, procarbazine, and busulfan. Some combination therapies can increase the risk of pulmonary toxicity.

Symptoms of pulmonary toxicity include dry hacking cough, complaints of dyspnea, and crackles in the lungs upon ausculation. Patients at risk for this complication include patients who smoke and patients with previous pulmonary conditions. Evaluation of high-risk patients involves a pulmonary function test. The chemotherapeutic drug should be discontinued at the first sign of this complication. Corticosteroids have been used in treatment of symptomatic relief of pulmonary toxicity (Jensen, Goel, & Venner, 1990).

Renal Toxicity

Renal toxicity is defined as an elevation of the BUN and creatinine levels. Agents that cause renal damage are cisplatin, methotrexate, mitomycin, and carboplatin.

✎ **NOTE:** Renal toxicity is a life-threatening complication. The risk of renal compromise versus renal toxic agents that could produce a meaningful tumor response must be weighed carefully. Vigorous hydration is required before administration of agents that are nephrotoxic.

Hypertonic sodium chloride solution helps to maintain a high renal flow. Mannitol and furosemide (Lasix) may be ordered in an effort to flush the kidneys. Accurate intake and output as well as frequent weights must be recorded.

The risk of hyperuricemia from tumor lysis syndrome is another factor that needs to be considered when administering nephrotoxic drugs. Alkalizing the urine prevents the precipitation of uric acid crystals, and the administration of allopurinol helps to prevent their formation. Prophylactic measures begin 12 to 24 hours before chemotherapy (Lydon, 1986).

ROUTES OF ADMINISTRATION

Chemotherapy is administered by a variety of routes. The route chosen is an important variable in optimal drug delivery within the body, in minimizing side effects, and in maintaining the person's level of functioning. The oral route is used for drugs that are well absorbed and nonirritating to the gastrointestinal tract.

521

Systemic Routes

Intravenous Route

The I.V. route is the most common route of chemotherapy administration and has two advantages. First, the I.V. route achieves a therapeutic blood level quickly. Second, most chemotherapeutic agents are not absorbed in the gastrointestinal tract, making the I.V. route more desirable. The subcutaneous and intramuscular routes, used commonly for delivery of other drugs, have limitations with anticancer drug therapy because of the chemotherapeutic drug's irritation of the tissues. Other methods are used that eliminate or reduce tissue irritation (Table 14–14).

Intrathecal Route

Other routes are used when delivery of a drug is required to pass the blood-brain barrier. The intrathecal route allows the drugs to be given directly into the cerebrospinal fluid. Methotrexate and cytosine arabinoside are most commonly given by this route in treating central nervous system leukemia and carcinomatosis meningitis (see Chapter 11).

Regional Routes

Intra-arterial Route

Chemotherapy administered through the intra-arterial route allows for high concentrations of antineoplastic agents to be delivered directly into tumor sites by means of arterial catheters or devices. A temporary catheter is placed via percutaneous angiography for carotid, brachial, femoral, or specific limb artery for short-term therapies (from hours to 5 days). This therapy is repeated by means of a new catheter insertion each time for 3 to 6 months of therapy.

An implantable arterial port is placed subcutaneously near the tumor site over a bony surface and sutured in place; the catheter is then threaded into the tumor artery site. The port is accessed via a noncoring needle, covered with a transparent dressing, and connected to a heparinized saline solution via an infusion pump (Stair & McNally, 1992).

✎ NOTE: Implantable arterial ports must be flushed with heparin weekly to maintain catheter patency if a continuous infusion solution is not being administered.

TABLE 14–14. **METHODS OF DELIVERING ANTINEOPLASTIC AGENTS**

Systemic Routes
    Intravenous
        Indwelling silastic catheters
        Peripherally inserted central lines
        Implanted ports
    Intrathecal

Regional Routes
    Intra-arterial
    Intraperitoneal
    Cerebrospinal reservoirs

KEY POINTS IN NURSING CARE OF INTRA-ARTERIAL INFUSIONS

Intra-arterial drug infusion requires astute clinical observations and interventions.

Percutaneous arterial catheters have the potential for restricting tissue perfusion.

Insertion site and affected extremity should be observed every 2 to 4 hours.

Monitor vital signs.

Femoral catheter placement requires bedrest with log-rolling to maintain catheter alignment.

Brachial catheter placement requires immobilizing the affected extremity.

All chemotherapy supplies should have Luer-lock connections, and infusion pumps may require a higher pounds per square inch PSI setting to overcome arterial flow resistance (ONS, 1989).

Intraperitoneal Route

Intracavitary drug administration instills drugs directly into body cavities, such as the bladder, peritoneum, pleura, and pericardium. This technique is used most frequently to control malignant effusions, but it is also used for localized malignancies (ONS, 1992).

Infusions via the intraperitoneal route (IP) involves the administration of therapeutic agents directly into the peritoneal cavity (Fig. 14–2). Many studies have confirmed the advantages of this approach to chemotherapeutic management of cancer (Dedrick, 1985; McClay & Howell, 1990).

The purpose of IP therapy is to increase the concentration of the antineoplastic agent at the tumor site, in this case the peritoneal cavity, to enhance its penetration and cell kill while limiting systemic effects. The peritoneal cavity acts as a reservoir for the drug. The goal is to decrease systemic toxic effects and increase the antitumor action of the antineoplastic agent (Zook-Enck, 1990). Chemotherapeutic agents that are delivered via the I.P. route include cisplatin, cytosine arabinoside, doxorubicin, and 5-FU.

✎ NOTE: For I.P. administration to be effective, the patient must have limited intra-abdominal adhesions.

KEY POINTS IN I.P. THERAPY

The disease must be limited to the body region in which the antineoplastic agent is administered.

There are three types of IP access devices: temporary indwelling catheter, IP implantable port, and indwelling Tenckhoff catheter (Table 14–15).

Nursing staff must be well prepared to care for an IP catheter.

Nurse and family must be familiar with the therapeutic effects of antineoplastic agents.

ADVANTAGES

When not in use, the IP device is invisible, enhancing a positive body image.

There is no catheter site care.

Cytotoxic drugs are administered directly to tumor area (Malloy, 1991).

DISADVANTAGES

It can be difficult to locate and access the port.

Catheter infections can occur.

Build-up of fibrin sheath can occur on the distal catheter tip (McClay & Howell, 1990).

Abdominal adhesions can cause spaces in the cavity, preventing the flow of the infusion.

523

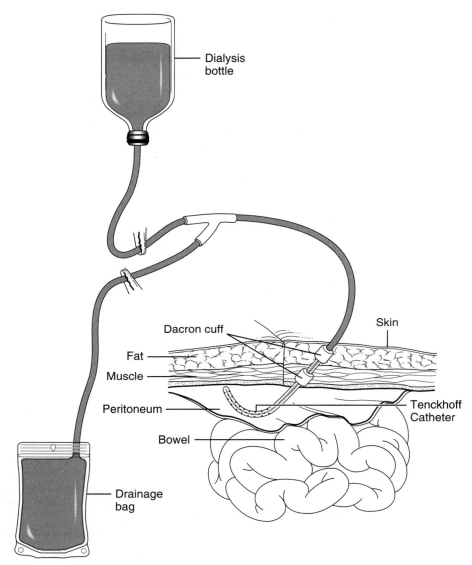

Figure 14–2. Intraperitoneal infusion via a Tenckhoff catheter directly into the peritoneal cavity.

KEY NURSING CONSIDERATIONS IN IP THERAPY
1. Maintain strict sterile technique; wash hands with antimicrobial solution before handling system.
2. Scrub all connectors with povidone-iodine.
3. Use sterile gloves when separating a connection.
4. Minimize accessing the system when possible.
5. Be aware that a fibrin sheath may build up on the distal catheter tip, resulting in a one-way flow problem. The injection of solution may be easily performed but withdrawal of solution is difficult (Howell, 1990).

TABLE 14–15. **ADVANTAGES AND DISADVANTAGES OF IP MANAGEMENT METHODS**

Advantages	Disadvantages
Temporary Catheter	
1. May be inserted at bedside	1. Increases risk of bowel or visceral
2. Does not require surgical procedure for removal	perforation
3. Is inexpensive	2. Requires extra precautions for removal to prevent displacement
4. Decreases risk of infection and bibrous sheath formation because it is temporary	when patient is mobile
IP Implantable Port	
1. Serves as a semipermanent access device	1. Requires use of the operating room for insertion
2. Decreases risk of bowel or visceral perforation when inserted during laparotomy	2. Requires surgical procedure for removal
3. Decreases risk of infection	3. Is expensive
4. Provides a greater chance of patient acceptance because there is no external catheter	4. Does not allow for high-pressure, forced irrigation or manipulation
	5. Requires a needle stick with each access
Indwelling Tenckhoff Catheter	
1. Serves as a semipermanent access device	1. Requires use of the operating room for insertion
2. Decreases the risk of bowel and visceral perforation	2. Increases the risk of infection
3. Is inexpensive	3. Requires catheter home care by the patient
4. Allows for high-pressure, forced irrigation, and manipulation to dislodge or loosen fibrin clots	4. May create body image changes with long-term use
5. Permits rapid instillation of fluid	
6. Permits rapid drainage of peritoneal fluid	
7. Is easy to remove without surgical procedure	
8. May be preferred for the obese patient	

Source: Adapted from Zook-Enck, D. (1990). Intraperitoneal therapy via the Tenckhoff catheter. *Journal of Intravenous Nursing, 13* (6), 375–382, with permission.

6. Irrigate catheter well before and after administering therapy or withdrawing or draining peritoneal fluid with 3 to 50 mL of normal saline (Piccart, Speyer, & Markman, 1985).
7. Ensure that administration and drainage tubing is free of kinks.
8. Maintain a sterile dressing in the hospital environment; for home care, maintain a clean and dry dressing.
9. Teach patient and family care of the dressing for home care.
10. If using Tenckhoff catheter, allow Dacron cuffs to heal for at least 1 to 2 weeks before initiating IP therapy.
11. Warm IP solution with dry heat to approximately 100°F before treatment. Approximately 200 mL drug or solution will infuse in 30 to 60 minutes.
12. Monitor vital signs and intake and output, measure abdominal girth, ascultate bowel sounds, and palpate the abdomen for rebound tenderness.

13. Observe catheter site for signs of infection and for peritonitis, which can be a significant concern (Otto, 1995).

Cerebrospinal Fluid Reservoirs

Intraventricular chemotherapy allows for the administration of antineoplastic agents into the cerebrospinal fluid via an Ommaya reservoir (Baxter, Illinois; Fig. 14–3). A physician must place the ventricular reservoir. The nurse administering medications into the reservoir must follow the Nurse Practice Act for the state in which he or she practices. An Ommaya reservoir is a silicone rubber device that is implanted surgically under the scalp and provides access to cerebrospinal fluid through a burr hole in the skull. Drugs are injected into the reservoir with a hypodermic syringe, then the domed reservoir is depressed manually to mix drug with the cerebrospinal fluid.

KEY POINTS IN DELIVERY OF CHEMOTHERAPY VIA A VENTRICULAR RESERVOIR
The patient should be taught the purpose of the reservoir.
When accessing the ventricular reservoir, wear sterile gloves and mask.
Use only preservative-free medications.

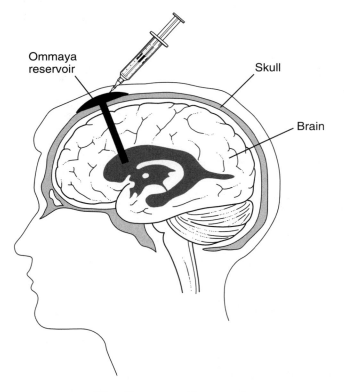

The Ommaya Reservoir.

Figure 14–3. Intraventricular chemotherapy administration (Source: Otto, S.E. [1995]. Advanced concepts in chemotherapy drug delivery regional therapy. *Journal of Intravenous Nursing, 18* (4), 170–176, with permission.)

Aspirate to check placement before drug delivery; spinal fluid should be present. Withdrawal of spinal fluid for diagnostic purpose is a medical act.

ADVANTAGES
Well tolerated
Eliminates need for multiple lumbar punctures

DISADVANTAGE
Increased risk of infection to spinal cord and brain

Infusion Pumps

Infusion pumps have been widely used in chemotherapy administration to provide continuous or intermittent drug delivery. These pumps are essential in intra-arterial administration, in which the drug must be given against arterial pressure, but they are used in delivery of antineoplastic agents by all routes.

Pumps are available as nonportable and portable. Nonportable pumps are usually designed to clamp onto an I.V. pole and are quite bulky; these are used in hospital or outpatient clinics. The compact, battery-operated portable pumps have enabled individuals to receive continuous chemotherapy on an outpatient or home care basis (Garvey, 1987).

When choosing an ambulatory infusion pump, several factors need to be considered for delivery of chemotherapy.

- The insurance coverage for ambulatory infusion therapy: cost pump, tubing, medication reservoirs
- Size and weight of pump
- Pump mechanism
- Delivery mode: continuous or intermittent
- Flow rate parameters
- Power source
- Access for individuals and families to health care provider on a 24-hour basis in the event of pump failure
- Pump choice dependent on the individual's manual dexterity, learning ability, and anxiety level (Schulmeister, 1992)

Pumps are covered in detail in Chapter 7.

SUMMARY OF KEY POINTS IN THE ADMINISTRATION OF ANTINEOPLASTIC AGENTS
1. Adequately assess the patient's venous status; examine both arms for phlebitis, bruises, or inflammation.
2. Discuss with patient any past problems experienced since last treatment.
3. Alternate arms with each chemotherapy administration.
4. Use sterile technique; be aware that the patient might have a compromised WBC count.
5. Meticulously prepare the site.
6. Do not use an extremity with compromised circulation, such as one with an invading neoplasm, existing phlebitis, varicosities, the side of a previous mastectomy, immobilized fracture, or inflamed areas.
7. Assess patency of vein with 10 to 20 mL of normal saline before infusing cytotoxic agent.
8. Mix chemotherapy drugs according to manufacturer's recommendations.
9. Tell the patient to inform you immediately if there is a feeling of burning or stinging at the infusion site.

527

10. Be constantly aware of a slow leak or insidious infiltration.
11. Use a final flush of 0.9% sodium chloride after the chemotherapeutic agent is infused to clear the drug from peripheral vein.
12. Follow OSHA 1995 standards for disposal of cytotoxic agents. See Appendix D for guidelines for personnel dealing with cytotoxic drugs. (Camp-Sorrell, 1991; Weinstein, 1993).

Nursing Plan of Care

ANTINEOPLASTIC THERAPY

Focus Assessment

Subjective	*Objective*
Interview patient regarding previous experience with chemotherapy.	Assess for nausea and vomiting.
Determine level of knowledge regarding chemotherapy and cancer.	Inspect oral cavity daily.
	Assess breath sounds.
	Monitor vital signs.
	Note type of cancer, length of illness, prognosis, previous chemotherapy.
	Assess nutritional status.
	Review laboratory data.
	Assess urinary output and hydration level.

Nursing Diagnoses

Altered nutrition less than body requirements, related to consequences of treatment

Risk for noncompliance with dietary restrictions of chemotherapy, related to no alcohol while on methotrexate, no foods high in tyramines while on procarbazine

Risk for fluid volume deficit related to excessive losses through vomiting, diarrhea, wounds, or impaired oral intake

Oral mucous membrane altered, related to side effects of chemotherapeutic agents (antimetabolites)

Risk for skin and tissue integrity impaired, related to effects of chemotherapy, immunologic deficit, altered nutritional state or anemia, or presence of lesions, drug extravasation

Risk for gas exchange impaired, related to alveolar membrane thickening (pulmonary fibrosis) altered blood flow or decreased circulation or altered oxygen carrying capacity

Fear and anxiety related to situational crisis, threat to or change in health and socioeconomic status, role functioning, interaction patterns, threat of death, separation from family

Knowledge deficit related to lack of exposure or recall, information misinterpretation, myths, unfamiliarity with resources

Outcome Criteria

The patient will:

Demonstrate stable weight or progressive weight gain toward goal and be free of signs of malnutrition

Demonstrate normalization of laboratory values

Demonstrate that antinausea medications are effective

Comply with dietary restrictions

Display adequate fluid balance

Display moist mucous membranes

Demonstrate techniques to maintain and restore integrity of oral mucosa

Continued on following page

Outcome Criteria
Identify interventions for specific condition; prevent complication promote healing as appropriate
Demonstrate adequate oxygenation of tissues by arterial blood gas values within patient's normal range
Be free of respiratory distress
Display appropriate range of feelings
Verbalize accurate information about diagnosis and treatment regimen
Initiate necessary lifestyle changes and participate in treatment regimen

Nursing Management: Critical Activities
Monitor for side effects and toxic effects of chemotherapeutic agent.
Institute neutropenic and bleeding precautions when necessary.
Offer bland, easily digested diet.
Administer antiemetic medication.
Administer chemotherapeutic drugs in the late evening so the patient may sleep at the time emetic effects are greatest.
Monitor for adequate fluid intake, dehydration, and electrolyte imbalance.
Monitor for effectiveness of measures to control nausea and vomiting; assist patient in obtaining a wig or other head covering device as appropriate.
Offer six small feedings daily.
Ascertain that I.V. is infusing well; dilute antineoplastic agents.
Administer appropriate antidotes per protocol and physician's orders if extravastion occurs.
Avoid use of commercial mouthwash products that contain alcohol or phenol and may increase mucous membrane discomfort; use mouthwash made from warm saline and dilute solution of hydrogen peroxide or baking soda and water.
Administer analgesics and topical xylocaine jelly, or antimicrobial mouthwash, or both (e.g., nystatin) as needed for stomatitis.
Monitor nutritional status and weight.
Minimize stimuli from noises, light, and odors, especially food.
Follow recommended guidelines for safe handling of parenteral antineoplastic drugs during drug preparation.

PATIENT EDUCATION

Inform the patient and family on how antineoplastic agents work on cancer cells.
Instruct patient and family about the effects of chemotherapy on bone marrow functioning.
Instruct patient and family on ways to prevent infection (e.g., avoiding crowds and using good hygiene and handwashing techniques).
Instruct on pretreatment hydration instruction sheet when appropriate.
Instruct to report promptly fever, chills, nosebleed, excessive bruising, tarry stools, severe headaches, or prolonged vomiting.
Inform to avoid aspirin products.
Instruct patient and family to monitor for signs and symptoms of stomatitis and to perform good oral hygiene.
Inform to avoid temperature extremes while receiving chemotherapy.
Inform that hair loss is expected as determined by type of chemotherapeutic agent.
Instruct to avoid hot, spicy foods.
Instruct patient and family to monitor for organ toxicity as determined by type of chemotherapeutic agent used.
Discuss with patient the possibility of sterility and other reproductive system impairments.

Inform long-term survivors and their families of the possibility of second malignancies and the importance of reporting increased susceptibility to infection, fatigue, or bleeding.
Instruct to avoid scratching skin.
(McCloskey & Bulechek, 1992)

HOME CARE ISSUES

In the past 10 to 15 years, treatment of cancer with chemotherapeutic agents have been done in the home setting (LaBell, O'Neil, & Bing, 1990). The most common antineoplastic agents given by the I.V. route for chemotherapy prescribed in the home are 5-FU and FUDR. Many other agents can be administered safely in the home care setting with the appropriate level of specialized clinical oncology support. Common issues of concern in delivery of chemotherapy in the home are as follows:

Patient and family education
Admixture
Transport of drug
Administration
Disposal
Monitoring
Disposal of excreta

Patient and Family Education

Family members must understand the nature of the risk of handling cytotoxic drugs. It is the professional health care team's responsibility on behalf of the agency to provide education regarding safe practices in handling these drugs. Potential risks to persons who come in contact with chemotherapy drugs and associated safety measures should be discussed with patient and family before the initial home chemotherapy treatment.

The Joint Commission for the Accreditation of Healthcare Organizations (JCAHO) 1995 has guidelines for home care, which address the use of hazardous substances in the home setting.

Admixture

Antineoplastic agents must be prepared in a biologic safety hood for protection during admixture; this task must be accomplished in a pharmacy.

Transport of Drug

In the home care situation, antineoplastic agents often are obtained by the family or nurse. The drugs are labeled as cytotoxic, capped securely, and sealed and packaged in an impervious packing material for transport. The outside of bags or bottles containing the prepared drug should be wiped with moist gauze. Entry ports should be wiped with moist alcohol pads and capped (OSHA, 1995). Transport should occur in sealed plastic bags and in containers designed to avoid breakage. The family should be cautioned to protect the package from breakage and taught the necessary procedures if a spill occurs. Spill kits should be available in the home care setting.

530

✎ **NOTE:** Personnel involved in transporting hazardous drugs should be trained in spill procedures, including sealing off the contaminated area and calling for appropriate assistance (OSHA, 1995).

Administration

The family member to administer the drug must be taught safe handling of chemotherapeutic agents, use of latex gloves, and how to handle the tubing or infusion pump during delivery of drug. The area of the patient's home designated for preparation of drug should be apart from the family activity area and food preparation. Ceiling fans, if present, should be turned off. A work surface area should be used which can be cleaned, such as a card table. All family members should remain outside the rooms in which the drugs are prepared and administered, if possible. Children should be cared for outside the home on the day of chemotherapy. All supplies should be assembled on a disposable, absorbent, plastic-backed pad that is taped over the work surface area. Only syringes, needles, and I.V. sets with Luer-lock fittings are used (Stair & McNally, 1992).

Administering aerosolized hazardous drugs requires special engineering controls to prevent exposure to health care workers and others (OSHA, 1995).

✎ **NOTE:** Handwashing should be stressed.

✎ **NOTE:** Peripheral access for administering vesicant agents in the home is discouraged.

Disposal

Needles, syringes, and breakable items not contaminated with blood or other infectious materials should be placed in a "sharps" container before being stored in the waste bag. Hazardous drug-related wastes should be handled separately from the trash and disposed of in accordance with the applicable Environmental Protection Agency (EPA) state and local regulations.

Monitoring

Clinical monitoring of the patient receiving chemotherapy at home demands close attention. Clinical monitoring should include laboratory values, physical status, fluid status, and drug-related side effects and toxicities (Grace & Tomaselli, 1995).

Disposal of Excreta

Cytotoxic activity of drugs and their metabolites can remain active in excreta for 48 hours or more. This special situation means that urine, feces, vomitus, and other excreta should be treated with caution, and the family should wear gloves when handling excreta, linens, or tissues. It is suggested that the dilution in most sewer systems is adequate to decrease risk to both family and environment. Sheets and other laundry soiled with excreta should be washed twice and kept separate from other family laundry (Stevens, 1989).

531

COMPETENCY CRITERIA: Administration of Antineoplastic Therapy

Competency Statement: The competent I.V. therapy nurse will be able to administer I.V. chemotherapy and follow guidelines for dealing with cytotoxic drug.

COGNITIVE CRITERIA

	Knowledgeable	Needs Education
1. Identifies 1995 OSHA standards for handling hazardous drugs.		
2. Identifies possible side effects: **Short Term:** Venous fragility Alopecia Diarrhea Altered nutritional status Anorexia and taste alterations **Acute Side Effects:** Hypersensitivity and anaphylaxis Extravasation Stomatitis Nausea and vomiting Myelosuppression		
3. Describes the procedure for treatment of extravasated drug.		

PERFORMANCE CRITERIA

	Skilled	Needs Education
1. Performs preinfusion assessment: Assesses previous response to drug therapy Laboratory data (WBC, AGC, platelet) Patient allergy history Physical assessment Assesses veins if I.V. access is to be established Calculates body surface area (BSA) or dose based on height and weight Explains procedure to patient		
2. Identifies correct dose, administration route, and rationale for administration: Verifies I.V. access patency		
3. Verifies physician order.		

532

4. **Differentiates vesicant and nonvesicant therapies.**

5. **Administers chemotherapy following set protocol:**
   Gathers supplies needed for chemotherapy administration

   Washes hands, dons gown and gloves, sets up work area.

   Checks patency by instilling 5–7 mL of saline

   Administers drug at prescribed rate

   Identifies frequency of I.V. patency checks

6. **Discontinues antineoplastic therapy safely:**
   Explains procedure, washes hands, gathers equipment

   States procedure for removing I.V. tubing from I.V.

   States procedure for removing and disposing of equipment

   Uses Luer-lock connections

7. **Documents performance of procedure and patient response**

SUGGESTED EVALUATION CRITERIA

Written test—cognitive

Return demonstration (administration techniques, management of extravasation)

Clinical preceptorship with demonstration and return demonstration

KEY POINTS

Role of clinician
   Certification available through ONS.
   Chemotherapy certification available at most institutions which deliver antineoplastic therapy
   Patient assessment and history
      Interview
         Knowledge of classification of cancer
         Symptoms
         Course of disease
         Past medical history
         Prior organ impairment
         Secondary diagnosis

533

Physical assessment
  Nutritional status
  Laboratory tests
  Diagnostic imaging studies
  Psychological state
  Spiritual state
Treatment objectives
  Curative goal—to successfully treat disease
  Palliative goal—to promote client comfort and quality of life
  Adjuvant goal—to enhance primary treatment

Cellular kinetics
Cell cycle
  G_0 Nonproliferative resting phase
  G_1 Presynthetic stage
  G_2 Interval after synthesis of DNA
  S Synthesis of DNA
  M Mitosis (G_2 cell divides into two cells)
Normal and malignant tissue growth
  Factors related during assessment of normal or tumor cells:
    1. Cell cycle time
    2. Growth fraction
    3. Total number of cells in population
    4. Rate of cell loss or number of cells that die or leave the cell population
Tumor cell kill
  Stem cells—regenerate the tumor cell population
  Non stem cells—differentiate and enter the maturing group of cells
As long as G_0 stem cells remain, a damaged cell population can be renewed. Certain drug doses destroy a constant fraction of tumor cells. (log-kill model)
  Drug resistance
    Factors
      Specific drug
      Specific tumor
      Specific host

Antineoplastic agents
Classifications
  Cell cycle-specific drugs
  Non–cell cycle-specific drugs
Drug dosing
  Based on
    Nomogram chart height and weight
  Body surface area (BSA)
Drug classes
  Alkylating agents
    Action: cell cycle-independent
    Major side effects: alopecia, bone marrow depression, nausea, vomiting, diarrhea
    Toxicity: cardiotoxicity (specific drugs), pancytopenia
  Antimetabolites
    Action: S phase of cell cycle
    Major side effects: gastrointestinal disturbances, stomatitis, esophagitis, elevated liver function tests, photosensitivity, severe nausea and vomiting
    Toxicities: myelosuppression

534

Natural products
> *Action:* cell cycle-specific
> *Major side effects:* tissue necrosis, neurotoxicities

Antibiotics
> *Action:* cell cycle-nonspecific
> *Major side effects:* cardiac toxicities, bone marrow suppression, arrhythmias, nausea, vomiting, stomatitis, hyperpigmentation of skin

Enzymes
> *Action:* G_1 phase of cell cycle
> *Major side effects:* fever, anorexia, nausea, vomiting, acute toxic reaction with elevated BUN and ammonia levels

Hormones and hormone antagonists
> Androgens
> Corticosteroids
> Estrogens
> Progestins
> Estrogen antagonist

Biologic response modifiers
> *Action:* bind to common receptors; role in inflammation; fever and tissue repair following injury
> *Major side effects:* usually dose-dependent; flu-like syndrome, cardiovascular complications, fluid overload

Colony-stimulating factors
> *Action:* Stimulate regrowth factor proliferative activity for bone marrow
> *Major side effects:* minimal; edema, hypertension in patients with renal failure

Monoclonal antibodies
> *Action:* Antibodies useful means of targeting cytotoxic radioisotopes, toxins or drugs to tumors.
> *Major side effects:* Hypotension, shortness of breath, risk of anapahylaxis.

Common side effects
Short-term complications
> Venous fragility
> Alopecia
> Diarrhea
> Constipation
> Altered nutritional status
> Anorexia and taste alteration

Acute side effects
> Hypersensitivity and anaphylaxis
> Extravasation
> Stomatitis and mucositis
> Nausea and vomiting
> Myelosuppression
>> Leukopenia
>> Thrombocytopenia
>> Anemia

Toxicities
> Neurotoxicity
> Cardiac toxicity
> Pulmonary toxicity
> Renal toxicity

535

Routes of administration
    Systemic route I.V.
    Intrathecal route
    Regional routes
        Intra-arterial
        Intraperitoneal
        Cerebrospinal fluid reservoirs

CRITICAL THINKING ACTIVITY

1. In your facility, locate the protocol for extravasation. Is there a specific extravasation kit available on your unit?

2. How does your facility deal with the neutropenic patient?

3. What criteria are used at your facility for competency in delivery of antineoplastic therapy?

4. Since cancer immunotherapy is still in a developmental stage, how is new information distributed in your facility?

Match the mode of action in column II to the antineoplastic class in column I.

Column I

1. _____ alkylating agents

2. _____ antimetabolites

3. _____ vinca alkaloids

4. _____ anthracycline antibiotics

5. _____ enzymes

Column II

A. Cell cycle-specific

B. Cell cycle-nonspecific

6. The goal of cancer immunotherapy is to:
   A. Produce remission
   B. Promote tumor-nonspecific immunity
   C. Stimulate immunocompetence in cancer patients
   D. Decrease the side effects of traditional chemotherapy

7. Mercaptopurine is an example of:
   A. Pyrimidine analogue
   B. Purine analogue
   C. Anthracycline antibiotic
   D. Alkylating agent

8. Identify key nursing interventions and assessments for patients receiving alkylating agents.

9. Identify key nursing interventions and assessment for patients receiving vinca alkaloids.

10. State two of the six short-term complications associated with antineoplastic therapy.

    A. _____

    B. _____

11. State the four toxicities associated with chemotherapy administration

    A. _____

    B. _____

    C. _____

    D. _____

12. A patient who is considered neutropenic has an absolute granulocyte count below:
    A. $10,000/\mu L$
    B. $4000/\mu L$
    C. $2000/\mu L$
    D. $1000/\mu L$

13. Pulmonary toxicity is associated with which of the following antineoplastic therapies?
    A. Bleomycin
    B. Paclitaxel
    C. Cisplatin
    D. Carboplatin

14. IP antineoplastic therapy delivers the drug directly into a/an:
    A. Artery
    B. Cavity
    C. Vein
    D. Ventricle

15. In a patient receiving doxorubicin (Adriamycin) via peripheral I.V. infusion, the nurse should monitor:
    A. ECG
    B. Uric acid levels
    C. Potassium levels
    D. Abdominal girth

16. When planning nursing care for a patient receiving vincristine intravenously, the following nursing intervention should be considered:
    A. Restirct fluids during treatment
    B. Limit dosage of acetaminophen
    C. Observe the I.V. site for drug infiltration
    D. Place patient on neutropenic precautions

17. When evaluating a patient for bone marrow depression related to BCNU therapy the nurse will do so:
    A. 2 days after the dose
    B. 14 days after the dose
    C. 3 to 6 weeks after the dose
    D. 2 months after the dose

18. Prior to administration of fluorouracil (5-FU), the nurse will check the following laboratory data:
    A. Sodium and potassium
    B. BUN and creatinine
    C. Liver enzymes and amylase
    D. WBC count and platelets

19. Cancer patients who experience anemia and thrombocytopenia have traditionally been treated with
    A. Antibiotic therapy
    B. Blood component therapy
    C. Corticosteroid therapy
    D. I.V. hydration therapy

20. Adverse effects of alkylating agents primarily are related to the:
    A. Gastrointestinal system
    B. Neurologic system
    C. Kidney
    D. Liver

ANSWERS TO CHAPTER 14

PRE-TEST

1. B
2. C
3. E
4. D
5. A
6. F
7. G_0 Nonproliferative phase
   G_1 Presynthesis phase
   G_2 Interval after synthesis
   S, Synthesis of DNA
   M, Mitosis cell divides

8. A
9. B
10. C
11. B
12. A
13. B
14. B
15. D
16. A
17. D
18. B

POST-TEST

1. B
2. A
3. A
4. B
5. A
6. C
7. B
8. Monitor I.V. sites for infiltration.
   Monitor CBC, platelets, liver enzymes.
   Administer antiemetics.
   Assess respiratory status if appropriate.
   Prehydrate.
   Assess oral cavity.
9. Assess oral mucosa.
   Assess infusion site for infiltration.
   Monitor CBC and platelets, cardiac
   enzymes, and ECG.
   Perform frequent neurologic checks when
   appropriate.
   Administer antiemetics.

10. Venous fragility
    Alopecia
    Diarrhea
    Altered nutritional status
    Anorexia and taste alterations
11. Neurotoxicity
    Cardiac toxicity
    Pulmonary toxicity
    Renal toxicity
12. D
13. A
14. B
15. A
16. C
17. C
18. D
19. B
20. A

REFERENCES

Angel, F.S. (1993). An overview of ondansetron for chemotherapy-induced nausea and emesis. *Journal of Intravenous Nursing, 16* (2), 84–89.

Angel, F.S. (1995). Current controversies in chemotherapy administration. *Journal of Intravenous Nursing, 18* (1), 16–23.

Baserga, R. (1981). The cell cycle. *New England Journal of Medicine, 301,* 454–459.

Camp-Sorrell, D. (1991). Controlling adverse effects of chemotherapy. *Nursing 91, 4,* 34–37.

Carter, S., Bakowski, H., & Hellman, K. (1987). *Chemotherapy of cancer,* 3rd ed. New York: John Wiley & Sons.

Dedrick, R. (1985). Theoretical and experimental bases of intraperitoneal chemotherapy. *Seminars in Oncology, 12* (3), 75–80.

Dollinger, M., Rosenbaum, E., & Cable, G. (1991). *Everyone's guide to cancer therapy.* Kansas City: Somerville House Books.

Doyle, M. (1995). Oncologic therapy. In Terry, J., Baranowski, L., Lonsway, R., & Hedrick, C. (eds.). *Intravenous therapy: Clinical principles and practice,* Intravenous Nurses Society. Philadelphia: W.B. Saunders.

Dundee, J., Ghaly, R., Bill, K. et al. (1990). Effect of stimulation of the P6 point on postoperative nausea and vomiting. *British Journal of Anaesthesia, 63,* 612–618.

Evans, B., Harvey, D., & Maki, L. (1991). Ondansetron controls carboplatin-induced vomiting resistant to standard antiemetics. *European Journal of Cancer, 27* (Suppl), 526.

Garvey, E.C. (1987). Current and future nursing issues in the home administration of chemotherapy. *Seminars in Oncology Nursing, 3,* 142–147.

Goodman, M. (1987). Management of nausea and vomiting induced by outpatient cisplatin (Platinol) therapy. *Seminars in Oncology Nursing, 3* (Suppl), 23–25.

Grace, L.A., & Tomaselli B.J. (1995). Intravenous therapy in the home. In Terry, J., Baranowski, L., Lonsway, R., Hedrick, C. (eds.). *Intravenous therapy: Clinical principles and practice,* Intravenous Nurses Society. Philadelphia: W.B. Saunders.

Groenwald, S.G., Frogge, M.H., Goodman, M.S., & Yarbro, C.H. (1990). *Cancer nursing: Principles and practice,* 2nd ed. Boston: Jones & Bartlett.

Holleb, A., Fink, D., & Murphy, G. (1991). *American Cancer Society textbook of clinical oncology.* Atlanta: American Cancer Society.

Howell, S.B. (1990). Intraperitoneal catheters for chemotherapy. *NAVAN, 1* (1), 8–9.

Jensen, J., Goel, R., & Venner, P. (1990). The effect of corticosteroid administration of bleomycin for lung toxicity. *Cancer, 65* 1291–1297.

Joint Commission on Accreditation of Healthcare Organizations. (1995). *Standards for the accreditation of home care.* Chicago: JCAHO.

Jordan, E. (1993). Preparing for hair loss. *Coping, 2,* 44–46.

LaBell, L., O'Neil, K., & Bing, C.M. (1990). An overview of home healthcare programs. *Journal of Pharmacy Practice, 3* (1), 4–10.

Lundquist, D., & Holmes, W. (1993). Documentation of neurotoxicity resulting from high-dose cytosine arabinoside. *Oncology Nursing Forum, 20,* 1409–1418.

Lydon, J. (1986). Nephrotoxicity of cancer treatment. *Oncology Nursing Forum, 13* (2), 68–77.

Malloy, J. (1991). Administering intraperitoneal chemotherapy: A new approach. *Nursing 91, 91* (1), 58–61.

Mathewson-Kuhn, M. (1994). *Pharmacotherapeutics: A nursing process approach,* 3rd ed. Philadelphia: F.A. Davis.

McClay, E.F., & Howell, S.B. (1990). A review: Intraperitoneal cisplatin in the management of patients with ovarian cancer. *Gynecology Oncology, 36,* 1–6.

McClosky, J.C. & Bulechek, G.M. (1992). *Iowa intervention project: Nursing interventions classification* (p. 167). St. Louis: Mosby-Year Book.

Oncology Nursing Society. (1989). *Cancer chemotherapy guidelines: Modules I–IV.* Pittsburgh:

Oncology Nursing Society News (1991). Scalp hypothermia devices: Current status. *ONS, 6* (8), 1, 3.

Oncology Nursing Society. (1992). *Cancer chemotherapy guidelines: Module V.* Pittsburgh:

OSHA. (1995). Controlling occupational exposure to hazardous drugs. Department of Labor Docket No. CPL 2-2.

Otto, S. (1995). Advanced concepts in chemotherapy drug delivery: Regional therapy. *Journal of Intravenous Nursing, 18* (4), 170–176.

Parkinson, D.R. (1995). Principles of therapy with biologic response modifiers and their role in cancer management. In Skeel, R.T., & Lanchant, N.A. (eds.). *Handbook of cancer chemotherapy,* 4th ed. Boston: Little, Brown, 34–45.

Pharmacia, Inc. (1995). *Package insert Zinecard* (dextrazoxane for injection). Ohio Pharmacia Adria, Inc.

Phillips, L.D., & Kuhn, M. (1996). *Manual of intravenous drugs.* Boston: Little, Brown.

Piccart, M.F., Speyer, J.L., & Markman, M. (1985). Intraperitoneal chemotherapy: Technical experience at five institutions. *Seminars on Oncology, 12* (3), 90–96.

Rostad, M. (1991). Current strategies for managing myelosuppression in patients with cancer. *Oncology Nursing Forum, 18,* 7–15.

Rowinsky, E., McGuire, W., Guarnieri, T., et al. (1991). Cardiac disturbances during the administration of taxol. *Journal of Clinical Oncology, 9,* 1704–1712.

Schulmeister, L. (1992). An overview of continuous infusion chemotherapy. *Journal of Intravenous Nursing, 15* (6), 315–321.

Skeel, R.T. (1995). Biologic and pharmacologic basis for cancer chemotherapy. In Skeel, R.T., & Lachant, N.A. (eds.). *Handbook of cancer chemotherapy.* Boston: Little, Brown.

Skeel, R.T., & Ganz, P.A. (1995). Systematic assessment of the patient with cancer and long-term medical complications of treatment. In Skeel, R.T., & Lachant, N.A. (eds.). *Handbook of cancer chemotherapy.* Boston: Little, Brown, 104–105.

Smith, M.R. (1995). Disorders of hemostasis and transfusion therapy. In Skeel, R.T., & Lachant, N.A. (eds.). *Handbook of cancer chemotherapy.* Boston: Little, Brown.

Stair, J., & McNally, J. (1992). Delivery systems for cancer care. Part VII In Groenwald, S.L., Goodman, M., Frogge, M.H., Yarbro, C.H. (eds.). *Cancer: Nursing principles and practice,* 2nd ed. Boston: Jones and Bartlett Publishers, 1124–1126.

Stevens, K.R. (1989). Safe handling of cytotoxic drugs in home chemotherapy. In Yarbro, C.H. (ed.). *Seminars in Oncology Nursing.* Philadelphia: W.B. Saunders.

Tipton, J.M., & Skeel, R.T. (1995). Management of acute side effects of cancer chemotherapy. In Skeel, R.T., & Lanchant, N.A. (eds.). *Handbook of cancer chemotherapy,* 4th ed. Boston: Little, Brown, 585.

Tsavaris, N.B., Komitsopolow, P., & Karagiaouris, P. (1990). Conservative approach to the treatment of chemotherapy-induced extravasation. *Journal of Dermatology Surgery and Oncology, 16:* 519–522.

Turbiana, M., & Malaise, E. (1976). Comparison of cell proliferation kinetics in human and experimental tumors: Response to irradiation. *Cancer Treatment, 60,* 1887–1895.

Turbiana, M., Richard, J.M., & Malaise, E. (1975). Kinetics of tumor growth and of cell proliferation in U.R.D.T. cancers: Therapeutic implications. *Laryngoscope, 85,* 1039–1052.

Weinstein, S. (1993). *Plumer's principles and practices of intravenous therapy,* 5th ed. Philadelphia: J.B. Lippincott, 445–507.

Zook-Enck, D. (1990). Intraperitoneal therapy via the Tenckhoff catheter. *Journal of Intravenous Nursing, 13* (6), 375–382.

CHAPTER 15

Nutritional Support

CHAPTER CONTENTS

GLOSSARY
LEARNING OBJECTIVES
PRE-TEST, CHAPTER 15
CONCEPTS OF NUTRITION
Nutritional Deficiency
NUTRITIONAL ASSESSMENT
History
Anthropometric Measurements
Diagnostic Tests
Physical Examination
Secondary Assessment Techniques
NUTRITIONAL REQUIREMENTS
Carbohydrates
Fat (Lipids)
Protein
Electrolytes
Vitamins
Trace Elements
Parenteral Nutrition Medication Additives
MODALITIES FOR DELIVERY OF NUTRITIONAL
    SUPPORT
Indications for Nutritional Support
Enteral Nutrition
Peripheral Parenteral Nutrition
Total Parenteral Nutrition
Total Nutrient Admixture
Cyclic Therapy
Specialized Parenteral Formulas

PARENTERAL NUTRITION IN THE PEDIATRIC
    PATIENT
Assessment
Indications
Monitoring
COMPLICATIONS AND NURSING
    CONSIDERATIONS
Metabolic Complications
Electrolyte Imbalances
Catheter-Related Complications
Admixture Complications
STANDARDS OF PRACTICE FOR NUTRITIONAL
    SUPPORT
Implementation Standards
Monitoring Standards
NURSING PLAN OF CARE: ADMINISTRATION
    OF TPN
PATIENT EDUCATION
HOME CARE ISSUES
COMPETENCY CRITERIA: NUTRITIONAL
    SUPPORT
KEY POINTS
CRITICAL THINKING ACTIVITY
POST-TEST, CHAPTER 15
ANSWERS TO CHAPTER 15
Pre-Test
Post-Test
REFERENCES

GLOSSARY

Amino acids   Chief organic component of protein
Anergy   Lack of immune response to an antigen
Anthropometry   Measurement of a part or whole of the body
BCAA   Branched-chain amino acid
Central parenteral nutrition   Total nutritional support via a central venous access device, tunneled catheter, implanted port, or subclavian entry.
C-TPN   Cyclic total parenteral nutrition
EFAD   Essential fatty acid deficiency

> **Fat emulsion** Natural product consisting of a mixture of neutral triglycerides of predominantly unsaturated fatty acids; permits inclusion of fat calories in the I.V. nutritional regimen.
> **HPN** Home parenteral therapy
> **Kwashiorkor** Malnutrition characterized by an adequate calorie intake with inadequate amount of protein
> **Marasmus** Malnutrition characterized by decreased intake of calories with adequate amounts of protein intake
> **Peripheral parenteral nutrition (PPN)** Nutritional support via a peripheral vein; glucose limited to 10%
> **Total parenteral nutrition (TPN)** Total I.V. nutritional support supplying glucose, protein, vitamins, electrolytes, trace elements, and sometimes fats to maintain the body's growth, development, and tissue repair
> **Total nutrient admixture (TNA)** A three-in-one formula of amino acids, fats, and dextrose in one container

LEARNING OBJECTIVES

Upon completion of this chapter, the reader will be able to:

- Define all terminology related to nutritional support.
- Identify the key elements of a nutritional assessment.
- List the six nutrients essential for total parenteral nutrition (TPN).
- Identify the key points in administration of glucose, protein, and fat emulsions.
- Describe the three major classifications of malnutrition.
- Identify early candidates for TPN.
- Describe the use of the additives heparin, insulin, and cimetidine, to parenteral nutrition.
- Describe three-in-one solutions.
- List the key concepts of cyclic therapy.
- Identify the TPN treatment plan for the patient with renal or liver disease.
- Identify key concepts of peripheral parenteral nutrition.
- State nursing considerations related to delivery of TPN.
- Identify the complications related to TPN.
- Use the nursing process in caring for a patient with TPN.

Match the following definitions in column II to the term in column I.

Column I

1. _____ EFAD
2. _____ anergy
3. _____ amino acids
4. _____ ketone bodies
5. _____ fat emulsion

Column II

A. Mixture of neutral triglycerides to provide fat calories

B. Lack of immune response to an antigen

C. Chief organic component of protein

D. Essential fatty acid deficiency

E. Substances formed by liver as a step in the combustion of fats

6. The most common carbohydrate used for parenteral nutrition is:
   A. Fructose
   B. Lactose
   C. Dextrose
   D. Invert sugar

7. Parenteral proteins are supplied as:
   A. Synthetic crystalline amino acids
   B. Casein amino acids
   C. Immunoglobulins

8. To treat or prevent essential fatty acid deficiency _____ is administered:
   A. Protein
   B. 10% dextrose
   C. Fat emulsion
   D. Trace elements

9. During times of stress, _____ metabolism is radically altered.
   A. Protein
   B. Fat
   C. Carbohydrate
   D. Vitamin C

10. Which of the following may be added to total parenteral solutions?
    A. Regular insulin, heparin, and cimetidine
    B. Iron, vitamin K, and cimetidine
    C. Iron, heparin, and neutral protamine Hagedorn (NPH) insulin
    D. Regular insulin, vitamin K, and cimetidine

11. A solution of total nutrient admixture refers to the combination of _____ ,
    _____ , and _____ in one solution container
    A. Fat emulsion, dextrose, and amino acids
    B. Fat emulsion, vitamins, and electrolytes
    C. Fat emulsion, heparin, and insulin
    D. Dextrose, amino acids, and trace elements

12. Components of a nutritional assessment include:
    A. Dietary history
    B. Anthropometric measurements
    C. Diagnostic tests
    D. Physical examination
    E. All of the above

13. Total parenteral nutrition includes which of the following key elements:
    A. Carbohydrates
    B. Protein
    C. Fats
    D. Electrolytes and vitamins
    E. All of the above

14. Total nutrient admixture solutions consists of a combination of:
    A. Platelets, plasma, and white blood cells
    B. Fats, carbohydrates, and protein
    C. Fats, electrolytes, and trace elements

15. The purpose of heparin added to the total parenteral nutrition (TPN) solution is:
    A. Enhance blood glucose levels
    B. Thin the TPN solution, so that it infuses easily
    C. Used to decrease incidence of subclavian vein thrombosis

16. The key points in delivery of cyclic therapy include:
    A. This therapy is indicated for patients receiving stabilized continuous TPN.
    B. This therapy is indicated for long-term parenteral nutrition.
    C. Cyclic TPN must be escalated to maintenance rate and tapered off to avoid abrupt changes in glucose levels.
    D. All of the above.

17. Patients with liver disease have elevated levels of aromatic amino acids and depressed levels of branched-chain amino acids. The patient with liver disease requires a TPN protein component that is:
   A. High in aromatic amino acids
   B. Equal in aromatic and branch chain amino acids
   C. High in branched-chain amino acids

18. Criteria for peripheral parenteral nutrition include:
   A. Good venous access
   B. No fluid restrictions
   C. Ability to tolerate fat emulsion therapy
   D. Expectation that patient will resume enteral feeding within 5 to 7 days
   E. All of the above

*Every careful observer of the sick will agree in this that thousands of patients
are annually starved in the midst of plenty, from want of attention to the
ways which alone make it possible for them to take food.*

FLORENCE NIGHTINGALE, 1859

Nutritional support nursing is the care of individuals with potential or known nutritional alterations. "Nurses who specialize in nutritional support use specific expertise to enhance the maintenance and/or restoration of an individual's nutritional health" (American Society for Parenteral and Enteral Nutrition [ASPEN], 1993). Nutrition support nursing encompasses all nursing activities that promote optimal nutritional health. Nursing interventions are based on scientific principles. The scope of practice includes but is not limited to direct patient care; consultation with nurses and other health professionals in a variety of clinical settings; education of patients, students, colleagues, and the public, participation in research; and administrative functions (ASPEN, 1993).

CONCEPTS OF NUTRITION

Nutritional balance occurs when nutrients are provided in sufficient quantities for the maintenance of body function and renewal of these components. Nutritional balance is based on three factors: (1) intake of nutrients (quantity and quality), (2) relative need for nutrients, and (3) ability of body to use nutrients (Knox, 1988).

Nutritional Deficiency

When nutritional deficiency exists, the body's components are used to provide energy for essential metabolic processes. For example, body stores of carbohydrates, fats, and protein are metabolized as energy sources in nutritional deficiency states. Carbohydrates are stored in the muscle and liver as glycogen. Adipose tissue is the body's long-term energy reserve of fat. Body protein is not stored in excess of the body's needs and therefore use without replacement adversely affects total body function (Ford & Vizcarra, 1995).

Malnutrition

Malnutrition is defined as a nutritional deficit associated with an increased risk of morbidity and mortality (Smith & Mullen, 1991). Starvation alters the distribution of carbohydrates, fats, and protein substrates. Brief starvation (24 to 72 hours) rapidly depletes glycogen stores and uses protein to produce glucose (gluconeogenesis) for glucose-dependent tissue. Prolonged starvation (longer than 72 hours) is associated with an increased mobilization of fat as the principal source of energy, reduction in the breakdown of protein, and increased use of ketones for central nervous tissue fuel. Stress in the form of pain, shock, injury, and sepsis intensifies the metabolic change seen in brief and prolonged starvation.

Three types of malnutrition have been defined and classified by an International Classification of Diseases (ICD) diagnostic code: marasmus, kwashiorkor, and mixed malnutrition. The outcome of nutritional assessment determines the category to which an undernourished person is assigned.

547

Marasmus

Marasmus is caused by a decrease in the intake of calories with adequate protein-calorie ratio. In this type of malnutrition, there is a gradual wasting of body fat and skeletal muscle with preservation of visceral proteins. The individual looks emaciated and has decreased anthropometric measurements and anergy to common skin test antigens.

Kwashiorkor

Kwashiorkor is characterized by an adequate intake of calories but a poor protein intake. This condition causes visceral protein wasting with preservation of fat and somatic muscle. It is seen during a period of decreased protein intake as seen with liquid diets, fat diets, and long-term use of I.V. fluids containing dextrose. Loss of body protein is due to depleted circulating proteins in the albumin. Individuals may appear obese and have adequate anthropometric measurements but decreased visceral proteins and depressed immune function.

Mixed Malnutrition

Mixed malnutrition is characterized by some aspects of both marasmus and kwashiorkor. The person presents with skeletal muscle and visceral protein wasting, depleted fat stores, and immune incompetence. The affected person appears cachectic and usually is in acute catabolic stress. This mixed protein-calorie disorder has the highest risk of morbidity and mortality.

Effects of Malnutrition

The hazards of malnutrition on bodily function are decreased protein stores, albumin depletion, and impaired immune status. Without protein stores in the body, a deficiency of total body protein results first in decreased strength and endurance (loss of muscle mass) and ultimately in decreased cardiac and respiratory muscle function. Skeletal muscle wasting occurs in a ratio of about 30:1 compared with visceral protein loss. The loss of gastrointestinal (GI) function follows skeletal muscle wasting and is associated with hypoalbuminemia. Protein-calorie malnutrition is one of the most common causes of impairment of immune function. Both B- and T-cell–mediated immune functions are impaired, causing enhanced susceptibility to infections.

NUTRITIONAL ASSESSMENT

A nutritional assessment of high-risk patients supplies the physician and nurse with invaluable information regarding a patient's nutritional status (Table 15–1). The nutritional assessment encompasses routine history taking with emphasis on dietary history, anthropometric measurements, diagnostic testing, and a complete physical examination (Farley, 1991).

History

The history is divided into three major components: medical, social, and dietary. The medical history should include a specific history of weight, chronic diseases, past surgical history; presence of increased losses, such as from draining wounds and fistulas; and factors such as age and drug, alcohol, and tobacco use. The social history

548

TABLE 15–1. COMPONENTS OF A NUTRITIONAL ASSESSMENT

1. History
     Medical
     Social
     Dietary
2. Anthropometric measurements
     Skinfolds
     Height and weight
     Midarm circumference
     Midarm muscle circumference
3. Diagnostic tests
     Anergy tests
     Bone radiologic tests
     Laboratory tests
          Serum electrolytes
          Total lymphocyte count
          Serum protein measurement
          Urine assays (creatinine, height index)
4. Physical examination

affecting nutrient intake includes income, education, ethnic background, and environment during mealtime, along with religious considerations (Kennedy-Caldwell & Guenter, 1988). The dietary history often provide clues as to the cause and degree of malnutrition. The components of a dietary history include appetite, GI disturbances, mechanical problems such as ill-fitting dentures, food allergies, medications, and food likes and dislikes (Farley, 1991).

Anthropometric Measurements

Anthropometry is the measurement of a part or whole of the body. It is a method of determining body composition. To estimate the size of the body fat mass, a skinfold test is done on the triceps of the nondominant arm using a caliper. Along with the skinfold measurement, a midarm circumference and midarm muscle circumference evaluation are performed. The height and weight are also part of this evaluation, with serial weights providing helpful information related to the protein-calorie status of the person. To calculate the current weight as a percentage of the usual weight, use the following calculation:

$$\% \text{ Usual weight} = [\text{Current weight} \div \text{usual weight}] \times 100$$

✎ **NOTE:** Mild malnutrition = 85% to 95%
     Moderate malnutrition = 75% to 84%
     Severe malnutrition = less than 75% (Kennedy-Caldwell & Guenter, 1988)

✎ **NOTE:** A loss of 10% of the usual weight, or a current weight less than 90% of ideal weight is considered to be a risk factor of nutrition-related complications (Ford & Vizcarra, 1995).

In simple starvation, 20% loss of body weight is associated with marked decreases in muscle tissue and subcutaneous fat, making the patient emaciated in appearance. Gross loss of body fat can be observed not only from appearance but also by palpating

549

a number of skinfolds. When the dermis can be felt between the fingers on pinching the triceps and biceps skinfolds, considerable loss from body stores of fat will have occurred. Protein stores can be assessed by inspection and palpation of a number of muscle groups, such as the triceps, biceps, and subscapular and infrascapular muscles. The long muscles in particular are profoundly protein-depleted when the tendons are prominent to palpation (Hill, 1991).

Diagnostic Tests

Several diagnostic tests are available to assess nutritional status. The anergy test is recommended for assessment of immunologic response and involves the intradermal injection of antigens. Proper nutrition is a key to an intact immune system, and a lack of response to antigens is considered anergic and possibly indicates, malnourishment. Radiologic findings as evidenced by osteoporosis, osteomalacia scurvy, and hypervitaminosis with widened sutures in the skull can help to determine severe prolonged deficiencies or excesses (Kennedy-Caldwell & Guenter, 1988).

Total lymphocyte count is also measured for the body's response immunologically. Serum protein measurements may indicate nutritional status and include albumin, transferrin, and prealbumin and retinol-binding protein tests (Farley, 1991).

Serum Albumin

Albumin is a major protein synthesized by the liver. Approximately 40% of protein mass is in circulation. The serum albumin concentration is normally between 3.5 and 5 g/dL. An albumin level of 2.8 to 3.2 g/dL represents mild protein depletion, 2.1 to 2.7 g/dL reflects moderate depletion, and less than 2.1 g/dL indicates severe depletion (Grant, 1992).

Serum Transferrin

Serum transferrin is a beta globulin that transports iron in the plasma and is synthesized in the liver. Transferrin is present in the serum in concentrations of 250 to 300 mg/dL. The serum levels are affected by nutritional factors and iron metabolism. Levels lower than 100 mg/dL indicate severe depletion (Smith & Mullen, 1991).

Prealbumin and Retinol-Binding Protein

Prealbumin functions in thyroxine transport and as a carrier for retinol-binding protein. Normal serum concentrations range from 15.7 to 29.6 mg/dL. Levels of 10 to 15 mg/dL reflect mild depletion, 5 to 9.9 mg/dL reflect moderate depletion, and a level lower than 5 mg/dL indicates severe depletion (Grant, 1992).

Total Lymphocyte Count

Immunologic testing is designed to assess nutritional deficiencies. The most common test used for the assessment of immunocompetence is the total lymphocyte count (TLC). The TLC is derived from the routine complete blood count (CBC) with differential. The TLC is calculated by means of the following formula.

$$TLC = \frac{5 \text{ lymph} \times WBC}{100}$$

A TLC between 1200 and 2000/μL indicates mild lymphocyte depletion; TLC between 800 and 1199/μL indicates moderate lymphocyte depletion; and a TLC lower than 800/μL indicates severe lymphocyte depletion (Grant, 1992).

✎ **NOTE:** TLC must be interpreted with caution, because many other nonnutritional factors may contribute to decreased lymphocyte counts.

Physical Examination

The final phase of nutritional assessment is a complete physical examination. Findings from a physical examination can reflect protein-calorie malnutrition along with vitamin and mineral deficiencies. The physical examination should include evaluation of the hair, nails, skin, eyes, oral cavity, glands heart, muscles, and abdomen along with neurologic evaluation and evaluation of delayed healing and tissue repair (Table 15–2).

Secondary Assessment Techniques

Additionally, several other tests have added to a proper physical exam. Other tests done include: objective measurements of wound healing, grip strength, skeletal muscle function, and respiratory muscle function (Windsor, 1988).

Nitrogen Balance

Other parameters are also used to assess overall nutrition. The nitrogen balance is a measure of daily intake of nitrogen minus the excretion. It is used to assess protein turnover.

✎ **NOTE:** A positive nitrogen balance indicates an anabolic state with an overall gain in body protein for the day. A negative nitrogen balance indicates a catabolic state with a net loss of protein.

Indirect Calorimetry

An indirect calorimetry is also used and is a technique used in the measurement of resting energy expenditure based on oxygen consumption and carbon dioxide production. In addition, multiparameter indices have been developed to improve nutritional assessments.

Prognostic Nutritional Index (PNI)

The most popular is the prognostic nutritional index (PNI). The PNI is based on four measures selected by analysis and computer-based stepwise regression that are then incorporated into a linear predictive model. The clinically important factors as determined by this analysis include the serum albumin concentration, serum transferrin, tricips skinfold thickness, and delayed hypersensitivity. This predictive model relates the risk of morbidity to nutritional status (Kaminski, 1985).

NUTRITIONAL REQUIREMENTS

Nutritional requirements are based on a basic formula that must contain all essential macro- and micronutrients for adequate energy production, support of synthesis, replacement, and repair of structural or visceral proteins, cell structure, production

TABLE 15–2. PHYSICAL FINDINGS ASSOCIATED WITH DEFICIENCY STATES

Physical Findings	Associated Deficiencies
Hair, Nails	
Flag sign (transverse depigmentation of hair)	Protein, copper
Hair easily pluckable	Protein
Hair thin, sparse	Protein, biotin, zinc
Nails spoon-shaped	Iron
Nails lackluster, transverse riding	Protein-calorie
Skin	
Dry, scaling	Vitamin A, zinc, essential fatty acids
Flaky paint dermatosis	Protein
Follicular hyperkeratosis	Vitamins A, C; essential fatty acids
Nasolabial seborrhea	Niacin, pyridoxine, riboflavin
Petechiae, purpura	Ascorbic acid, vitamin K
Pigmentation, desquamation (sun-exposed area)	Niacin (pellagra)
Subcutaneous fat loss	Calorie
Eyes	
Angular blepharitis	Riboflavin
Corneal vascularization	Riboflavin
Dull, dry conjunctiva	Vitamin A
Fundal capillary microaneurysms	Ascorbic acid
Scleral icterus, mild	Pyridoxine
Perioral	
Angular stomatitis	Riboflavin
Cheilosis	Riboflavin
Oral Cavity	
Atrophic lingual papillae	Niacin, iron, riboflavin, folate, vitamin B_{12}
Glossitis (scarlet, raw)	Niacin, pyridoxine, riboflavin, vitamin B_{12}, folate
Hypogeusesthesia (also hyposmia)	Zinc, vitamin A
Magenta tongue	Riboflavin
Swollen, bleeding gums (if teeth present)	Ascorbic acid
Tongue fissuring, edema	Niacin
Glands	
Parotid enlargement	Protein
Sicca syndrome	Ascorbic acid
Thyroid enlargement	Iodine
Heart	
Enlargement, tachycardia, high output failure	Thiamine ("wet" beriberi)
Small heart, decreased output	Calorie
Sudden failure, death	Ascorbic acid

TABLE 15–2. **PHYSICAL FINDINGS ASSOCIATED WITH DEFICIENCY STATES** (*Continued*)

Physical Findings	Associated Deficiencies
Abdomen	
Hepatomegaly	Protein
Muscles, Extremities	
Calf tenderness	Thiamine, ascorbic acid (hemorrhage into muscle)
Edema	Protein, thiamine
Muscle wastage (especially temporal area, dorsum of hand, spine)	Calorie
Bones, Joints	
Bone tenderness (adult)	Vitamin D, calcium, phosphorus (osteomalacia)
Neurologic	
Confabulation, disorientation	Thiamine (Korsakoff's psychosis)
Decreased position and vibratory senses, ataxia	Vitamin B_{12}, thiamine
Decreased tendon reflexes, slowed relaxation phase	Thiamine
Ophthalmoplegia	Thiamine, phosphorus
Weakness, paresthesias, decreased fine tactile sensation	Vitamin B_{12}, pyridoxine, thiamine
Other	
Delayed healing and tissue repair (e.g., wound, infarct, abscess)	Ascorbic acid, zinc, protein

Source: From Nutritional assessment of critically ill patients by J. Morgan, 1984, *Focus on critical care*, 11, pp. 32–33. Copyright 1984 by Mosby–Year Book, Inc. Reprinted by permission.

of hormones and enzymes, and maintenance of immune function. The basic design contains carbohydrates, protein, fat, electrolytes, vitamins, trace elements, and water.

Carbohydrates

The I.V. source of carbohydrates is predominantly dextrose. Other sources of carbohydrate calories can be provided by glycerol, sorbitol, or fructose. These are considered nondextrose carbohydrates and do not require insulin for metabolism. However, these nondextrose carbohydrates may require more energy in the metabolism process. Other sources of carbohydrate calories are provided by invert sugar and xylitol.

✎ **NOTE:** 1 g carbohydrate = 4 kcal

553

Glucose

The major purpose of carbohydrate is to provide energy. Glucose provides calories in parenteral solutions. Carbohydrates also spare body protein. When glucose is supplied as a nutrient, it is stored temporarily in the liver and muscle as glycogen. When glycogen storage capacity is reached, the carbohydrate is stored as fat. When glucose is provided parenterally, it is completely bioavailable to the body without any effects of malabsorption.

When dextrose is administered rapidly, the solution acts as an osmotic diuretic and pulls interstitial fluid into the plasma for subsequent renal excretion. The nurse must be aware that when infusing 20% to 50% dextrose solutions the rate must be kept within 10% of the prescribed order (Table 15–3). The pancreas secretes extra insulin to metabolize infused glucose. If 20% to 50% dextrose is discontinued suddenly, a temporary excess of insulin in the body may cause symptoms of hypoglycemia (Metheny, 1996).

✎ **NOTE:** During the critical phase of illness or injury, carbohydrate metabolism is radically altered; hyperglycemia is a hallmark of stress.

Fructose

Fructose has been used in 5% and 10% solutions combined with glucose and xylitol in Europe, but its use has not gained popularity in the United States. Fructose offers several advantages over dextrose. Fructose does not require insulin for initial uptake. Since most adult tissues cannot utilize fructose directly but require its conversion to glucose in the liver, this advantage is limited. Fructose also is associated with a lower incidence of hyperglycemia and glycouria than glucose. Fructose has disadvantages, such as lactic acidosis, hypophosphatemia, elevated serum bilirubin and uric acid levels, and depletion of hepatic adenine nucleotides. Fructose is contraindicated in patients with fructose intolerance (Singh, 1983; Friedman, 1980).

Invert Sugar

Invert sugar consists of equal parts of dextrose and fructose. Both 5% and 10% solutions of invert sugar are commercially available. Clinical experience using invert sugar is limited (Torosian & Daly, 1991).

Sorbitol and Xylitol

Sorbitol and xylitol are alcohol sugars and are only partially insulin-dependent. Both require conversion to glucose in the liver. Severe toxic effects can occur with these

TABLE 15–3. **DEXTROSE SOLUTIONS FOR TOTAL PARENTERAL NUTRITION**

Solution (%)	g/liter	kcal/liter	mOsm/liter
5	50	170	252
10	100	340	505
20	200	680	1010
30	300	1020	1515
40	400	1360	2020
50	500	1700	2525
60	600	2040	3030
70	700	2380	3535

alcohol sugars, including lactic acidosis, hepatic failure, hyperuricemia, and depletion of liver adenosine triphosphate and inorganic phosphate (Ahnefeld, Bassler, &
Bauer, 1975).

Fat (Lipids)

Fat is the primary source of heat and energy. Fat provides twice as many energy
calories per gram as either protein or carbohydrate. Fat is essential for structural
integrity of all cell membranes. Linoleic acid and linolenic acid are the only fatty
acids essential to man. These two acids prevent essential fatty acid deficiency (EFAD).
Linoleic acid is necessary as a precursor of prostaglandins, regulates cholesterol metabolism, and maintains integrity of the cell wall. Signs and symptoms of EFAD
include desquamating dermatitis, alopecia, brittle nails, delayed wound healing,
thrombocytopenia, decreased immunity, and increased capillary fragility.

✎ **NOTE:** To prevent EFAD, 2% to 4% of the total calorie requirement should come
from lineolic acid (25 to 100 mg/kg/day). Ten percent of calories from soy or
safflower oil emulsions should provide adequate linoleic acid to prevent EFAD
(Skipper & Marian, 1993).

Complications associated with EFAD include impaired wound healing, platelet dysfunction, increased susceptibility to infection, and development of fatty liver. In patients with respiratory failure, the administration of fat can help decrease carbon
dioxide excretion (Table 15–4). The primary purpose of fat emulsions in total parenteral nutrition (TPN) is to prevent or treat EFAD with infusion of two to three 500-
mL bottles of 10% to 20% fat emulsions per week (Kennedy-Caldwell & Guenter,
1988).

✎ **NOTE:** Use of fat can help control hyperglycemia in stress states.

✎ **NOTE:** A 1.2-micron filter should be used when adding lipid mixtures to total
nutrient admixtures. This filter was found to remove *Candida albicans* and to
prevent passage of particulates and precipitates (Whitbread, Jarres, & Brandwein, 1994).

TABLE 15–4. **LIPID EMULSIONS FOR TOTAL PARENTERAL NUTRITION**

Manufacturer	Emulsion	Percentages Available	Osmolarity (mOsm/L)
Abbott			
Liposyn II 10%	50/50 safflower oil, soybean oil	10% (1.1 kcal/mL)	276
Liposyn II 20%	50/50 safflower oil, soybean oil	20% (2.0 kcal/mL)	258
Liposyn III 10%	Soybean oil	10% (1.1 kcal/mL)	284
Liopsyn III 20%	Soybean oil	20% (2.0 kcal/mL)	292
Clintec			
Intralipid 10%	Soybean oil	10% (1.1 kcal/mL)	280
Intralipid 20%	Soybean oil	20% (2.2 kcal/mL)	330
Kendal McGaw			
NutriLipid 10%	Soybean oil	10% (1.1 kcal/mL)	280
NutriLipid 20%	Soybean oil	20% (2.0 kcal/mL)	330

Source: Data from *Facts and Comparisons*, Philadelphia: J.B. Lippincott, 1992.

555

The use of I.V. fat has increased in recent years owing to decreased cost and greater availability of the product. When fat is used as a calorie source in parenteral nutrition, there is less problem with glucose homeostasis, CO_2 production is lower, and hepatic tolerance to I.V. feedings may improve. Primarily, I.V. fats are supplied by safflower or soybean oil, with egg yolk phospholipids and glycerol to provide tonicity. Fat emulsions provide 1.1. to 2.0 kcal/mL for the 10% to 20% concentrations, respectively (Metheny, 1996).

✎ **NOTE:** 1 g fat = 9 kcal

Protein

Protein is a body-building nutrient that functions to promote tissue growth, repair, and replacement of body cells. Protein is also a component in antibodies, scar tissue, and clots. Amino acids are the basic unit of protein. The eight amino acids essential for adults are isoleucine, leucine, lysine, methionine, phenylalanine, threonine, tryptophan, and valine. Parenteral proteins are elemental, providing a synthetic crystalline amino acid that does not cause an antigenic reaction. These proteins are available in concentrations of 3% to 15% and come with and without electrolytes (Metheny, 1996). Some amino acid solutions are presented in Table 15–5.

Enzymes, hormones, and carrier substances also require protein for development. Protein contributes to energy needs; however, this is not its major purpose.

✎ **NOTE:** Protein requirements for healthy adults are 0.8% g/kg/day in critical illness, 1.2 to 2.5 g/kg/day. Protein sparing can be accomplished by administration of 100 to 150 g of carbohydrate daily.

Protein hydrolysate solutions of either casein or fibrin origin were used initially for parenteral nutrition. Because of their high ammonia content and unfavorable microbial growth characteristics, these products have been replaced by synthetic amino acids. Modifications of amino acid have been recommended in situations of renal or liver disease.

Increased need for protein by the body is usually reflected by an increase in excretion of urinary nitrogen, as evidenced by laboratory values.

Newborn infants require another amino acid—histidine. Premature infants also require cystine and tyrosine.

Electrolytes

Electrolytes are infused either as a component already contained in the amino acid solution or as a separate additive. Electrolytes are available in several salt forms and are added based on the patient's metabolic status.

The electrolytes necessary for long-term TPN include potassium, magnesium, calcium, sodium, chloride, and phosphorus. Potassium is needed for the transport of glucose and amino acids across the cell membrane. Approximately 30 to 40 mEq of potassium are necessary for each 1000 calories provided by the parenteral route. Potassium may be given as potassium chloride, potassium phosphate, or potassium acetate salt. Serum potassium levels must be closely monitored during TPN.

✎ **NOTE:** Patients with impaired renal function may need decreased amount of potassium.

TABLE 15–5. **AMINO ACID SOLUTIONS FOR TOTAL PARENTERAL NUTRITION**

Solution	Protein Concentration (%)	Nitrogen (g/100 mL)	Osmolarity (mOsm/L)
Abbott			
Aminosyn	3.5	0.55	357
Aminosyn II	3.5	0.55	308
Aminosyn II	4.25	0.65	894
Aminosyn	5	0.786	500
Aminosyn II	5	0.786	438
Aminosyn	7	1.10	700
Aminosyn II	7	1.10	869
Aminosyn	8.5	1.33	850
Aminosyn II	8.5	1.3	742
Aminosyn	10	1.57	875
Aminosyn II	10	1.57	1000
Aminosyn II	15	2.3	1300
Stress formulation			
Aminosyn-HBC	7	1.12	665
Clintec Nutrition			
Travasol	2.75	0.46	530
Travasol	3.5	0.591	450
Travasol	4.25	0.7	680
Travasol	5.5	0.924	575
Travasol	8.5	1.42	890
Travasol	10	1.68	970
Novamine	11.4	1.8	1057
Novamine	15	2.37	1388
Stress formulation			
BranchAmin	4	0.443	316
Kendal McGaw			
FreAmine III	3	0.46	300
FreAmine III	8.5	1.42	810
FreAmine III	10	1.57	950
FreAmine III with electrolytes	3	0.46	405
TrophAmine	6	0.93	525
TrophAmine	10	1.55	875
ProcalAmine	3	0.46	735
Stress formulation			
FreAmine HBC	6.9	0.97	620
Hepatic formulation			
HepatAmine	8	1.2	785

Source: Data from *Drug facts and comparisons*, Philadelphia: J. B. Lippincott, 1992.

The other electrolytes include magnesium sulfate, at 10 to 20 mEq every 24 hours; calcium gluceptate, gluconate, or chloride at 10 to 15 mEq in 24 hours; sodium chloride, acetate, lactate, or phosphate at 60 to 100 mEq in 24 hours; and phosphorus sodium or potassium at 20 to 45 mM in 24 hours. Chloride is provided based on acid-base status. Electrolytes must be individually compounded and can be highly variable in the patient receiving TPN. Choice of each of the above salts depends on renal and cardiac functioning, disease-specific needs, acid-base balance, and any abnormal losses during the course of illness.

TABLE 15–6. **DAILY VITAMIN RECOMMENDATIONS FROM THE AMA**

Vitamin	Amount
A	3300 IU
D	200 IU
E	10 IU
Ascorbic acid (C)	100 mg
Folic acid	400 µg
Niacin (B_3)	40 mg
Riboflavin (B_2)	3.6 mg
Thiamin (B_1)	3.0 mg
Pyridoxine (B_6)	4.0 mg
Cyanocobalamin (B_{12})	5.0 µg
Pantothenic acid (B_5)	15 mg
Biotin (B_7)	60 µg

Source: Adapted from American Medical Association Department of Foods and Nutrition, 1979.

Vitamins

Vitamins are necessary for growth and maintenance, along with multiple metabolic process. The fat- and water-soluble vitamins are needed for the patient requiring TPN. The Nutritional Advisory Group of the American Medical Association (AMA) has developed recommendations for the daily administration of I.V. multivitamins (AMA, 1979) (Table 15–6).

There is controversy over the exact parenteral vitamin requirements for patients receiving TPN. Certain disease states can alter vitamin requirements, and the sequelae of vitamin deficiency can be catastrophic to the very ill person. Vitamin K is not a component of any of the vitamin mixtures formulated for adults. Maintenance requirements can be satisfied by administering vitamin K, 5 mg per week, intramuscularly (Torosian & Daly, 1991).

Trace Elements

Trace elements are found in the body in minute amounts. Basic requirements are very small, measured in milligrams. Each trace element is a single chemical and has an associated deficiency state.

The many functions of trace elements are often synergistic (Metheny, 1996). The AMA has also established guidelines for the daily administration of four trace elements (AMA, 1979) (Table 15–7).

TABLE 15–7. **DAILY TRACE ELEMENTS RECOMMENDED BY THE AMA**

Zinc, 2.5–40 mg
Copper, 0.5–1.5 mg
Chromium, 10–15 µg
Manganese, 0.15–0.8 mg

Zinc contributes to wound healing by increasing the tensile strength of collagen; copper assists in iron's incorporation of hemoglobin. The other trace elements—selenium, iodine, fluorine, cobalt, nickel, and iron—all have been identified as beneficial; however, there are no guidelines established for TPN (Kennedy, Caldwell & Guenter, 1988).

Parenteral Nutrition Medication Additives

Compatibility is always an issue whenever two agents are combined. Parenteral solutions should be used immediately after mixing or else refrigerated. Stability of the admixed component dictates the appropriate length of time that the solution may be refrigerated. The parenteral solutions must be infused within 24 hours or discarded (INS, 1996). In addition to combining amino acids, dextrose, fats, electrolytes, vitamins, and trace elements, medications such as insulin, heparin, and cimetidine can be added to the TPN solution.

Insulin

Hyperglycemia is the most common complication of TPN therapy, which is due to the high concentration of glucose in the TPN solutions (Johndrow, 1988). Insulin is considered to be chemically stable in parenteral nutrition. By adding regular insulin to the parenteral admixture, some patients benefit from the enhanced blood glucose levels. Insulin is responsible for adequate metabolism of carbohydrates. Insulin also has a lipolytic effect and increased muscle uptake of amino acids (Dolan, 1991).

Heparin

Heparin in doses of 100 to 300 U/L has been routinely used to decrease the incidence of subclavian vein thrombus. This is controversial because recent studies disprove this claim. It is thought that larger doses of heparin, up to 20,000 U/liter, may be needed to significantly reduce the risk of thrombosis (Schilling, 1988; Suzuki, 1986).

Cimetidine

Cimetidine can be added to the TPN solution as a prophylactic measure against development of stress ulcers. Concentrations of 900 to 1300 mg/liter are compatible with TPN (Baptista, Palombo, & Tahan, 1985; Tsallas & Allen, 1982).

Other Medications

Other medications currently being studied to reduce the volume of fluid administration are the combination of antibiotics and corticosteroids with TPN (Dolan, 1991).

MODALITIES FOR DELIVERY OF NUTRITIONAL SUPPORT

Modalities for nutritional support include enteral nutrition, peripheral, parenteral nutrition (PPN), total parenteral nutrition (TPN), total nutrient admixtures (TNA), and cyclic therapy. There are also specialized parenteral formulas that can be used for patients in renal or liver failure or in stress formulas.

559

Indications for Nutritional Support

Patients who would be good candidates for nutritional support are those who suffer from a multiplicity of problems. Their clinical course can be complicated by malnutrition and depletion of body protein (Fig. 15–1). The leading use of nutritional support in the pediatric population is for the support of infants with inadequate absorptive surface owing to congenital defect or loss from necrotizing enterocolitis (Fischer, 1991). Primary therapy in adults has shown efficacy for those with short gut syndrome, enterocutaneous fistulas, renal failure, hepatic failure, and burns (Table 15–8; Fig. 15–2).

Enteral Nutrition

Patients who are unable to eat regular diets have two alternatives to nutritional support: enteral therapy or parenteral therapy. Enteral nutrition has certain advantages over parenteral: it is less expensive and more physiologic, it is easier to achieve a positive nitrogen balance, and it makes use of the GI tract. If the patient has a functioning GI tract, enteral nutrition should be used; otherwise, the parenteral route is indicated (Farley, 1991).

KEY POINTS IN DELIVERY OF ENTERAL NUTRITIONAL SUPPORT
1. GI tract must be functioning.
2. Several approaches may be used to deliver enteral feedings.
3. There are three methods by which enteral nutrition can be delivered: bolus, intermittent, or continuous.
4. Six different categories of enteral formulas are available:
   Blenderized

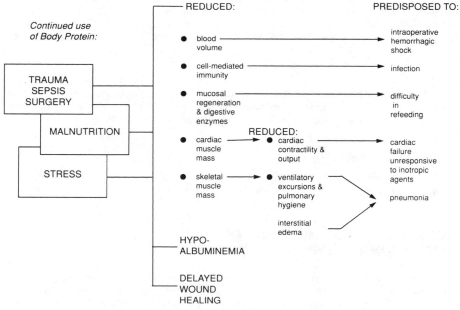

Figure 15–1. Body protein depletion.

TABLE 15–8. INDICATIONS FOR TOTAL PARENTERAL NUTRITION

Primary Therapy
  Efficacy shown
    Short gut syndrome
    Enterocutaneous fistula
    Renal failure due to acute tubular necrosis
    Hepatic failure
    Burns
  Efficacy not shown
    Inflammatory bowel syndrome
    Anorexia nervosa

Supportive Therapy
  Efficacy shown
    Acute radiation enteritis
    Chemotherapy enteritis
    Perioperative support of the clearly malnourished
  Efficacy not shown
    Chronic pancreatitis
    Perioperative support in "cardiac cachexia"
    Chronic protein loss from wounds or disease in excess of enteral repletion
    Prolonged respiratory support with ileus

Under Investigation
  Cancer support
  Sepsis and trauma
  General perioperative support

Source: From Sax, H. C., & Hasselgrew, P. (1991). *Total parenteral nutrition*, 2nd ed. (3–4). Boston: Little, Brown.

  Meal replacement
  Elemental or chemically defined
  High-calorie and high-protein
  Specialty
  Modular
5. The patient must be monitored for:
  Formula intolerance (gastric residuals every 4 to 8 hours)
  Stools (frequency and consistency)
  Tube tolerance (placement and maintenance checks)
  Effectiveness (weight gain, nutrient intake)
  Laboratory tests (Kennedy-Caldwell & Guenter, 1988)

COMPLICATIONS OF ENTERAL NUTRITION
1. Incorrect tube placement
2. Occlusion of feeding tube
3. Aspiration of feeding
4. Tracheoesopheageal fistula
5. Acute sinusitis
6. Otitis media
7. Diarrhea
8. Metabolic imbalances: hypoglycemia, hyperglycemia, hyperosmolar nonketotic dehydration, EFAD

561

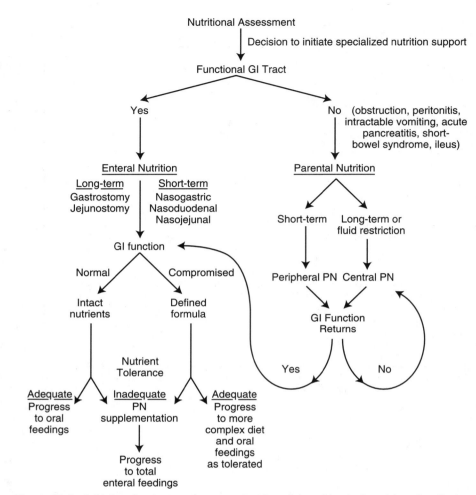

Figure 15–2. Guidelines for the use of parenteral and enteral nutrition in the adult and pediatric patient. (Reprinted from the American Society for Parenteral and Enteral Nutrition (A.S.P.E.N). Guidelines for the use of parenteral and enteral nutrition in adult and pediatric patients, *JPEN,* 17(4), ISA-52SA.)

Peripheral Parenteral Nutrition

Peripheral parenteral nutrition (PPN) was first proposed in the early 1970s as a "nitrogen-sparing" therapy. This parenteral nutrition is designed for mildly stressed patients who fall into the following categories:

1. Patients in whom central venous access is either impossible or contraindicated
2. Patients with no fluid restrictions
3. Patients able to tolerate fat emulsions
4. Patients expected to resume enteral feeding within 7 to 10 days (Kennedy-Caldwell & Guenter, 1988)

562

The ASPEN (1993) practice guidelines may be used to provide partial or total nutrition support for up to 2 weeks in selected patients who cannot ingest or absorb oral or enteral tube-delivered nutrients or in those for whom central vein parenteral nutrition is not feasible.

Generally, PPN provides dextrose in percentages below 20% with 500 mL of amino acids and fat emulsions via a peripheral line. PPN is used for therapies of less than 3 weeks. This therapy maintains the nutritional state in patients who can tolerate relatively high fluid volume, those who usually resume bowel function and oral feeding within a few days, and those who are susceptible to catheter-related infection of central venous TPN. PPN can be delivered by an over-the-needle catheter or by a peripherally inserted central line. Osmolarity factors of the solution must be considered when delivering PPN. It is recommended that TPN not exceed 900 mOsm to prevent phlebitis (INS, 1990).

✎ **NOTE:** A commercial product designed for peripheral nutrition, Procal Amine, provides 3% amino acids and 3% glycerol and electrolytes and has an osmolarity of 735. Glycerol is used as a carbohydrate source in this product instead of dextrose (Miller, 1991). Table 15–9 shows standard PPN solution.

The delivery of PPN involves both advantages and disadvantages.

ADVANTAGES
1. Avoids insertion and maintenance of central catheter
2. Delivers less hypertonic solutions than central venous TPN
3. Reduces the chance of metabolic complications from that of central venous TPN
4. Increases calorie source, along with fat emulsion

DISADVANTAGES
1. Cannot be used in nutritionally depleted patients
2. Cannot be used in volume-restricted patients, since higher volumes of solution are needed to provide adequate calories
3. Does not usually increase a patient's weight
4. May cause phlebitis owing to the osmolarity of the solution

Total Parenteral Nutrition

Total parenteral nutrition (TPN) by central line reverses starvation and adequately achieves tissue synthesis, repair, and growth. TPN solutions are usually administered through a central vein because of the high concentration of dextrose and the hypertonicity and hyperosmolarity of the solution. By infusing this solution into the central venous system, there is a decreased incidence of phlebitis, and the highly concentrated formula can be rapidly diluted. Table 15–10 gives an example of standard total parenteral nutrition solution.

TABLE 15–9. **STANDARD PERIPHERAL VEIN NUTRITION SOLUTIONS/LITER**

Dextrose, 5–10% Crystalline amino acids, 2.75–4.25% Electrolytes, trace elements, and vitamins, as ordered Lipid emulsion, 10% or 20% Heparin or hydrocortisone, as ordered

TABLE 15–10. **STANDARD CENTRAL
PARENTERAL NUTRITION SOLUTION**

> 500 mL of 8.5–10% amino acids
> 500 mL of 50–70% dextrose at 3 liters/day
> Addition of 500 mL of 10–20% fat emulsion/day
> Multivitamins, electrolytes, and trace elements,
>   as needed
> Heparin and insulin, as prescribed

The delivery of total parenteral nutrition involves both advantages and disadvantages.

ADVANTAGES
1. Dextrose solution of 20% to 70% administered as a calorie source
2. Useful for long-term (usually longer than 3 weeks)
3. Useful for patient with large caloric and nutrient needs
4. Provides calories, restores nitrogen balance, replaces essential vitamins, electrolytes, and minerals
5. Promotes tissue synthesis, wound healing, and normal metabolic function
6. Allows bowel rest and healing
7. Improves tolerance to surgery
8. Is nutritionally complete

DISADVANTAGES
1. Requires a minor surgical procedure for insertion
2. May cause metabolic complications: glucose intolerance, electrolyte imbalances, EFAD
3. Fat emulsions possible not used effectively in severely stressed patient (especially burn patients)
4. Risk of pneumothorax or hemothorax with central line insertion procedure

TPN solutions infused through a central vein are highly concentrated and range from 1800 to 2000 mOsm/kg with final additives, compared with 300 mOsm/kg in plasma.

Total Nutrient Admixture

Total nutrient admixtures (TNAs) are systems that describe combinations of dextrose, amino acids, and fat emulsions in one container. Referred to as total nutritional admixture, all-in-one, or three-in-one, this new product combines fat, amino acids, and dextrose in one container. The formula is provided in a 3-liter container that infuses over 24 hours. Lipids are mixed with dextrose and amino acid solution in the pharmacy. This solution is white and has a nonreflective surface, making precipitation difficult to observe (Driscoll, 1990).

These admixtures have been shown to be stable and well tolerated by patients via central line administration (Andrusko, 1987; Deitel, 1987). Compounding of lipids, amino acids, and dextrose solutions raises the pH of the formula.

TNAs must be administered through a 1.2-micron filter because of the mean particle size of fat droplets. There is a potential that cholestasis may develop and that long-chain triglycerides may depress the immune system. Catheter occlusion resulting from fat deposits has been reported with long-term use of this therapy. Limited data exist on the compatibility and stability of TNA with various products and concentration (Warshawsky, 1992).

✎ **NOTE:** Bacterial growth may be enhanced by admixture of fat emulsions with dextrose and amino acid solutions (Green & Baptista, 1985). The solutions should be observed for pink discoloration and for separation of oils in the three-in-one admixture (Kennedy-Caldwell & Guenter, 1988).

Cyclic Therapy

For patients requiring long-term parenteral nutritional support, cyclic TPN (C-TPN) is widely used. This therapy delivers concurrent dextrose, amino acids, and fat over a regimen of reduced time frame, usually 12 to 18 hours, versus a 24-hour continuous infusion.

KEY POINTS IN DELIVERY OF C-TPN
1. This therapy is indicated for patients stabilized on continuous TPN.
2. This therapy is indicated for long-term parenteral nutrition.
3. The patient's cardiovascular status must be able to accommodate large fluid volume during the cyclic phase.
4. For patients without complications such as glucose intolerance or a precarious fluid balance, a 12-hour cycling regimen can be used (McClary-Bennett & Rosen, 1990).
5. To avoid abrupt changes in glucose, there must be a period of escalating to maintenance rate as well as tapering down from maintenance rate. Tapering rates vary from 1 to 2 hours (McClary-Bennett & Rosen, 1990).

✎ **NOTE:** The patient who is septic or metabolically stressed is not a good candidate for C-TPN.

ADVANTAGES
1. Prevents or treats hepatotoxicity induced by continuous TPN
2. Prevents or treats EFAD in patients on fat-free TPN (Baker & Rosenberg, 1987)
3. Improves quality of life by encouraging normal daytime activities and enhances psychological well-being

DISADVANTAGES
1. Patients must be observed for symptoms of hypoglycemia, hyperglycemia, dehydration, excessive fluid administration, and sepsis associated with central-line manipulation.
2. Patients must be carefully monitored for rebound hypoglycemia after cessation of C-TPN.
3. Hyperglycemia can develop during the peak C-TPN flow rate. Blood glucose levels should be checked whenever the patient displays symptoms of nausea, tremors, sweating, anxiety, or lethargy.

✎ **NOTE:** Blood glucose should be checked 1 hour after tapering off C-TPN.

Dehydration can occur when fluid requirements are not met. Monitoring should include pulse, orthostatic blood pressures, examination of mucous membranes, skin turgor, and laboratory tests such as blood urea nitrogen (BUN), creatinine, hematocrit, and albumin.

Symptoms of excess fluid administration should be monitored, such as weight gain, resulting in edema or infusion-related shortness of breath. If too much fluid is

TABLE 15–11. **SPECIALIZED PARENTERAL FORMULAS**

Disease State	Parenteral Formulas	Treatment Plan
Renal failure	Nephramine 5.4% (Kendall-McGaw) Aminosyn RF 5.2% (Abbott) Amines 5.2% (Clintec) RenAmin 6.5% (Clintec)	Administer formulas high in essential amino acids. Administer electrolytes based on patient's clinical status. Restrict fluids based on status.
Liver disease	Hepatamine 8% (Kendall-McGaw)	Administer formulas high in BCAA. Restrict total protein intake in encephalopathy.
Cardiac disease	Basic formula	Provide nutrients in as high a concentration as possible without precipitating fluid overload. Administer I.V. lipid emulsions cautiously in severe cardiac disease. Restrict fluids. Administer electrolytes based on patient's clinical status, especially potassium and magnesium.
Trauma	FreAmine HBC 6–9% (Kendall-McGaw)	Administer formulas high in BCAA. Administer insulin based on patient's status.
Pulmonary disease	Basic formula	Nonprotein calories should be supplied in the following amounts: Carbohydrates 40–50% Lipids 30–50% Administer fluids and sodium cautiously to avoid causing fluid overload. Administer electrolytes based on patient's clinical status, especially phosphorus, magnesium, potassium and calcium.
Burns	Basic formula	Administer higher concentrations of carbohydrates than lipids. Administer formulas high in amino acids. Administer fluid based on
Sepsis	Heptamine 8%	Administer formulas high in BCAA. Administer lipids as 30–50% of the total nonprotein calories. Administer insulin based on patient's clinical status. Restrict the administration of iron.
Stress formula	FreAmine HBC 6.9% BranchAmine 4% Aminosyn HBC 8%	

administered during the cyclic period, the time frame should be extended. Using the C-TPN regimen requires twice the manipulations as continuous TPN; therefore, the risk of sepsis associated with central line manipulation must be considered.

Specialized Parenteral Formulas

Some parenteral formulas are designed to meet the needs of patients with specific disease states such as renal and liver failure and general stress conditions such as trauma, burns, and sepsis (Table 15–11).

Renal Failure

Formulas used for patients in renal failure contain high amounts of essential amino acids. The high amounts of essential amino acids increase nephron repair in renal failure. The amino acid L-histidine enhances amino acid utilization in uremia (Fischer, 1972).

Liver Failure

Solutions high in branched-chain amino acids (BCAA) are designed for liver disease. Patients with chronic liver disease have elevated levels of aromatic amino acids and depressed levels of BCAA. The administration formulas high in BCAA would seem to be beneficial; however, as with formulas for renal failure, controversy exists.

Stress Conditions

Formulas high in BCAA have also been recommended in the care of the trauma patient. This group of patients has a predilection to break down BCAA in the muscles (Schmidt, Ahnefeld, & Burri, 1983). The use of formulas with high BCAA replenish those depleted in the trauma patient. To offset the increased rate of nitrogen excretion, the protein intake should be increased (Ford & Vizcarra, 1995).

PARENTERAL NUTRITION IN THE PEDIATRIC PATIENT

TPN must be monitored in the pediatric patient to meet the demands of growth and development. Children have a high basal metabolic rate per unit of body weight, an increased evaporative fluid loss, and immature kidneys. Infants and young children need additional amino acids, which are nonessential in adults. The amino acids required for infants and children include histidine, tyrosine, cystine, and taurine. Special amino acid formulas are available to meet these needs (Ford & Vizcarra, 1995).

Assessment

Nutritional assessment of the pediatric patient uses standard growth curves. Calculation of the ratio of weight to height indicates wasting, and calculation of the ratio of height to age indicates stunting of growth. Anthropometric measurements are used as gauges of somatic protein and fat stores. Visceral protein stores are evaluated by determining serum albumin, serum transferrin, prealbumin, and retinol-binding protein levels (Taylor, 1991).

567

Indications

Pediatric patients requiring parenteral nutrition fall into three major categories:

1. Those with congenital or acquired anomalies of the GI tract, such as abdominal wall defects and intestinal atresias
2. Those with intractable diarrhea syndromes, such as inflammatory bowel disease, necrotizing enterocolitis, and complicated meconium ileus
3. Those with other conditions, such as burns, sepsis, hepatic disease, and renal disease

Monitoring

Many children require long-term support at home. Monitoring includes many of the same parameters as for adults. The monitoring during initiation of parenteral nutrition includes daily weights, strict intake and output, daily electrolytes until stable, serum glucose measurements every 8 to 12 hours, serum triglyceride and free fatty acid levels weekly, and liver function test biweekly.

In addition, children require evaluation of growth determinations including weight, height, head circumference, and anthropometric measurements for the duration of the therapy.

✎ **NOTE:** The predominant complication associated with parenteral nutrition in infants is cholestasis.

COMPLICATIONS AND NURSING CONSIDERATIONS

Complications associated with parenteral nutrition are classified as metabolic, catheter-related, or related to precipitation formation (Table 15–12). Complications may be minimized by appropriate monitoring.

Metabolic Complications

The complications associated with metabolic imbalances when administering TPN are either avoidable or controllable.

Hyperglycemia and Hyperosmolar Syndrome

Hyperglycemia is a common metabolic occurrence with TPN because of the high dextrose concentrations included in the admixture. Other factors that put the patient at risk for hyperglycemia are the presence of overt or latent diabetes mellitus, increased age, sepsis, hypokalemia, and hypophosphatemia. Conditions of stress result in decreased glucose tolerance and hyperglycemia in up to 25% of patients on TPN. Infusion of large amounts of glucose can also unmask latent diabetes, making hyperglycemia one of the most common complications encountered with parenteral nutrition. Other considerations when infusing formulas containing high concentrations of TPN solution is the potential effect of carbohydrate metabolism on respiration. Metabolism of carbohydrates results in increased production of carbon dioxide that must be compensated for by increased minute ventilation. This could precipitate respiratory failure in patients with preexisting respiratory disease or interfere with weaning from mechanical ventilation (Allmen & Fischer, 1991).

568

TABLE 15–12. COMPLICATIONS OF PARENTERAL NUTRITION

Complication	Possible Etiology	Symptoms	Treatment	Prevention
		Metabolic Complications		
Hypervolemia	Excess fluid administration Renal dysfunction Congestive heart failure Hepatic failure	Dyspnea, bounding pulse, moist rales, edema, weight gain	Restrict fluid Use diuretics Dialysis in extreme cases	Initiate PN once fluid balance stable Monitor input/output Monitor serum and urine osmolarity
Hypovolemia	Inadequate fluid administration Overdiuresis	Dehydration, thirst, dry mucous membranes, low urine output, weight loss	Increase fluid intake	Monitor daily intake/output Monitor serum and urine osmolality
Hyperkalemia	Renal dysfunction Excessive potassium administration Metabolic acidosis Use of potassium-sparing medications (ie, aldactone)	Diarrhea, tachycardia, cardiac arrest, oliguria, paresthesias	Decrease potassium intake Use potassium binders	Monitor serum levels for trends Assess for drug-nutrient interactions, especially potassium-sparing diuretics
Hypokalemia	Inadequate potassium provision Increased potassium losses (diarrhea, diuretics, intestinal fistulas)	Nausea, vomiting, confusion, arrhythmias, cardiac arrest, respiratory depression	Increase PN potassium or provide intravenously	Give 40 mEq of potassium daily unless contraindicated 3 mEq of potassium per gram of nitrogen needed with anabolism
Hypernatremia	Inadequate free water administration Excessive sodium intake Excessive water losses (fever, burns, hyperventilation)	Thirst, decreased skin turgor, mild irritability in some cases, elevated serum sodium, BUN and hematocrit	Decrease sodium intake Replenish fluids	Avoid excess sodium intake Monitor fluid status Monitor urine sodium

TABLE 15–12. **COMPLICATIONS OF PARENTERAL NUTRITION** (*Continued*)

Complication	Possible Etiology	Symptoms	Treatment	Prevention
Metabolic Complications				
Hyponatremia	Excessive fluid administration Nephritis and/or adrenal insufficiency Dilutional states (congestive heart failure, SIADH, cirrhosis of the liver with ascites)	Confusion, hypotension, irritability, lethargy, seizures	Restrict fluid intake Increase sodium intake as dictated by clinical status	Avoid overhydration Provide 60 to 100 mEq/d unless contraindicated by cardiac, renal, or fluid status Monitor urine sodium
Hyperglycemia	Rapid infusion of concentrated dextrose solution Sepsis, pancreatitis, postoperative stress Chromium deficiency Use of steroids Advanced age Multiple sources of dextrose from both oral and intravenous routes	Blood glucose >200 mg/dL Metabolic acidosis Polyuria, polydipsia	Use insulin Reduce dextrose concentration in PN	Slow initiation and advancement of PN Use mixed substrate solution
Hypoglycemia	Abrupt discontinuation of PN Insulin overdose	Weakness, sweating, palpitations, lethargy, shallow respirations	Administer dextrose	Taper PN solution With abrupt discontinuation of TPN, hang 10% dextrose at the same rate as the TPN to prevent rebound hypoglycemia Monitor serum glucose levels with use of insulin

	Causes	Signs/Symptoms	Treatment	Prevention
Hypertriglyceridemia	Lipid provision exceeds ability to clear lipids from bloodstream (>4 mg/kg per minute) Sepsis, multisystem organ failure, pathologic hyperlipidemia, lipoid nephrosis Medication usage alters fat metabolism (ie, cyclosporin)	Serum triglyceride level 300 to 350 mg/dL 6 hr past lipid initiation Elevated levels in previously stable patients (ie, sepsis)	Decrease lipid volume administered Lengthen infusion time Simultaneously infuse glucose	Assess for preexisting history of hyperlipidemia before initiation of PN Avoid lipid administration >2.5 g/kg per day or >60% of total calories
Hypercalcemia	Renal failure, tumor lysis syndrome Bone cancer Excess vitamin D administration Prolonged immobilization and stress Hyperparathyroidism	Confusion, dehydration, muscle weakness, nausea, vomiting, coma	Administer isotonic saline Inorganic phosphate supplementation Administration corticosteroids, mithramycin	Encourage weight bearing activity Evaluate vitamin D intake
Hypocalcemia	Decreased vitamin D intake Hypoparathyroidism Citrate binding of calcium due to excessive blood transfusions Hypoalbuminemia (use correction factor to determine if patient truly hypocalcemic; [correction factor = (normal albumin − observed albumin) × 0.8]	Parasthesias, tetany, irritability, ventricular arrhythmias	Calcium supplementation	Provide 15 mEq of calcium daily

571

TABLE 15–12. COMPLICATIONS OF PARENTERAL NUTRITION (*Continued*)

Metabolic Complications

Complication	Possible Etiology	Symptoms	Treatment	Prevention
Hypermagnesemia	Excessive magnesium administration Renal insufficiency	Respiratory paralysis, hypotension, premature ventricular contractions, lethargy, cardiac arrest, coma, liver dysfunction	Decrease magnesium provision	Monitor serum levels for trends
Hypomagnesmia	Refeeding syndrome Alcoholism Diuretic usage Increased losses (eg, diarrhea) Medication usage (eg, cyclosporin) Diabetic ketoacidosis Chemotherapy	Cardiac arrhythmias, tetany, convulsions, muscular weakness	Magnesium supplementation	Monitor serum levels for trends
Hyperphosphatemia	Excess phosphate administration Renal dysfunction	Parasthesias, flaccid paralysis, mental confusion, hypertension, cardiac arrhythmias, tissue calcification with prolonged elevated levels	Decrease phosphate administration Phosphate binders	Monitor serum levels for trends
Prerenal azotemia	Dehydration Excess protein provision Inadequate nonprotein calorie provision with mobilization of own protein stores	Elevated serum BUN	Increase fluid intake Decrease protein load Increase nonprotein calories	Monitor serum BUN for trends Perform nitrogen balance study

Overfeeding	Excess carbohydrate and/or protein administration	Excess carbohydrate: CO_2 retention, cardiac tamponade, liver dysfunction. Excess protein: elevated BUN, excess nitrogen excretion, elevated BUN/Cr ratio	Decrease carbohydrate/protein provision as needed	Avoid excess carbohydrate/protein administration
Essential fatty acid deficiency	Inadequate fat intake	Dermatitis, alopecia, alterations in pulmonary, neurologic, and red cell membranes	Lipid administration	Provide 2–4% of calories as linoleic acid, or 8–10% of calories from fat, especially in patients severely malnourished or expected not to take food by mouth for more than 3 wk
Catheter-Related Complications				
Pneumothorax	Catheter placement by inexperienced personnel	Tachycardia, dyspnea, persistent cough, diaphoresis	A small pneumothorax may resolve untreated, a larger pneumothorax may require chest tube placement	Catheter placement by experienced personnel
Air embolism	Occurs when line is interrupted and air is inspired while the line is uncapped	Cyanosis, tachypnea, hypotension, churning heart murmur (classic sign)	Immediately place patient on the left side and lower the head of the bed; this may keep the air within the apex of the right ventricle until it is reabsorbed	Line placement by appropriately trained personnel
Catheter embolization	Pulling the catheter back through the needle used for insertion	Cardiac arrhythmias	Surgically remove the catheter tip	Avoid withdrawing the catheter through the insertion needle

TABLE 15–12. COMPLICATIONS OF PARENTERAL NUTRITION (*Continued*)

Complication	Possible Etiology	Symptoms	Treatment	Prevention
		Catheter-Related Complications		
Venous thrombosis	Mechanical trauma to vein Hypotension Solution osmolality Hypercoagulopathy, sepsis	Swelling or pain in one or both arms, shoulders, or neck	Anticoagulation therapy with urokinase or streptokinase Remove catheter	Use of silicone catheter Addition of heparin to PN Low-dose warfarin therapy
Catheter occlusion	Hypotension Failure to maintain line patency Formation of fibrin sheath outside the catheter Solution precipitates	Increasing need for greater pressure to maintain a continuous infusion rate	Anticoagulation therapy with urokinase or streptokinase	Use of a large-diameter catheter as appropriate Routine flushes of catheter Monitor for solution precipitation
Improper tip location	Venous vasculature anomalies Catheter placement by inexperienced personnel	Phlebitis, severe cardiorespiratory distress, possible thrombosis	Remove catheter	Proper catheter placement by properly trained personnel
Phlebitis	Peripheral administration of hypertonic solution (osmolarity ≥900 mOsm/kg) Line infiltration	Redness, swelling, pain at peripheral site	Change peripheral line site, start central PN if appropriate	Minimize osmolarity of peripheral solution by using lipids as primary source of calories Reduce addition of electrolytes and other PN additives as possible
Catheter-related sepsis	Inappropriate technique in line placement Poor catheter care Contaminated solution	Unexplained fever, chills; red, indurated area around catheter site; possible catheter tip	Remove catheter and replace at another site	Development of strict protocols for line placement and catheter care

*Cr = creatinine, PN = parenteral nutrition; SIADH = syndrome of inappropriate antidiuretic hormone.

Source: From Skipper, A., & Marian, M. (1993). Parenteral therapy. In Gottschlich, M. M., Matarese, L. E., & Shronts, E. P. (eds.). *Nutrition support dietetics: Core curriculum,* 2nd ed. Baltimore, MD: American Society for Parenteral Therapy and Enteral Nutrition (ASPEN) with permission.

NURSING CONSIDERATIONS
1. Begin TPN infusion at a slow rate (40 to 60 mL/hour).
2. Gradually increase the rate 25 mL/hour until maximal infusion rate is achieved.
3. Maintain a steady state of infusion (TPN must stay within 10% of prescribed rate).
4. Use a rate control device to monitor the infusion.
5. Monitor serum blood sugar every 6 hours, particularly during the first week of infusion.
6. Record fluid intake and output accurately very 8 hours.
7. Measure hourly urine output if urinary losses are above 250 mL/hour.
8. Check body weight daily using same scale. The ideal weight gain for patients receiving TPN is approximately 2 lb/week.
9. Monitor vital signs at regular intervals. Look for signs of hypovolemia.

Postinfusion Hypoglycemia

Postinfusion hypoglycemia due to hyperinsulinism can occur if the TPN solution is abruptly discontinued.

NURSING CONSIDERATION
1. Wean the patient from the TPN solution gradually in decreased increments of 25 to 40 mL/hour over 24 to 48 hours.
2. If using C-TPN, gradually initiate and decrease the solution.

Essential Fatty Acid Deficiency

Fat administration is important for delivery of essential fatty acids. If the regimen for nutritional support does not include a calorie source from fats, the patient is at risk for EFAD. Fats may be administered in amounts that supply 30% to 50% of the calories. By adding fats to the nutritional support, CO_2 production can be decreased and other metabolic complications may be avoided (Farley, 1991).

Hyperammonemia

An elevated blood ammonia level is a common finding in infants and children receiving TPN. High protein intake may lead to elevated ammonia levels. Arginine is important in the urea cycle, and a deficiency of this amino acid may contribute to the development of hyperammonemia (Seashore, Seashore, & Rily, 1972).

✎ **NOTE:** In adults, the most common laboratory finding is that of elevated transaminase levels; the most common abnormality is liver steatosis. Cholestasis and gallbladder disease are potential complications of long-term TPN.

Electrolyte Imbalances

Major electrolyte imbalances associated with TPN can occur if excessive or deficient amounts of electrolytes are supplied in the daily fluid allowance. These include imbalances of sodium, potassium, magnesium, phosphate, or calcium.

Hypophosphatemia

Adenosine triphosphate (ATP) is required for all cell energy production. Protein synthesis begins when TPN is administered and phosphate is driven into the intracellular space as a component of ATP. Therefore, a deficiency of phosphate can occur.

575

Hypokalemia

Potassium is also driven into the intracellular space during TPN. Serum potassium can become depleted with an inadequate supply of this electrolyte along with the use of insulin in the TPN solution. Insulin administration further intensifies intracellular potassium.

Hypomagnesemia

The magnesium electrolyte also is driven into the intracellular space during TPN administration. Therefore, this electrolyte must also be included in TPN solution compounding.

Hypernatremia

To maintain homeostasis the sodium ion is driven from the intracellular space into the extracellular space. This compensatory mechanism tries to combat the extracellular anion loss (Metheny, 1996). This shift can cause hypernatremia.

> **NURSING CONSIDERATIONS**
> 1. Observe for signs and symptoms of hypophosphatemia, hypokalemia, hypomagnesemia, and hypernatremia. (See Chapter 4 for a review of signs and symptoms.)
> 2. Chemistry panel should be drawn every 3 days to check electrolyte levels.

Catheter-Related Complications

Pneumothorax

Pneumothorax results when injury occurs during catheter placement. Blood, air, or infusion of fluid collects in the pleural cavity. Care must be taken to assess catheter placement before infusion of TPN. Assess for sharp chest pain, decreased breath sounds, changes in vital signs, and respiratory status. If pneumothorax has occurred, it is evident on a chest x-ray.

Air Embolism

Passage of air into the heart can occur during insertion of the central line or during catheter maintenance. All connections should be taped and procedures strictly followed for tubing changes along with dressing management techniques. Change tubing during patient's expiratory respiratory phase. Apply an occlusive dressing over the site after the catheter has been removed.

Vein Thrombosis

Long-term central catheterization can cause vein thrombosis in the superior vena cava or its tributaries. Use of a silicone catheter decreases the risk of thrombogenic factors. Pulmonary emboli can be a secondary complication of vein thrombosis. Thrombolytic therapy is of benefit when flow rates are affected owing to thrombus formation, as is the use of heparin added to the infusate to prevent thrombosis. The physician should be notified if thrombosis is suspected.

Catheter Malposition

This complication can occur during introduction of the catheter. If there is difficulty in passage of the catheter, cardiac arrhythmias during insertion along with irregularities of flow of infusate could indicate malposition of the catheter. Check dressing at least every 4 hours for signs of inadvertent displacement. Report suspected catheter malposition to the physician promptly.

Infection

When TPN is provided by a central line there are concerns related to the contamination of the central venous catheter as discussed in Chapter 13. Catheter-related sepsis is a serious complication of central TPN therapy. This complication is preventable with strict aseptic technique.

TPN patients are often immune-compromised as a result of malnutrition; these patients are highly susceptible to infection. The origin of TPN catheter-related sepsis is most often the site itself; infection related to contaminated infusates is rare (Kennedy-Caldwell & Guenter, 1988).

NURSING CONSIDERATIONS
1. Maintain aseptic technique in catheter maintenance and administration of TPN.
2. Aseptic dressing changes should be done every 48 to 72 hours if nontransparent occlusive dressing is used; every 4 to 7 days, depending on institutional policy, if transparent dressing is used. See Chapter 13 for dressing management.
3. Use of a 0.22-micron inline antimicrobial filter is recommended for TPN lines, except when lipid emulsion is added to these solutions, at which time a 1.2-micron filter should be used (INS, 1990).

Admixture Complications

Admixture complications involve the formation of precipitates in the formula. The Food and Drug Administration (FDA) has issued a safety alert regarding the hazards of precipitation associated with parenteral nutrition (April, 1994). Two deaths and at least two cases of respiratory distress have been reported as being related to infusion of three-in-one TPN admixtures containing precipitate of calcium phosphate. Because of the potential life-threatening events, caution should be taken to ensure that precipitates have not formed in any parenteral nutritional admixtures. The FDA suggests the following steps to decrease the risk of additional injuries:

1. The amounts of phosphorus and calcium added to the admixture are critical. The solubility of the added calcium should be calculated from the volume at the time the calcium is added and should not be based on the final volume.
2. Some amino acid injections for TPN admixtures contain phosphate ions. These phosphate ions and the volume at the time the phosphate is added should be considered.
3. The line should be flushed between the addition of any incompatible components.
4. A lipid emulsion in a TNA admixture obscures the presence of a precipitate. Add calcium before the lipid solution.
5. A filter should be used when infusing either central or peripheral parenteral nutrition. Standards of practice vary, but the following is suggested: 1.2-micron air-eliminating filter for lipid-containing admixtures; a 0.22-micron air-eliminating filter for non–lipid-containing admixtures
6. Parenteral nutrition admixture should be administered within the following time frames:
   If stored at room temperature, start within 24 hours after mixing.
   If stored at refrigerated temperatures, start within 24 hours of rewarming.

577

7. If symptoms of acute respiratory distress, pulmonary embolus, or interstitial pneumonitis develop, stop the infusion immediately and thoroughly check solution for precipitates.

STANDARDS OF PRACTICE FOR NUTRITIONAL SUPPORT

Standards of practice related to nutritional support have been addressed by ASPEN (1993) and the INS (1990). Presented here are the accepted Standards of Practice related to nutritional support.

Implementation Standards

Parenteral formulations shall be prepared according to established guidelines for safe and effective nutritional therapy (Fig. 15–3).

1. Parenteral formulations shall be sterile.
2. Parenteral formulations should be stored at 4°C.
3. Policies should be established limiting additions to the parenteral feeding formulations after they are infusing.
4. Patient or responsible person shall receive education and demonstrate competence in access route care in home care situations.

Monitoring Standards

Patients should be monitored for therapeutic efficacy, adverse effects, and clinical changes that might influence specialized nutritional support.

1. Protocols shall be developed for periodic review of the patient's clinical and biochemical status.
2. Routine monitoring should include nutrient intake; review of current medications; signs of intolerance to therapy; weight changes; biochemical, hematologic and other pertinent data, including clinical signs of nutrient deficiencies and excesses; adjustment of therapy; changes in lifestyle; psychosocial problems; and changes in home environment.
3. Assessment of patient's major organ functions should be made periodically (ASPEN, 1993).

A summary of monitoring standards is presented in Table 15–13.

Metabolic

Monitor the following:

Blood or urine glucose levels several times daily
Electrolytes (daily during the first 2 to 3 days and three times weekly thereafter
Blood urea nitrogen (BUN) creatinine three times a week
Fluid balance daily for the duration of therapy
Calcium, aspartate transaminase (AST), alanine transaminase (ALT), and alkaline phosphatase weekly
Phosphorus and magnesium one to two times the first week, then weekly

TOTAL PARENTERAL NUTRITION (TPN) ORDER FORM

Date _____ Time _____

ATTENTION DOCTORS: Please order electrolyte content in **mEq/24 hours.** Pharmacy will supply a 24 hour amount. Please fill out for any ingredient or rate changes. They will be initiated with the next bag unless otherwise indicated.

Protein Source:	
Aminosyn 7% (35 grams/500 ml)	mls/24 hours
Aminosyn 10% (50 grams/500ml)	mls/24 hours

Carbohydrate Caloric Source:	
Dextrose 50% (850 kcal/500ml)	mls/24 hours
Dextrose 70% (1190 kcal/500ml)	mls/24 hours

Total Volume: _____ mls/24 hours,   Rate: _____ mls/hour

Electrolyte Additions:	
Sodium Chloride	mEq/24 hours
Potassium Chloride	mEq/24 hours
Potassium Phosphate	mEq/24 hours
Calcium Gluconate	mEq/24 hours
Magnesium Sulfate	mEq/24 hours

Multivitamin-12 (10 ml = 1 vial/24 hours)	mls/24 hours
Trace Elements (1 ml = 1 vial/24 hours)	ml/24 hours
Regular Insulin (Humulin-R, 100 units/ml)	Units/24 hours

Fat Emulsion 10 % (550 kcal/500 ml unit)®	Unit every ____ day(s)
Fat Emulsion 20% (1,000 kcal/500 ml unit)®	Unit every ____ day(s)
Normal Serum Albumin 25% (50ml and 100ml)*	

® Each unit will be piggybacked below filter and infused over 4 to 8 hours.

* All albumin shall be infused separately below final filter over no more than 4 hours as recommended by CDC and FDA since it is a blood product.

Refer to I.V. Therapy P/P for standard nursing care of TPN patients (Pol. #10-A,B,C)
* □ Blood glucose fingerstick _____ times per day.
  □ Urine S & A every _____ hours. Report 2+ or over.
  □ Baseline lab if not obtained in last 48 hours including: CBC, Chem Profile-20, Serum Magnesium, Protime & Urinalysis.
  □ Daily lab tests: Blood Sugar, Electrolytes or
  □ Ongoing lab tests including: □ Chem. Profile-20 & Serum Magnesium 3x weekly,
      □ CBC twice weekly, □ Protime weekly.

TO/VO_____ M.D. / _____ R.N./Pharm.D
(Circle one)   (Circle one)

(Addressograph) | Roseville Community Hospital
                                         | Roseville, California 95661
                                         | Daily TPN Order Form

Figure 15–3. Total parenteral nutrition order form.

579

TABLE 15–13. **SUMMARY OF MONITORING OF PARENTERAL NUTRITION THERAPY**

> Before initiation of therapy by central line:
>   Check placement of catheter tip by x-ray.
> After initiation of parenteral nutrition therapy:
>   Start TPN infusion slowly.
>   Check temperature and vital signs every 6 hours.
>   Monitor blood sugar every 6 hours.
>   Maintain strict intake and output.
>   Check weight daily.
>   Decrease TPN solutions gradually.
>   Change TPN and lipid administration sets every 24 hours.
> Laboratory parameters to check twice weekly:
>   Liver function
>   Electrolyte profile
>   Serum profiles weekly: calcium, AST, ALT, alkaline phosphatase
>   BUN and creatinine
> Nutritional
>   Evaluate nitrogen balance weekly.
>   Check albumin, transferring, prealbumin, or retinol-binding protein
>   Check total lymphocyte count and anergy panels
>   Check creatinine height index to monitor protein.

Nutritional

Weigh the patient daily (may be decreased to two to three times per week in stable patients)

Evaluate nitrogen balance weekly (or as needed to determine adequacy of protein intake).

Albumin, transferrin, transthyretin (prealbumin) or retinol-binding protein may be measured as needed to assess visceral protein status.

Total lymphocyte count and anergy panels may be used to monitor changes in immune function.

Creatinine height index may be used to monitor somatic protein status.

For patients receiving modified amino acid solutions, plasma aminograms may be helpful if available (INS, 1990).

Nursing Plan of Care

ADMINISTRATION OF TPN

Assessment

Subjective	Objective
History of weight loss	Vitals signs, especially temperature
History of disease state and malnourished state	Level of consciousness
	Skin turgor assessment
Biographic data	Weight gains or losses
Past health history	Tissue edema
Allergies and medications	Ratios of urinary output to intake
	Oral mucous membranes
	Serum blood glucose levels

Continued on following page

Patient Outcome Criteria

The patient will:
1. Stabilize weight and gradually increase to within 10% of ideal weight
2. Gain weight at a rate of 1 lb every 3 weeks, increasing to 1 lb every 2 weeks
3. Display moist skin and mucous membranes, stable vital signs, individually adequate urinary output, and no edema
4 Verbalize understanding of condition or disease process and individual nutritional needs
5. Correctly perform necessary procedures and explain reasons for the actions

Nursing Diagnoses

Altered nutrition less than body requirements related to chewing or swallowing difficulties; anorexia; nausea; vomiting; difficulty or inability to procure foods
Altered health maintenance related to poor dietary habits, with perceptual or cognitive impairment
Altered nutrition (greater than body requirement) related to imbalance of intake versus activity expenditure
Altered tissue perfusion (peripheral) related to infusion of irritating solution

Nursing Management: Critical Activities

Assist with insertion of central line
Insert peripheral intravenous central catheter per agency protocol
Ascertain correct placement of intravenous central catheter by x-ray prior to beginning TPN
Maintain central line patency and dressing per agency protocol
Monitor for infiltration and infection
Check the PPN or TPN solution to ensure correct nutrients are included as ordered
Maintain sterile technique when perparing and hanging TPN solution
Keep infusion within 10% of prescribed rate
Use an infusion pump for delivery of TPN solutions
Avoid rapidly replacing lagging TPN solutions
Monitor daily weight
Monitor intake and output
Monitor serum albumin, total protein, electrolyte, glucose and chemistry profile
Monitor vital signs
Monitor blood sugar every 6 hours.
Administer insulin as ordered, to maintain serum glucose in the designated range as appropriate.
Report abnormal signs and symptoms associated with TPN to the physician and modify care accordingly.
Maintain universal precautions.
(McCloskey & Bulechek, 1992)

PATIENT EDUCATION

The patient receiving enteral nutrition, PPN, or TPN will need education, periodic assessment, and retraining as needed.

Inform the patient about the purpose and duration of the projected nutritional support.
Instruct the patient on the product hang time.
Educate the patient and caregiver about management of the access device.
Instruct the patient receiving enteral feedings about clean techniques for handling the tube, maintaining the access site, and flushing the tube to maintain patency.

581

Inform the patient about complications associated with TPN administration, including:

    Metabolic complications such as: hypoglycemia, electrolyte imbalances (recognize and respond to these complications)

    Mechanical or procedural problems (catheter or tube occlusion, leakage, breakage, or dislodgment)

    Equipment malfunction or breakage

    Infusion contamination precipitate or inhomogeneity (recognize and report signs and symptoms of localized or systemic infectious process)

Provide 24-hour phone numbers for home care agency or physician so that patient or caregiver can access professional help.

HOME CARE ISSUES

Home parenteral nutrition (HPN) has been well established over the past 10 years and should be instituted and supervised by a multidisciplinary team with knowledge and expertise (ASPEN, 1993). Clients and their families can be taught to safely administer I.V. admixtures, and they can be monitored in a home setting. Hospital-to-home transition can be a difficult task. Keep in mind that the day of discharge is usually physically and emotionally stressful; the home care nurse should be in attendance for starting the TPN infusion at home. Before home therapy for nutritional support is initiated, a baseline electrolyte chemistry panel, magnesium and phosphorus levels, and a CBC should be obtained within 7 days of discharge. Home safety must be determined before discharge from the hospital (Wiseman, 1985).

Successful home therapy depends on several factors:

1. Medical stability
2. Emotional stability
3. Patient's lifestyle
4. Intellectual ability (client or primary caregiver)
5. Visual acuity
6. Manual dexterity
7. Home environment:
   Dry storage space for supplies
   Refrigerator large enough to store admixtures
   Clean, low-traffic area for procedure preparation
   Electronic outlets for any electronic equipment

The patient or caregiver and home environment should be suitable for safe delivery and monitoring of HPN (ASPEN, 1993).

Advantages of home treatment for nutritional support are that it involves lesser expense than treatment in the hospital; it allows the patient to remain in a familiar, comfortable surrounding, thereby decreasing the confusion associated with age-related environment changes; it allows the patient to return to normal activities in many cases; and it is associated with a lesser risk of acquiring a nosocomial infection. HPN is usually cycled or given over a 12- to 16-hour period, and most of the administration occurs during the sleeping hours (Grace & Tomeselli, 1995). In addition, a person's control over his or her body and the self-care responsibility increase self-esteem (Weinstein, 1993).

The home education process should include but not be limited to:

1. Verbal and written instructions of appropriate procedures
2. Demonstration and return demonstration of procedures by primary caregiver
3. Evaluation and documentation of competency

582

4. Self-monitoring instruction
5. Limitations of physical activity
6. Emergency intervention and problem-solving techniques
7. Care of infusion equipment, solutions, and supplies
8. Disposal of supplies
9. Expectations of home care and medical and nursing follow-up (Kennedy-Caldwell & Guenter, 1988)

Home care training must be individually designed according to the individual's capabilities. Assessment of the patient's physical and emotional status before each teaching session aids in determining goals for that session. A minimum number of people should be involved with each teaching session to limit distractions and anxiety.

COMPETENCY CRITERIA: Nutritional Support

Competency Statement: The nurse will demonstrate competency in administration of nutritional support.

COGNITIVE CRITERIA

	Knowledgeable	Needs Education
1. Identifies proper placement of central line catheter tip:		
Superior vena cava		
Radiology confirmation		
2. Recognizes critical abnormal laboratory values:		
Serum albumin		
Total protein		
Serum glucose		
Serum electrolytes		
Chemistry profile		
3. Identifies basic formula for nutritional support:		
Carbohydrates		
Amino acids		
Lipids		

PERFORMANCE CRITERIA

	Skilled	Needs Education
1. Initiates TPN:		
Verifies correct TPN solution		
Prepares appropriate equipment, including filter		
Follows procedure for accessing system		
Verifies blood return and irrigates with 0.9% sodium chloride		
2. Maintains TPN Infusion:		
Irrigates catheter with correct solution at appropriate intervals		
Ensures the TPN/lipid I.V. tubing are changed		

584

Ensures that only TPN will infuse via the TPN lumen of the vascular assess device

Ensures that blood glucose monitoring is documented every 6 hours

Ensures that the physician is notified if temperature is $> 38°C$

3. **Assesses patient for development of potential complications:**

Hyper/hypo glycemia

Electrolyte imbalance

Catheter-related infection/sepsis

4. **Discontinues therapy safely:**

Weans patient from TPN as prescribed by physician

During weaning continues to monitor patient for complications

Suggested Evaluation Criteria

Written test—Cognitive criteria

Observation of initiation and discontinuation of TPN

Review of documentation of assessments

Return demonstration of simulation model

KEY POINTS

Concepts of nutrition
Nutritional deficiencies
Types of malnutrition
Marasmus
Kwashiorkor
Mixed malnutrition
Effects of malnutrition
Decreased protein stores
Albumin depletion
Impaired immune status

Nutritional assessment
History
Medical
Social
Dietary
Anthropometric measurements

585

Diagnostic tests
　　Serum albumin
　　Serum transferrin
　　Prealbumin and retinol-binding protein
　　Total lymphocyte count
Physical examination

Nutritional requirements
Carbohydrates (energy source)
　　Dextrose in 5%, 10%, 20%, 50%, and 70%
　　Other potential sources—fructose, invert sugar, and sorbitol and xylitol
Lipids (fats) (energy source)
　　Prevents EFAD. Use of fat emulsions can help control hyperglycemia.
Protein (amino acids)
　　Solutions of eight essential amino acids, 3.5% to 10%
Electrolytes
　　Potassium: 30 to 40 mEq per 1000 mL
　　Magnesium sulfate: 10 to 20 mEq every 24 hours
　　Calcium gluceptate, calcium gluconate, or calcium chloride: 10 to 15 mEq
　　　in 24 hours
　　Sodium chloride: 60 to 100 mEq in 24 hours
　　Phosphorus sodium or phosphorus potassium: 20 to 45 mEq in 24 hours
　　Chloride provided related to acid-base balance
Vitamins
　　A, D, E, C, B_1, B_2, B_3, B_5, B_6, B_{12}, folic acid, biotin
　　Vitamin K, 5 mg given intramuscularly
Trace elements
　　Zinc, copper, chromium, manganese
Medication additives
　　Insulin
　　Heparin
　　Cimetidine
　　(Antibiotics and corticosteroids are being studied.)

Modalities for delivery of nutritional support
Indications for
　　Infants with inadequate absorptive surface
　　Adults with short gut syndrome, enterocutaneous fistulas, renal failure, hepatic
　　　failure, burns
Enteral nutrition
　　Advantages over parenteral nutrition
　　　Makes use of the GI tract (if patient's GI tract is functioning)
　　　Easier to achieve a positive nitrogen balance
　　　Less expensive
Peripheral parenteral nutrition
　　PPN provides nutritional support in patients with mild stress and is used
　　　for short term duration, usually less than 3 weeks.
　　　Combination of 5% to 10% dextrose, with amino acids ranging from
　　　　2.75% to 4.25% along with electrolytes, trace elements, and vitamins
　　　Maximum osmolarity 900 mOsm/liter.
Total parenteral therapy (TPN)
　　Provides calories for weight gain, growth and development, and wound
　　　healing
　　Osmolarity 1800 to 2000 mOsm/liter

586

Total nutrient admixture (TNA)
    Combination of carbohydrate, protein and fats in one 3-liter solution, or all-in-one system bag to infuse over 24 hours
Cyclic therapy (C-TPN)
    Indicated for patients on long-term nutritional support
    Administered over 12 to 18 hours, usually at night, thus leaving the patient free to lead an active lifestyle
    Patient must escalate and taper the solution so as not to cause dramatic changes in blood glucose levels.
Specialized parenteral formulas
    Renal failure
        Special amino acid formula that contains high amounts of essential amino acids to aid in nephron repair
    Liver failure
        Solutions high in BCAA
    Stress formula
        Solutions high in BCAA for trauma patient

Parenteral nutrition in the pediatric patient
Nutritional assessment
    Growth curves
    Ratio of weight to height; to age height
    Anthropometric measurements
    Visceral protein stores
Indications
    Congenital or acquired anomalies of the GI tract (e.g., abdominal wall defects, intestinal atresias)
    Intractable diarrhea syndromes (e.g., inflammatory bowel disease, necrotizing enterocolitis, meconium ileus
    Other conditions (e.g., burns, sepsis, hepatic disease, renal disease)
Monitoring
    Same as for adults
    Growth evaluation
    Anthropometric measurements

Complications
Metabolic
    Hyperglycemia and hyperosmolar syndrome
    Postinfusion hypoglycemia
    EFAD
    Hyperammonemia
    Electrolyte imbalances
        Hypophosphatemia
        Hypokalemia
        Hypomagnesemia
        Hypernatremia
Catheter-related
    Pneumothorax
    Air embolism
    Vein thrombosis
    Catheter malposition
    Infection
Admixture-related
    The FDA has a safety alert regarding the hazards of precipitation associated with parenteral nutrition containing calcium phosphate.

CRITICAL THINKING ACTIVITY

1. Check your agency policy and procedure manual for guidelines for monitoring the patient on TPN. Is there a set policy and how are these procedures documented?

2. You check your patient on TPN at the beginning of the shift and find that the fat emulsion has a 0.22-micron filter attached in the line in which it is infusing. What do you do?

3. A patient has had a blood glucose level of 100 mg/dL during the course of the first 48 hours of TPN. The next time you check the blood sugar, it is 240 mg/dL. What could be the reason for this sudden increase in blood sugar? How would you begin to check for the problem?

4. The physician has ordered C-TPN for 12 hours for your patient who has been stabilized on nutritional support for 2 weeks. How would you explain this therapy to the patient? Upon discharge, what kind of guidelines would you provide?

POST-TEST, CHAPTER 15

Match the definition in column II with the term in column I.

Column I

1. _____ BCAA
2. _____ Kwashiorkor
3. _____ HTPN
4. _____ Marasmus
5. _____ EFAD

Column II

A. Essential fatty acid deficiency
B. Branched-chain amino acid
C. Malnutrition caused by decreased intake of calories with adequate amount of protein
D. Malnutrition caused by adequate intake of calories with inadequate amount of protein
E. Home total parenteral nutrition

6–10. List five types of patients who would benefit from TPN.

_____

_____

_____

_____

_____

11–16. Identify the six nutrients essential for TPN.

_____

_____

_____

_____

_____

17. In addition to multiple vitamins, it is recommended that _____ be given intramuscularly weekly.
    A. Heparin 1000 U
    B. Vitamin K 5 mg
    C. Zinc 2.5 mg
    D. Biotin 60 μg

18. Cimetidine is added to parenteral nutrition for what purpose?
    A. To decrease incidence of vein thrombosis
    B. As a prophylactic measure against development of stress ulcers
    C. To increase muscle uptake of amino acids
    D. To increase tensile strength of the collagen

19. Insulin is added to parenteral nutrition for:
    A. Enhancing blood glucose levels
    B. Metabolism of carbohydrates
    C. Lipolytic effect
    D. All of the above

589

20. A disadvantage of TNA solutions is:
    A. Solution must be changed every 8 hours.
    B. Precipitation may be difficult to observe.
    C. Fats coagulate when mixed with dextrose.
    D. Risk of contamination increases owing to multiple adds to the mixture.

21. Nurses must be aware of which of the following when using C-TPN:
    A. Blood sugar can drop 1 hour after tapering off C-TPN.
    B. The patient who is metabolically stressed is not a good candidate for this therapy.
    C. Dehydration can occur if the fluid requirements are not met in 24 hours.
    D. All of the above.

22. Key points in delivery of PPN would be:
    A. Patient will resume enteral feeding within 5 to 7 days.
    B. PPN maintains patient nutritional state only.
    C. The osmolarity of the solution is a major consideration.
    D. All of the above.

23. Advantages of home care nutritional support include:
    A. Increased control of one's body
    B. Decreased risk of acquiring a nosocomial infection
    C. Continuation of normal routine
    D. All of the above

24. Identify the nursing considerations for TPN administration.

ANSWERS TO CHAPTER 15

Pre-test

1. D	6. C	11. A	16. D
2. B	7. A	12. E	17. C
3. C	8. C	13. E	18. E
4. E	9. C	14. B	
5. A	10. A	15. C	

Post-Test

1. B
2. D
3. E
4. C
5. A
6–10. Patients with delayed wound healing, postoperative complications, predisposition to intraoperative hemorrhage, GI problems, trauma, severe burns, anorexia nervosa, or cancer cachexia; also any patient with difficult in refeeding
11–16. Carbohydrates
Protein
Fats
Electrolytes
Trace Elements
Vitamins
17. B
18. B
19. D
20. B
21. D
22. D
23. D

24. Check catheter tip placement before starting TPN.
Begin administration of TPN slowly.
Gradually increase TPN at the rate of 25 mL/hour until maximal infusion rate is achieved.
Use rate control device to monitor the infusion.
Blood glucose monitoring must be done every 6 hours.
Chart intake and output accurately every 8 hours.
Check body weight daily using the same scale.
Monitor vital signs every 4 hours, especially temperature.
Wean patient off TPN gradually.
Observe for signs and symptoms of electrolyte imbalances.
Check chemistry panel every 3 days.
Maintain aseptic technique in catheter maintenance and in the administration of TPN.
Use Luer-lock connector or tape all connections.
Use 0.22 in-line filter for TPN solutions without fats added.

REFERENCES

Ahnefeld, F.W., Bassler, K.H., & Bauer, B.L. (1975). Suitability of nonglucose carbohydrates for parenteral nutrition. *European Journal of Intensive Care Medicine, 1*, 105.

American Medical Association. (1979). Guidelines for essential trace element preparation for parenteral use: A statement by the Nutrition Advisory Group. *Journal of Parenteral and Enteral Nutrition, 3*, 263.

American Medical Association Department of Foods and Nutrition. (1979). Multivitamin preparations for parenteral use: A statement by the Nutrition Advisory Group. *Journal of Parenteral and Enteral Nutrition, 3*, 259.

American Society for Parenteral and Enteral Nutrition. (1993). Guidelines for the use of parenteral and enteral nutrition in adult and pediatric patients. *Journal of Parenteral and Enteral Nutrition, Suppl 17*, 1SA–52SA.

Andrusko, K. (1987). Advantages and disadvantages of total nutrient admixtures in the home care patient. *Hospital Pharmacy, 22.*

Baker, A.L., & Rosenberg, I.H. (1987). Hepatic complications of total parenteral nutrition. *American Journal of Medicine, 82*, 489–97.

Baptista, R.H., & Rosenberg, I.H. (1987). Hepatic complications of total parenteral nutrition. *American Journal of Hospital Pharmacy, 42*, 2208.

Dietel, M. (1987). Total nutrient admixtures. An NSS symposium in three parts. *Nutrition Support Services, 7*, (13).

Dolan, J.T. (1991). *Critical case nursing: Clinical management through the nursing process.* Philadelphia: F.A. Davis.

Driscoll, D.F. (199). Clinical issues regarding the use of total nutrient admixtures. *DICP, 24*, 296–303.

Farley, J.M. (1991). Nutritional support of the critically ill patient. In Dolan, J.T. *Critical care nursing* (1125–1149). Philadelphia: F.A. Davis.

Fischer, (1991). *Total parenteral nutrition*, 2nd ed. Boston: Little, Brown.

Ford, C.D. & Vizcarra, C. (1995). Parenteral nutrition. In Terry, J., Baranowski, L., Lonsway, R., & Hedrick, C. (eds.). *Intravenous therapy: Clinical principles and practices* (505–534). Philadelphia: W.B. Saunders.

Friedman, G.J. (1980). Diet in the treatment of diabetes mellitus. In Goodhart, R.S., Shils, M.E. (eds.). *Modern nutrition in health and disease*. Philadelphia: Lea & Febiger.

Grant, J.P. (1992). *Handbook of Parenteral Nutrition, 2nd ed*. Philadelphia; W.B. Saunders, 15–47

Grace, A. & Tomaselli, B. (1995). Intravenous therapy in the home. In Terry, J., Baranowski, L., Lonsway, R. & Hedrick, C. (eds.). *Intravenous therapy: Clinical principles and practices* (505–534). Philadelphia: W.B. Saunders.

Hill, G.L. (1991). Nutritional assessment In Fischer, J.E. (ed.). *Total parenteral nutrition*, 2nd ed. (142–144) Boston: Little, Brown.

Intravenous Nursing Society. (1990). *Revised standards of practice*. Philadelphia: J.B. Lippincott.

Johndrow, P.D. (1988). Making your patient and his family feel at home with T.P.N. *Nursing 88, 10*, 65–69.

Kaminski, M.V. (1985). *Hyperalimentation: A guide for clinicians*. New York: Marcel Dekker, 23–45.

Kennedy-Caldwell, C., & Guenter, P. (1988). *Nutrition society nursing core curriculum*. Baltimore: ASPEN.

Knox, L.S. (1988). Nutritional requirements. In Kennedy-Caldwell, C., & Guenter, P. (eds.). *Nutrition support nursing*, 2nd ed. Baltimore: ASPEN, 5–28.

Mathewson-Kuhn, M. (1994). *Pharmacotherapeutics: A nursing process approach*, 3rd ed. Philadelphia: F.A. Davis.

McClary-Bennett, K., & Rosen, G.H. (1990). Cyclic total parenteral nutrition. *Nutrition in Clinical Practice, 5*(4), 163–165.

McCloskey, J.C., & Bulechek, G.M. (1992). Iowa intervention project: Nursing interventions classification (NIC), (501). St. Louis: Mosby-Year Book.

Metheny, N.M. (1996). *Fluid and electrolyte balance: Nursing considerations*, 3rd ed. Philadelphia: J.B. Lippincott.

Miller, S.J. (1991) Peripheral parenteral nutrition: Theory and practice. *Hospital Pharmacy, 26*(9), 796–801.

Sax, H.C. & Hasselgren, P. (1991). In Fischer, J.E. (ed.). *Total parenteral nutrition*, 2nd ed. (3–4) Boston: Little, Brown.

Schilling, C.G. (1988). Compatibility of drugs with a heparin-containing neonatal total parenteral nutrition. *American Journal of Hospital Pharmacy, 45*, 313.

Schmidt, J.E., Ahnefeld, F.W., & Burri, C. (1983). Nutritional support of the multiple trauma patient. *World Journal of Surgery, 7*, 132–142.

Singh, V.N. (1983). Non-glucose carbohydrate as an alternative energy source. (Abstract). Presented at the 7th Clinical Congress, Washington, DC: ASPEN.

Skipper, A., & Marian, M. (1993). Parenteral therapy. In Gottschlich, M.M., Matarese, L.E., & Shronts, E.P. (eds.). *Nutrition supports diatetics core curriculum*, 2nd ed. (117–122) Baltimore: ASPEN.

Smith, L.C., & Mullen, J.L. (1991). Nutritional assessment and indications for nutritional support. *Surgical Clinics of North America, 71*, 449–458.

Suzuki, N. T. (1986). Heparin in peripheral parenteral nutrition. *Drug Intell. Clinical Pharmacy, 11*, 714.

Torosian, M.H., & Daly, J.M. (1991). In Fischer, J.E. (ed.). *Total parenteral nutrition*, 2nd ed. (13–23). Boston: Little, Brown.

Tsallas, G., & Allen, L. (1982). Stability of cimetidine hydrochloride in parenteral nutrition solutions. *American Journal of Hospital Pharmacy, 39*, 484.

Warshawsky, K.Y. (1992). Intravenous fat emulsion. *Nutrition in Clinical Practice, 7*, 187–196.

Weinstein, S.M. (1993). *Plumer's principles & practice of intravenous therapy*. Philadelphia: J.B. Lippincott.

Whitbread, J., Jarres, L., & Brandwein, H. (1994). *Removal of Candida albicans from total nutrient admixtures by 1.2 micron filters*. New York: Pall Corporation Scientific and Laboratory Services.

Wiseman, M. (1985). Setting standards for home I.V. therapy. *American Journal of Nursing, 85*(4), 421–423.

APPENDICES

APPENDIX A
Nomogram of Body Surface Areas

APPENDIX B
Physical and Chemical Compatibility Chart

APPENDIX C
Normal Laboratory Reference Values

APPENDIX D
OSHA Guidelines 1995: Controlling Occupational Exposure to Hazardous Drugs

APPENDIX E
Dilution of Intravenous Drugs

APPENDIX F
Resource List of National Organizations

APPENDIX G
Survey of Scope of Intravenous Practice by State for Licensed Practical and Vocational Nurses

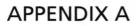

APPENDIX A

Nomogram of Body Surface Areas

HEIGHT		SURFACE AREA	WEIGHT	
feet	centimeters	in square meters	pounds	kilograms

			440	200
			420	190
			400	180
			380	170
			360	160
			340	150
		3.00	320	140
7′	220	2.90	300	
	215	2.80	290	130
10″	210	2.70	280	
8″	205	2.60	270	120
6″	200	2.50	260	
4″	195	2.40	250	
2″	190	2.30	240	110
	185	2.20	230	
6′	180		220	100
10″	175	2.10	210	95
8″	170	2.00	200	90
6″	165	1.95 / 1.90	190	85
4″	160	1.85	180	80
2″	155	1.80 / 1.75	170	
5′	150	1.70		75
10″	145	1.65 / 1.60	160	70
8″	140	1.55 / 1.50	150	
6″	135	1.45	140	65
4″	130	1.40 / 1.35	130	60
2″	125	1.30	120	55
4′	120	1.25	110	50
10″	115	1.20 / 1.15		
		1.10	100	45
8″	110	1.05	90	40
6″	105	1.00		
4″	100	.95	80	35
2″	95	.90		
3′	90	.85	70	30
		.80		
10″	85	.75	60	
8″	80	.70		25
		.65	50	
6″	75	.60		20

595

HEIGHT		SURFACE AREA	WEIGHT	
feet	centimeters	in square meters	pounds	kilograms

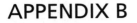

APPENDIX B

Physical and Chemical Compatibility Chart*

***Source:** From *Pharmacotherapeutics: A Nursing Process Approach*, third edition by M. M. Kuhn (1994), Philadelphia: F. A. Davis Company. Copyright 1993 by F. A. Davis Company. Reprinted with permission.

	Aminophylline	Ampicillin	Atropine sulfate	Bretylium	Calcium chloride	Calcium gluconate	Cefazolin	Cimetidine	Diazepam	Diazoxide	Digoxin	Dobutamine	Dopamine	Epinephrine HCl	Furosemide	Gentamicin	Heparin	Hydralazine
Aminophylline		P	N	D	N	P	S	I	N	N	P	B	P	I	B	P	P	I
Ampicillin	P		N	N	N	I	S	A	N	N	N	N	N	I	N	I	H	I
Atropine sulfate	N	N		N	N	N	N	P	N	N	N	P	N	D	N	N	P	N
Bretylium	D	N	N		C	D	N	N	N	N	D	I	C	N	N	M	N	N
Calcium chloride	N	N	N	C		N	N	N	N	N	P	I	D	I	N	N	N	N
Calcium gluconate	P	I	N	D	N		I	N	N	N	N	I	P	I	N	N	P	N
Cefazolin	S	S	N	N	N	I		P	N	N	N	N	N	N	N	I	S	N
Cimetidine	I	A	P	N	N	N	P		N	N	M	P	P	P	P	P	P	N
Diazepam	N	N	N	N	N	N	N	N		N	N	N	N	N	N	N	N	N
Diazoxide	N	N	N	N	N	N	N	N	N		N	N	N	N	N	N	N	I
Digoxin	P	N	N	D	P	N	N	M	N	N		N	N	N	N	N	N	H
Dobutamine	B	N	P	I	I	I	N	P	N	N	N		S	D	I	B	D	S
Dopamine	P	I	N	C	D	P	N	P	N	N	N	S		P	N	A	P	N
Epinephrine HCl	I	I	D	N	I	I	N	P	N	N	N	D	P		I	P	D	N
Furosemide	B	N	N	N	N	N	N	P	N	N	N	I	N	I		N	P	I
Gentamicin	P	I	N	M	N	N	I	P	N	N	N	B	A	P	N		I	N
Heparin	P	H	P	N	N	P	S	P	N	N	N	D	P	D	P	I		P
Hydralazine	I	I	N	N	N	N	N	N	N	I	H	S	N	N	I	N	P	
Insulin reg	I	N	N	P	N	N	N	A	N	N	I	I	N	N	N	N	P	P
Isoproterenol	I	P	N	I	P	P	N	P	N	N	N	P	P	N	N	P	P	P

Insulin reg	Isoproterenol	Lidocaine	Morphine sulfate	Netilmicin	Nitroglycerin	Nitroprusside	Norepinephrine	Phenytoin	Phytonadione	Potassium chloride	Procainamide	Propranolol	Quinidine	Sodium bicarbonate	Streptokinase	Tobramycin	Verapamil
I	I	P	I	N	G	N	I	N	N	P	N	N	N	B	N	N	P
N	P	P	N	N	N	N	P	N	I	P	N	N	N	N	N	N	P
N	N	N	P	P	N	N	N	N	N	P	P	N	N	I	N	N	P
P	I	C	N	N	G	N	N	N	N	P	I	N	P	C	N	N	P
N	P	P	I	N	N	N	P	N	N	P	N	N	N	I	N	I	P
N	P	D	N	N	N	N	P	N	P	P	N	N	N	I	N	I	P
N	N	I	N	P	N	N	N	N	N	S	N	N	N	N	N	N	P
A	P	D	N	N	N	N	D	N	P	D	N	N	P	P	N	N	P
N	N	N	N	N	N	N	N	N	N	N	N	I	N	N	N	N	N
N	N	N	N	N	N	N	N	N	N	N	N	I	N	N	N	N	N
I	N	P	N	N	N	N	N	N	N	Y	N	N	N	N	N	N	P
I	P	P	N	N	N	N	P	N	I	I	P	N	N	I	N	N	I
N	P	P	N	N	G	N	H	N	P	P	N	N	N	I	N	N	P
N	N	I	N	N	N	N	P	N	I	P	N	N	N	I	N	N	P
N	N	N	N	N	G	N	N	N	N	P	N	N	I	N	N	N	P
N	P	P	H	N	N	N	P	N	N	N	N	N	N	N	N	N	P
P	P	P	I	N	N	N	P	N	P	P	P	N	I	P	N	I	P
P	P	P	N	N	G	N	N	N	N	Y	N	N	N	N	N	N	S
	N	L	N	N	N	N	N	N	N	N	N	N	I	N	N	P
N		I	N	P	N	N	P	N	N	P	N	N	N	I	N	N	P

	Aminophylline	Ampicillin	Atropine sulfate	Bretylium	Calcium chloride	Calcium gluconate	Cefazolin	Cimetidine	Diazepam	Diazoxide	Digoxin	Dobutamine	Dopamine	Epinephrine HCl	Furosemide	Gentamicin	Heparin	Hydralazine
Lidocaine	P	P	N	C	P	D	I	D	N	N	P	P	P	I	N	P	P	P
Morphine sulfate	I	N	P	N	I	N	N	N	N	N	N	N	N	N	N	H	I	N
Netilmicin	N	N	P	N	N	N	P	N	N	N	N	N	N	N	N	N	N	N
Nitroglycerin	G	N	N	G	N	N	N	N	N	N	N	N	G	N	G	N	N	G
Nitroprusside	N	N	N	N	N	N	N	N	N	N	N	N	N	N	N	N	N	N
Norepinephrine	I	P	N	N	P	P	N	D	N	N	N	P	H	P	N	P	P	N
Phenytoin	N	N	N	N	N	N	N	N	N	N	N	N	N	N	N	N	N	N
Phytonadione	N	I	N	N	N	P	N	P	N	N	N	I	P	I	N	N	P	N
Potassium chloride	P	P	P	P	P	P	S	D	N	N	Y	I	P	P	P	N	P	Y
Procainamide	N	N	P	I	N	N	N	N	N	N	N	P	N	N	N	N	P	N
Propranolol	N	N	N	N	N	N	N	N	N	I	N	N	N	N	N	N	N	N
Quinidine	N	N	N	P	N	N	N	P	I	N	N	N	N	N	I	N	I	N
Sodium bicarbonate	B	N	I	C	I	I	N	P	N	N	N	I	I	I	N	N	P	N
Streptokinase	N	N	N	N	N	N	N	N	N	N	N	N	N	N	N	N	N	N
Tobramycin	N	N	N	N	I	I	N	N	N	N	N	N	N	N	N	N	I	N
Verapamil	P	P	P	P	P	P	P	P	N	N	P	I	P	P	P	P	P	S

C = Physically and chemically compatible
P = Physically compatible
D = Physically compatible only in D5W.
S = Physically compatible only in 0.9% NaCl.
G = Physically compatible only in a glass bottle.
H = Physically compatible for 24 hours.
A = Physically compatible for 4–8 hours.
B = Physically compatible for 4–8 hours only in D5W.
Y = Physically compatible through Y-site for at least 6 hours.
L = Regular insulin compatible with preservative free lidocaine solution.
M = Manufacturer claims medication should not be mixed with other medications but some compatibility data are available.
I = Incompatible.
N = Information on compatibility is not available.
Source: Zeller, FP, et al: Compatibility of IV drugs in a coronary intensive care unit. Drug Intell Clin Pharm 20(5):352, 1986, with permission.

Insulin reg	Isoproterenol	Lidocaine	Morphine sulfate	Netilmicin	Nitroglycerin	Nitroprusside	Norepinephrine	Phenytoin	Phytonadione	Potassium chloride	Procainamide	Propranolol	Quinidine	Sodium bicarbonate	Streptokinase	Tobramycin	Verapamil
L	I		N	N	G	N	I	N	N	P	P	N	N	D	N	N	P
N	N	N		N	N	N	N	N	N	P	N	N	N	I	N	N	P
N	P	N	N		N	N	P	N	P	P	P	N	N	N	N	N	N
N	N	G	N	N		N	N	N	N	N	N	N	N	N	N	N	P
N	N	N	N	N	N		N	N	N	N	N	N	N	N	N	N	N
N	P	I	N	P	N	N		N	N	P	N	N	N	I	N	N	P
N	N	N	N	N	N	N	N		N	N	N	N	N	N	N	N	N
N	N	N	N	P	N	N	N	N		P	N	N	N	N	N	N	N
N	P	P	P	P	N	N	P	N	P		P	P	N	P	N	N	P
N	N	P	N	P	N	N	N	N	N	P		N	N	N	N	N	P
N	N	N	N	N	N	N	N	N	N	P	N		N	N	N	N	P
N	N	N	N	N	N	N	N	N	N	N	N	N		N	N	N	P
I	I	D	I	N	N	N	I	N	N	P	N	N	N		N	N	P
N	N	N	N	N	N	N	N	N	N	N	N	N	N	N		N	N
N	N	N	N	N	N	N	N	N	N	N	N	N	N	N	N		P
P	P	P	P	N	P	N	P	N	N	P	P	P	P	P	N	P	

601

Normal Laboratory Reference Values*

SERUM BLOOD VALUES

Determination	Reference Range
Albumin	3.5–5.0 g/100 mL
Ammonia	12–55 μmol/liter
Amylase	4–25 U/mL
Bilirubin	Direct: up to 0.4 mg/100 mL
	Total: up to 1.0 mg/100 mL
Calcium	8.5–10.5 mg/100 mL
	(slightly higher in children)
Carbon dioxide content	24–30 mEq/liter
Chloride	100–106 mEq/liter
Creatinine	0.6–1.5 mg/100 mL
Globulin	2.3–3.5 g/100 mL
Glucose	70–110 mg/100 mL
Lactic acid	0.6–1.8 mEq/liter
Lipids:	
Cholesterol	120–220 mg/100 mL
Triglycerides	40–150 mg/100 mL
Magnesium	1.5–2.0 mEq/liter
Osmolality	280–296 mOsm/kg
Oxygen saturation	96–100%
P_{CO_2}	35–45 mm Hg
pH	7.35–7.45
P_{O_2}	75–100 mm Hg
Phosphorus	3.0–4.5 mg/100 mL
Potassium	3.5–5.0 mEq/liter
Protein total	6.0–8.4 g/100 mL
Serum glutamic-pyruvic transaminase (SGPT)	1–21 U/liter
Sodium	135–145 mEq/liter
Urea nitrogen (BUN)	8–25 mg/100 mL
Uric acid	3.0–7.0 mg/100 mL

*Source: Adapted from information appearing in *NEJM*. Case Records of the Massachusetts General Hospital by R.E. Scully, 1986, The New England Journal of Medicine, 324, pp. 39–49. Copyright 1986 by The New England Journal of Medicine, by permission.

URINE VALUES

Determination	Reference Range
Amylase	24–76 U/mL
Calcium	300 mg/day or less
Catecholamines:	
Epinephrine	< 20 μg/day
Norepinephrine	< 100 μg/day
Copper	1–100 μg/day
Creatinine	15–25 mg/kg of body weight per day
Hemoglobin	0
pH	5–7
Protein	<150 mg/24 hours
Glucose	0

HEMATOLOGIC VALUES

Determination	Reference Range
Coagulation screening tests	
Bleeding time	3–9.5 minutes
Prothrombin time	<2-second deviation from control
Partial thromboplastin time	25–38 seconds
Whole blood clot lysis	No clot lysis in 24 hours
Thrombin time	Control +5 seconds
Complete blood count	
Hematocrit	Males: 45–52 percent
	Females: 37–48 percent
Hemoglobin	Males: 13–18 g/100 mL
	Females 12–16 g/100 mL
Leukocyte count	4300–10,800/μL
Erythrocyte count	4.2–5.9 million/μL
Platelet count	150,000–350,000/μL
Reticulocyte count	0.5–2.5 percent red cells

IMMUNOLOGIC TESTS

Determination	Reference Range
Rheumatoid factor	<60 IU/mL
Anti-DNA antibodies	Negative at 1:8 dilution of serum
Complement, total hemolytic	150–250 U/mL
Cryoprecipitate proteins	None detected
Immunoglobulins:	
IgG	639–1349 mg/100 mL
IgA	70–312 mg/100 mL
IgM	86–352 mg/100 mL

APPENDIX D

OSHA Guidelines 1995: Controlling Occupational Exposure to Hazardous Drugs

The Occupational Safety and Health Administration (OSHA) established guidelines for the management of cytotoxic (antineoplastic) drugs in the workplace in 1986. At that time engineering controls and personal protective equipment (PPE) were not standardized. Practices have improved, but the problems associated with administration of chemicals still exist.

In 1995, OSHA revised its work practice guidelines to incorporate hazardous drugs (HDs) in addition to the cytotoxic drugs covered in the 1986 guidelines. The recommendations apply to all practice settings in which employees are occupationally exposed to HDs. Anesthetic agents are not included in the review. There are four drug characteristics that are considered hazardous:

1. Genotoxicity
2. Carcinogenicity
3. Teratogenicity or fertility impairment
4. Serious organ other toxic manifestations at low doses

TABLE 1 **Drugs Considered as Hazardous**

Altretamine	Cytarabine
Aminoglutethimide	Dacarbazine
Azathioprine	Catinomyin
L-Asparaginase	Daunorubicin
Bleomycin	Diethylstilbestrol
Busulfan	Doxorubicin
Carboplatin	Estradiol
Carmustinel	Estramustine
Chlorambucil	Ethnyl estradiol
Chloramphenicol	Etoposide
Chlorotrianisene	Floxuridine
Chlorozotocin	Fluorouracil
Cyclosporine	Flutamide
Cisplatin	Ganciclovir
Cyclophosphamide	Hydroxyurea

604

Idarubicin
Ifosamide
Interferon-A
Isotretinoin
Leuprolide
Levamisole
Lomustine
Mechlorethamine
Medroxyprogesterone
Mestrol
Melphalan
Mercaptopurine
Methotrexate
Mitomycin
Mitotane
Mitoxantrone

Nafarelin
Pipobroman
Plicamycin
Procarbazine
Ribavirin
Streptozocin
Tamoxifen
Testolactone
Thioguanine
Thiotepa
Uracil mustard
Vidarabine
Vinblastine
Vincristine
Zidovudine

I. Environmental Protection

A. Risks to personnel working with HDs are by three main routes: aerosols, dermal absorption, and ingestion.

B. Manipulations that can cause splattering, spraying, and aerosolization include withdrawal of needles from drug vials, drug transfer via syringes and needles or filter straws, breaking open ampules, and expulsion of air from a drug-filled syringe.

C. HD preparation should be performed in a restricted, preferably centralized area.

D. Signs restricting the access of unauthorized personnel are to be prominently displayed.

E. Smoking, drinking, applying cosmetics, chewing gum, and eating where these drugs are prepared, stored, or used also increases the chance of exposure.

F. The use of Class II or III Biologic Safety Cabinets (BSC) that meet the current National Sanitation Foundation Standard should minimize exposure to HDs during preparation. If a BSC is unavailable (such as in private practice office), the sharing of a cabinet or sending the patient to a center where HDs can be prepared in a BSC is an alternative solution. Alternatively, preparation can be performed in a facility with a BSC and the drugs transported to the area of administration.

✎ NOTE: Use of a dedicated BSC where only HDs are prepared is prudent medical practice. Use of a horizontal BSC is contraindicated in the preparation of HDs.

G. The cabinet should be cleaned according to the manufacturer's recommendations. Decontamination most frequently is done weekly, as well as whenever spills occur or when cabinet requires moving.

H. Decontamination should consist of surface cleaning with water and detergent followed by thorough rinsing. The use of detergent is recommended because there is no single accepted method of chemical deactivation for all agents.

✎ NOTE: Avoid use of quaternary ammonium cleaners, ethyl alcohol, or 70% isopropyl alcohol. Spray cleaners should also be avoided because of the risk of spraying the HEPA filter.

I. Cleaning should proceed from the least to the most contaminated areas. All materials from the decontamination process should be handled as HDs and disposed of in accordance with federal, state, and local laws.

J. Procedures for spills and emergencies, such as skin or eye contact, should be available to workers.

II. PERSONAL PROTECTIVE EQUIPMENT

A. Basic precautions
1. All PPE must be donned before work is started in the BSC.
2. All items necessary for drug preparation should be placed within the BSC before work is started.
3. Extraneous items should be kept out of the work area.

B. Gloves
1. The thickness of gloves used in handling HDs is more important that the type of material. Latex gloves are best and should be used for preparation of HDs unless the drug product manufacturer specifically stipulates that some other glove provides better protection. Thicker, longer latex gloves that cover the gown cuff are recommended for use with HDs.
2. Gloves with minimal or no powder are preferred, since the powder may absorb contamination.
3. Individuals with latex allergy should consider the use of vinyl or nitrile gloves or glove liners.
4. Double-gloving is recommended if it does not interfere with an individual's technique.
5. All gloves are permeable to some extent. They should be changed regularly (hourly) or immediately if they are torn.

C. Gowns
1. A protective disposable gown made of lint-free, low-permeability fabric with a closed front, long sleeves, and elastic or knit cuffs should be worn.
2. The cuffs should be tucked under the gloves.

D. Respiratory protection
1. A NIOSH approved respirator should be worn when a BSC is not currently available.
2. The use of respirators must comply with OSHA's Respiratory Protection Standard, including selection, fit testing, and worker training.

✎ **NOTE:** Surgical masks are not appropriate, since they do not prevent aerosol inhalation.

E. Eye and face protection
1. Eyeglasses with temporary side shields are inadequate protection.
   a. Use a respirator with a full face piece.
   b. Use a plastic face shield or splash goggles complying with American National Standards Institute regulations.
2. Eyewash facilities should be made available.

F. Disposal of PPE
1. All gowns, gloves, and disposable materials used in preparation should be disposed of according to the hospital's hazardous drug waste procedures.
2. Goggles, face shields, and respiratory equipment may be cleaned with mild detergent and water for reuse.

G. Work equipment
1. Syringes and I.V. sets with Luer-lock fittings should be used for HDs.
2. Syringe size should be large enough so as not to be full when the entire drug dose is present.
3. All syringes and I.V. bags containing HDs should be labeled with a distinctive warning label such as:

✎ **NOTE:** The following are special handling/disposal precautions

4. A covered disposable container should be used to contain excess solution. A covered sharps container should be in the BSC.
5. Labeled HD-labeled plastic bags must be available for all contaminated materials (including gloves, gowns, and paper liners).
6. Preparation of HDs must be carried out in a BSC on a disposable plastic-backed paper liner.
7. All needles used in the course of preparation must be placed in "sharps" containers for disposal without being crushed, clipped or capped.
8. Drug administration sets should be primed within the BSC.
9. Vials
   a. The use of large-bore needles (No. 18 or 20) avoids high-pressure injections through syringes of solution in vials; however many large-bore needles are more likely to drip. Multi-use dispensing pins are recommended to avoid these problems.
   b. Venting devices such as filter needles or dispensing pins permit outside air to replace the withdrawn liquid.
   c. Another technique is to add diluent slowly to the vial by alternatively injecting small amounts and allowing displaced air to escape into the syringe. This air should not be expelled into room air because it may contain drug residue. It should either be injected into a vacuum vial or left in the syringe to be discarded.
   d. The drug should be cleared from the needle and hub of the syringe before separating to reduce spraying or separation.
10. Ampules
    a. Ampules with dry material should be "gently tapped down" before opening to move any material in the top of the ampule to the bottom quantity.
    b. A sterile gauze pad should be wrapped around the ampule neck before breaking the top.
    c. If adding a diluent, inject *slowly* down the inside wall of the ampule. Tilt the ampule to ensure that all the powder is wet before agitating.
    d. After the solution is withdrawn from the ampule with a syringe, the needle should be cleared of solution by holding it vertically with the point upward; the syringe should be tapped to remove air bubbles.
11. Transport of HDs
    a. The outside of bags or bottles containing the prepared drug should be wiped with moist gauze.
    b. Entry ports should be wiped with moist alcohol pads and capped.
    c. Transport should occur in sealed plastic bags and transported in containers designed to avoid breakage.
    d. Any HDs that are shipped are subject to EPA regulation as hazardous waste.

III. DRUG ADMINISTRATION
A. Personal protective equipment
   1. The National Study Commission or Cytotoxic Exposure has recommended that personnel administering HDs wear gowns, latex gloves, and chemical splash goggles or equivalent safety glasses.
   2. NIOSH-approved respirators should be worn when administering aerosolized drugs.
B. Administration kit
   1. Protective and administration equipment may be packaged together and labeled as a HD administration kit. The kit should include:
      a. Personal protective equipment
      b. Gauze (4 × 4) for cleanup

      c. Alcohol wipes

      d. Disposable plastic-backed absorbent liner

      e. Puncture-resistant container for needles and syringes

      f. Thick sealable plastic bag (with warning label)

      g. Accessory warning labels

C. Work practices

  1. Hands should be washed before donning and after removing gloves.

  2. Gowns or gloves that become contaminated should be changed immediately.

  3. Employees should be trained in proper methods to remove contaminated gloves and gowns.

  4. Infusion sets and pumps that should have Luer-lock fittings should be observed for leakage during use.

  5. A plastic-backed absorbent pad should be placed under the tubing during administration to catch any leakage.

  6. Sterile gauze should be placed around any push sites.

  7. Tubing connection sites should be taped.

  8. Priming I.V. sets or expelling air from syringes should be carried out in a BSC.

  9. Syringes, I.V. bottles, and bags and pumps should be wiped clean of any drug contamination with sterile gauze.

  10. Dispose of administration sets intact.

  11. Waste bag should follow HD disposal requirements.

  12. Protective goggles should be cleaned with detergent and properly rinsed.

  13. Nursing stations where cytotoxic drugs will be administered should have spill and emergency skin and eye decontamination kits available.

✎ **NOTE:** The increased use of HDs in the home environment necessitates special precautions. Employees involved in home care delivery should follow the above work practices and, employers should make administration and spill kits available.

D. Aerosolized drugs

  1. In the case of pentamidine, engineering controls include treatment booths with local exhaust ventilation designed specifically for its administration.

  2. Ribavirin can be administered in isolation rooms with separate HEPA-filtered ventilation systems via endotracheal tube.

  3. Both isolation and ventilation are used for volatile HDs.

E. Caring for patients receiving HDs

  1. The Bloodborne Pathogens Standard provides guidelines for universal precautions which must be observed to prevent contact with blood or other potentially infectious materials.

  2. Personnel dealing with excreta, primarily urine, from patient who have received HDs in the last 48 hours should be provided with and wear latex or other appropriate gloves and disposable gowns, to be discarded after each use of whenever contaminated.

  3. Eye protection should be worn if splashing is possible.

  4. Linen soiled with blood or other potentially infectious materials as well as contaminated with excreta must be managed according to the Bloodborne Pathogens Standard. Linen should be placed in specially marked laundry bags and placed in a labeled impervious bag.

  5. Any reusable item should be washed twice with detergent by personnel wearing double latex gloves and a gown.

IV. WASTE DISPOSAL
A. Equipment
1. Thick, leakproof plastic bags, colored differently from other hospital trash bags, should be used for routine accumulation and collection of used containers, discarded gloves, gowns, and other disposable material.
2. Needles, syringes, and breakable items not contaminated with blood or other potentially infectious materials should be placed in a sharps container before being stored in the waste bag. Those contaminated with blood *must* be placed in a "sharps" container.
3. The waste bag should be kept inside a covered waste container clearly labeled **"HD Waste Only."**
B. Handling
1. Personnel disposing of HD waste should wear gowns and protective gloves when handling waste containers.
C. Disposal
1. Hazardous drug-related wastes should be handled separately from other hospital trash and disposed of in accordance with applicable EPA, state, and local regulations.
2. Disposal can occur at either an incinerator or a licensed sanitary landfill for toxic wastes.
D. Spills

✎ **NOTE:** Incidental spills and breakage's should be cleaned up immediately by a properly protected person.

1. *Personnel contamination cleanup*
   a. Immediately remove the gloves or gown.
   b. Immediately cleanse the affected area with soap and water.
   c. Flood an affected eye at an eyewash station for 15 minutes.
   d. Obtain medical attention.
   e. Document the exposure in the employee's medical file.
2. *Cleanup of small spills* (less than 5 mL)
   a. Liquids should be wiped with absorbent gauze pads; solids with wet absorbent gauze.
   b. Spills areas should be cleaned three times using detergent solution followed by clean water.
   c. Any broken glass fragments should be picked up with a small scoop (never the hands) and placed in a sharps container.
   d. Contaminated reusable items, such as glassware and scoops, should be treated as previously outlined under reusable items.
3. *Cleanup of large spills*
   a. The area should be isolated.
   b. For spills larger than 5 mL liquid, spread is limited by gently covering with absorbent sheets or spill-control pads or pillows.
   c. If powder is involved, damp cloths or towels should be used.
   e. Protective apparel including respirators should be used as with small spills when there is any suspicion of airborne powder or that an aerosol has been or will be generated.
   f. All contaminated surfaces should be thoroughly cleaned three times with detergent and water.
4. *Spills in the BSC*
   a. Extensive spills within a BSC necessitate decontamination of all interior BSC surfaces after completion of the spill cleanup.

609

5. *Spill kits*
   a. Spill kits should be clearly labeled.
   b. The American Society of Hospital Pharmacists (ASHP) recommendations:
      (1) Chemical splash goggles
      (2) Two pairs of gloves
      (3) A low-permeability gown
      (4) Two sheets (12 × 12 inches)
      (5) 250-mL and 1-liter spill control pillows
      (6) sharps container
      (7) Small scoop to collect glass fragments
      (8) Two large HD waste-disposal bags

V. STORAGE AND TRANSPORT

A. Storage areas
   1. Limit authorized personnel to access to areas where HDs are stored.
   2. Facilities used for storing HDs should not be used for other drugs.
   3. Warning labels should be applied to all HD containers.
B. Receiving damaged HD packages
   1. Damaged shipping cartons should be opened in an isolated area or a BSC by a designed employee wearing double gloves, a gown, goggles, and appropriate respiratory protection.
   2. Broken containers and contaminated packaging mats should be placed in a sharps container and then into HD disposal bags.
C. Transport
   1. HDs should be securely capped or sealed and placed in sealed clear plastic bags.
   2. Personnel involved in transporting HDs should be trained in spill procedures, including sealing off the contaminated area and calling for appropriate assistance.

VI. MEDICAL SURVEILLANCE

A. Medical examinations
   1. Employees who will be working with HDs in the workplace should have a preplacement medical examination including an initial evaluation consisting of history, physical examination, and laboratory studies.
   2. Examinations should be updated on a yearly basis or every 2 to 3 years.
   3. Postexposure evaluation is tailored to the type of exposure.
      a. For cytotoxic drugs, the skin and mucous membranes
      b. For aerosolized HDs, the pulmonary system
   4. Exit examinations and laboratory evaluation should be guided by the individual's history of exposures.
   5. The examining physician should consider the reproductive status of employees and inform them regarding relevant reproductive issues.

✎ **NOTE:** Spontaneous abortion and congenital malformation excesses have been documented among workers handling some hazardous drugs without currently recommended engineering controls and precautions.

VIII. HAZARD COMMUNICATION

Employers shall develop, implement, and maintain at the workplace a written hazard communication program for employees handling or otherwise exposed to chemicals, including drugs that represent a health hazard to employees.

VII. TRAINING AND INFORMATION DISSEMINATION

A. Employees must be informed of the requirements of the Hazard Communication Standard, including:
   1. Any operation or procedure in their work area where drugs that present a hazard are present
   2. Location and availability of the written hazard communication
B. Employee training
   1. Methods and observations that may be used to detect the presence or release of HDs
   2. Physical and health hazards of the covered HDs in the work area
   3. The measures employees can take to protect themselves from hazards
   4. The details of the hazards communication program developed by the employer, including an explanation of the labeling systems.

Source: US Department of Labor (1995). Controlling occupational exposure to hazardous drugs. Occupational Safety and Health Administration, Instruction CPL 2-2, 21-1 to 21-31.

POSITION STATEMENT

The Handling of Cytotoxic Agents by Women Who Are Pregnant, Attempting to Conceive, or Breastfeeding

There are substantial data regarding the mutagenic, teratogenic, and abortifacient properties of certain cytotoxic agents both in animals and humans who have received therapeutic doses of these agents. In addition, the scientific literature suggests a possible association of occupational exposure to certain cytotoxic agents during the first trimester of pregnancy with fetal loss or malformation. These data suggest the need for caution when women who are pregnant or are attempting to conceive handle cytotoxic agents. Incidentally, there is no evidence relating male exposure to cytotoxic agents with adverse fetal outcome. There are no studies that address the possible risk associated with the occupational exposure to cytotoxic agents and the passage of these agents into breast milk. Nevertheless, it is prudent for women who are breastfeeding to exercise caution in handling cytotoxic agents.

If all procedures for safe handling, such as those recommended by the Commission are complied with, the potential for exposure will be minimized.

Personnel should be provided with information to make an individual decision. This information should be provided in written form, and it is advisable that a statement of understanding be signed.

It is essential to refer to individual state right-to-know laws to ensure compliance.

Source: From Recommendations for Handling Cytotoxic Agents, National Study Commission on Cytotoxic Exposure, September 1987. For additional information, contact the Commission's Chairman.

Dilution Rates of Intravenous Drugs

Drug	Type and Amount of Diluent to Use
Adrenocorticotropic hormone (ACTH) (corticotropin for injection) (Acthar)	D$_5$W* or NSS† At least 250 mL for whatever diagnostic dose physician orders; dilution is often 500 mL (do not mix in Soluset)
Alteplase, recombinant (Activase)	Sterile water only *without preservatives* 50 mg in 50 mL 100-mg dose; 60 mg in 1 h, 20 mg/h for 2 h
Amikacin sulfate (Amikin)	D$_5$W or NSS 5 mg/mL (500 mg in 200 mL of diluent)
Aminocaproic acid (Amicar)	D$_5$W or NSS or Ringer's injection 1 g in 50 mL of diluent
Aminophylline (multisource)	D$_5$W or NSS 250 mL or more (do not mix in a Soluset)
Amphotericin B (Fungizone)	Reconstitute as follows: 1. With sterile needle and syringe, rapidly inject 10 mL sterile water for injection (without additives). 2. Shake vial well until clear. 3. Dilute with D$_5$W (with pH of above 4.2) 1 mg/10 mL. Do not use NSS (suspension will precipitate). Do not filter (filter may block passage of antibiotic dispersion). Wrap bottle in foil to protect from exposure to light
Ampicillin (Omnipen, Polycillin, others)	Sterile water or NSS D$_5$NS, D$_5$W 2–30 mg/mL over 10–15 min
Anistreplase (APSAC, Eminase)	Sterile water 5 mL to 30 U over 2–5 min; do not shake
Aztreonam (Azactam)	Most solutions 1 g in 100 mL over 20–60 min 1 g in 6–10 mL bolus over 3–5 min
Calcium disodium edetate (Calcium Disodium Versenate)	D$_5$W or NSS 1 g in 250–500 mL

Drug	Type and Amount of Diluent to Use
Carbenicillin disodium (Geopen, Pyopen)	Most solutions 1 g in 10–20 mL of sterile water for direct I.V. administration; may be added to large volume of most solutions, including 50–100 mL additive bottles
Cefamandole naftate (Mandol)	D_5W or NSS 1 g in 10 mL (I.V. push) 1 or 2 g in 50 mL (infusion)
Cefotaxime sodium (Claforan)	D_5W, NSS, or other compatible solution 1 g 30 to 90 min
Cefotetan (Cefotan)	D_5W or NSS 1–2 g in 10–20 mL over 3–5 min direct or 50–100 mL intermittent
Cefoxitin sodium (Mefoxin)	D_5W, NSS, sterile water for injection, lactated Ringer's solution 1 to 2 g in 50 mL
Ceftazidime (Fortaz)	D_5W 1 g diluted in 50–100 mL
Ceftizoxime sodium (Cefizox)	D_5, $D_{10}W$, D/NS, invert sugar, or lactated Ringer's solution 1 g in 50–100 mL bolus over 2–3 min or 30 min intermittent
Ceftriaxone (Rocephin)	D_5W, $D_{10}W$, NSS 250 mg diluted with 50–100 mL
Cephapirin sodium (Cefadyl)	D_5W or NSS 1 g in 50 mL; 2 g in 100 mL
Cimetidine (Tagamet)	D_5W 300 mg in 100 mL
Cortisol sodium succinate (Solu-Cortef, A-hydroCort)	D_5W or NSS At least 1 ml of diluent/mg
Dexamethasone phosphate (Decadron, Hexadrol)	D_5W, NSS, D_5NS, or lactated Ringer's solution 1 mg–40 mg in 500 mL
Erythromycin gluceptate (Ilotycin Gluceptate)	D_5W or 0.9% sodium chloride injection less than 500 mg in 100 mL 500 mg in 250 mL 1 g in 1000 mL (Reconstitute with sterile water, no preservatives. Add 2.5 mL sodium bicarbonate to 100 mL of I.V. solution and 5 mL sodium bicarbonate to 250 mL. Without sodium bicarbonate, solution remains stable for only 4 h and is extremely irritating to the vein wall; solution *must* run over 1 h).
Famotidine (Pepcid)	0.9% NSS, D_5W, or lactated Ringer's solution 2 mL in 100 mL infused over 15–30 min (20 mg in 2 mL)
Heparin sodium (multisource)	Usually D_5W or NSS or lacated Ringer's injection At least 250 mL and usually 500 mL or 1000 mL depending on physician's order; heparin is given by I.V. push bolus or slow I.V. infusion (do not mix in Soluset)
Imipenem-cilastatin sodium (Primaxin)	Most solutions 250 mg in 100 mL over 20–30 min 1 g over 40–60 min

613

Drug	Type and Amount of Diluent to Use
Iron dextran (Imferon, Chromagen D, Dextraron-50)	Administer undiluted (drug comes already reconstituted with NSS) by slow I.V. push bolus (1 min/mL). Drug is sometimes mixed with at least 250 mL NSS and given by slow I.V. infusion (over 1–3 h), but this is not a manufacturer's recommendation. Physician should give initial test dose to check for adverse reactions.
Methicillin (Staphcillin, Celbenin)	D_5W, NSS, or sterile water for injection: 1 g in 50 mL 2 g in 100 mL
Methyldopate (Aldomet Ester)	D_5W 100 mL Usual dosage is 250–500 mg, but up to 1 g can be given in 100 mL; solution usually runs over 30–60 min
Methylprednisolone sodium succinate (Solu-Medrol, A-Methapred)	D_5W or NSS mix-o-vial Less than 1 g in 50 mL 1 g or more in 100 mL For initial reconstitution of drug in manufacturer's vial, use *only* the diluent provided by the manufacturer.
Metronidazole (Flagyl I.V.)	D_5W, NSS, or lactated Ringer's solution 1. Reconstitute with 4.4 mL of diluent. 2. Add to I.V. solution in concentration not to exceed 8 mg/mL. 3. Neutralize with 5 mEq sodium bicarbonate for each 500 mg of metronidazole.
Mezlocillin sodium (Mezlin)	0.9% NSS 10–100 mg/mL Lactated Ringer's solution 10–100 mg/mL 0.9% NSS 250 mg/mL
Nafcillin sodium (Nafcil, Unipen, Nallpen)	Sterile water, NSS, Ringer's injection, D_5W 1 g in 15–30 mL bolus over 10–15 min
Oxacillin sodium (Prostaphlin)	NSS or sterile water 1 g in 10–20 mL bolus over 10 min
Oxytocin (Pitocin, Syntocinon)	D_5W or NSS 10 to 40 U in 1000 mL.
Penicillin G sodium	D_5W or NSS 3 million U or less in 50 mL More than 3 million U in 100 mL
Piperacillin sodium (Pipracil)	Sterile water, NSS, D_5W 1 g in 50–100 mL over 30 min or as bolus over 3–5 min
Potassium chloride (multisource)	Any standard diluent (D_5W, NSS, Ringer's lactate, and so on) as ordered by physician; do not mix in Soluset (too great a concentration can cause cardiac irritability and phlebitis)
Potassium phosphate (multisource)	Any standard diluent as ordered by physician. At least 500 mL. Use vials once only; do not store used vial (solution does not contain a bacteriostatic agent.) Do not mix in Soluset.

614

Drug	Type and Amount of Diluent to Use
Ranitidine (Zantac)	0.9% NSS, D_5W, $D_{10}W$, lactated Ringer's solution 50 mg in 20 mL injected over 5 min
Streptokinase (Streptase)	NSS, D_5W 5 mL to vial. Do not shake. Withdraw and dilute with additional 45 mL. 15 mL/h over 30 min; 3 mL/h maintenance dose.
Ticarcillin disodium (Ticar)	D_5W, NSS, or sterile water for injection 1.0 g to 5.0 g in 100 mL
Tobramycin sulfate (Nebcin)	D_5W or NSS 40 mg or less in 50 mL; 41–100 mg in 100 mL; more than 100 mg; 1 mg/mL
Vancomycin (Vancocin)	D_5W or NSS less than 500 mg in 100 mL 500 mg in 200 mL
Vitamins (Folate, 5 mg; Betalin-5, 100 mg; Berocca C, 1 amp; Hexabetalin)	All common diluents in amounts ordered by physician Added to 500 mL or more of solution, usually 1 L.

*D_5W = 5% dextrose in water; $D_{10}W$ = 10% dextrose in water.
†NSS = Normal saline solution; D_5NS = 5% dextrose in normal saline.
Source: From When You Have to Reconstitute Meds by R. Hickman, 1981, *RN, 4*, pp. 40–43. Copyright 1981 by Medical Economics Co. Adapted by permission.

APPENDIX F

Resource List of National Organizations

AMERICAN ASSOCIATION OF
CRITICAL CARE NURSES (AACN)
101 Columbia Avenue
Aliso Viejo, CA 92656-1491

AMERICAN SOCIETY OF PAIN
MANAGEMENT NURSES
11512 Allecingie Parkway
Richmond, VA 23235

AMERICAN SOCIETY FOR
PARENTERAL AND ENTERAL
NUTRITION—NURSE'S
COMMITTEE
8630 Fenton Street, Suite 412
Silver Springs, MD 20910–3803

ASSOCIATION OF NURSES IN AIDS
CARE
704 Stoney Hill Road, Suite 106
Yardley PA 19067
(215) 321-2371

ASSOCIATION FOR
PROFESSIONALS IN INFECTION
CONTROL AND EPIDEMIOLOGY
1061 16th Street NW
Washington, DC 20016

ASSOCIATION OF PEDIATRIC
ONCOLOGY NURSES
Suite 3A
11512 Allecingie Parkway
Richmond, VA 23235

CENTERS FOR DISEASE CONTROL
AND PREVENTION
1600 Clifton Road
Atlanta, GA 30333
(404) 639-3311

INTRAVENOUS NURSES SOCIETY
Fresh Pond Square
10 Fawcett Street
Cambridge, MA 01238
(617) 441-2909

NATIONAL ASSOCIATION FOR
PRACTICAL NURSE EDUCATION
AND SERVICE, INC. (NAPNES)
1400 Spring Street, Suite 310
Silver Springs, MD 20910

ONCOLOGY NURSING SOCIETY
501 Holiday Drive
Pittsburgh, PA 15220

SOCIETY FOR VASCULAR NURSING
(SVN)
309 Winter Street
Norwood, MA 02062

616

Survey of Scope of Intravenous Practice by State for Licensed Practical and Vocational Nurses

In a follow-up to the original survey in 1991, this survey, completed in June 1995, identifies the role of the LPN/LVN related to I.V. therapy. The results are as follows.

The role of LPN/LVN has changed over the past few years. Certification for the LPN/LVN in I.V. therapy will be available for the first time in September 1996. Each state still addresses the issue and identifies the scope of practice for the practical and vocational nurse. Twenty-six states have clearly defined expanded role guidelines established. Nineteen states have identified that the LPN/LVN has a designated role in I.V. therapy; however, the scope of practice is decided by each individual agency. Four states clearly state that the role of the LPN/LVN is not in the maintenance or initiation of I.V. therapy

STATES WITH EXPANDED ROLE GUIDELINES

Alabama
Alaska
Arizona
California
Colorado
Connecticut (home health care agencies, long-term care facilities; scope not defined in acute care facilities)
Delaware
Florida
Idaho
Kansas
Kentucky
Louisiana
Maine
Maryland
Mississippi
Missouri
Nevada
New Hampshire
New York
North Carolina
Ohio
Oregon
Pennsylvania
South Carolina
South Dakota (limited to adult and geriatric population)
Wyoming

617

STATES THAT IDENTIFY THAT THE ROLE OF THE LPN/LVN INCLUDES I.V. THERAPY, BUT DELEGATES THE RESPONSIBILITY OF EDUCATION, COMPETENCY, AND ROLE DELINEATION TO EACH AGENCY

Arkansas
Georgia
Illinois
Indiana
Massachusetts
Michigan
Minnesota
Montana
New Mexico
Oklahoma

Rhode Island
Tennessee
Texas
Utah
Vermont
Virginia
Washington
West Virginia
Wisconsin

STATES THAT DO NOT INCLUDE INITIATION OF I.V. THERAPY IN THE ROLE OF THE LPN/LVN

Hawaii

Iowa

Nebraska (limited role—may discontinue; temporarily may slow and regulate flow rate)

New Jersey

INDEX

An "f" following a page number indicates a figure; a "t" following a page number indicates a table.

Abdomen, nutritional assessment using, 553t
ABO system
  compatibility chart, 444t
  description of, 443
  grouping of, 443t
Acid-base
  balance
    chemical buffer systems, 99–100
    pH values, 99
    regulation by lungs, 54
    renal regulation, 100
    respiratory regulation, 100
  imbalances
    metabolic
      acidosis. See Metabolic acidosis
      alkalosis. See Metabolic alkalosis
    respiratory
      acidosis. See Respiratory acidosis
      alkalosis. See Respiratory alkalosis
Acidosis
  metabolic
    alkalizing fluids for, 131–132
    diagnostic tests, 101
    etiology of, 100–101
    signs and symptoms, 101
    summary of, 104t
    treatment, 101
  respiratory
    diagnostic tests, 103
    etiology of, 102
    signs and symptoms, 102
    summary of, 104t
    treatment, 103

Acthar. See Adrenocorticotropic hormone
Activase. See Alteplase, recombinant
Active transport, 53
Acylovir (Zovirax), 376t
Add-on devices
  microbore extension tubing, 216–217
  T, J, or U shaped port devices, 216
Adenine arabinoside (Vidarabine), 376t
Adenoids, role in immune system, 154t
Administration sets
  basic type of, 191f
  components of, 191–192
  filters, 467
  large bore, 196
  OSHA guidelines for, 607
  primary, 192f, 193
  primary Y, 193–194, 196
  secondary
    piggyback, 193
    volume-controlled, 193, 194f
  standards of practice for, 194
  transfusion therapy, 467
Admixture
  antineoplastic therapy, 530
  infection prevention, 166
  parenteral nutrition, 577–578
  total nutrient, 564–565
Adrenal gland, role in fluid balance, 54–55
Adrenocorticotropic hormone (ACTH), 612T
Adsorption
  disadvantages of, 354

619

Adsorption—*Continued*
  factors that affect, 354–355
  polyvinylchloride bags, 355
Agglutinins. *See* Antibodies
A-hydroCort. *See* Cortisol sodium
    succinate
Air embolism
  description of, 294–295
  documentation, 296
  parenteral nutrition and, 573t
  peripherally inserted central catheters
      and, 410
  prevention, 295
  signs and symptoms, 295
  treatment, 296
  tunneled catheters and, 417
Albumin
  administration of, 462
  characteristics of, 139t
  in colloid solutions, 135, 461, 465t
  compatibility, 462
  serum levels, nutritional assessment
      using, 550
  uses of, 461
Aldomet Ester. *See* Methyldopa
Aldosterone, role in fluid balance, 54–55
Alkalosis
  metabolic
    acidifying parenteral solutions, 132
    diagnostic tests, 102
    etiology of, 101–102
    signs and symptoms, 102
    summary of, 104t
    treatment, 102
  respiratory
    diagnostic tests, 103–104
    etiology of, 103
    signs and symptoms, 103
    summary of, 104t
    treatment, 104
Alkylating agents
  action, 501
  description of, 500
  drug types, 501t
  side effects, 501
Allergic reactions, from transfusion
      therapy, 476–477
Alopecia, chemotherapy-induced, 510
Alteplase, recombinant (Activase), 612t
American Nursing Association (ANA),
      21
A-Methapred. *See* Methylprednisolone
    sodium succinate
Amicar. *See* Aminocaproic acid
Amikacin sulfate (Amikin), 279t, 612t

Amino acids
  essential types, 556
  solutions for total parenteral
      nutrition, 557t
Aminocaproic acid (Amicar), 612t
Aminoglycosides, characteristics of, 374t
Aminophylline, 612t
Amphotericin B (Fungizone), 279t, 375t,
      612t
Ampicillin (Omnipen, Polycillin), 612t
Anaphylaxis, chemotherapy-induced,
      512–513
Ancef. *See* Cefazolin
Androgens, 505
Anemia, chemotherapy-induced, 520
Anions, in body fluids, 76t
Anistreplase (APSAC, Eminase), 612t
Anorexia, chemotherapy-induced, 512
Antebrachial vein, 235t
Antecubital vein, 236t
Anthracycline agents
  cardiac toxicities, 520–521
  types, 504
Anthropometric measurements, 549–550
Antibiotics. *See also specific drug*
  categories of, 374t
  compatibility issues, 373
  home therapy, 381
  nursing considerations, 373
  strategies to improve use, 159t
Antibodies, 444–445
Antidiuretic hormone, 55
Antifungals, 374. *See also specific drug*
Antigens
  ABO system, 443
  HLA system, 444
  Rh system, 443–444
Antimetabolites, chemotherapeutic use
      of
  action, 502
  categories of
    folic acid analogues, 502
    purine analogues, 503
    pyrimidine analogues, 502
  description of, 502
  side effects, 503
Antimicrobial therapy
  selection for nosocomial pathogens,
      160t
  stages of, 160
Antineoplastic therapy
  agents
    alkylating agents, 500–501
    androgens, 505
    anthracycline antibiotics, 504

620

antimetabolites, 502–503
classifications, 500
corticosteroids, 505
cytokines, 507–508
dosing, 500
enzymes, 504–505
estrogens, 506
progestins, 506
vinca alkaloids, 503
cellular kinetics
cell cycle, 496–497, 497f
drug resistance, 499
normal and malignant tissue
growth, 497–498
tumor cell kill, 498–499
clinician's role
patient assessment and history, 495,
496t
treatment objectives, 495–496
contraindications, 496
home care considerations
administration, 531
admixture, 530
disposal of excreta, 531
monitoring, 531
transportation, 530–531
nursing plan of care, 528–529
OSHA guidelines, 30–31
patient and family education,
529–530
Antiseptics, cutaneous, 170
Antiviral agents, 374, 376t. See also
specific drug
APSAC. See Anistreplase
Aquavene, 198
Arm
veins for I.V. use, 235t
venous structures, 394, 395f
Arteries, 233t. See also specific artery
Arteriovenous (AV) fistula, 372
Ativan. See Lorazepam
Atropine, 511t
Autologous blood donation
advantages and disadvantages, 449
definition of, 449
patient selection, 449
types of, 449–450
Azactam. See Aztreonam
AZT. See Zidovudine
Aztreonam (Azactam), 612t

Bacterial pathogens, common types in
intravascular devices, 165t
Bacterial phlebitis, 279

Base bicarbonate
deficit. See Acidosis
excess. See Alkalosis
Basilic vein
description of, 394
illustration of, 395t
insertion site, 235t–236t
Bastedo's rule, 327
Benzodiazepines, 517t
Berocca C, 615t
Betalin-5, 615t
Biologic hazards
precautions for, 32
universal symbol of, 33f
Biologic response modifiers,
chemotherapeutic use of
colony-stimulating factors, 508
cytokines, 507–508
monoclonal antibodies, 508–509
toxicities, 509
Biologic safety cabinets (BSC), 605
Blood banks, 7, 447, 469–470
Bloodborne pathogens, 32–33
Blood component therapy
administration, steps for
checklist preparation, 470, 471f
equipment selection and
preparation
administration sets, 467
blood warmers, 467–468
cannula, 466
electronic monitoring devices,
468
filters, 467
solution, 467
obtaining blood product from
blood bank, 469–470
patient preparation, 469
physician's order, 466
antibodies, 444–445
antigens, 443–444
blood components
cryoprecipitate, 460–461, 465t
fresh frozen plasma, 459–460,
464t
granulocytes, 456–457, 463t
overview, 451
platelets
administration, 458
compatibility, 458
description of, 457, 464t
storage, 457f
uses of, 457–458
red blood cells
deglycerolized, 456, 463t

Blood component therapy, blood
components, red blood cells—
Continued
    packed. *See* Packed red blood
      cells
    washed, 455–456, 463t
    whole blood, 452, 453f
  blood preservatives, 447–448
  blood substitutes, 462, 466
  colloid volume expanders. *See* Colloid
    volume expanders
  compatibility testing, 446–447
  complications of
    allergic reactions, 476–477
    circulatory overload, 477
    hemolytic reactions, 474–475
    hypocalcemia, 478
    hypothermia, 478
    nonhemolytic febrile reactions, 476
    potassium toxicity, 477
  discontinuation of, 472–473
  donor blood testing, 445–446, 446t
  in home setting, 480–481
  initiation of, 470–471
  key advances
    in 19th century, 4–5, 9t
    in 20th century, 7, 9t
  monitoring, 471–472
  nursing plan of care, 479–480
  patient education, 480
  risks of, 478, 478t
Blood count, in newborns, 317t
Blood donors
  collection methods
    autologous
      advantages and disadvantages,
        449
      definition of, 449
      patient selection, 449
      types of, 449–450
    designated, 449–451, 451f
    homologous, 448
  testing of, 445–446, 446t
Blood filters
  leukocyte depletion, 206–207, 207f
  microaggregate, 206, 467
  standard clot, 206
  for transfusion therapy, 467
Blood laboratory values, 602
Blood preservatives, 447–448
Bloodstream infections
  cannula-related, 167f, 167–168
  infusate contamination
    common pathogens, 165t
    mechanisms of, 169–170

    preventive measures
      cutaneous antiseptics, 170
      dressings, 170–171
      reporting to proper agency, 170
    sources of, 165
Blood substitutes, 462, 466
Blood warmers, 467–468
Body fluid
  anions, 76t
  cations, 76t
  composition of, 48
  distribution of, 48–50
  function of, 50
  percentages of, in relation to age and
    sex, 48t, 49f
  transportation
    active, 53
    passive. *See* Passive transport
  water sources, 49
Body surface area
  description of, 327
  nomogram of, 595–596
Body weight, evaluation of, for fluid
    imbalances, 58
Bone marrow
  chemotherapy-induced depression,
    520
  role in immune system, 154t
Breach of duty, 22
Buffer systems, 99–100
Buprenorphine, 377t
Burns, parenteral formulas for, 566t
Butorphanol, 377t
Butyrophenones, 517t

Calcium
  deficit. *See* Hypocalcemia
  excess. *See* Hypercalcemia
  functions, 85
  normal values, 85
Calcium disodium edetate (Calcium
    Disodium Versenate),
    612t
Cancer treatment. *See* Antineoplastic
    therapy; chemotherapy
Cannabinoids, 518t
Cannulas
  culturing techniques, 168t, 168–169
  infections related to
    common pathogens, 167–168
    culturing techniques, 168t, 168–169
    sources of, 167f, 167–168
  procedure for. *See* Cannulation
  transfusion therapy, 466

Cannulation
  catheter stabilization, 245t, 245–246
  dressing management, 246
  in geriatric patients, 334
  gloving, 242–243
  needle selection, 242
  procedure to discontinue, 253–254
  site preparation, 243
  summary of, 249–250
  vein entry, 243–244
Carbenicillin disodium (Geopen,
      Pyopen), 613t
Carbohydrates
  dextrose. See Dextrose
  fructose. See Fructose
  nutritional requirements, 553
  in parenteral solutions, 123
Cardiac arrhythmias, 409
Cardiac failure, parenteral formulas for,
      566t
Cardiovascular system evaluation, for
      fluid imbalances, 55–56, 59t
Care standards. See Standards of care
Catheters
  bacterial pathogens commonly found
      in, 165t
  cannula. See Cannulas
  CDC recommendations for use, 253
  dual-lumen peripheral
    description of, 199
    illustration of, 200f
  embolism, 297–298
  embolizations, 573t
  Groshong
    blood sampling, 415
    composition of, 414
    description of, 414
    flushing procedure, 415
    illustration of, 415f
    insertion of, 414
    management of, 416
  inside-the-needle
    advantages and disadvantages,
        195t
    description of, 198
  midclavicular, 204
  midline, 198, 199f
  over-the-needle
    advantages and disadvantages,
        195t
    guide for use of, 198t
    materials, 197–198
  stabilization of, 245t, 245–246
  tunneled
    advantages and disadvantages, 412

complications, 416–417
  composition of, 411
  description of, 411
  development of, 9, 411
  dressing management, 416
  flushing procedure, 412–413
  injection cap change, 416
  insertion of, 411–412
  nursing management, 414
  placement, 412f
  repair, 413, 413f
Cations, in body fluids, 76t
Cefadyl. See Cephapirin sodium
Cefamandole naftate (Mandol), 613t
Cefazolin, 279t
Cefizox. See Ceftizoxime sodium
Cefotan. See Cefotetan
Cefotaxime sodium (Claforan), 613t
Cefotetan (Cefotan), 613t
Cefoxitin sodium (Mefoxin), 613t
Ceftazidime (Fortaz), 613t
Ceftizoxime sodium (Cefizox), 613t
Ceftriaxone (Rocephin), 613t
Celbenin. See Methicillin
Cell cycle
  illustration of, 497f
  phases, 497, 498t
Cellular kinetics
  cell cycle, 496–497, 497f
  drug resistance, 499
  normal and malignant tissue growth,
      497–498
  tumor cell kill, 498–499
Centers for Disease Control
      (CDC)
  catheter recommendations, 253
  isolation guidelines, 162–163
Central infusion devices, 199
Central venous access devices
  catheters
    materials
      coatings, 396
      elastomeric hydrogel, 396
      lumens, 396, 397f
      polyurethane, 396
      silicone elastomers, 395–396
      vialon, 396
    percutaneous catheters
      advantages and disadvantages,
          399t
      dressing management, 398
      insertion site, 398
      patient positioning, 398
      sterile gauze and tape, 401
      TSM dressings, 401–402

623

Central venous access devices,
      catheters—*Continued*
   peripherally inserted. *See*
      Peripherally inserted central
      catheters
   tunneled
      Broviac, 201f, 201–202
      Groshong, 202, 202f
      Hickman, 200–201, 201f
      implantable ports, 202, 203f
   home care issues, 427
   nursing plan of care, 426
   occlusions
      description of, 421
      mechanical, 421–422
      nonthrombotic, 424–425, 425f
      thrombotic
         fibrin sleeve and tail, 422, 422f
         intraluminal occlusion, 422, 422f
         management of, 423–424
         portal reservoir, 423, 423f
         venous thrombosis, 423
   patient education, 427
Cephalic vein
   description of, 394
   illustration of, 395f
   insertion site, 235t
Cephalosporin, 374t
Cephapirin sodium (Cefadyl), 613t
Cerebrospinal fluid reservoirs
   description of, 526–527
   Ommaya, 524f, 526f
Chain of infection
   breaking of, 158–160
   elements of
      agent, 157
      host, 158
      transmission, 157–158
Chemical buffer systems, 99–100
Chemical incompatibility, of drugs, 358,
      598–601
Chemical phlebitis
   contributing factors, 278, 357
   drugs that can cause, 279t
   prevention of, 278
Chemoreceptors, 233
Chemotherapy
   administration routes
      cerebrospinal fluid reservoirs,
         526–527
      infusion pumps, 527–528
      intra-arterial, 522–523
      intraperitoneal, 523–526
      intrathecal, 522
      intravenous, 522

agents
   alkylating agents, 500–501
   androgens, 505
   anthracycline antibiotics, 504
   antimetabolites, 502–503
   classifications, 500
   corticosteroids, 505
   cytokines, 507–508
   dosing, 500
   enzymes, 504–505
   estrogens, 506
   progestins, 506
   vinca alkaloids, 503
cellular kinetics
   cell cycle, 496–497, 497f
   drug resistance, 499
   normal and malignant tissue
      growth, 497–498
   tumor cell kill, 498–499
clinician's role
   patient assessment and history, 495,
      496t
   treatment objectives, 495–496
considerations for, 496
contraindications, 496
dosage determinations, 500
home care considerations
   administration, 531
   admixture, 530
   disposal, 531
   disposal of excreta, 531
   monitoring, 531
   transportation, 530–531
nursing plan of care, 528–529
objectives of, 495–496
OSHA guidelines, 30–31
patient and family education, 529–530
side effects
   acute
      anaphylaxis, 512–513
      anemia, 520
      extravasation, 513
      hypersensitivity, 512–513
      mucositis, 514–515
      myelosuppression. *See*
         Myelosuppression
      nausea, 515–516
      stomatitis, 514
      vomiting, 515–516
   short-term
      alopecia, 510
      altered nutritional status, 512
      anorexia, 512
      constipation, 511–512
      diarrhea, 510–511

624

taste alterations, 512
venous fragility, 510
toxicities
cardiac, 520–521
neurologic, 520
pulmonary, 521
renal, 521
Chest, venous structures, 394–395,
395f
Chloramphenicol, characteristics of,
374t
Chloride
deficit. *See* Hypochloremia
excess. *See* Hyperchloremia
functions, 93
normal values, 92
Chromagen D. *See* Iron dextran
Chvostek's sign, 87f
Cimetidine (Tagamet)
description of, 279t
dilution rate, 613t
in parenteral solutions, 559
Circulatory overload, 293, 477
Circulatory system
arteries. *See* Arteries
divisions of, 233
veins. *See* Veins
Citrate, as blood preservative, 447
Claforan. *See* Cefotaxime sodium
Clark's rule, 327
Coatings, of central venous catheters,
396
Colloid solutions
albumin, 135
dextran, 135
hetastarch, 136
mannitol, 136
Colloid volume expanders
albumin, 461–462, 465t
description of, 461
plasma protein fraction, 461–462,
465t
Colonization, of bacteria, 156
Colony-stimulating factors,
chemotherapeutic use of, 508
Compatibility
of donor blood for transfusion
therapy
cryoprecipitate, 461
fresh frozen plasma, 460
granulocytes, 457
packed red blood cells, 455
platelets, 458
washed red blood cells, 456
whole blood, 452

drug
chemical, 358, 598–601
description of, 357
physical, 357–358, 598–601
therapeutic, 358
factors that affect, 354
Compazine. *See* Prochlorperazine
Competency standards
development of, 27
educational programs
development of, 27–28
three-part model, 29, 30t
JCAHO, 28t
Complement system, role in immune
system functioning, 155
Complete blood count, normal values
for, 603
Complications. *See also specific
complication*
erratic flow rate, 300–301
home care issues, 302–303
local. *See* Local complications
patient education, 302
prevention of, 301–302
systemic. *See* Systemic complications
Constipation, chemotherapy-induced,
511–512
Continuous infusion, 359
Continuous quality improvement (CQI)
description of, 34
guidelines for evaluation, 36–37
programs, 159
Continuous subcutaneous infusion
advantages and disadvantages, 365
pain management, 364
procedure, 365, 365f
Corticosteroids, chemotherapeutic use
of, 505
Cortisol, role in fluid balance, 55
Cortisol sodium succinate (Solu-Cortef,
A-hydroCort), 613t
Cowling's rule, 327
Cryoprecipitate, for transfusion therapy,
460–461, 465t
Crystalloid solutions
acidifying fluids, 132
alkalizing fluids, 131–132, 139t
description of, 125
dextrose
and sodium chloride, 126t, 128–129
in water
advantages and disadvantages, 127
contents, 126t
description of, 125
infusion rates, 127–128

625

Crystalloid solutions—*Continued*
  hydrating fluids, 126t, 129
  multiple electrolyte fluids
    advantages, 138t
    balanced hypertonic, 130
    balanced hypotonic, 130
    balanced isotonic, 130
    contents, 126t
    lactate fluids, 131
    side effects, 138t
    uses of, 138t
  potassium chloride, 132
  sodium chloride, 128, 137t
Cubital vein, insertion site, 236t
Culturing techniques, for cannulas,
      168t, 168–169
Cycling cells, 498
Cytokines, 507. *See also specific cytokine*
Cytotoxic agents. *See* Antineoplastic
      therapy
Cytovene. *See* Ganciclovir

Decadron. *See* Dexamethasone
Defense mechanisms, of immune
      system
  description of, 153
  nonspecific, 154
  primary elements, 155
  specific, 155
Delivery systems. *See* Infusion delivery
      systems
Dermis
  aging effects, 331
  description of, 232
Dexamethasone (Decadron, Hexadrol),
      518t, 613t
Dexrazoxane (Zinecard), 521
Dextran fluids, 135, 139t
Dextraron-50. *See* Iron dextran
Dextrose, fructose and, comparison, 554
Dextrose solutions
  advantages, 137t
  pH, 354
  side effects, 137t
  and sodium chloride, 126t, 128–129,
      138t
  for total parenteral nutrition, 554t
  uses of, 137t
  in water
    advantages and disadvantages, 127
    contents, 126t
    description of, 125
    infusion rates, 127–128

Diarrhea, chemotherapy-induced,
      510–511, 511t
Diethylhexyphthalate, adsorption of,
      355
Diffusion
  definition of, 51
  factors that increase, 51
Diflucan. *See* Fluconazole
Digital vein, 234t
Diphenoxylate and atropine (Lomotil),
      511t
Direct injection
  advantages and disadvantages,
      363–364
  procedure for, 364
Disease transmission
  airborne, 158
  common vehicle, 158
  contact, 157–158
  vectorborne, 158
Documentation, for risk management,
      26–27
Donor blood testing, 445–446, 446t
Dopamine, 279t
Dopastat. *See* Dopamine
Doxycycline, 279t
Dressing management, 246
Dronabinol (Marinol), 518t
Drug compatibility
  chemical, 358, 598–601
  description of, 357
  physical, 357–358, 598–601
  therapeutic, 358
Drug interactions
  considerations for, 354
  factors that affect, 354
Drugs. *See* Medications
Dual-lumen peripheral catheters
  description of, 199
  illustration of, 200f

ECF. *See* Extracellular fluid
Edema
  fluid imbalances and, 57
  scales, 57f
EID. *See* Electronic infusion devices
Elastomeric hydrogel, 396
Elderly, therapy for. *See* Geriatric
      therapy
Electrolytes
  calcium. *See* Calcium
  chloride. *See* Chloride
  definition of, 76
  in extracellular fluid, 77

imbalances
home care issues, 95
overview of, 96t
patient education, 95
plan of care, 94–95
in intracellular fluid, 77
magnesium. *See* Magnesium
in newborns, 317t
phosphorus. *See* Phosphorus
potassium. *See* Potassium
sodium. *See* Sodium
for total parenteral nutrition, 556–557
Electronic infusion devices
controllers, 208–209
mechanical infusion pumps
elastomere balloons, 212–213,
213f
implantable, 213
nurse's education regarding, 207
positive-pressure infusion pumps
ambulatory, 210–211, 211f
commonly used terminology, 209
dual-channel, 211
multichannel, 211
patient-controlled analgesia,
211–212
peristaltic, 209–210
syringe, 210
volumetric, 209
programming of, terminology
associated with, 214–215
types of, 207
Electronic monitoring devices, 468
Embolism, catheter, 409
Eminase. *See* Anistreplase
EMLA cream
application of, 258f
pre-venipuncture use, 257–258
Emporiatics, 160
Enteral nutrition
complications of, 561
delivery of, 560–561
guidelines for, 562f
parenteral nutrition and, comparison,
560
Epidemiology, basic principles of
chain of infection
breaking of, 158–160
elements of
agent, 157
host, 158
transmission, 157–158
colonization, 156
dissemination, 156
nosocomial infections, 156

Epidermis, 232
Epidural administration
advantages and disadvantages, 367
catheter insertion and maintenance,
367–368, 368f
complications, 372
dressing management, 370
medication infusion, 370
nursing care, 368, 369f
patient selection, 366
site care, 369–370
Epidural space, 366
Erratic flow rate
factors that influence, 300t
prevention, 300–301
treatment, 301
Erythromycin (Ilotycin Gluceptate)
characteristics of, 374t
dilution rate, 613t
Erythropoietin, 508
Essential fatty acid deficiency (EFAD),
555, 573t
Estrogen, chemotherapeutic use of,
506
External jugular vein
description of, 395
illustration of, 395f
Extracellular fluid
deficit. *See* Fluid volume deficit
definition of, 48
electrolyte composition, 77
excess. *See* Fluid volume excess
Extravasation
antidotes, 286, 287t
chemotherapy-induced, 513
description of, 283, 357
documentation, 286
illustration of, 283–284f
kits for, 514t
prevention, 285
procedure for, 514t
risk factors, 284t
signs and symptoms, 284
treatment, 285–286
Eyes, nutritional assessment using,
552t

Famotidine (Pepcid), 613t
FDA. *See* Food and Drug
Administration
Filters
blood. *See* Blood filters
inline solution. *See* Inline solution
filters

Filtration, 53
5-HT3 antagonists, 518t
Flagyl. *See* Metronidazole
Fluconazole (Diflucan), 375t
Fluid imbalances
  fluid volume
    deficit. *See* Fluid volume deficit
    excess. *See* Fluid volume excess
  physical assessment to evaluate for
    body weight, 58
    cardiovascular, 55–56
    integumentary, 58
    neurologic, 55
    respiratory, 57
    special senses, 58
Fluid requirements, in pediatric patients
  factors that affect levels, 319–320
  formulas to determine
    caloric method, 319
    meter square method, 318–319
    weight method, 319
Fluid transportation
  active, 53
  passive. *See* Passive transport
Fluid volume deficit
  causes of, 60t–61t
  characteristics of, 60
  description of, 59–60
  home care issues, 63
  laboratory findings, 60
  patient education, 63
  plan of care, 62–63
Fluid volume excess
  causes of, 60t–61t
  home care issues, 64
  patient education, 64
  plan of care, 63–64
  signs and symptoms, 60, 62
Fluid warmer, 215
Fluoroquinolones, 374t
Flushing methods
  heparin lock
    advantages and disadvantages, 255
    INS recommendations, 255
    saline lock flush and, comparison, 254t
  saline lock
    advantages and disadvantages, 255
    description of, 254–255
    heparin lock flush and, comparison, 254t
Folate, 615t
Folic acid analogues, 502

Food and Drug Administration (FDA)
  in-line filter device recommendations, 204
  responsibilities of, 21
Foot
  superficial veins of, 321f
  venipuncture site, 322
Forearm, superficial veins of, 238f
Fortaz. *See* Ceftazidime
Foscarnet (Foscavir), 376t
Foscavir. *See* Foscarnet
Fresh frozen plasma (FFP)
  administration of, 459
  description of, 464t
  for transfusion therapy, 459–460
Fried's rule, 327
Fructose
  description of, 127
  dextrose and, comparison, 554
Fungemia
  factors that contribute, 166
  incidence of, 165
Fungizone. *See* Amphotericin B

Ganciclovir (Cytovene), 376t
Garamycin. *See* Gentamicin
Gastrointestinal secretions, 78
Gentamicin, 279t
Geopen. *See* Carbenicillin disodium
Geriatric therapy
  fluid balance, 331, 332t
  home care considerations, 339
  immune system changes, 331
  nursing plan of care, 337
  patient education, 338
  physiologic changes, 330–331
  special considerations
    edema, 336
    hard sclerosed vessels, 335
    obesity, 336
    skin surface alterations, 334–335
    tangential lighting, 335f
  venipuncture techniques
    administration equipment, 332
    cannulation, 334
    vascular access device selection, 332
    vein selection, 332–333
Glands, 552t
Glass delivery systems
  advantages and disadvantages, 187t
  checking for clarity, 186, 188
  illustration of, 187f

Glucose
  characteristics of, 554
  conversion of, 119
  parenteral therapy use, 119
  potassium deficiency and, 119
Granisetron (Kytril), 518t
Granulocyte colony-stimulating factor
    (G-CSF), 508
Granulocytes
  compatibility of, 457
  description of, 463t
  transfusion therapy use, 456–457
Groshong catheter
  blood sampling, 415
  composition of, 414
  description of, 414
  flushing procedure, 415
  illustration of, 415f
  insertion of, 414
  management of, 416

Haldol. *See* Haloperidol
Haloperidol (Haldol), 517t
Hand
  superficial veins of, 237f, 321f
  veins for I.V. use, 234t
  venipuncture site, 322
Handwashing, for prevention of
    infection
  description of, 161
  reasons for noncompliance, 161
Hazardous drugs
  management guidelines, 31
  OSHA guidelines
    communication among employees,
      610
    drug administration, 607–608
    drug types, 604t–605t
    environmental protection, 605–606
    information dissemination, 611
    medical surveillance, 610
    personal protective equipment,
      606–607
    storage and transportation, 610
    training, 611
    waste disposal, 609–610
    for women who are pregnant,
      breastfeeding, or attempting
      to conceive, 611
Heart
  nutritional assessment using, 552t
  role in fluid balance, 54
Hematologic laboratory values, 603

Hematoma
  causes, 272
  documentation, 274
  illustration of, 273f
  prevention, 273
  signs and symptoms of, 273
  treatment, 273
Hemolytic reactions, from transfusion
    therapy
  acute, 474–475
  delayed, 475
Heparin
  dilution rate, 613t
  in parenteral solutions, 559
Heparin lock flush
  advantages and disadvantages,
    255
  INS recommendations, 255
  saline lock flush and, comparison,
    254t
Hetastarch, 136, 139t
Hetastarch (HES), 461
Hexabetalin, 615t
Hexadrol. *See* Dexamethasone
Home care
  antineoplastic therapy. *See*
    Antineoplastic therapy,
    home care considerations
  central venous access devices, 427
  chemotherapy. *See* Chemotherapy
  complication prevention, 302–303
  electrolytes imbalances, 95
  fluid imbalances, 63–64
  geriatric therapy, 339
  infections, 172
  medications
    antibiotic therapy, 381
    pain management, 381
  parenteral nutrition, 582–583
  parenteral therapy, 142
  pediatric patients, 338–339
  peripheral intravenous therapy, 219,
    259–260
  transfusion therapy, 480–481
Homeostatic mechanisms
  glands, 54–55
  heart and blood vessels, 54
  kidneys, 54
  lungs, 54
Homologous blood donation, 448
Human immunodeficiency virus (HIV),
    478
Human leukocyte antigens, 155, 444
Hydromorphone, 377t

Hyoscyamine, 511t
Hyperammonemia, 575
Hypercalcemia
  conditions associated with, 87
  diagnostic tests, 88
  etiology of, 87–88
  parenteral nutrition and, 571t
  signs and symptoms, 88
  treatment, 88
Hyperchloremia, 93–94
Hyperglycemia, 570t
Hyperkalemia
  definition of, 82
  diagnostic tests, 83
  ECG tracings, 84
  etiology of, 82–83
  hypotonic multiple electrolyte
      solutions and, 130
  parenteral nutrition and, 569t
  signs and symptoms, 83
  treatment of, 83, 84t
Hypermagnesemia
  diagnostic tests, 90
  etiology of, 90
  parenteral therapy and, 572t
  signs and symptoms, 90
  treatment, 91
Hypernatremia
  definition of, 79
  diagnostic tests, 80
  etiology of, 79–80
  hypertonic multiple electrolyte
      solutions and, 130
  parenteral nutrition and, 569t
  signs and symptoms, 80
  treatment, 80
Hyperphosphatemia
  diagnostic tests, 92
  etiology of, 92
  parenteral therapy and, 572t
  signs and symptoms, 92
  treatment, 92
Hypersensitivity, chemotherapy-
      induced, 512–513
Hypertonic solutions
  effect of fluids shifts, 52
  multiple electrolyte, 130
  osmolarity of, 52–53, 53
Hypertriglyceridemia, 571t
Hypervolemia, 569t
Hypocalcemia, 478
  definition of, 85
  etiology of, 85
  parenteral nutrition and, 571t

signs and symptoms, 85–86
  treatment, 87
Hypochloremia
  diagnostic tests, 93
  etiology of, 93
  signs and symptoms, 93
  treatment, 93
Hypodermic needle, 4
Hypoglycemia, 570t
Hypokalemia
  definition of, 81
  diagnostic tests, 81
  ECG tracings, 82
  etiology of, 81
  parenteral nutrition and, 569t
  signs and symptoms, 81
  treatment of, 82
Hypomagnesemia
  description of, 89
  diagnostic tests, 89
  etiology of, 89
  parenteral therapy and, 572t
  signs and symptoms, 89
  treatment, 89, 90t
Hyponatremia
  definition of, 78
  diagnostic tests, 79
  etiology of, 78
  parenteral nutrition and, 570t
  signs and symptoms, 79
  treatment, 79
Hypophosphatemia
  diagnostic tests, 91–92
  etiology of, 91
  signs and symptoms, 91
  treatment, 92
Hypothermia, 478
  scalp, for chemotherapy-induced
      alopecia, 510
  during transfusion therapy, 478
Hypotonic multiple electrolyte
      solutions, 130
Hypotonic solutions
  effect of fluids shifts, 52
  osmolarity of, 52, 53, 124
  in parenteral therapy, 124
Hypovolemia, 569t

ICF. See Intracellular fluid
Ilotycin Gluceptate. See Erythromycin
Imferon. See Iron dextran
Imipenem-cilastatin sodium (Primaxin),
      613t

630

Immune system
  defense mechanisms
    description of, 153
    nonspecific, 154
    primary elements, 155
    specific, 155
  function of, 153
  impaired host resistance, 155–156
  organs of, 153, 154t
Immunoglobulins
  description of, 445
  role in immune system functioning, 155
Imodium. *See* Loperamide
Implanted ports
  advantages and disadvantages, 400t, 418
  assessment of, 419–420
  blood sampling, 420
  chemotherapy administration, 525t
  complications, 420–421
  description of, 417
  flushing procedure, 420
  illustration of, 417f–418f
  insertion of, 418–419
Indirect calorimetry, 551
Infants. *See* Pediatric patients
Infections
  chain of
    breaking of, 158–160
    elements of
      agent, 157
      host, 158
      transmission, 157–158
  home care issues, 172
  infusate-related
    common pathogens, 165t
    mechanisms of, 169–170
    preventive measures
      cutaneous antiseptics, 170
      dressings, 170–171
      reporting to proper agency, 170
  I.V.-related
    cannula. *See* Cannula, infections related to
    fungemia, 165–166
    phlebitis, 163–164
    septicemia, 165–166
  nursing plan of care for, 171–172
  patient education, 172
  preventive strategies
    correct contaminations immediately, 162
    handwashing procedures, 161

isolation guidelines. *See* Isolation guidelines
  know what is clean, disinfected, and sterile, 161–162
  know what is dirty, 162
  technologic advances, 172–173
Inflammatory process, 155
Informed consent
  components of, 25t
  validity of, criteria for, 24
Infusate-related infections
  common pathogens, 165t
  mechanisms of, 169–170
  preventive measures
    cutaneous antiseptics, 170
    dressings, 170–171
    reporting to proper agency, 170
Infusion delivery systems
  glass
    advantages and disadvantages, 187t
    checking for clarity, 186, 188
    illustration of, 187f
  peripheral. *See* Peripheral intravenous therapy, infusion devices
  plastic
    advantages and disadvantages, 189t
    flexible *vs.* rigid, 188–189
    illustration of, 187f–188f
    spiking of, 189f
    use-activated containers, 190, 190f
  slowed delivery, steps for checking, 275t
Infusion pumps
  chemotherapy administration, 527–528
  mechanical
    elastomere balloons, 212–213, 213f
    implantable, 213
  nonportable *vs.* portable, 527
  positive-pressure
    ambulatory, 210–211, 211f
    commonly used terminology, 209
    dual-channel, 211
    multichannel, 211
    patient-controlled analgesia, 211–212
    peristaltic, 209–210
    syringe, 210
    volumetric, 209
Infusion therapy
  key advances
    in 19th century, 5
    in 20th century, 7–8
  technological advances, 172–173

Inline solution filters
    FDA recommendations, 204
    function of, 205t
    particulate matter removal, 204
    set saver, 206
    types of
        depth, 204
        membrane, 204–206, 205f
    uses of, 205
Innominate veins
    description of, 395
    illustration of, 395f
Inside-the-needle catheters
    advantages and disadvantages, 195t
    description of, 198
Insulin
    binding to plastic containers, 355
    in parenteral solutions, 559
Integument system, evaluation of, for
            fluid imbalances, 58, 59t
Interferon-alpha, 507
Interferon-beta, 507
Interleukin-1 (IL-1), 507
Interleukin-2 (IL-2), 507
Interleukin-3 (IL-3), 508
Interleukin-4 (IL-4), 507
Interleukin-6 (IL-6), 507
Interleukin-7 (IL-7), 507
Interleukin-12 (IL-12), 507
Intermittent infusion
    description of, 359
    piggyback, 361
    piggyback through primary pathway,
            360f, 361
    simultaneous, 360f, 361
    through locking device, 362–363
    volume-control, 361–362, 362f
    volume control chamber, 362f, 363
Internal jugular vein
    description of, 395
    illustration of, 395f
Intracellular fluid
    definition of, 48
    electrolyte composition, 77
Intraperitoneal delivery, of
            antineoplastic agents
    advantages and disadvantages,
            523–525, 525t
    illustration of, 524f
    purpose of, 523
Intraspinal infusion
    description of, 366
    epidural administration. See Epidural
            administration
    indications, 366

intrathecal administration, 370–371
    medications commonly used for, 371t
    side effects of, 371–372
Intrathecal catheter
    advantages and disadvantages, 371
    medication administration, 371
Intrathecal space, 366
Intravenous therapy
    complications of
        local types. See Local complications
        systemic types. See Systemic
            complications
    delivery systems. See Infusion
            delivery systems
    infections related to. See Infections,
            I.V.-related
    initiation of
        cannulation. See Cannulation
        postcannulation. See
            Postcannulation
        precannulation. See Precannulation
    key advances in
        Renaissance era, 4, 5t
        in 19th century, 8t
        in 20th century, 7–11, 11t–12t
    national support organizations, 616
    nursing teams, 37
    pediatric. See Pediatric patients,
            intravenous therapy
    during 1950s, 118
    trends for 21st century
        bloodborne pathogens, 13
        education, 13
        health care reform, 11, 13
        technology, 13
Invert sugar, 127, 554
Ions, 76
Iron dextran (Imferon, Chromagen D,
            Dextraron-50), 614t
Isolation guidelines, for prevention of
            infection
    body substance, 162
    CDC system, 162–163
    government regulations, 162–163
    Universal Precautions, 162
Isotonic solutions
    effect of fluids shifts, 52
    osmolarity, 52, 53
I.V. push, 363–364

Joint Commission on Accreditation of
            Healthcare Organizations
            (JCAHO)
    antibiotic recommendations, 159

632

competency standards of, 28t
infection control guidelines, 163
nursing standards and, 21
quality management monitoring and
evaluation steps, 35t
risk management and, 19
Jugular vein distention, 56, *57*

Kaopectate, 511t
Kidneys
acid-base balance, 100
role in fluid balance, 54
sodium regulation, 78
Kwashiorkor, 548
Kytril. *See* Granisetron

Laboratory values
hematologic, 603
immunologic, 603
serum blood, 602
urine, 603
β-Lactamase agents, 374t
characteristics of, 374t
Lactate fluids, 131
L-asparaginase, chemotherapeutic use
of, 504
Latex allergies, 31–32
Latex resealable locks
advantages and disadvantages, 254
description of, 215–216, 254
illustration of, 216f
Leukocytes, 155
Leukopenia, 155
Levophed. *See* Norepinephrine
Levorphanol, 377t
Licensed practical nurse (LPN), 13,
617–618
Licensed vocational nurse (LVN), 13,
617–618
Lidocaine, 256–257
Linoleic acid, 555
Linolenic acid, 555
Lipids
nutritional requirements, 555–556
in total parenteral nutrition, 555, 555t
Liver
failure, parenteral nutrition formulas
for, 566t
role in immune system, 154t
Local complications
extravasation
antidotes, 286, 287t
description of, 283

documentation, 286
illustration of, 283–284f
prevention, 285
risk factors, 284t
signs and symptoms, 284
treatment, 285–286
hematoma
causes, 272
documentation, 274
illustration of, 273f
prevention, 273
signs and symptoms of, 273
treatment, 273
infiltration
illustrations of, 282f–283f
signs and symptoms, 281
site assessment, 281–282
local infection
description of, 286–287
documentation, 287
prevention, 287
signs and symptoms, 287
phlebitis
description of, 275
documentation, 280
formation of, factors that affect,
276, 276t
illustration of, 276f
prevention, 280
scale, 277t
signs and symptoms, 276
treatment, 280
types of
bacterial, 279
chemical, 278
mechanical, 277–278
postinfusion, 279
thrombophlebitis
description of, 280
documentation, 281
prevention, 280–281
treatment, 281
thrombosis
causes of, 274
documentation, 275
prevention of, 274
slowed infusion as cause of, steps
for checking, 275f
treatment, 274
tips to prevent, 289
types of, 272t
venous spasm, 288–289
Local infection
description of, 286–287
documentation, 287

633

Local infection—*Continued*
  prevention, 287
  signs and symptoms, 287
Lomotil. *See* Diphenoxylate and
    atropine
Loperamide (Imodium), 511t
Lorazepam (Ativan), 517t
Lumens, of central venous catheters,
    396, 397f
Lungs
  acid-base regulation, 54
  disease, 566t
  edema, 293–294
  role in fluid balance, 54
  role in immune system, 154t
  toxicity, chemotherapy-induced, 521
Lymph nodes, 154t

Macrophage colony-stimulating factor
    (CSF-1), 508
Magnesium
  deficit. *See* Hypomagnesemia
  excess. *See* Hypermagnesemia
  function of, 88–89
  normal values, 88
Maintenance therapy, 118–119
Malnutrition
  chemotherapy-induced, 512
  description of, 547
  effects of, 548
  types of
    kwashiorkor, 548
    marasmus, 548
    mixed, 548
Malpractice cases
  negligence and, 23
  nurse's role as expert witness, 23
Mandol. *See* Cefamandole naftate
Mannitol, 136, 139t
Marasmus, 548
Marinol. *See* Dronabinol
Mechanical infusion pumps
  elastomere balloons, 212–213, 213f
  implantable, 213
Mechanical phlebitis, 277–278
Mechanoreceptors, 233
Medical devices
  FDA inspection of, 25
  problems associated with, when to
    report, 25–26
Medications. *See also specific medication*
  administration methods
    arteriovenous fistula, 372
    continuous infusion, 359

continuous subcutaneous infusion,
    364–365, 365f
  direct injection, 363–364
  intermittent infusion. *See*
      Intermittent infusion
  intraspinal infusion. *See* Intraspinal
      infusion
  key advances in, 10
  nursing plan of care, 379–380
  pediatric patients. *See* Pediatric
      patients
  adsorption, 354–355, 355t
  advantages, 353, 353t
  antibiotics
    categories of, 374t
    compatibility issues, 373
    nursing considerations, 373
  antifungal agents, 374
  antiviral agents, 374
  compatibility
    chemical, 358
    description of, 357
    factors that affect, 354
    physical, 357–358
    therapeutic, 358
  disadvantages, 353, 354t
  drug interactions, 354
  extravasation, 357
  home care issues
    antibiotic therapy, 381
    pain management, 381
  investigational, 378–379
  key advances, in 19th century, 6–7
  mixing errors, 355–356
  narcotics
    description of, 375–376
    patient-controlled analgesia,
        376–377
  parenteral additives
    cimetidine, 559
    heparin, 559
    insulin, 559
  patient education, 380
  speed shock, 356
Mefoxin. *See* Cefoxitin sodium
Meperidine, 377t
Metabolic acidosis
  alkalizing fluids for, 131–132, 139t
  diagnostic tests, 101
  etiology of, 100–101
  signs and symptoms, 101
  summary of, 104t
  treatment, 101
Metabolic alkalosis
  acidifying parenteral solutions, 132

diagnostic tests, 102
etiology of, 101–102
signs and symptoms, 102
summary of, 104t
treatment, 102
Metacarpal vein, 234t
Methicillin (Staphcillin, Celbenin), 614t
Methotrexate, 502
Methyldopa (Aldomet Ester), 614t
Methylprednisolone sodium succinate
         (Solu-Medrol, A-Methapred),
         614t
Metoclopramide (Reglan), 517t
Metronidazole (Flagyl), 614t
Mezlocillin sodium (Mezlin), 614t
Miconazole (Monostat IV), 375t
Midclavicular catheters, 204
Midline catheters
   CDC recommendations for use, 253
   description of, 198, 199f
Mixed malnutrition, 548
Mixing, of drugs
   adequate, recommendations for, 356
   inadequate, factors that contribute to,
      356
Monoclonal antibodies,
         chemotherapeutic use of,
         508–509
Monostat IV. See Miconazole
Morphine, 279t, 377t
Mucous membranes, 58
Multiple electrolyte fluids
   advantages, 138t
   balanced hypertonic, 130
   balanced hypotonic, 130
   balanced isotonic, 130
   contents, 126t
   lactate fluids, 131
   side effects, 138t
   uses of, 138t
Muscles, nutritional assessment using,
      553t
Myelosuppression, chemotherapy-
         induced
   description of, 516
   neutropenia, 516, 518
   thrombocytopenia, 519

Nafcillin sodium (Nafcil, Unipen,
         Nallpen), 279t, 614t
Nalbuphine (Nubain)
   guidelines for use, 377t
   intraspinal infusion use, 371–372

Nallpen. See Nafcillin sodium
Naloxone (Narcan), 371
Narcotics
   description of, 375–376
   patient-controlled analgesia, 376–377
Nausea, chemotherapy-induced
   antiemetics, 517t–518t
   description of, 515
   nursing interventions, 516
   patient assessment, 515–516
Nebcin. See Tobramycin sulfate
Needleless systems, 217, 218f
Needle protector systems, 217
Needle-stick injuries, 29
Neonate
   definition of, 316
   laboratory values, 317t
   renal function, 316
Neurologic system
   chemotherapeutic side effects, 520
   fluid imbalances and, 55, 59t
   nutritional assessment using, 553t
Neutropenia
   chemotherapeutic complications, 516,
      518
   precautions, 518
Nitrogen balance, 551
Nitroglycerin, topical, pre-venipuncture
      use, 258
Nociceptors, 233
Nondividing cells, 498
Nonhemolytic febrile reactions, from
         transfusion therapy, 476
Nonthrombotic occlusions, 424–425,
      425f
Norepinephrine, 279t
Nosocomial infections, 156
Nurse, as expert witness, 23
Nursing
   laws that apply to, 20
   standards in, 21
Nutritional assessment
   anthropometric measurements,
      549–550
   components of, 549t
   diagnostic tests, 550–551
   history, 548–549
   physical examination, 551, 552t–
      553t
   secondary technique
      indirect calorimetry, 551
      nitrogen balance, 551
      prognostic nutritional index, 551
Nutritional deficiencies. See
         Malnutrition

Nutritional requirements
    carbohydrates, 553–555
    electrolytes, 556–557
    fats, 555–556
    proteins, 556
    trace elements, 558–559
    vitamins, 558
Nutritional support
    cyclic therapy, 565, 567
    enteral. *See* Enteral nutrition
    key advances
        in 19th century, 6
        in 20th century, 9–10
    parenteral. *See* Total parenteral
        nutrition
    standards of practice
        implementation, 578
        monitoring, 578, 580, 580t
    total nutrient admixture, 564–565

Occlusions, of vascular access devices
    description of, 421
    mechanical, 421–422
    nonthrombotic, 424–425, 425f
    parenteral therapy, 574t
    thrombotic
        fibrin sleeve and tail, 422, 422f
        intraluminal occlusion, 422, 422f
        management of, 423–424
        portal reservoir, 423, 423f
        venous thrombosis, 423
Occupational risks
    abrasions and contusions, 29
    biologic hazards, 32
    chemical exposure, 30–31
    latex allergies, 31–32
    needle-stick injuries, 29
Occupational Safety and Health
        Administration (OSHA)
    bloodborne pathogens exposure
        guidelines, 32–33
    hazardous drug exposure guidelines
        communication among employees,
            610
        drug administration, 607–608
        drug types, 604t–605t
        environmental protection, 605–606
        information dissemination, 611
        medical surveillance, 610
        personal protective equipment,
            606–607
        storage and transportation, 610
        training, 611
        waste disposal, 609–610

for women who are pregnant,
        breastfeeding, or attempting
        to conceive, 611
Occurrence reports, 23–24
Octreotide, 511t
Ommaya reservoir
    description of, 526–527
    illustration of, 524f, 526f
Omnipen. *See* Ampicillin
Oncology Nursing Service (ONS), 495
Ondansetron (Zofran), 518t
Opioids, 376
Oral cavity, nutritional assessment
        using, 552t
Oral mucosa, chemotherapeutic
        complications
    description of, 514
    management, 514–515, 515t
Organizations, national, 616
OSHA. *See* Occupational Safety and
        Health Administration
Osmolarity
    of body fluids, 51
    definition of, 51
Osmosis
    definition of, 51
    schematic of, 52
Over-the-needle catheters
    advantages and disadvantages, 195t
    guide for use of, 198t
    materials, 197–198
Oxacillin sodium (Prostaphlin), 614t
Oxytocin (Pitocin, Syntocinon), 614t

Packed red blood cells (PRBC)
    administration of, 454, 455f
    advantages of, 454
    compatibility, 455
    description of, 463t
    uses of, 454
Pain management, 381
Pain medication, administration of
    epidural. *See* Epidural administration
    key advances in, 10
Parathyroid gland, 55
Parathyroid hormone, 85
Paregoric, 511t
Parenteral therapy
    administration of, 141
    home care issues, 142
    hypertonic solutions, 125
    hypotonic solutions, 124
    isotonic solutions, 125
    patient education regarding, 142

pediatric patients
  assessment, 567
  indications, 568
  monitoring, 568
  overview, 567
reasons for
  maintenance therapy, 118–119
  replacement therapy, 119–120
  restoration therapy, 120–121
solutions
  components of
    carbohydrates, 123
    electrolytes, 124
    pH, 124
    protein, 123
    vitamins, 123
    water, 123
  types of
    colloid solutions. *See* Colloid
      solutions
    crystalloid solutions. *See*
      Crystalloid solutions
  total. *See* Total parenteral nutrition
Passive transport
  diffusion, 51
  filtration, 53
  mechanisms, 51t
  osmosis, 51–53
Patient-controlled analgesia (PCA)
  concepts of, 378
  description of, 376–377
  ideal candidates, 378
  pumps, 211–212
Pediatric patients
  body composition, 316
  intravenous therapy
    administration routes
      intraosseous
        advantages and disadvantages,
          329
        contraindications, 329–330
        illustration of, 328f
        insertion technique, 329
        nursing management, 330
        umbilical veins and arteries,
          330
      based on physical and
        psychological development,
        325t
    equipment selection, 322–323
    home care considerations, 338–339
    laboratory values, 317t
    medication administration
      formulas for delivery, 326–327
      intermittent infusions, 326

retrograde infusion, 326
syringe pump, 326
needle selection, 323
patient education, 338
physical assessment
  components of, 318t
  fluid requirements. *See* Fluid
    requirements, in pediatric
    patients
  risk factors, 318
physiologic characteristics of,
  316–317
venipuncture
  site selection
    factors that influence, 320
    foot, 322
    hand and forearm, 322
    scalp veins, 320–321, 321f
  techniques, 235t, 323–324, 324f
parenteral therapy
  assessment, 567
  indications, 568
  monitoring, 568
  overview, 567
Penicillin G sodium, 614t
Pentam 300. *See* Pentamidine
  isethionate
Pentamidine isethionate (Pentam 300),
  376t
Pentazocine, 377t
Pepcid. *See* Famotidine
Percutaneous catheters
  advantages and disadvantages, 399t
  dressing management, 398
  insertion site, 398
  patient positioning, 398
  sterile gauze and tape, 401
  TSM dressings, 401–402
Perioral region, nutritional assessment
  using, 552t
Peripheral intravenous therapy
  CDC recommendations, 253
  controversial practices
    lidocaine, 256–257
    topical nitroglycerin, 258
    transdermal analgesia, 257–258
  home care issues, 259–260
  infusion devices
    central infusion devices. *See* Central
      infusion devices
    central venous tunneled catheters.
      See Tunneled catheters
    dual-lumen peripheral catheters
      description of, 199
      illustration of, 200f

Peripheral intravenous therapy, infusion devices—*Continued*
  home care issues, 219
  inside-the-needle catheters
    advantages and disadvantages, 195t
    description of, 198
  midclavicular catheters, 204
  midline catheters, 198, 199f
  nursing plan of care, 218–219
  over-the-needle catheters
    advantages and disadvantages, 195t
    guide for use of, 198t
    materials, 197–198
  patient education, 219
  scalp vein needles
    advantages and disadvantages, 195t
    types of, 196f, 196–197
  types of, 195t
  patient education, 259
  recommendations for use, 253
  venipuncture. *See* Venipuncture
Peripherally inserted central catheters (PICC)
  advantages and disadvantages, 399t, 403
  blood administration, 408
  blood sampling, 408
  CDC recommendations, 405
  complications
    insertion
      bleeding, 408
      cardiac arrhythmias, 409
      embolism, 409
      malpositioning of catheter, 409
      tendon or nerve damage, 408–409
    postinsertion
      air embolism, 410
      cellulitis, 410
      declotting of line, 411
      phlebitis, 410
      sepsis, 410
      thrombophlebitis, 410
      thrombosis, 410
      Twiddler's syndrome, 410
  description of, 202–203
  dressing management, 405–406
  flushing procedure, 406, 407t, 408
  illustration of, 203f
  indications, 403

  infections, 167
  infusion pumps, 408
  nursing management of, 405–406
  placement, 404f, 404–405
  repair, 408
  vein selection, 403
Peripheral parenteral nutrition (PPN)
  advantages and disadvantages, 563
  indications for, 562
Peripheral vein filling, 56
Personal protective equipment (PPE), 606–607
Peyer's patches, 154t
pH
  drug interactions and, 354
  mechanisms to maintain, 99
  regulation of
    chemical buffer systems, 99–100
    kidneys, 100
    lungs, 100
  scale of, *99*
Phagocytic cells, 155
Phenobarbital, 511t
Phenothiazines, 517t
Phlebitis
  description of, 275
  documentation, 280
  factors that influence development, 163–164
  formation of, factors that affect, 276, 276t
  illustration of, 276f
  parenteral therapy and, 574t
  peripherally inserted central catheters and, 410
  prevention, 280
  risk factors, 164t
  scale, 277t
  signs and symptoms, 276
  treatment, 280
  types of, 164
    bacterial, 279
    chemical, 278, 357
    mechanical, 277–278
    postinfusion, 279
Phosphorus
  deficit. *See* Hypophosphatemia
  excess. *See* Hyperphosphatemia
  function of, 91
  normal values, 91
Physical assessment, for evaluation of fluid imbalances
  body weight, 58
  cardiovascular, 55–56

integumentary, 58
neurologic, 55
respiratory, 57
special senses, 58
Physical incompatibility, of drugs
absorption, 357
chart, 598–601
description of, 357–358
insolubility, 357
recommendations, 358
Piggyback infusions, 360f, 361
Piperacillin sodium (Pipracil), 614t
Pitocin. *See* Oxytocin
Plasma protein fraction (PPF)
administration of, 462
compatibility, 462
description of, 461, 465t
uses of, 461
Plastic delivery systems
advantages and disadvantages, 189t
flexible *vs.* rigid, 188–189
illustration of, 187f–188f
spiking of, 189f
use-activated containers, 190, 190f
Platelets, transfusion therapy
administration, 458
compatibility, 458
description of, 457, 464t
storage, 457f
uses of, 457–458
Pneumothorax, 573t
Polycillin. *See* Ampicillin
Polyvinylchloride (PVC) bags,
adsorption in, 355
Positive-pressure infusion pumps
ambulatory, 210–211, 211f
commonly used terminology, 209
dual-channel, 211
multichannel, 211
patient-controlled analgesia, 211–212
peristaltic, 209–210
syringe, 210
volumetric, 209
Postcannulation, steps for
documentation, 248–249
equipment disposal, 247
labeling, 246–247
patient education, 247
rate calculations
amount of solution to be infused,
248
conversion chart, 248t
drip rate, 247–248
summary of, 250

Postinfusion phlebitis, 279
Potassium
acid-base imbalance and,
relationship between,
80–81
administration of, guidelines for,
83t
deficiencies from glucose infusions,
119
deficit. *See* Hypokalemia
dietary intake of, 119
excess. *See* Hyperkalemia
function of, 80–81
normal values, 80
parenteral solution use, 132
toxicity, 477
Potassium chloride, 614t
Potassium phosphate, 614t
Prealbumin, 550
Precannulation, steps for
checking physician's order, 239
equipment preparation, 239–240
handwashing, 239
patient assessment and psychological
preparation, 240
site selection, 240–241
summary of, 249
vein dilation, 241–242
Prerenal azotemia, 572t
Primaxin. *See* Imipenem-cilastatin
sodium
PRN device. *See* Latex resealable lock
Prochlorperazine (Compazine), 517t
Product problem reporting system,
25–26
Progestins, chemotherapeutic use of,
506
Prognostic nutritional index (PNI),
551
Prostaphlin. *See* Oxacillin sodium
Protein
amino acids, 556
body depletion of, 560f
daily requirements, 556
function of, 556
in parenteral solutions, 123
Pulmonary disease, 566t
Pulmonary edema, 293–294
Pulmonary toxicity, chemotherapy-
induced, 521
Pumps. *See* Infusion pumps
Purine analogues, 503
Pyopen. *See* Carbenicillin disodium
Pyrimidine analogues, 502

Quality management
  approaches
    continuous quality improvement,
      34–35
    JCAHO monitoring and evaluation
      steps, 35t
    performance improvement, 34
  components of, 33
  example of, 37t
  intravenous therapy nursing teams,
    37
  types of standards, 35–36

Ranitidine (Zantac), 615t
Red blood cells (RBC)
  antigens, 443–444
  for transfusion therapy
    deglycerolized, 456, 463t
    packed. *See* Packed red blood cells
    washed, 455–456, 463t
Reglan. *See* Metoclopramide
Renal failure, 566t
Renal toxicity, chemotherapy-induced,
  521
Replacement therapy
  description of, 119–120
  indications for, 119
Respiratory acidosis
  diagnostic tests, 103
  etiology of, 102
  signs and symptoms, 102
  summary of, 104t
  treatment, 103
Respiratory alkalosis
  diagnostic tests, 103–104
  etiology of, 103
  signs and symptoms, 103
  summary of, 104t
  treatment, 104
Respiratory system
  acid-base balance, 100
  evaluation of, for fluid imbalances,
    57, 59t
Restoration therapy
  documentation of, 120
  sample schedule for, 121t
  selection of fluid, 120
Retinol-binding protein, 550
Ringer's injection, 131
Risk management
  for breaking chain of infection, 159
  classification of, 19
  competency standards
    development of, 27

educational programs
  development of, 27–28
  three-part model, 29, 30t
  JCAHO, 28t
documentation, 26–27
historical origins, 19
law sources, 19–20
occupational risks
  abrasions and contusions, 29
  biologic hazards, 32
  chemical exposure, 30–31
  latex allergies, 31–32
  needle-stick injuries, 29
product problem reporting system,
  25–26
standards of care
  agencies that influence, 22t
  breach of duty, 21–22
  evolution of, 20–21
  informed consent, 24–25, 25t
  nurse's role as expert witness, 23
  nursing, 21
  screenings, 24t
  unusual occurrence reports, 23–24
  strategies of, 19t
Rocephin. *See* Ceftriaxone
Rochester needle, development of, 8
Rubber gloves
  OSHA guidelines, 606
  surgical use, history of, 6
Rubber latex allergies, 31–32

Saline lock flush
  advantages and disadvantages, 255
  description of, 254–255
  heparin lock flush and, comparison,
    254t
Scalp veins
  needles
    advantages and disadvantages,
      195t
    types of, 196f, 196–197
    pediatric use as venipuncture site,
      320–321, 321f
Scopolamine, 511t
Sensory receptors, 233
Sepsis
  parenteral formulas for, 566t
  parenteral therapy and, 574t
  tunneled catheters and, 416
Septicemia
  common pathogens, 165t
  description of, 165
  documentation, 292

incidence of, 291
prevention, 292
risk factors, 291t
signs and symptoms, 292
sources of, 165–166
treatment, 292
Silastic, 395–396
Site selection, for venipuncture, 240t, 240–241
Skin
  aging effects, 331
  barrier protection, 154
  illustration of, 232f
  layers of, 232–233
  nutritional assessment, 552t
Sodium
  cellular fluid and, relationship between, 78
  deficit. See Hyponatremia
  excess. See Hypernatremia
  functions of, 77–78
Sodium chloride fluids, 137t, 354
Solubility, factors that affect, 354
Solu-Cortef. See Cortisol sodium succinate
Solu-Medrol. See Methylprednisolone sodium succinate
Solutions. See Colloid solutions; Crystalloid solutions
Sorbitol, 554–555
Speed shock, 296–297, 356
Spleen, 154t
Standards of care
  agencies that influence, 22t
  breach of duty, 21–22
  evolution of, 20–21
  informed consent, 24–25, 25t
  nurse's role as expert witness, 23
  nursing, 21
  screenings, 24t
  unusual occurrence reports, 23–24
Staphcillin. See Methicillin
Starvation
  anthropometric measurements, 549–550
  physiologic effects of, 547
Steroids, 518t
Streptase. See Streptokinase
Streptokinase (Streptase), 615t
Subclavian vein
  description of, 394
  illustration of, 395t
Superior vena cava
  description of, 395
  illustration of, 395f

Syntocinon. See Oxytocin
Systemic complications
  air embolism. See Air embolism
  catheter embolism, 297–298
  circulatory overload, 293
  pulmonary edema, 293–294
  septicemia. See Septicemia
  speed shock, 296–297

Tagamet. See Cimetidine
Tangential lighting, for veins of geriatric patients, 335f
Taste alterations, chemotherapy-induced, 512
TBW. See Total body water
Tetracycline, 374t
Therapeutic incompatibility, of drugs, 358
Thermoreceptors, 233
Thiethylperazine (Torecan), 517t
Thrombocytopenia, 519
Thrombophlebitis, 280–281
Thrombopoietin (TPO), 508
Thrombosis
  causes of, 274
  documentation, 275
  peripherally inserted central catheters and, 410
  prevention of, 274
  slowed infusion as cause of, steps for checking, 275f
  treatment, 274
  tunneled catheters and, 416
  venous, from parenteral nutrition, 574t
Thymus, 154t
Ticarcillin disodium (Ticar), 615t
Tigan. See Trimethobenzamide
Tobramycin sulfate (Nebcin), 615t
Tongue, 58, 59t
Tonicity, of solutions, 51–52
Tonsils, 154t
Topical nitroglycerin, pre-venipuncture use, 258
Torecan. See Thiethylperazine
Total body water
  distribution of, 48
  intake and output of, 50t
  sources of, 49
Total lymphocyte count (TLC), 550–551
Total nutrient admixture (TNA), 564–565
Total parenteral nutrition (TPN)
  advantages and disadvantages, 564

Total parenteral nutrition (TPN)—
Continued
amino acid solutions, 557t
complications of
admixture, 577–578
catheter-related
air embolism, 573t, 576
embolization, 573t
improper tip location, 574t
infection, 577
malposition, 576–577
occlusions, 574t
phlebitis, 574t
pneumothorax, 573t, 576
sepsis, 574t
venous thrombosis, 574t, 576
hyperglycemia, 568, 569t, 575
hyperosmolar syndrome, 568, 575
metabolic
essential fatty acid deficiency,
573t, 575
hyperammonemia, 575
hypercalcemia, 571t
hyperglycemia, 570t
hyperkalemia, 569t
hypermagnesemia, 572t
hypernatremia, 569t, 576
hyperphosphatemia, 572t
hypertriglyceridemia, 571t
hypervolemia, 569t
hypocalcemia, 571t
hypoglycemia, 570t, 575
hypokalemia, 569t, 576
hypomagnesemia, 572t, 576
hyponatremia, 570t
hypophosphatemia, 575
hypovolemia, 569t
overfeeding, 573t
prerenal azotemia, 572t
cyclic, 565, 567
dextrose solutions, 554t
electrolytes, 556–557
enteral nutrition and, comparison,
560
guidelines for, 562f
home, 582–583
hypophosphatemia and, 91
indications for, 560, 561t
medication additives
cimetidine, 559
heparin, 559
insulin, 559
nursing plan of care, 580–581
order form, 579f

origins of, 9–10
patient education, 581–582
peripheral, 562–563
solutions, 563t–564t
components of
carbohydrates, 123
electrolytes, 124
pH, 124
protein, 123
vitamins, 123
water, 123
types of
colloid solutions. *See* Colloid
solutions
crystalloid solutions. *See*
Crystalloid solutions
specialized formulas, 566t, 567
Total quality management (TQM),
34–35
Trace elements
AMA recommendations, 558t
description of, 558–559
Transferrin, serum levels, nutritional
assessment using, 550
Transfusion therapy
administration, steps for
checklist preparation, 470, 471f
equipment selection and
preparation
administration sets, 467
blood warmers, 467–468
cannula, 466
electronic monitoring devices,
468
filters, 467
solution, 467
obtaining blood product from
blood bank, 469–470
patient preparation, 469
physician's order, 466
antibodies, 444–445
antigens, 443–444
blood components
cryoprecipitate, 460–461, 465t
fresh frozen plasma, 459–460,
464t
granulocytes, 456–457, 463t
overview, 451
platelets
administration, 458
compatibility, 458
description of, 457, 464t
storage, 457f
uses of, 457–458

red blood cells
  deglycerolized, 456, 463t
  packed. *See* Packed red blood
    cells
  washed, 455–456, 463t
  whole blood, 452, 453f
blood preservatives, 447–448
blood substitutes, 462, 466
colloid volume expanders. *See* Colloid
    volume expanders
compatibility testing, 446–447
complications of
  allergic reactions, 476–477
  circulatory overload, 477
  hemolytic reactions, 474–475
  hypocalcemia, 478
  hypothermia, 478
  nonhemolytic febrile reactions, 476
  potassium toxicity, 477
discontinuation of, 472–473
donor blood testing, 445–446, 446t
in home setting, 480–481
initiation of, 470–471
key advances
  in 19th century, 4–5, 9t
  in 20th century, 7, 9t
monitoring, 471–472
nursing plan of care, 479–480
patient education, 480
risks of, 478, 478t
Transmission, disease
  airborne, 158
  common vehicle, 158
  contact, 157–158
  vectorborne, 158
Trauma, 566t
Trimethobenzamide (Tigan), 517t
Trousseau's sign, *86*
Tumor growth
  antineoplastic therapy, 498–499
  cell changes, 498
  factors that affect, 498
Tunica adventitia, 234
Tunica intima, 234–235
Tunica media, 234
Tunneled catheters
  advantages and disadvantages, 399t,
    412
  complications, 416–417
  composition of, 411
  description of, 411
  development of, 9, 411
  dressing management, 416
  flushing procedure, 412–413
  with Groshong valve
    blood sampling, 415
    composition of, 414
    description of, 414
    flushing procedure, 415
    illustration of, 415f
    insertion of, 414
    management of, 416
  injection cap change, 416
  insertion of, 411–412
  nursing care of, 407f
  nursing management, 414
  placement, 412f
  repair, 413, 413f
Twiddler's syndrome, 410

Unipen. *See* Nafcillin; Nafcillin sodium
Universal Precautions, 162
Urine laboratory values, 603
Urokinase
  complications, 424
  contraindications, 424
  incompatibilities, 424
  thrombosis treatment, 275, 423–424

Vancocin. *See* Vancomycin
Vancomycin (Vancocin), 615t
Veins. *See also specific vein*
  anatomy of, 233, 237f
  artery and, comparison, 233t
  chemotherapeutic effects, 510
  dilation of, 241–242
  fragility of, 510
  in geriatric patients, 332–333
  of hands and arm, 234t–235t, 235
  layers of
    tunica adventitia, 234
    tunica intima, 234–235
    tunica media, 234
  procedure for entry, 243–244,
    244t–245t
  troubleshooting, 245t
Venipuncture
  cannulation, steps for
    catheter stabilization, 245t, 245–246
    dressing management, 246
    gloving, 242–243
    needle selection, 242
    site preparation, 243
    vein entry, 243–244
  controversial practices
    lidocaine, 256–257

Venipuncture, controversial practices—
  Continued
    topical nitroglycerin, 258
    transdermal analgesia, 257–258
  geriatric patients
    administration equipment, 332
    cannulation, 334
    vascular access device selection,
      332
    vein selection, 332–333
  nursing plan of care, 258–259
  pediatric patients
    site selection
      factors that influence, 320
      foot, 322
      hand and forearm, 322
      scalp veins, 320–321, 321f
    techniques, 235t, 323–324, 324f
  Phillips 15-step approach, 238t, 239
  postcannulation, steps for
    documentation, 248–249
    equipment disposal, 247
    labeling, 246–247
    patient education, 247
    rate calculations
      amount of solution to be infused,
        248
      conversion chart, 248t
      drip rate, 247–248
  precannulation, steps for
    checking physician's order, 239
    equipment preparation, 239–240
    handwashing, 239
    patient assessment and
        psychological preparation,
        240
    site selection, 240–241
    vein dilation, 241–242
  procedure for, 243, 244t–245t

Venous spasm, 288–289
Venous system. *See* Arteries; Veins
Vesicant agents, 513
Vialon, 198, 396
Vibramycin. *See* Doxycycline
Vidarabine. *See* Adenine arabinoside
Vinca alkaloids, 503
Vitamin K, 558
Vitamins
  AMA recommendations, 558t
  in parenteral solutions, 123, 558
Vomiting, chemotherapy-induced
  antiemetics, 517t–518t
  description of, 515
  nursing interventions, 516
  patient assessment, 515–516

Water
  maintenance requirements, 123
  in parenteral solutions, 123
White blood cell count, 155
Whole blood
  administration of, 452
  compatibility, 452
  components of, 452
  derivation of, 453f
  description of, 463t
  uses of, 452

Xylitol, 554–555
Xylocaine hydrochloride. *See* Lidocaine

Zantac. *See* Ranitidine
Zidovudine (AZT), 376t
Zinecard. *See* Dexrazoxane
Zofran. *See* Ondansetron
Zovirax. *See* Acylovir